CW01583067

ENCYCLOPAEDIA
OF
INDIAN MEDICINE

लोकाः समस्ताः
सुखिनो भवन्तु ॥

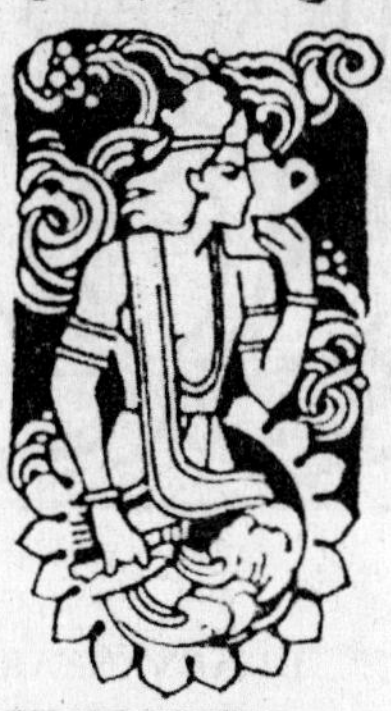

SRI DHANVANTARI

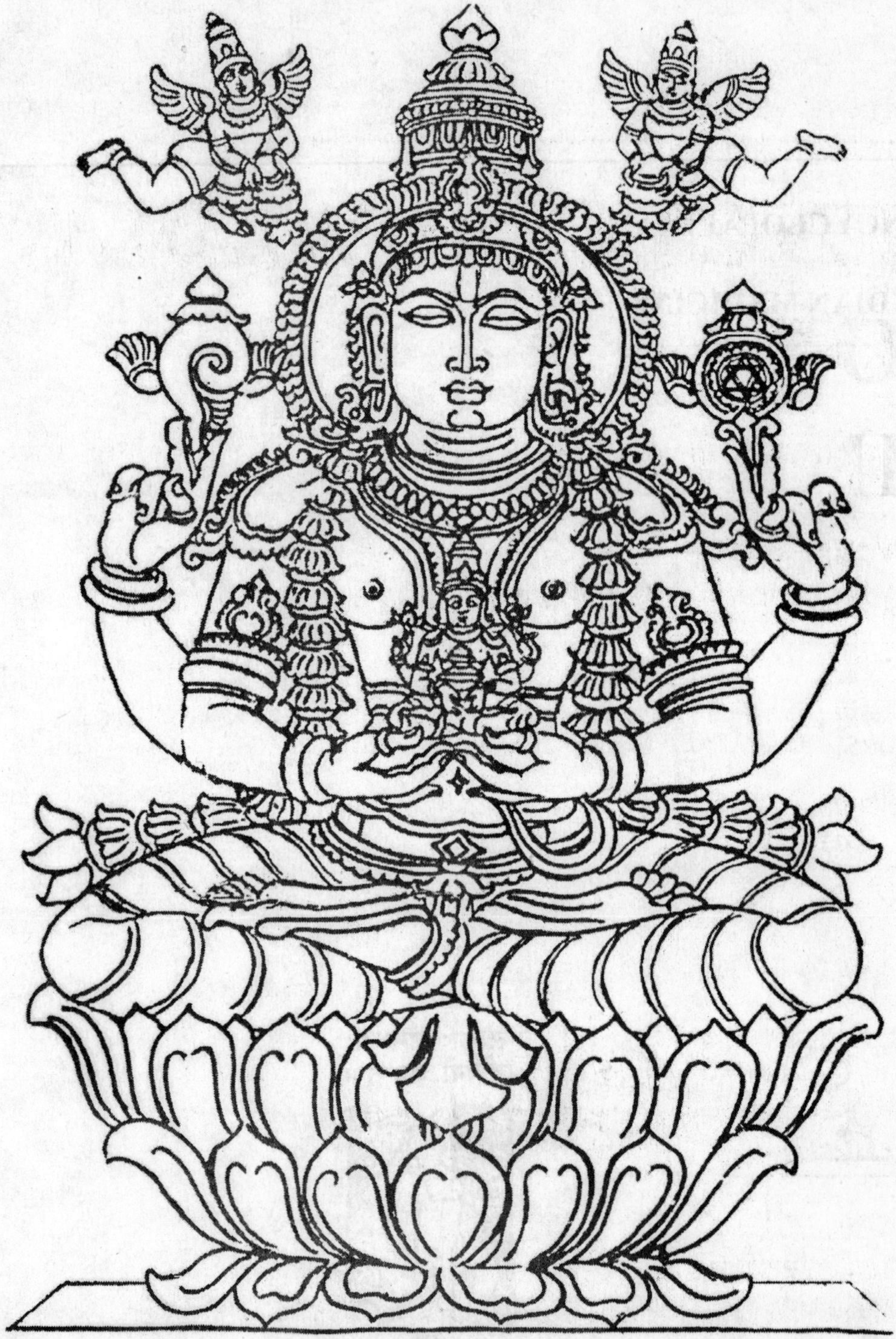

DHANVANTARI

Drawing from a temple icon in Tamil Nadu
(Courtesy : Regional and Technical Development Centre, Bangalore)

ENCYCLOPAEDIA OF INDIAN MEDICINE

VOLUME SIX
Diseases and Their Cures

Editor
Dr. S. R. SUDARSHAN

Popular Prakashan

On behalf of
Dr. V. PARAMESHVARA CHARITABLE TRUST, Bangalore

ENCYCLOPAEDIA OF INDIAN MEDICINE PROJECT

VOLUME SIX

Sponsored by

Dr. V. P. Parameshvara Charitable Trust Bangalore

Chairman

Dr. V. Parameshvara

M.B.B.S.,F.R.C.P. (London), F.A.C.C.,F.C.C.P.,F.I.C.A., F.I.S.E.,F.A.I.I.D.,M.S.A.,F.I.A.M.S.,F.I.C.N.

Editor

Dr. S. R. Sudarshan

© Dr. PARAMESHVARA CHARITABLE TRUST, Bangalore

First published 2005

ISBN : 81-7154-862-8

(3603)

Printed in India by:
Tarun Enterprises
20, Jaina Building,
Roshan Ara Road,
Delhi - 110 007

Published by RAMDAS BHATKAL for
Popular Prakashan Pvt. Ltd.
35-C Pandit Madan Mohan Malaviya Marg,
Tardeo, Mumbai-400 034

PREFACE

Indian religions are well known in the world. The philosophical systems that emerged on the Indian soil have also engaged the attention of scholars all over the world. India's achievements in the field of science and technology have also been recognised. However, the fact that India developed a system of medicine, thousands of years ago, has not received wide coverage in the world. And that the system thus developed is still prevalent among the masses of India is likewise not generally known, even to historians of medicine.

There are manifold reasons for this general ignorance of Indian medicine among historians of medicine, medical practitioners outside the country and intelligentsia interested in the problems of health and disease. One is absence of authoritative and well documented publications in English by Indians, dealing with this branch of medicine. The European indologists who have taken an interest in Indian medicine and have written on the subject do not seem to carry much credibility, because they are alien to the traditional details which are indispensable to the understanding of the spirit, outlook and value of Indian medicine. The literature available on this topic written in the traditional style of Indian languages have proved to be enigmatic to the modern reader. A great need is, therefore, felt for an authentic publication which communicates to the modern mind the traditional wisdom of India concerning medical practice.

The *Encyclopaedia of Indian Medicine* has been planned in six volumes to fulfill this need. The first three volumes have come out already (1985 and 1987), and the next three volumes are now being released. The first volume provided the historical perspective as well as an acquaintance with the classical medical literature in India. The second volume dealt with the basic ideas in Ayurvedic theory and practice. The third volume gave a detailed account of clinical examination and diagnostic methods in Ayurveda. These volumes were prepared by Vidyalankara, Sastra-chudamani, Vachaspati Prof. S.K.Ramachandra Rao who hails from a family of traditional physicians and has been conversant with Ayurvedic texts from his boyhood. He was the president of the Ayurvedic Academy, Bangalore. He has also been a scientist, having headed the Department of Clinical Psychology in the National Institute of Mental Health and Neurosciences, where he was instrumental in opening a department in Ayurveda. He was also a visiting Professor at the

Centre for Theoretical Studies, Indian Institute of Science, and is a Senior Fellow of National Institute of Advanced Studies, Bangalore.

The three subsequent volumes which are now seeing the light of day were prepared by his son, Dr. S.R.Sudarshan, who is an alumnus of the Government. College of Indian Medicine, Bangalore, and who has been a successful and popular Ayurvedic physician and Consultant in Bangalore. He has also been an author of several volumes dealing with Ayurvedic theory and practice. The three volumes that have been included in the *Encyclopaedia of Indian Medicine* pertain to the Materia Medica of herbal and mineral drugs used in Ayurveda, and to the diseases and the therapeutic practices in Ayurveda.

It is hoped that the comprehensive and factual knowledge of Ayurveda, enshrined in these volumes of *Encyclopaedia of Indian Medicine*, will now be available to the world for the more efficient health-care programmes that are afoot. We are grateful to Prof. S.K.Ramachandra Rao and to Dr. S.R.Sudarshan for having spared their time and energy to complete the volumes we undertook. We also acknowledge the help of Messers Popular Prakashan, Mumbai in bringing out these volumes. We regret that due to several factors beyond our control the publication of the three later volumes which were ready for publication more than fifteen years ago was delayed beyond our expectation.

Bangalore

Dr.V.Parameshvara
Chairman
Dr. V. Parameshvara Charitable Trust,
Bangalore.

INTRODUCTION

The first three volumes of the *Encyclopaedia of Indian Medicine* edited by Prof. S. K. Ramachandra Rao and published in 1985 deal with the historical perspective, the basic concepts, and clinical examination and diagnostic methods respectively.

Of the subsequent volumes, the fourth one deals with the herbal drugs that have been described in the texts of Ayurveda. The information regarding the rasa, guna, virya, vipaka and the medicinal action has been taken from various nighantus and the samhitas; however the main text that has been referred to is the *Saligrama-nighantu*. All the herbs have been given the botanical names excepting those plants that have not been accurately identified, such as meda, mahameda and other plants that form the ashta-varga. I have tried to adopt a clinical approach by giving the therapeutic applications of numerous herbs that have been gleaned from the ancient classical texts like *Charaka-samhita* and *Susruta-samhita*.

The names of diseases have been given in English so as to make it more accessible, but they are only approximate. Thus dyspnoea and asthma are used as synonyms for the disease svasa while toxicosis refers to visha and drugs useful in toxicosis are those which are vishahara or vishaghna.

The fifth volume consists of the description and analysis of the metallic and mineral drugs that are used in Ayurveda, as well as an account of the animal products that have been mentioned in the Ayurvedic texts. The sixth volume contains a detailed account of the aetiology, pathogenesis, prodromal symptoms, symptomatology and treatment of all diseases that find a mention in the texts.

I am grateful to Dr. V. Parameshvara for having sponsored this work. I thank Mr. Prasad for the neat line drawings of the plants.

Dr. S. R. Sudarshan

CONTENTS

ABBREVIATIONS & MAJOR REFERENCES

AHṛ Ashṭanga-hṛdaya (Vagbhata, ed.A.M.Kunte, NS, Bombay, 1891).

AMD Āyurveda-rnahodadhi- an- napana-vidhi (Sushena, ed. S. Venkatasubrahmanya Sastri).

AP Āyurveda-prakaśa (ed. with comm. by Gulraj Sharma Miśra, C, Varanasi, 1962).

ARH Āyurveda-rasāyana (Hemadri on AHṛ).

AS Ashṭanga-samgraha (Vagbhaṭa, ed. Atrideva Gupta, NS, Bombay, 1951, with Hindi translation).

ASK Āyurvedīya-śabda-kosha (Veṇimādhav-śastri Joshī, Nārayaṇaharī Joshī, Bombay, 1968, in 2 volumes).

ASS Ānandaśrama Sanskrit Series, Puṇe.

BP Bhāva-prakaśa (Bhāvamiśra).

BPN Bhāva-prakaśa-nighaṇṭu.

BR Bhaishjya-ratnavali (ed. Govindadasa, Calcutta, 1893).

C Chowkhambha Series, Varanasi.

Chkp. Chakrapaṇi-datta (comm. on CS).

CS Charaka-samhita (ed. Yadavji Trikumji Acharya, NS, Bombay, 1941).

CSS Chikitsa-sāra-samgraha (Vanga sena, Calcutta, 1884).

CSSS Charaka-samhita: a scientific synopsis (P.Ray, et.al.. Indian National Science Academy, New Delhi, 1965, 1980).

DN Dhanvantari-nighantu (ASS, Pune, 1927, includes RN).

HHC History of Hindu Chemistry (P.C.Ray, Calcutta, 1902 and 1925, in 2 volumes).

HS Hārīta-samhita (Calcutta, 1887).

IMM Indian Materia Medica (N.M. Nadkarni, Popular Prakashan, Mumbai, revised and enlarged, 1976, in 2 volumes).

KS Kaśyapa-samhita (ed. Hemraj Sharma, C, Varanasi, 1953).

MI Minerals of India (D.N. Wadia, National Book Trust, India, Reprint Edition, 1988).

MMH Materia Medica of the Hindus (U.C.Dutta, Calcutta, 1922).

MPN Madana-pala-nighaṇṭu (Madana-pala).

NiS Nibandha-samgraha (Dalhana, on SS, NS, Bombay, 1915).

NS Nirṇaya-sāgar-press, Bombay RJN Rasa-jala-nidhi (Bhudev Mookerjee, Calcutta, 1926).

RN Rāja-nighantu (Abhidhāna chintāmani, ASS, Pune).

RRS Rasa-ratna-samucchaya (ed. Dattātreya Ananta Kulkarni, New Delhi, 1982, Vol.I, Dharmānanda Sharma, Motilal Banarsidass, 1958).

RSS Rasendra-sara-samgraha (ed. Naren-dranath Mitra, Motilal Banarsidass, 1976).

RT Rasa-tarangini

SaS Sārngadhara-samhita (ed. Paraśurama-sāstrī, NS, Bombay, 1931).

SdS Siva-daṣa-sena

SN Śāligrama-nighantu (Lālā Śāligram, Varanasi, 1891).

SS Suśruta-samhita (ed. Yadavji Trikumjee Acharya, C, 1960).

SSS Suśruta-samhita : a scientific synopsis (P.Ray, et. al., Indian National Science Academy, New Delhi, 1980).

VSS Vaidyaka-śabda sindhu (Umesh Chandra Gupta, Calcutta, 1894).

YR Yoga-ratnākara (ASS, Pune, 1889; Mysore, 1899 in Kannada ch., with Kannada and Telugu Translations).

ENCYCLOPAEDIA
OF
INDIAN MEDICINE

Diseases and Their Cures

Abhyantarāyāma

Synonyms: Antarāyāma (CS), Dhanuh-stambha, (SS).

Western Nosology: Emprosthotonus; Parkinsonism.

Causes:

External: Factors which aggravate vāta.

Internal: Vāta

Pathogenesis:

1. The aggravated vāta affects the ligaments, tendons and nerves of the toes, ankles, abdomen, chest and neck (SS).
2. The aggravated vāta localises in the side of the neck (manyā) and spreads to the deeper vessels (CS).

Symptoms:

1. Spasms which bend the body forwards, like a bow, fixed and staring eyes, frothing at the mouth, and stiffness of the jaw (SS).
2. Spasms which bend the body forwards, like a bow, stiffness and flexing forward of the neck, contraction of the back, stiffness of the head (muscles), grinding or clenching of the teeth, spasmodic yawning and salivation (CS).
3. Grinding of teeth, pain in the sides, and inability to speak (AHr).

Prognosis: Difficult to cure. Incurable if spasms are continuous.

Related Diseases: Bāhyāyāma, Apatantraka, Ākshepaka, Vāta roga.

Treatment: See Ākshepaka.

Ref.: SS, nidāna, 1, 54-56; CS, chikitsa, 28, 43-44: AHṛ, nidāna, 15, 22-23.

Ādhmāna

Western Nosology: Flatulent distension of the abdomen.

Causative Factors:

Extrinsic: All factors which aggravate vāta.

Intrinsic: Vāta, apāna vāta.

Pathogenesis: The normal passage of flatus is blocked either due to constipation or as a result of emesis.

Symptoms: Distension, pain, uneasiness and rumbling in the abdomen, obstruction of flatus.

Prognosis: Easily curable.

Related Subjects: Āṭopa, Agnimāndya, Pratyādhmāna, Ānāha.

Ref.: SS, nidāna, 1, 88; AHṛ, nidāna, 11; CS, siddhi, 6.

Treatment: Fasting, intake of food that is easily digested, application of suppositories (phala-vartayah), drugs that are appetizing and digestive, massaging of warm oil on the abdomen followed by mild, hot fomentation (the palms can be employed for this purpose), enemata (śodhana basti).

Drugs such as jiraka, etc. can be taken either alone or with gruel.

Hot water is to be used for drinking. Food that is easy to digest is taken in a limited quantity.

Ref.: CSS, page.329; CD, 22, 387; SS, chikitsā, 5, 26.

Classical Prescriptions: Hinguvachādi - chūrna; Hingvādi-chūrṇa; Kalyāṇa-kshāra; Panchasama-chūrṇa; Śatapushpārka; Tālisādi-chūrṇa; Vaisvānara-chūrṇa; Yavakshāra.

Agnirohini

Western Nosology: Bubonic plague ?

Causative Factors: All three doshas, predominantly pitta.

Constituents Affected: Blood and flesh.

Symptomatology: Deep suppurating swellings (buboes ?) in the axillae, which have the hue of glowing embers of coal.

Fever, and severe burning, pains.

Prognosis: This is a fatal disease which brings about death in 7, 10 or 15 days, (SS).

Ref.: SS, nidāna, 13, 19-20.

Ajagallika

Type: A disease affecting only children.

Causative Factors: Intrinsic: Kapha and vāta.

Constituents Affected: Skin and flesh. The stratum granulosum (the śveta layer of skin)

Symptoms: Smooth, skin-coloured nodular painless eruptions of the size of māsha (black-gram) or mudga (green-gram).

Prognosis: Easily curable.

Ref.: SS, nidāna, 13, 4; AHṛ, uttara, 31, 1.

Line of Treatment:

1. If the eruptions are still immature, a paste of śukti, svarjika and yava-kshāra is applied.
2. Leeches can be later employed, if required.
3. If the eruptions have begun to suppurate, treatment as given for vraṇa is to be employed. (SS).

Ref.: SS, chikitsā, 20, 3-4; AHṛ, uttara, 32, 1.

Ahipūtana

Synonyms: Pṛshṭāru, Gudakuṭṭa, Anāmika (AHṛ.); Guda-kīṭa, Gudapāka, (RRS).

Western Nosology: Diaper rash, intertrigo, ulcerating eruption of perineum.

Type: A disease affecting children.

Causative Factors: Intrinsic: Kapha and pitta (SS, AHṛ.); kapha and vitiated blood (RRS).

Extrinsic: Uncleanliness, excessive perspiration and unhealthy breast-milk (SS, AHṛ); uncleanliness and excessive sweating (RRS).

Symptomatology:

1. There will be itching in the perineal region and around the anus, followed by a moist copper coloured eruption which later ulcerates (SS, AHṛ.)
2. The anal region is covered over by a vraṇa (ulcer) (RRS).

Prognosis: Easily curable.

Ref.: SS, nidāna, 13, 56; AHṛ, uttara, 2, 69; MN, 55; RRS, 22, 147.

Treatment:

1. The affected area is smeared with a paste of rock-salt and bark of badara. The child is given either ghee medicated with triphala, rasānjana and paṭola leaves or a decoction of khadira, kola and triphala (SS).
2. If the child is being breast fed, the mother or wet-nurse is to be administered drugs which alleviate kapha and pitta (AHṛ.)
3. Rasānjana is particularly useful in this disease. The affected area is to be kept clean and periodically washed with a decoction of triphala and khadira (CD).
4. The vraṇa has to be smeared with a paste of śileya, lūka (tanduliya), honey and cold water. The area should be washed with the decoction of triphala and badara leaves. If these measures do not relieve the condition, leeches are used to remove the vitiated blood. Other measures used in pittaja-vraṇa are also beneficial.

The child should be administered goats' milk boiled with jīraka, rasānjana and juice of jāti leaves (RRS).

Ref.: SS, chikitsā, 20, 57-59; AHṛ, uttara, 2, 71-75; CD, 55, 25; RRS, 22, 148-152.

Ajīrṇa

Western Nosology: Indigestion, dyspepsia.

Causes:

Extrinsic: Fasting or overeating; irregular and untimely intake of food; intake of unaccustomed, raw, dirty, dry, cold, heavy, fried, spoiled food; and food for which one has an aversion; excessive intake of water; change of climate and routine; travelling; suppressing the natural urges; other diseases; sleeplessness or sleeping during the day; emotions such as anger, fear, jealousy, depression; and purgatives and emetics improperly administered, (SS).

Intrinsic: Vāta, pitta and kapha individually.

Constituents Affected: The food juice, the digestive fire.

Types: Āmājirṇa (caused by kapha)
Vidagdhājīrṇa (caused by pitta)
Vishṭabdhājīrṇa (caused by vāta)
Rasaśeshājirṇa (SS)
Dinapāki-ajīrṇa
Prākṛtājīrṇa

Pathogenesis: The digestive fire is affected, and is not capable of digesting the food. The improperly digested food turns into poison, known as Anna-visha. When this poison is acted upon by pitta the person experiences burning pains, thirst, diseases of the mouth, etc. and may suffer from amlapitta. When acted upon by kapha, it may engender tuberculosis (rāja-yakshma), repeated attacks of coryza, urinary disorders, etc. When influenced by vāta, it causes many diseases. It may also localize in the bladder causing urinary complaints and in the abdomen causing abdominal troubles. It may also localize in the dhatus, (CS).

Symptoms: Common symptoms are- constipation, flatulence, weakness, headache, syncope, vertigo, stiffness of the back and waist, yawning, body-pain, thirst, fever, vomiting, anorexia, indigestion and difficulty in urination and defaecation (CS).

Āmājīrṇa: The causative factor is kapha.

Symptoms: Sweet taste in the mouth; nausea; salivation; eructations of food; swelling around the eyes; heaviness of the body.

Vidagdhājīrṇa: The causative factor is pitta.

Symptoms: Syncope; vertigo; burning in the mouth; thirst ; burning and sour eructations.

Vishtabdhājīrṇa: The causative factor is vāta.

Symptoms: Pain and distension of the abdomen; constipation, vertigo; pain and stiffness of the body.

Rasaśeshājīrṇa

Symptoms: Loss of appetite despite normal eructations; salivation; heaviness of the chest (SS).

Dinapāki-ajirṇa: This category is found only in MN. This is not considered to be a disease category. It refers to such cases where the food takes a longer time for digestion.

Prākratājīrṇa: This is also not a disease condition and occurs in all persons immediately after the intake of food (MN).

Complications: Syncope, vertigo, incoherent speech, salivation, vomiting, body pain, death. (SS)

Prognosis: Curable.

Ref.: CS, chikitsā, 15, 41-49; SS, sūtra, 46, 498-506; AHr, sūtra, 8, 25-32; MN, 6, 5-13.

Treatment:

1. Sleeping during the day after applying a paste of hingu, trikaṭu and rock-salt on the abdomen (CSS, CD)
2. Administering the powders of harītaki and pippali with suvarchala salt and hot water (CD)
3 If a person has partaken of excess of oily food, indigestion may be prevented by taking, ginger and harītaki, early in the morning.

4 Other useful preventives of ajīrṇa are: ginger powder with hot water, in the early morning (BR); harītāki, ginger and rock salt with cold water, in the early morning (BP, BR).

5 A yavāgu (gruel) prepared from chitraka, pippali, chavika and ginger is also useful in ajīrṇa (CSS).

6 Ghee medicated with dhānyaka and jīraka or with dhānyaka alone is also beneficial (CSS)

7 For ajīrṇa which occurs after partaking of certain types of food, suitable antidotes are to be administered. A few antidotes mentioned in BR are given below:

Food	Antidote
Panasa (Jack fruit)	Fruit of kadali
Kadali	Ghee
Ghee	Juice of jambīra or seeds of nimba
Mango fruit	Milk
Takra (butter-milk)	Seeds of nimba
Kharjūra	Seeds of nimba
Kapittha	Seeds of nimba
Rice	Milk
Milk	Ajamoda
Wheat	Seeds of dhattūra
Black gram	Seeds of dhattūra
Green-gram	Seeds of dhattūra
Kulattha	Curd-water
Pishṭānna (sweets)	Cold-water

Treatment of Āmājirṇa:

1. Fasting.
2. Powders of ginger, harītaki and pippali are to be taken with jaggery, (BR, CD).
3 Powders of ginger and pippali are to be administered with dāḍima and jaggery, (BR).
4. Vomiting can be induced by vachā and salt water, (CD).

Treatment of Vidagdhājirṇa:

1. Emetics can be administered with hot salt water.
2. A linctus of drākshā and harītaki is to be administered with honey.
3. Powder of harītaki can be given with honey, (SS).
4. Plenty of cold water is to be given internally, (CD, SS).

Treatment of Vishṭabdājīrṇa:

1. Inducing perspiration (svedana), (SS).
2. Salt-water is also useful when taken internally, (CD).

Treatment of Rasaśeshājīrṇa:

1. Sleep during the day-time.
2. Fasting or eating food that is easily digested.
3. Avoiding the factors that aggravate vāta,(CD).

Diet:

1. Food that is hard to digest is to be avoided.
2. Meals should not be taken after nightfall, (CD)

Ref.: SS sūtra, 46, 505-512; CD, 6; CSS; AHṛ, sūtra, 8; BR.

Classical Prescriptions: Ajamodārka; Bilvādi-guṭika; Bṛhat-nṛpavallabha-rasa; Daśamūla-shatpala-ghṛta; Gandhaka-vati; Laśunādi-vaṭi; Mustākarishta; Sanjivani-vaṭi; Śankha-bhasma; Vajra-kshāra.

Ākshepaka

Definition: Ākshepaka is a disease where there is jerking of the limbs similar to that which occurs while riding a horse, (comm. on MN 22).

Western Nosology: Tetanus

Causes:

Extrinsic: All factors which aggravate vāta including trauma.

Intrinsic: Vāta, vāta and kapha or vāta and pitta, (SS).

Constituents Affected: Nerves, blood vessels and hard fibrous structures like tendons and ligaments, (CS, SS).

Pathogenesis: The extrinsic causative factors aggravate vāta, which in turn may provoke pitta and kapha, or may itself cause this diseases, (SS, CS).

Symptoms: Repeated, paroxysmal, spasmodic, contractions or jerking of the limbs. The patient is well in between the episodes. There may be emaciation of the hands and feet.

Prognosis: Difficult to cure.

Ref.: SS, nidāna, 1, 50-51; CS, chikitsā, 28, 50; AHr, nidāna, 15, 16; MN, 22.

Treatment: See general line of treatment of vāta-roga, and apatānaka.

Related Subjects: Abhyantarāyāma, Bāhyāyāma, Apatānaka, Ḍaṇḍāpatānaka.

Alasa

Western Nosology: Tinea pedis, Athlete's foot

Causative Factors:

Extrinsic: Lack of cleanliness; walking in mud, and damp places.

Intrinsic: Kapha

Constituents Affected: Blood

Symptoms: Moisture between the toes, itching and burning between the toes.

Prognosis: Easily curable.

Ref.: SS, nidāna, 13, 30; AHṛ, uttara, 31, 25.

Treatment:

1. The feet are to be washed with sour kānji (aranāla). Application of a paste of neem, tila seeds, kāsisa (green vitriol) and rock-salt, or of juice of lāksha and harītaki. This may be followed if necessary by blood-letting. Application of juice of kaṇṭakāri or mustard oil. Rubbing with fine powders of kāsīsa, rochana and manahśila (SS).
2. Application of a paste of the leaves of jāti (CD).

Ref.: SS, chikitsā, 20, 20-22; CD, 55, 422.

Alasaka

Synonyms: Alasa (AHr)

Western Nosology: Intestinal obstruction

Causes:

Extrinsic: Intake of food which is too dry, pungent, cold, and hard to digest, overeating, improper digestion, and suppression of natural urges (CS).

Intrinsic: All the doshas.

Pathogenesis: The food is not digested due to the vitiation of the doshas. The channels of the body being blocked by the aggravated kapha, food is also not eliminated, (CS).

Symptoms:

1. The patient is found moaning, suffering from rumbling and severe pain in the abdomen, flatulence, obstructed flatus, constipation, thirst and eructations (SS).
2. The patient suffers from flatulence, severe pain in the abdomen, thirst, bruised pain all over the body, dryness of the mouth, vertigo, syncope, stiffness of the waist, back and sides, fever with chill or internal heat, incoherent and rambling speech, lethargy, heaviness of the body, loss of appetite and contractions of limbs, (CS).

Complications: If this condition is not quickly attended to, a condition known as Dandālasaka occurs wherein the body turns as rigid as a rod, (CS).

Treatment:

1. The patient is first made to vomit by administering hot salt water. Then the patient is made to sweat and is given a rectal suppository. Fasting is mandatory in this condition (CS, vimāna, 2, 13)
2. Emesis can even be done by administering hot water medicated with vacha, salt and fruit of madana, (AHṛ, sutra, 8, 15) or by administering water with pippali and salt (ARH on ibid). If the limbs are contracted, they are fomented and firmly bound with a cloth, (AHṛ).
3. The severe pain in the abdomen can be relieved by applying a paste of buttermilk, yava and yavakshāra on the abdomen. It can also be relieved by hot fomentation, (CD).
4. The severe thirst can be alleviated by administering a decoction of lavanga, (CSS).

References: CS, vimāna, 2, 7-12, SS, uttara, 56, 7-8, AHṛ, sutra 8, 4-16; CD, 6, 95, CSS.

Āmavāta

Western Nosology: Rheumatism

Causative Factors:

Extrinsic: Intake of incompatible food, faulty habits of living, chronic indigestion, lack of adequate exercise, exertion after partaking of rich food.

Intrinsic: Vāta, pitta and kapha.

Pathogenesis: The undigested food (āma-visha) localises primarily in the region of kapha (such as the stomach, chest, joints, etc.) It is then vitiated by the three doshas, and circulates all over the body, spreading diseases.

Symptoms: General debility, heaviness in the chest; pain in the sacrum; breaking pain all over the body; loss of appetite; thirst, lethargy and heaviness of the body; fever; indigestion; swelling of the body; stiffness of the joints.

Complications: Painful swelling of the joints; biting pain in the regions affected; loss of appetite and bad taste in the mouth; feeble digestion; salivation; heaviness of body; lethargy, burning pains, polyuria, stiffness and pain in the flanks, sleeplessness, thirst, vomiting, vertigo and unconsciousness, clutching pain in the heart, constipation, rumbling in the abdomen, distension of abdomen, contractions and deformities.

Prognosis: Good when only one dosha is mainly involved. Can be palliated when two doshas are involved. Difficult to treat when all doshas are involved, and when all the joints are swollen.

Ref.: MN, 25, 1-12.

Treatment:

I. General line of healing: Fasting, fomentation (sudation), administration of drugs and diet which are bitter, pungent and appetizing; purgation, oleation and enemata.

Administration of the paste of śaṭi and sunṭhi with the decoction of punarnava.

A decoction of ginger or daśamūla drugs is administered with castor oil. This is particularly beneficial in pain in the abdomen, sides and bladder.

A decoction of rāsna, guḍūchi, eraṇḍa, devādaru and ginger is also useful.

A decoction of śuṇṭhi and gokshura can also be administered early in the morning.

The powder of harītaki can also be regularly administered with castor oil.

One karsha of ginger powder is to be administered along with kānji.

The powder of panchakola, if taken with hot water is also of benefit in this disease.

The powders of śatapushpa, viḍanga, rock salt and maricha, if taken with hot water, are useful in loss of appetite and feeble digestion.

Ghee medicated with guḍuchi and ginger is also useful in this disease.(CD)

II. Castor oil is very useful in the disease.

The patient can be purged with powders and a decoction of trivrit.

A decoction of rasona (garlic), ginger and nirguṇḍi is very efficacious.

Equal quantities of pippali, hingula and visha (ativisha) are triturated in a mortar, and administered in a dosage of half gunja with honey in this disease (BR).

Diet: The following substances are beneficial: Vāstuka, punarnava, paṭola, rasona, vārtāka, kāravellaka, śigru, yavānna, old rice, shāshṭika-śāli, the flesh of lavaka, with butter-milk, soup of kulattha, kalaya and chaṇaka, gokshura, bitter substances (CD, BR).

These are better avoided - curds, fish, jaggery, milk, māsha, impure water, bathing in cold water, keeping awake at night, flesh of aquatic animals, food which is hard to digest and abhishyandi (CD, BR).

Ref.: CD, 25, BR, Āmavāta.

Classical Prescriptions: Ajamodādi-chūrṇa, Amṛta-ghṛta, Ānanda-bhairava-ghṛta, Bṛhat-saindhavādya-taila, Daśamūla-harītaki, Jirakādi-modaka, Kottamchukkādi-taila, Daśamūla-harītaki, Jīrakādi-modaka, Mahālakshmi-vilāsa-rasa, Nimbādi-chūrṇa, Panchasama-chūrṇa, Rāsnādi-kvātha-chūrṇa, Rasa-parpaṭi, Simhanāda-guggulu, Svarṇa-bhūpati-rasa, Vaishvānara-chūrṇa, Vātari-guggulu, Vyoshadi-guggulu, Yogarāja-guggulu.

Amla-pitta

Synonyms: Śuktaka (KS), Amla-śūla, Jarat-pitta (Āḍhamalla on SaS, 1, 7, 42).

Western Nosology: Pyrosis, dyspepsia; food poisoning.

Causative Factors:

Extrinsic: Food which is incompatible (MN, KS), food which is spoilt, sour and heat producing (MN, KS). All factors which aggravate Pitta (MN). Overeating and eating when the food previously taken is not yet digested. Starchy food, and food which is hard to digest, abhishyandi, too hot, too oily and too dry. Excessive intake of sugarcane products, molasses, kulattha, fried grains and cereals, parched and flattened rice, and cold milk. Sleeping after meals, and excessive bathing. It is common in aquatic and damp areas (KS).

Intrinsic: Pitta.

Pathogenesis: The vitiated doshas cause a dimunition in the power of digestion. As a result, the food partaken becomes fermented (śukta) and sour (amla), and localises in the stomach (KS).

Symptoms: Diarrhoea, heaviness of the body, sour eructations, headache, chest pain, distension and rumbling of the abdomen, weakness of the limbs, burning in the chest and throat, and goose-flesh (KS).

Sour eructations, vomiting, burning of the palms, soles, and in the chest and abdomen, bitter taste in the mouth, sharp pain in the abdomen and loss of appetite (RRS).

Indigestion, lethargy, nausea, bitter and sour eructations, heaviness of the body, burning in the chest and throat and loss of appetite (MN).

When vāta is involved there is weakness of limbs (KS, MN); pains of various kinds (KS, MN); yawning (KS); amelioration by oily, unctuous food (KS); twitchings, irrelevant speech, unconsciousness, horripilation, blindness, vertigo and formication of skin (MN).

When pitta is involved there is vertigo, burning pains and amelioration by sweets and cold (KS).

When kapha is involved there is heaviness of body (KS, MN); vomiting (KS, MN); amelioration by dry food and heat (KS); lethargy, loss of appetite, chilliness, weakness, itching of skin, sleepiness, salivation, sweet taste in the mouth, feeling of uncleanliness, and hawking of mucus (MN).

The vitiated doshas sometimes take a downward course. In such a condition, the symptoms are: Thirst, burning pains, unconsciousness, vertigo, nausea, urticaria, gooseflesh, perspiration, yellow discolouration of body and stools which are green, yellow, black or red.

If the doshas move upwards, the symptoms are: Vomiting of very sour matter which may be green, yellow, blue, black or reddish. The vomitus may also be very slimy and may resemble water in which meat has been washed. Vomiting of sour and bitter substances may occur before, during or after digestion, eructations of bitter and sour taste, burning in the chest, throat and abdomen, headache, heat and burning in soles and palms, fever, loss of appetite and itching eruptions (MN).

Complications: Fever, diarrhoea, anaemia, sharp pain in abdomen, swelling, anorexia and vertigo (KS).

Prognosis: Curable in the early stages (MN). Can be palliated or cured with difficulty when advanced. Incurable if all the complications are present (KS).

Ref.: KS, khila, 16; RRS, 18, 196; MN, 51.

Treatment:

1. This is a disease mainly concerning the stomach, and therefore emesis is to be done first, in a patient who is not weak and not emaciated. It can be done by administering salt water, warm milk, sugar cane juice, or decoction of madhuyashṭi KS), or a decoction of paṭola, nimba, madanaphala, honey and rock-salt (CD) or decoction of patola and nimba (RRS).
2. The patient is then made to fast, and to partake of only food which is easily digested. He is also advised some exercise (KS).
3. The following medicines are then to be administered: ginger, ativisha and musta, or ginger, ativisha and harītaki, or trāyamāṇa, leaves of paṭola and kaṭukarohiṇi, or a decoction of kirātatikta or rohini (KS).
4. The patient may then be administered a mild purgative, such as trivrit, honey and the juice of āmalaki (CD, RRS, KS). If necessary, enemata (anuvāsana and later āsthāpana) may also be administered (CD, CSS)
5. Generally the condition where the doshas move upwards is treated with emetics, while purgatives are useful where the doshas move downwards (CS).
6. Barley (yava) is dehusked, made into a decoction with vāsa, āmalaki and the group-trisugandhi. This is administered with honey to the patient, who is on a diet of mudga soup.

A decoction of fresh ginger and paṭola is appetizing, digestive, alleviates kapha and pitta and relieves vomiting, fever, burning and pruritus.

A decoction of paṭola, ginger and dhānyaka is beneficial in diseases of kapha and pitta and indigestion.

A decoction of barley, pippali and paṭola, if taken with honey relieves amlapitta and vomiting.

Powders of harītaki and bhṛngarāja are given with old jaggery in amlapiṭa and vomiting.

A decoction of guḍūchi, khadira, madhu-yashṭi and dāru-haridra, taken with honey, or the powders of draksha and haritaki taken with honey and jaggery are very useful (CD).

7. Laśuna (garlic), pippali, harītaki, cow's ghee and old madira are useful in amlapitta and improves digestion and strength (KS).
8. Powders of kaṭuki and sugar-candy, or a decoction of paṭola and ginger with honey are also very efficacious.

Ghee medicated with jīraka and dhānya is useful in diseases of kapha and pitta, indigestion, loss of appetite and vomiting.

Ghee medicated with pippali and honey should

be administered in the early morning.

Ghee medicated with śatāvari and milk is also useful (CD).

9. A concoction is prepared by heating gently 100 palas each of the juice of kūshmāṇḍa and milk with 8 palas each of āmalaki powder and sugar candy and 1/2 pala of guḍūchi powder. This is very useful in amlapitta (RRS).

Diet: These are beneficial: Bitter substances, barley, wheat, green gram, old rice, red rice, masūra, boiled and cooled water, sugar, cow's ghee, cow's milk, karkoṭaka, kāravellaka, paṭola, kalāya śāka, flowers of vāsa, flesh of animals living in desert areas, hilamochika, ripe kūshmāṇḍa, bananas, flowers of vāstuka, kapittha, daḍima and āmalaki (KS,CD).

These are to be avoided: New rice, all substances which aggravate kapha and pitta, tila, black gram, kulattha, oily substances, curds, alcoholic beverages and food which is sour, pungent, salty and hard to digest (CD).

Ref.: KS, khila, 16; RRS, 18, 197-204; CD, 52, CSS.

Classical Prescriptions: Amla-pīttāntaka rasa, Avipattikara-chūrṇa; Chaturmukha-rasa; Dhātri-louha; Jīrakādi-modaka; Kuṭajāvaleha; Lauha-parpaṭi; Loha-bhasma; Nārikela-khaṇḍa; Mahā-tiktaka-ghṛta; Pūga-khaṇḍa; Punarnavāsava; Śankha-bhasma; Saptāmṛta-lauha; Śūla-vajrini-vaṭika; Svarṇa-bhasma; Sūta-śekhara-rasa.

Amśa-śosha

Causative Factors:

Extrinsic: All factors which aggravate vāta.

Intrinsic: Vāta

Pathogenesis and Symptomatology: The aggravated vāta localises in the shoulder and brings about emaciation of the muscles and ligaments present therein.

Complication: Avabāhuka

Ref.: SS, nidāna, 1, 82.

Treatment: See general line of treatment in vāta roga.

Amśu-ghāta

Western Nosology: Sun stroke

Causative Factors: Extrinsic: Exposure to severe rays of the sun. Working or going out in summer without protecting the feet and head.

Symptoms: Intense thirst; unconsciousness; vertigo, blood-shot eyes; nausea; vomiting; involuntary urination; irregular pulse; dryness of skin, numbness, convulsions.

Prognosis: The disease is to be considered incurable when these symptoms are present: intermittent pulse, blueness of palms and soles and convulsions.

Ref.: BR, p. 695, 1-5.

Treatment: The patient is to be divested of his clothing and shifted to a shady place where there is plenty of fresh air, fragrance of fresh flowers and where the chirping of birds can be heard. The patient is then to be fanned with the leaves of tāla, kamala or kadali. Even if the patient is very thirsty, he should only be allowed to sip water medicated with chandana. He should then be covered with a cloth dipped in cold water and cold water should be sprinkled on the head. A shower bath is also of benefit in this disease.

Mild purgation with the oil extracted from danti is also beneficial.

If the body temperature falls down to subnormal levels, and if the pulse is abnormal, the patient is subjected to svedana (formentation) and administered mṛta-sanjīvini sura.

In this disease, measures are to be adopted which relieve unconsciousness, haemorrhages (rakta-pitta), which are a heart-tonic, strength-giving, refreshing and cooling.

Even after recovering from this disease, the patient is advised to take plenty of rest and to remain calm.

Diet: Food which is strength-giving, laxative, unctuous and nourishing, is beneficial.

Ref.: BR, pages 694-695.

Ānāha

Western Nosology: Flatulence

Causative Factors:

Extrinsic: All factors which aggravate vāta.

Intrinsic: Vāta.

Pathogenesis: The aggravated vāta blocks the channels of either āma (the undigested food) or the faeces and localises in the abdomen (SS, CS).

Symptomatology: The obstructed flatus does not move either upward or downwards (CS).

Symptoms: When the ama is involved there is thirst, coryza, burning pain in the head, sharp pain and heaviness in the stomach, nausea and difficult belching (CS).

Where the faeces is obstructed there is rigidity of loins and back, constipation, retention of urine, sharp pain in the loins, unconsciousness, vomiting of faeces, dyspnoea and symptoms of alasaka (SS).

Symptoms in Children: Dilated and fixed eyes, breaking pain in joints, restlessness, lethargy, constipation and obstruction of urine and flatus (KS).

Prognosis: Curable.

Ref.: SS, uttara, 56, 20-25; CS, sūtra, 18, 32; KS, sūtra, 25, 19.

Treatment:

1. Emesis is useful in cases where āma is involved. It is to be followed by drugs such as pippali, etc. which are appetizing.

In cases where the faeces is obstructed, if there is no vomiting of faeces, fomentation (svedana) is administered, followed by drugs which are digestive.

Anal suppositories of drugs used in visūchika are introduced along with cow's or buffalo's urine, after svedana. Enemata (nirūha and anuvāsana) are also useful (SS).

2. In cases where āma is involved, fasting, and drugs which are digestive are useful. The treatment which is given for udāvarta is also to be carried out.

Fine powders of hingu, vacha, kushtha, suvarchika and viḍanga are to be administered with warm water.

A suppository made of manahśila, soot, viḍa, trikaṭu, jaggery and cow's urine is to be introduced into the rectum (CD).

3. Small pills made of trivṛt, pippali and jaggery, are administered in constipation (BR).

Diet: The same diet is to be followed as in udāvarta, (BR).

Ref.: SS, uttara, 56, 20-27; CS, sūtra, 18, 32; CD, 29; BR.

Classical Prescriptions: Abhaya-lavaṇa; Āśvakanchuki-rasa; Bṛhat-saindhavādya-taila; Chandraprabha-vaṭi; Changeri-ghṛta; Danti-haritaki; Dadhika-ghṛta; Icchabhedi-rasa; Triphala-chūrṇa; Yava-kshāra.

Andhālaji

Synonyms: Antrālaji (MN)

Western Nosology: Phlegmonous Abscess.

Causative Factors: Intrinsic: Kapha and vāta.

Symptomatology: The vitiated doshas engender eruptions which are without a vent, circular, thick, raised above the skin, and of the colour of unripe figs. These eruptions have very little pus, do not itch and are localised mainly in hard fibrous structures such as ligaments, tendons, etc. (SS).

Prognosis: Curable

Ref.: SS, nidāna, 13, 6.

Treatment:

The affected area is subjected to fomentation (svedana). A paste of manahśila, haratāla, kushṭha and devadāru is then to be applied over it. (SS)

A paste of devadāru, manahśila and kushṭha can also be applied (CD).

When the eruptions begin to suppurate and break open, they are to be treated as in vraṇas, (SS).

Ref.: SS,chikitsā, 20, 5-6; CD, 55, 8.

Annadrava śūla

Synonyms: Jarat pitta (SaS, I, 7, 44)

Western Nosology: Gastritis.

Causative Factor:

Extrinsic: Same factors which engender śūla.

Intrinsic: All three doshas

Symptomatology: Abdominal pain which is sharp and which may occur during, before or after digestion, and which is not influenced by change in diet or by fasting. It is also ameliorated after bile is vomited out.

Ref.: MN, 26, 21-22.

Prognosis: Curable

Treatment:

1. Emetics are to be administered until the patient vomits bile and later purgation is done until phlegm (mucus) is eliminated. The same treatment is administered as for amlapitta. (CD)
2. The powders of āmalaki and loha bhasma are administered with honey. The powders of āmalaki and madhu-yashti are to be administered with honey. (BR)
3. Food is to be taken in limited quantities. (CD)

Diet: These are beneficial: Māsha which is boiled with ghee along with the husk. Godhūma (wheat) which is treated with jaggery and ghee, or with sugar-candy and cold milk. Then warm gruel with old rice. Sugar followed by boiled milk. Soup prepared from leaves of paṭola with chaṇaka, (CD).

Ref.: CD, 27, 83-87; BR.

Anuśayi

Causative Factors: Intrinsic: Kapha

Symptomatology: A slight inflammatory swelling on the head which suppurates internally, and is not discoloured. (SS)

Prognosis: This is a grave disease, difficult to cure. (SS, nidāna, 13, 23)

Treatment:

The same line of treatment as for kapha-vidradhi (SS, CD)

Ref.: SS, chikitsā, 20,11; CD, 55,3.

Apachi

Definition: Tumors which increase in number and growth and are not discoloured are known as Apachi, (SS).

Western Nosology: Diseased lymph nodes; lymphadenopathy

Causative Factors:

Extrinsic: All factors which aggravate kapha and medas (fat) (SS).

Intrinsic: Kapha, (SS).

Constituents Affected: Medas (SS, AHṛ).

Pathogenesis: Same as for granthi

Symptomatology: Knotty tumors of the size of the stone of the āmalaki fruit, in the regions of the jaws, axillae, clavicle, chest, shoulder joint, neck and throat, which are firm, rounded or elongated, unctuous, with itching and slight pain. A few of these tumors suppurate and disappear while others make their appearance. This process may continue for years, (SS, MN).

Prognosis: Cases of apachi with the symptoms of catarrh, pain in the sides, cough, fever, vomiting, severe pain and dyspnoea are to be considered incurable (MN, AHṛ).

Ref.: SS, nidāna, 11, 10-12; AHṛ, uttara, 29, 23-25; MN, 38.

Treatment:

1. The patient is administered emesis and purgation and is later given ghee medicated with danti, dravanti, trivṛt, jālini and devadālika. He should then regularly use dhūma (fumigation), gargle and take errhines of drugs which alleviate kapha and fat. Venesection can also be performed. Rasānjana is also to be administered with cow's urine. (AHṛ).
2. Ghee medicated with devadālī, kaṭu-koshātaki, danti, dravanti and trivṛt is useful.

The patient is administered an emetic composed of nirguṇḍi, jāti, bālaka, jīmutaka (devadali), honey and rock salt.

An oil medicated with kaiḍarya, bimbi, and karavīra or the juice of śakhoṭaka is used as an errhine.

Avapīḍa nasya can be used employing an extract of madhuka and seeds of śigru and apāmārga.

The region of the wrist should be branded with three lines, each one finger apart. (SS)

3. The roots of girikarṇika should be collected during pushya, and administered with cow's ghee. This will eradicate even advanced cases of apachi, (RRS).
4. The leaf-juice of alambusha is also very efficacious. A cake (pupika) prepared from the roots of vana-kārpāsika and rice is also of use in apachi.

A paste of bark of śigru, devadāru and kānji is applied, luke warm to the affected areas.

Oil medicated with chandana, harītaki, lāksha, vacha and kaṭurohini, is very useful when given internally. A paste of sarshapa, nimba, bhallātaka and goat's urine can also be applied in apachi, (CD).

Ref.: SS, chikitsa, 18, 20-23, 27; AHṛ, uttara, 30, 23-24; CD, 41, 23, 28, 29, 36; RRS, 24, 140.

Classical Prescriptions: Kānchanāra-guggulu; Vachādi-taila; Vraṇa-rākshasa-taila.

Apasmāra

Western Nosology: Epilepsy

Definition:

1. Epilepsy is defined as a disease caused by derangement of intelligence and mind, characterised by loss of memory, unconsciousness and violent spasms of the body (CS, chikitsā, 10,3)
2. The epileptic stage is attended by the loss of consciousness and fearful paroxysmal movements of the body which are produced by the perversion of memory, understanding and other mental functions (CS,nidāna,8,5)
3. The loss of both self-identity(smṛiti) and contact with reality is called apasmāra which is a defect in mindfulness (SS, uttara, 6l, 3).

Causes and Pathogenesis:

1. Persons of the following description are prone to epilepsy-those in whom excess passion and ignorance have overpowered the consciousness, in whom doshas change to other tracts, in an imbalanced state, those who have neglected the rules of dietary regimen and use unclean and wrongly

prepared food, those who neglect the hygenic way of living, those who resort to wrong activities and those persons who are extremely emaciated. In such persons the doshas get aggravated and the vitiated doshas enter the heart which is the supreme seat of life and the sense faculties in a person whose thoughts have been overcome by rajas and tamas (CS, nidāna, 8, 4).

The doshas, being aggravated due to intake of unwholesome and contaminated food, obstruct the passage (of the heart) thus causing passion and ignorance. The mind is preoccupied with passion,fear, anger, grief and anxiety whereafter epilepsy exhibits itself. Although the blocking of passages has been mentioned in general, the channels pertaining to the heart are to be considered in particular. The main precipitating cause for both insanity and epilepsy is intake of unwholesome and contaminated food and incompatible diet (ibid, chikitsā, 10, 4).

2. `The doshas of the psycho-physical body *viz.* vāta, pitta, kapha, rajas and tamas are excited and disturbed by the following causes:

(i) Perverted and excess sensual and physical activities.
(ii) Intake of unhealthy, unclean, and incompatible food.
(iii) Suppression of the natural urges.
(iv) Overloading of the mind with passion, ignorance, lust, fear, excitement, anger, grief, etc.

These excited and distrubed doshas affect the consciousness and cause apasmāra, (SS, uttara, 61, 4-6).

Epilepsy is of four types viz. epilepsy caused by vāta, pitta, kapha and all combined.

Prodromal Symptoms:

1. The premonitory symptoms and signs are spasms of the eyebrow, continuous distortion of the eyes, hearing sounds not present, dribbling of saliva, nasal discharge, disinclination for food, indigestion, catch in the chest, distension of the abdomen, general weakness, cracking pain in the bones, pains in the body, delusion, a feeling as if entering into darkness, swooning, giddiness and frequent dreams of scenes of intoxiation, dancing, acting, murdering, trembling, falling and so on, (CS,. nidāna, 8, 6).

2. Palpitation, feeling of emptiness in the heart, perspiration, unconsciousness, vacuity of mind, dullness, and sleeplessness are the premonitory symptoms of apasmāra, (SS, uttara, 61, 7).

Symptomatology:

1. The person's channels of cognition are affected by the excited psycho-physical doshas and whose consciousness has been overclouded with passion and lethargy has convulsive movements of his hands and legs, and distortion of his eyes and eyebrows. The person also gnashes his teeth, and foams at the mouth. His eyeballs will be fixed and starting. Finally, the patient falls down unconscious, and revives after a short while. These are the general symptoms of apasmāra, (SS, uttara, 61, 8-10). Incoherent speech, moaning and distress are common in all forms of apasmāra, (SS).

2. Since the passages are occluded by the morbid doshas the person is enveloped by stupor and anxiety. He sees things which do not exist and falls down with violent spasms. His tongue, eyes and eye brows become distorted, he secretes excess saliva, and throws his limbs about into awkward postures. As the passages clear he regains consciousness as if awakening from sleep, (CS, chikitsā, 10, 6-8).

Vāta-apasāra:

1. Sudden loss and regaining of consciousness,

bulging of the eyes, incoherent speech, vomiting of froth, heaviness and stiffness of the neck, bending of the head to one side, irregularly clenched fingers, tightly clenched teeth, trembling of the hands and feet, reddish or brown discolouration of the nails, eyes, face and skin, aura of flickering, rough, moving and dry objects, and aggravation from things which vitiate vāta and amelioration from these which alleviate it, (CS).

2. Tremors, grinding of the teeth, vomiting of froth, pricking pain in the heart, a sensation of being pursued by black creatures and incoherent speech, (SS).

Pitta apasmāra:

1. Sudden loss and regaining of consciousness, groaning, scratching the ground (with hands and feet), thirst, green, yellow or coppery discolouration of nails, eyes, face, and skin, feeling of heat, aura of bleeding, terrifying, cruel, burning objects, aggravation from things which vitiate pitta and amelioration from those which alleviate it, (CS).
2. Thirst, fever, perspiration, loss of consciousness, convulsions of extremities, and a feeling of being pursued by yellow objects (SS).

Kapha apasmāra:

1. Delayed loss of regaining of consciousness, absence of much distortion, horripilation, vomiting of saliva, white discolouration of nails, eyes, face and skin, aura of white, heavy and unctuous objects, heaviness of body, aggravation by things which vitiate kapha and amelioration by those which alleviate it, (CS).
2. Coldness, nausea, drowsiness, falling to the ground and vomiting of phlegm, and a feeling of being pursued by white objects (SS).

Prognosis: Cases of apasmāra engendered by the vitiated three doshas, which are chronic, and which occur in debilitated persons are incurable (CS).

Note: The attacks of apasmara recur once a month, or once in twelve or fifteen days, as the morbid matter accumulates. (CS)

Ref.: CS, nidāna, 8; chikitsā, 10; uttara, 61; AHṛ . uttara, 7.

Treatment:

1. The channels of the heart and mind which have been occluded by the vitiated doshas should first be cleansed or opened up by means of drastic purificatory procedures such as emesis, etc. The patients suffering from vāta, pitta and kapha apasmāra should be subjected to enemata, purgation and emesis respectively.

Later, the patient can be administered these recipes: old ghee medicated with the juice of brāhmi, vacha, kushṭha and śankhapushpi; ghee boiled with four times its quantity of urine of bull or goat, along with rock salt and hingu; one droṇa of cow's milk boiled with one prastha of til oil, one prastha of ghee and one pala of each of the drugs of the jīvaniya group; one prastha of ghee boiled with one āḍhaka of milk and sugarcane juice and eight times the amount of juice or a decoction of kāśmari and paste of one karsha each of the drugs of the jīvaniya group; (especially in vāta and pitta apasmara), and, one prastha of ghee boiled with one droṇa of juice of āmalaka and paste of two palas of yashṭi-madhu, in case of pitta-apasmāra.

The formulations known as pancha-gavya ghṛta, mahā-pancha-gavya-ghṛta, and vachādya-ghṛta are also useful.

The patient can also be massaged with mustard oil (sarshapa taila) boiled with four times its quantity of goat's urine, or with kaṭabhyādi-taila or palankashādya-taila.

The patient can be exposed to fumigation by burning the paste of pippali, rock salt, chitraka, hingu, kākoli, hingu-śivatika, sarshapa, kākanāsa, kaiṭarya, chandana, bones of the shoulder-girdle, nails and ribs of dog, and goat's urine.

The patient can also be massaged with a paste of tulasi, kushṭha, harītaki, jaṭāmāmsi and cow's urine.

A paste of bhārngi, vacha, nāgadanti and cow's urine; of śveta, white vishanika, and cow's urine, and of jyotishmati, nāgadanti and cow's urine can be used as nasya. The oil medicated with goat's urine, triphala, trikaṭu, devadāru, yavakshāra, phaṇijjaka, śyāma (trivṛt), apāmārga, and karanja fruits is also useful when employed as nasya. The powder of pippali, vṛschikāli, kushṭha, bhārngi and the salts can be used as snuff.

A paste of ela, mudga harvested in the autumn, musta, uśira, yava, trikaṭu and goat's urine can be applied as collyrium. The formulation known as mustadya-varti can also be used in the form of collyrium. (CS)

2. The remedial measures indicated in unmāda can be employed after due consideration, in apasmāra also.

The patient should be massaged with old ghee, while potions of it should be given internally also. Oil medicated with four times its quantity of cow's urine and a paste or the juice of śigru, kaṭvanga, kiṇihi, and nimba can also be used for massaging the body. Later, the patient can be subjected to purificatory procedures. Patients suffering from vātaja, pittaja and kaphaja apasmāra should be subjected to enemata, purgation and emetics respectively.

Ghee boiled with goat's urine, and a decoction of kulattha, yava, kola, śana seeds, guggulu, jaṭamāmsi, daśamūla drugs and harītaki can be administered in vāta-apasmāra. Ghee medicated with drugs of the kākolyadi group and vidārigandhādi group can be given with milk, honey and sugar in pitta-apasmāra. Ghee medicated with drugs of pippalyādi, vachādi and mustakādi groups, and decoction of drugs of āragvadhādi group, and urines can be administered in kapha-apasmāra.

The formulations known as siddhārtaka-ghṛta, and panchagavya-ghṛta are also useful. (SS)

3. The following formulations are useful in apasmāra: milk medicated with the decoction of kāśa, vidāri, kuśa and sugarcane juice and one prashtha of ghee medicated with a paste of yashṭi-madhu and eighteen parts of juice of kūshmānāa; The patient should regularly partake of oil medicated with lasuṇa (garlic), milk boiled with śatāvari, juice of brāhmi with honey, juice or a decoction of kushṭha with honey and paste of vacha and honey, (AHṛ).

4. The following preparations can be usefully employed in apasmāra : the regular intake of two gunjas of parpaṭi-rasa with the expressed juice of brahmi; regular intake of the root of nirgundi; the formulation known as apasmāra-nāśana-rasa; pārada bhasma taken with ghee medicated with hingu, souvarchala, trikaṭu and cow's urine; a paste of pārada bhasma, madhuka, kunati (manah-śila), rasānjana, and dung of pārāvata applied as collyrium; nasal drops comprised of seeds of white aparājita, and seeds of vijaya (bhanga) and human urine, or of brahmyādi-nasya or gavakshyādi-nasya; and external use of root of white aparājita. (RRS)

Ref.: CS, chikitsa, 10, SS, uttara, 61; AHṛ, uttara, 8; RRS, 21, 52-58; 30, 60-61.

Classical Prescriptions:

Asvagandhādyarishṭa; Balā-taila; Brāhmi-ghṛta; Chandanādi-taila; Chaturbhuja-rasa; Chaturmukha-rasa; Kalyāṇaka-ghṛta; Kayasthadya-varti; Kumaryāsava; Haratāla-bhasma; Mahā-Kalyāṇaka-ghṛta; Mahā-panchagavya-ghṛta; Mānasa-mitra-vataka; Mṛta-sanjivani-guṭika; Mṛgānka-rasa; Navaratna rāja; Pancha-gavya-ghṛta;Rajata-bhasma; Sāraswatarishṭa; Śiva-guṭika; Śvarṇa-bhasma; Svarna-mākshika-bhasma; Vātakulāntaka-rasa; Yogendra-rasa.

Apatānaka

Western Nosology: Repeated convulsions ; Status Epilepticus.

Causative Factors:

Extrinsic: All factors which aggravate vatā.

Instrinsic: vāta and kapha

Symptomatology: Paroxysms of falling unconscious to the ground, (SS, CS). Darkness before the eyes and production of hoarse cries. (CS).

Prognosis: Apatānaka which occurs after abortion, or severe haemorrhage or after injuries is incurable, (SS).

Note: Apatānaka is said to be of three kinds, i.e. Daṇḍāpatānaka, Abhyantarāyama and Bahirāyama. (SS)

Ref.: SS, nidāna, 1, 52, 59; CS, siddhi, 9.

Treatment:

The patient should be massaged with warm oil and then subjected to fomentation. He is later administered avapīḍa kind of errhine.

Ghee medicated with a decoction of vidāri group of drugs, meat-juices, milk and curds are administered internally.

Ghee medicated with souvarchala salt, harītaki, śunṭhi, maricha and pippali is also useful.

A gruel prepared from yava, kola, kulattha, mūlaka, curds, til oil and ghee is to be administered.

The patient can also be administered sour curds, vacha and maricha on an empty stomach.

In severe cases the patient is made to stand neckdeep in a pit which is heated with cow dung and burning husks.

A stone slab is heated and sprinkled with wine (sura). Palāśa leaves are then placed over it, and the patient is made to lie down on them. After the attack subsides, the patient is administered avapīḍa errhine. If the paróxysms do not subside even after ten days, oily purgatives and āsthapana and anuvāsana kinds of enemata are administered, (SS).

Ref.: SS, chikitsā, 5; AHṛ, chikitsā, 21, 31.

Apatantraka

Western Nosology: Grand mal.

Causative Factors:

Extrinsic: All factors which aggravate vāta

Intrinsic: Vāta and kapha

Pathogenesis: The deranged vāta surges upwards and affects the heart, head and temples, (SS; CS).

Symptomatology: Clonic and tonic spasms of limbs, closed and fixed eyes, moaning, difficult breathing, gasping and unconsciousness. These symptoms are transitory, and vanish when the vāta resumes its normal activities. (CS, SS, AHṛ)

Prognosis: Same as for Apatānaka

Ref.: SS, nidāna, 1, 64-66; AHṛ, nidāna, 15, 17-19; CS, siddhi, 9, 12-13.

Treatment:

1. Apatarpana, emesis and āsthāpana and anuvāsana kinds of enemata are contra indicated, (SS).
2. Pradhamana type of errhine is to be administered with drugs which are sharp (tīkshṇa), (SS). Drugs such as maricha, seeds of śigru, viḍanga etc. can be used, (CS).
3. Treatment is to be carried out which alleviates kapha and vāta and is useful in hṛdroga, (CS).
4. The patient is to be administered a decoction of yava which is medicated with tumburu, pushkara, hingu, amla vetasa, harītaki and the three salts, (SS). CS has

given the same prescriptions, omitting only amlavetasa.

5. Ghee medicated with harītaki, souvarchala and milk is useful in this disease, (SS).
6. Ghee medicated with souvarchala, harītaki, śuṇṭhi, pippali and maricha is also beneficial, (CS).
7. A decoction of ginger, hingu, amlavetasa, souvarchala and daḍima is also effective, (CS).
8. Svalpa rasona pinda: the bulbs of garlic (laśuna) (six tolas) are crushed well and mixed with the powders of one masha each of hingu, jīraka, saindhava, souvarchala, śuṇṭhi, pippali and maricha. This mixture is to be taken with the decoction of the root of eraṇḍa (castor) in the morning with due consideration to the digestive power. If this is taken regularly for one month, it cures all diseases caused by deranged vāta including Apatantraka, (CD).
9. A decoction of śālaparṇi with milk is also useful, (CD).

Classical Prescription: Rasa-rāja-rasa.

Ref.: SS, chikitsā, 5, 21; CS, siddhi, 9, 16-20; CD, 22, 29, 31-34.

Arakīlaka

Western Nosology: Warts; condylomata

Causative Factors:

Extrinsic: Regular application over the body of powder of burnt bricks, or intake of seeds of trapuśa and aervāru, food which increases the fatty tissues (medas) and sleeping during daytime.

Intrinsic: Vāyu

Constituents Affected: Medas (fat)

Pathogenesis and Symptomatology: The deranged vāta and medas engender the formation of polypi on the outer surface of the body. These will gradually increase in size. Emaciation will also be present.

Treatment:

1. Cauterisation with hot oil or of jaggery.
2. They can also be excised, and the area smeared over with kshāras.
3. Kshāra-sūtras can also be employed.

Ref.: KS, chikitsā, p.128.

Arbuda

Western Nosology: Tumours

Causative Factors: Intrinsic: Vāta, pitta and kapha.

Constituents Affected: Flesh (māmsa).

Pathogenesis: The doshas localise in a particular area in the body and engender disease in the flesh (māmsa) in that region. The disease may be caused by vāta, pitta, kapha and by the diseased state of blood, flesh and fat, (SS).

Symptomatology: General: A circular, firm, extensive and deep rooted swelling in the fleshy regions, which is slow in growth, does not suppurate, and pains only slightly, (SS). The arbuda caused by vāta, pitta, kapha and fat has symptoms similar to granthi caused by these agents.

Pathogenesis and Symptoms: Of arbuda engendered by blood: The vitiated dosha causes a disturbance in the blood and constricts the blood vessels. A fleshy tumour which bleeds continuously, has rapid growth and suppurates only slightly, forms in such regions. A patient suffering from this disease soon becomes anaemic due to the steady loss of blood.

Pathogenesis and Symptoms: Of arbuda engendered by flesh: Any injury or bruises in a particular region vitiate the flesh and engender in that region, a stony hard, oily, painless, immobile and non-suppurative tumour which is not discoloured.

Prognosis: Arbuda caused by vitiated blood is considered incurable.

Arbuda engendered by flesh is incurable in a person who partakes of meat.

Arbudas which occur in vital organs or in any body channels and which are characterised by any discharge are incurable.

An arbuda which is found upon a pre-existing one, arbudas which are contiguous, which crop up simultaneously or one after another are incurable, (SS).

Note: The arbudas do not suppurate because of the predominance of kapha and medas (fat), (SS).

Ref.: SS, nidāna, 11, 13-21.

Line of Treatment:

1. Arbuda should be treated along the same lines as granthi, because the regions involved, the causative factors, the doshas responsible and the constituents affected are the same, (CD).
2. Tumours which are superficial are covered with thin sheets of zinc, copper, lead or iron and subjected to cautery.

Arbuda engendered by vāta: A hot poultice of kushmānda, ervaru, coconut, priyāla, eranda seeds, milk, ghee, oil and water is to be applied.

Poultices of boiled meat or of vesavāra are also useful. The blood of that area can also be let out by means of a horn.

The patient should also be administered a decoction of trivṛt and other drugs which alleviate vāta. (SS)

Arbuda engendered by pitta: Mild fomentation and poultices are to be used. Purgation should also be administered.

The arbuda is to be rubbed with the leaves of udumbara, śāka, or goji, and smeared with the paste of sarja rasa, priyangu, patanga, lodhra and yashṭi-madhu and honey.

Ghee medicated with yashṭi-madhu is also to be administered internally. (SS)

Arbuda engendered by kapha: The patient is administered śodhana therapy and is then subjected to blood letting. The tumour is then plastered with drugs which are both emetic and purgative. (SS)

A paste of powders of śankha and ash of mūlaka is useful. (BR)

Arbuda engendered by medas (fat): The tumour is fomented and later incised. It is later smeared with the paste of haridra, soot, lodhra, patanga, manahśila, haritāla and honey.

Oil medicated with karanja can also be applied, (SS).

Ref.: SS, chikitsā, 18, 29-42; CD, 41, 49; BR.

Classical Prescriptions: Chandrodaya-varti; Khadirarishṭa; Kānchanāra-guggulu; Madhusnuhi-rasāyana; Mahā-triphalādya-ghṛta; Triphala-ghṛta; Vajra-bhasma.

Ardita

Synonyms: Sanskrit - Ekāyama (AHṛ)

Western Nosology: Facial palsy ; Bell's Palsy

Causative Factors:

1. All factors which aggravate vāta.
2. Constant talking in a loud tone, chewing hard substances, loud and immoderate laughter, excessive yawning, carrying heavy loads, sleeping in awkward positions. (SS)
3. Carrying heavy loads on the head, immoderate laughing and talking, bending heavy bows, sleeping on hard and lumpy pillows, chewing hard substances. (AHṛ)

Dosha Involved: Vāta

Pathogenesis: The vāta gets vitiated and localises in the head, nose, lips, chin, forehead, eyes and the joints therein, (SS). The vitiated vāta affects one side of the body. (CS)

Prodrome: Gooseflesh, tremors, obscuration of vision, numbness, pricking pain and stiffness of jaws and neck, (SS).

Symptoms: Partial distortion of the face and neck, tremors of the head, inability to speak, distortion of eyes, eyebrows, forehead, eyes, jaw and mouth, staring eyes, fits of sneezing, low, rapid, broken and indistinct speech, hoarseness, chattering of teeth, deafness, pain in the legs, hands, eyes, thighs, temples, ears and cheeks. Sometimes only one side of the face will be affected, (CS).

(The main difference between ardita and ardhānga vāta is that the former is spasmodic, while the latter is not.- Chkp.).

Partial distortion of mouth, obscuration of sight, indistinct speech, spasmodic laughter, trembling of head, loss of speech, staring eyes, chattering of teeth, hoarseness, deafness, loss of sense of smell, fits of sneezing, confused memory, trembling in the affected part, ptosis of the eyelid of the affected side, flow of saliva from a corner of the mouth, intense pain below or above the clavicles, (AHṛ).

Prognosis: This disease is incurable in

1. Emaciated persons
2. Where there is inability to blink
3. Where there is compulsive and incoherent speech
4. Where severe tremors have continued for more than three years, (SS).

Ref.: SS, nidāna, 1, 68-73; CS, sūtra, 11, 49; chikitsā, 28, 40; AHṛ, nidāna, 15, 32-37; CSS, vāta-vyādhi-adhikära, 556-559.

Note: CSS enumerates three varieties of ardita- (1) ardita caused by vitiated vāta, where there will be salivation, uneasiness, pain, stiffness of jaw, pulsation, trembling and swelling of lips and inability to speak. (2) ardita engendered by vitiated pitta, characterized by yellow discolouration of face, fever, thirst and burning; and (3) ardita brought about by vitiated kapha, characterized by swelling of cheeks and neck and stiffness.

This disease is said to affect the middle path (madhyama-roga-mārga) (CS, sūtra, 11, 49).

Treatment:

1. Ardita is to be treated along the same lines as other disease of vāta (see Vāta-roga). In particular, sirovasti, nasya, dhūmapana, upanāha, svedapāna, nādisveda etc. are to be carried out. Akshitarpaṇa with a particular medicated oil is also beneficial, (SS).
2. In cases where there is swelling, emetics are beneficial while presence of burning and redness necessitates blood letting, (AHṛ).
3. A dish ((māshandari) prepared from māsha is to be administered with fresh cow's butter. The patient is to partake of a diet of milk, and meat-juice, followed by a decoction of the daśamūla.Massags with oils, śirobasti, and oily errhines are also useful. Cow's ghee is particularly useful, (CD).
4. The paste of rasona is to be administered with fresh cow's butter in ardita, (BR).
5. Svalpa-rasona-pinda(see treatment of apatantraka) is also useful in this disease.

Milk medicated with bala or pancha-mūla or a decoction of mātulunga or a decoction of daśamūla is useful in ardita caused by vitiated vāta. Mashed meat moistened with fresh butter is also beneficial.

Cold applications, oily substances, ghee, sprinkling of milk, oily enemata and oily errhine are useful in ardita engendered by vitiated pitta.

Patients who have symptoms of distortion of the face, inability to speak and burning pains are treated with drugs, etc. which alleviate vāta and pitta.

A paste of rasona administered with til oil is very effective in ardita, (CSS).

Note: See treatment of vāta roga.

Ref.: SS, chikitsā, 5, 22; AHṛ, chikitsā, 21, 43-44; CD, 22, 17; CSS, vāta-vyādhi-adhikāra; BR, 325.

Classical Prescriptions: Bṛhat-māsha-taila; Bṛhat-saindhavādya-taila; Ekāngavīra-rasa; Karpasāsthyādi-taila; Mahā-nārāyaṇa-taila; Prabhanjana-vimardana-taila; Rasa-rāja-rasa.

Arochaka

Definition and Synonyms: Some physicians consider the terms Abhakta-cchanda and Anna-dvesha as synonyms for arochaka. Some others, however, define arochaka as tastelessness, anna-dvesha as aversion to the sight, thought and even mention of food, and abhaktha-cchanda as loss of appetite. (NiS on SS, uttara, 57, 3).

Causative Factors: Arochaka can be caused by the vitiation of any one of the doshas or of all three. It can also be engendered by emotions such as grief, fear, greed, anger, etc. and exposure to unpleasant sights, smell or food, (SS, CS).

Symptomatology:

Arochaka Caused by Vāta: Excessive sensitiveness of teeth, astringent taste in the mouth, pain and discomfort in the chest and tastelessness, (CS, SS).

Arochaka Caused by Pitta: Pungent, sour, bitter or salty taste and bad odour of the mouth, burning in the chest, unconsciousness, and thirst, (SS, CS).

Arochaka Caused by Kapha: Sweet taste, sliminess and itching in the mouth, heaviness of the body, chilliness, lethargy, body ache, and salivation, (CS, SS).

Ref.: SS, uttara, 57; CS, chikitsā, 26, 124-126.

Treatment:

1. Medicated gargles, inhalations, brushing and cleaning the mouth, pleasant food and drink, inducing gaiety and reassurance are beneficial.

Enemata, purgation and emesis are useful in cases of arochaka engendered by vāta, pitta and kapha respectively, (CS).

2. The patient is administered emesis by means of a decoction of vacha in arochaka caused by vāta, by water medicated with jaggery or sweet drugs in arochaka caused by pitta, and by a decoction of nimba in arochaka engendered by kapha.

The patient is administered food which is easily digestible, dry and tasty.

The mouth is to be washed with drugs which are bitter and pungent, such as haridra, triphala, etc.

Arochaka caused by mental disequilibrium is to be treated by reassuring and cheering up the patient, (SS).

3. The patient is made to gargle with dālchini, dhānyaka, musta and ela, or pippali and chavya, or musta, āmalaki and dālchini.

The patient suffering from abhakta-cchanda is made to gargle with amlika, jaggery water, dālchini, ela and maricha.

Long and chronic cases of arochaka can be cured by gargling with the juice of dāḍima mixed with vida lavaṇa, or with the juice of fresh daḍima mixed with jiraka and śarkara, (CD).

Ref.: CS, chikitsā, 26, 215-220; SS, uttara, 57; CD, 14.

Classical Prescriptions: Āmalakyādi-chūrṇa; Bīlvādi-lehya; Danti-harītaki; Daśamūla-haritaki; Dasāmūlarishṭa; Gandharva-hastādi-kvātha-chūrṇa; Chaturjāta-chūrṇa; Chitrakādi-chūrṇa; Jātiphalādi-chūrṇa; Jaṭāmāmsyārka; Karpurādyarka; Maṇḍūra-vaṭaka; Nārikela-khaṇḍa; Pippalayādi-ghṛta; Śankha-vaṭi; Sitopalādi-chūrṇa; Saubhagya-vaṭi; Viḍanga-lauha.

Arśa

Synonyms: Dur nāma

Western Nosology: Haemorrhoids, piles.

Causative Factors:

1. Lack of self-control, partaking of incompatible food, over-eating, excessive sexual stimulation, improper postures (squatting, according to NiS), riding horses, etc, and suppression of natural urges, in a person with weak digestive power (SS).
2. Partaking of food which is hard to digest, sweet, dry, unclean, cold, abhishyandi, heat-producing, incompatible, indigestible, that which disagrees with the person concerned, eating at irregular timing in too limited a quantity, excessive indulgence in meat, delicacies, milk, curds, tila, jaggery, sweet dishes, dishes prepared from māsha, sugar-cane, juice, pinyānka, piṇḍāluka, dry leafy vegetables, alcoholic drinks, laśuna, etc., sleep during the day-time, excessive exertion and coitus, improperly administered enemata, frequent abortions, improperly conducted parturition, pregnancy, etc, (SS).
3. Debility consequent upon fever, abdominal tumours, diarrhoea, indigestion, sprue, swelling, anaemia, etc. (AHṛ).

Constituents Affected: Rasa (body fluids), blood, flesh and fat.

Pathogenesis: The causative factors vitiate the doshas which either singly or together localise in the mucous folds of the rectum (guda-vali) and bring about fleshy growths, (SS).

Location: The disease manifests itself in the guda which is the lower end of the intestine, measuring four and a half angulas in length, and which has three mucous folds which lie one and a half angulas distant from each other. These three folds cover an area of four angulas, (SS).

According to CS, fleshy growths which occur in other parts of the body such as the penis, vagina, throat, nose, eyelids, etc. are known as adhimāmsa.

Classification: CS classifies arśa into two main types, that which is congenital (sahaja) and that which occurs due to the vitiation of the doshas. According to SS, there are six kinds of arśa: Arśa engendered by the three doshas individually, arśa caused by vitiated blood, arśa brought about by the vitiation of all three doshas together, and that which is congenital.

Premonitary Symptoms:

1. Loss of appetite, slow digestion, sour and acid eructations, thirst, weakness of thighs, rumbling in the abdomen, emaciation, excessive eructations, swelling around the eyes, cutting pain in the rectum, and symptoms which lead one to think of tuberculosis, cough, and dyspnoea; debility, vertigo, lethargy and weakness of the sense organs, (SS).

2. Weak digestion, heaviness of limbs, weakness of thighs, cramps in the calf, vertigo, lethargy, swelling of the eyes, constipation or loose stools, rumbling and movements of flatus below the umbilicus, cutting pain in the rectum, flatulent distention of the abdomen, profuse urination, scanty stools, sour and burning eructations, pain in the head, back and chest, lethargy, discolouration of the skin, weakness of sense organs, irritability, and symptoms of sprue, anaemia, abdominal tumours and ascites, (CS, AHṛ).

Symptoms: General Symptoms: Emaciation, loss of enthusiasm, depression, hoarseness, loss of lustre, cough, thirst, bad taste in the mouth, dyspnoea, catarrh, body ache, shortness of breath, vomiting, sneezing, swelling, fever, deafness, impotence, urinary calculi, loss of appetite, salivation, pain in the joints, chest, umbilicus, groin and rectum, oozing of moisture from the rectum, and variation in the colour and consistency of stools. (AHṛ)

Symptoms of Arṭa caused by Vāta:

1. The growths will be dry, rose coloured, uneven, tubular or needle shaped, resembling the flowers of kadamba or tuṇḍikeri. The stools will be very hard, dry and can be evacuated only with difficulty. There will be pain and discomfort in the waist, back, sides, rectum, umbilicus and penis, and black discolouration

of the skin, eyes, nails, mouth, face and faeces. There will also be present some symptoms seen in abdominal tumours, ashṭhila, enlargement of spleen and ascites, (SS).

2. The piles will be dry, withered, hard, rough, blackish and sharp with a cracked tip and ragged edges. There will be pain, tremors, pricking pain, pulsation, horripilation and formication, and general amelioration from unctuous and hot substances. There will be flatulent distension of the abdomen, pravāhika, retraction of testes, stiffness of the penis, groins and chest, body-ache, palpitation, constipation, and obstruction of flatus and urine, pain in the thighs, waist, back, sacrum, sides, abdomen, nose, ears, temples and bladder, heat at the vertex, sneezing, belching, coryza, cough, emaciation, swelling, syncope, tastelessness, a bad taste in the mouth, clouded vision, pruritus, hoarseness, and brown or black discolouration and roughness of the nails, eyes, face, skin, urine and faeces, (CS).

3. The piles resemble the fruits of bimbi, karkaṇḍu, kharjūra and kārpasi, or sarshapa. There will also be defaecation of frothy, slimy, hard stools with pain and sound, in small quantities, (AHṛ).

Symptoms of Arṭa Caused by Pitta:

1. The piles will be slender, blue tipped, shifting, yellowish in colour, thick in the middle (like grains of yava), and secrete a slimy fluid. There will be diarrhoea with burning in the anus and bloody stools. There will also be fever, burning pains, thirst, unconsciousness, and yellow discolouration of the skin, nails, eyes, face, mouth, urine and faeces, (SS).

2. The piles will be soft, extremely tender, red, yellow, blue or blackish in colour, and foul odoured. There will be discharge of a foul smelling, yellow, thin, blood-streaked fluid. There will also be burning, itching, pain, pricking pain and inflammation and general amelioration from cold substances. The stools will be loose and yellowish or green in colour and foul smelling. The patient will also suffer from thirst, fever, dyspnoea, confusion of the mind, aversion to food and yellow discolouration of nails, eyes, skin, urine and faeces, (CS).

Symptoms of Arśa Caused by Kapha:

1. The piles will be deep rooted, firm, thick, rounded, whitish in colour, and resemble the fruits of panasa, karīra or a cow's teat. There will be exudation and severe itching. The patient will also suffer from diarrhoea with the stools resembling water with which meat has been washed, swelling, chilliness, fever, tastelessness, indigestion, heaviness of the head and, white discolouration of the skin, nails, eyes, mouth, face, urine and faeces, (SS).

2. The protrusion will be big, firm, smooth, slimy, white in colour, heavy, swollen, numb and painless, with intense itching. The exudation will be continuous, slimy and tawny or whitish red in colour. The stools and urine will also be slimy, heavy and white in colour. There will be amelioration from dry substances. The patient also suffers from pravāhika, swelling in the groins, cutting pain in the rectum, flatulence, nausea, salivation, cough, tastelessness, coryza, heaviness of the body, vomiting, dysuria, emaciation, swelling, anaemia, fever with chills, urinary calculi, feeling of dullness or obstruction in the chest, sense organs and mouth, sweet taste in the mouth, urinary disorders, impotency, and severe indigestion, white discolouration of the nails, skin, face, mouth, urine and faeces. This variety of arśa is chronic, (CS).

3. There will be cutting pain in the rectum and bladder. There will not be any exudation, (AHṛ).

Symptoms of Arśa Engendered by Vitiated Blood:

1. The protrusion resembles the shoots of vaṭa, pearls, or fruits of kākanantika. The passage of hard stools will be accompanied by flow of profuse, foul blood. When the flow of blood is excessive, the complications of haemorrhage

supervene. The patient will also experience other symptoms of vitiation of pitta, (SS).

2. The blood can be vitiated either by the aggravated vāta or by the aggravated kapha. If vāta is mainly involved, the stools will be blackish, hard, dry and frothy. There will also be obstructed flatus, pain in the waist, thighs and rectum and weakness. The protrusion will be reddish in colour. If kapha is mainly involved, the stools will be unctuous, whitish-yellow, heavy and unformed. The protrusion will be thick, unctuous and whitish in colour. There will also be moisture around the rectum, (CS).

3. The patient experiences loss of strength, enthusiasm and complexion, and weakness of sense faculties, (AHṛ).

Symptoms of Congenital Arśa:

The protrusions will be of different appearances and sizes. The patient is excessively emaciated and weak, with a hoarse voice and unclear skin, and will suffer from urinary calculi. He will have excessive and obstructed flatus, urine, and faeces. The stools will be changeable in colour, and consistency. The patient also suffers from severe cutting pain in the regions of the umbilicus, bladder and groins, pain in the rectum, pravāhika, formication, urinary disorders (including diabetes), constipation, rumbling in the abdomen, udāvarta, dullness of the sense faculties, excessive, difficult, sour and bitter eructations, debility, weak digestion, impotence, irritability, cough, dyspnoea, thirst, nausea, vomiting, tastelessness, indigestion, coryza, sneezing, blurred vision, frequent bouts of headache, hoarseness and diseases of the ears, swelling of the extremities, face and eyelids, fever, body-ache, pain in the joints and bones, and frequent episodes of stiffness of the sides, abdomen, bladder, back and sacrum, depression and lassitude. (CS).

Prognosis:

1. Cases of arśa where the five kinds of vāta are involved along with kapha and pitta, and where all the three mucous folds (guda-vali-trayam) are involved are difficult to treat.

Cases where there is swelling of the extremities, face, umbilicus, rectum, and testes, and pain in the chest and sides, confusion of mind, vomiting, body-pain, fever, thirst and inflammation of rectum are incurable.

Arśa which are congential, where all the doshas are involved and where the innermost mucous fold is affected are also incurable, (CS).

Note: Three diseases are engendered by the same causative factor, weak digestion, viz. arśa, atisāra and grahaṇi, (CS).

Ref.: CS, chikitsā, 14; SS, nidāna, 2; AHṛ, nidāna 7.

Treatment:

I. Arśa caused by vāta and kapha are dry (śushka) whereas those caused by pitta and vitiated blood are accompanied by bleeding. The treatment for the former cases should be as follows :

a) If there is swelling and pain around the rectum, the area is to be fomented first, and later smeared with the oil prepared from bilva and kshara of chitraka, and massaged with a ball of cloth which encloses the warm paste of yava, māsha and kulattha, or the warm paste of vachā and śātāvari, or the paste of dry mūlaka. The area is later sprinkled with a decoction of the leaves of vāsa, arka, eraṇḍa and bilva. If there is intense pain , the affected area is immersed in a decoction of kola, or bilva or in butter-milk or sour kānji or cow's urine. The area is then exposed to fúmigation by burning the root of arka or the leaves of śāmi. Aśvagandha, bṛhati, pippali, surasa and ghee can also be employed for this purpose. A paste of haridrā and sudhākshīra can also be applied. All these measures relieve the itching, pain and swelling. Blood letting can also be done in order to eliminate the vitiated blood. Drugs which are digestive are useful in this condition.

Harītaki can be taken with jaggery before meals. The fine powder of trivṛt can also be administered with a decoction of triphala, or can be used after soaking it in cow's urine for one night. Harītaki can be used with butter-milk. Yavāni can also be administered with chitraka, bilva and nāgara. The patient can also be administered butter-milk with panchakola or with chitraka, hapusha and hingu.

Takra (butter-milk) is considered to be very useful in arśa engendered by vāta and kapha. An earthen vessel is smeared within with the paste of the root bark of chitraka. Buttermilk which is obtained in such a vessel is to be used. Patients with dry arśa can be benefitted by subsisting mainly on butter-milk for a week, ten days, fifteen days or a month, depending on their age, state of digestion etc. Persons with very weak digestion should partake of buttermilk only, morning and evening. When there is an improvement in the digestion, the patient can partake of lāja (fried or parched rice) and saktu (flour of dehusked and fried barley) with takra, in the evening. When the digestion further improves, the patient can partake of gruel (peya) with takra and rock salt and rice with takra, in the evening. After a few days, meat-juices, soup (yūsha), etc. can be taken in the evening with takra. This diet must not be continued for more than a month nor should intake of takra be abruptly discontinued. There is no medicine which is as effective in arśa caused by vāta and kapha as takra.

Yavāgu medicated with śāti and palāśā or with pippali or nāgara is also useful. Soup (Yūsha) prepared with dry mūlaka or kulattha or kulattha and makushṭhaka is also beneficial.

The medicines and diet are particularly useful where there is a tendency to diarrhoea.

In cases where the patient suffers from constipation and hard stools, the following medicines are of use: guḍa with nāgara, pāṭha and phalāmla, or with ghee and yava-kshāra; pāṭha with bilva or dussparśa, or yavāni or nāgara; madirā with guḍa and nāgara; ghee medicated with root of pippali, curds, dāḍima and dhānyaka; ghee medicated with chitraka, bilva and harītaki; decoction of kaṇṭakāri or of nāgara and dhānyaka.

b) The treatment for bleeding piles is as follows; purificatory treatment or langhana(fasting) is indicated. In the initial stages, bleeding should not be checked by astringents, etc. Its suppression aggravates the vāta, and causes diseases such as fever, rakta pitta, thirst, tastelessness, weak digestion, jaundice, swellings, pain in the rectum and groins, pruritus, skin eruptions, anaemia, retention of urine, constipation, obstructed flatulence, headache, heaviness of body and disease of vitiated blood. Therefore a competent physician who is aware of the aetiology, symptoms, duration of the disease and normal colour of blood should not check the bleeding until the vitiated blood is eliminated, and dangerous signs appear. Later, when further blood loss would be injurious, bitter substances are administered to stop the bleeding. These drugs will also strengthen the digestion.

A general principle to be followed is that bleeding should be checked at once in arśa engendered by pitta, and later in that engendered by vāta and kapha. The drugs which check bleeding are : a decoction of the bark of kuṭaja with nāgara, or of the bark of dāḍima or of nāgara and chandana, or of chandana, kirātatikta, dhanvayāsa and nāgara or of uśira, bark of dāru-haridrā and nimba. In severe bleeding, ghee medicated with the juice of dāḍima and yava-śuka or kaṇṭakāri and dugdhika is efficacious.

If these measures are not successful, the patient is administered unctuous and warm meat-juices, ghee after meals, massaged with warm ghee and oil and sprinkled with warm milk, ghee and oil, (CS).

II. Arśa of recent origin can be treated with medicines alone, while chronic cases necessitate the employment of medicines, alkali (kshāra), cautery (agni) and surgery (śastra). Protrusions which are deep seated, soft and markedly elevated (external) should be treated with kshāras and those which are rough, firṃ, thick and hard require cauterization. Protrusions which are raised, slender at the roots and exuding need to be surgically removed.

Application of Kshāra: The patient who is reasonably strong should be anointed (snehana) and fomented (svedana), and should partake of warm and unctuous semi-solid food. He should then be placed in a knee-chest position, with his head resting on the lap of an attendant. The thighs should be firmly secured. A straight and slender-mouthed speculum, lubricated with ghee is gently introduced into the rectum, the patient being asked to strain down. The protrusion is then scraped well and cleaned with a cotton swab after which the kshāra is applied over it. The kshāra is to be in contact with the protrusion for about one minute. The polypus is then cleaned and washed with fermented rice gruel, curd cream, and ghee medicated with yashṭi-madhu is applied over it. Further application should be done after due consideration of the state of the vitiated dosha.

Cauterization: Polypi engendered by vitiated vāta and kapha should be cauterized with fire or alkali while those caused by vitiated pitta and blood should be treated with alkali alone. Excessive cauterization causes cracking in the region of the anus, a burning sensation in the area, fainting, fever, thirst, profuse haemorrhage, etc.

Certain plasters can be applied locally in arśas: powdered haridra with the milky exudation of snuhi; pippali, rock-salt, seeds of sirīsha and kushtha with milky exudation of arka or snuhi; etc.

The following medicines are useful in internal piles: Harītaki with guḍa, in the early morning; a paste of the roots of apāmarga with rice water and honey; a paste of śātāvari with milk; powder of bhallātaka with fried and dehusked barley, gruel and takra without salt; etc.

Oleation (snehana), sudation, emetics, purgation and enemata such as anuvāsana and asthāpana are indicated in arśa engendered by vāta. Purgatives are useful in cases caused by deranged pitta while soothing measures (samśamana) are indicated in arśa caused by vitiated blood. Śṛngavera (fresh ginger) and kulattha are beneficial in arśa caused by vitiated kapha.

Bhallātaka Yoga: The patient should be administered purificatory procedures such as emetics and purgatives and should reside in a house protected from draughts of wind. He should then be given the oil extracted from bhallataka in the appropriate dosage. A meal of boiled rice, milk, ghee, etc. should be taken after digestion of the oil. The diet should be continued for three months, the patient being advised to remain tranquil during this period. This treatment will radically cure even complicated cases of arśa.

Drugs which are extremely useful in arśa are kuṭaja and bhallātaka, (SS).

III. A patient of arśa suffering from constipation and retention (or suppression) of urine is to be sprinkled with or immersed in a warm decoction of varuṇa, alambushā, eraṇḍa, punarnava, sushavi, etc. or milk mixed with oil or ghee, or oil which alleviates vāta. He should also partake of food which is laxative, unctuous, appetizing and alleviates vāta.

Fumigation with aśvagandhā, surasā, bṛhati, pippali and ghee and application of a paste of milky exudation of snuhi, and haridrā are useful as they facilitate the elimination of the vitiated blood from the polypus.

The powder of the root of kovidāra when administered with pure buttermilk is very beneficial in arśa. Buttermilk which has been kept overnight in a vessel smeared with the paste of fruits of kaṇṭakāri is also beneficial. These two recipes are particularly useful in patients disposed to diarrhoea. Constipated patients of arśa can take the following medicines with benefit: The tender leaves of karanja fried with oil and ghee, with the powder of fried and dehusked barley, before meals: or dry ginger and pāṭhā with jaggery, or jaggery, yava-kshāra and ghee.

The patient can also take a paste of the root of ajaśṛngi with goat's urine while partaking of a diet of jaggery and vārtāku.

The powders of trivṛt with a decoction of triphala; of harītaki with buttermilk; of harītaki and pippali fried in ghee with jaggery are useful in arśa especially when there is constipation.

The patient can also be administered sīdhu or gauḍam with chitraka and śunthi, or pāṭhā with kaṇṭakāri or bilva or yavāni or nāgara. The latter recipe is particularly useful in relieving pain.

Palāṇḍu (onion) taken alone or added to gruel, etc. is efficacious in arśa engendered by vitiated blood and vāta.

Bhallātaka is very efficacious in dry arśa while the bark of kuṭaja is useful in bleeding piles, (AHṛ).

IV. Parada bhasma given puṭapāka in tubers of sūraṇa, fried with til oil and administered with rock-salt is very efficacious in arśa, (RRS, 13, 33).

If fresh leaves of kusumbha are fried with kanji and taken regularly as a vegetable, it alleviates arśa, (ibid, 15, 81).

A paste of the seeds of devadāli, rock-salt and kānji is to be applied over the polyps, (ibid, 15, 82).

The rectum is to be washed regularly with a decoction of devadāli. This proves to be very useful in rectal prolapse also, (ibid, 15, 84).

The application of a paste of the root bark of śigru and leaves of arka; or of seeds of kaṭu-tumbi, kānji and jaggery is beneficial in arśa. (ibid, 85, 88).

V. The regular use of fresh butter and tila, or of nāga-kesara, fresh butter and sugar or of curds which has been churned is beneficial in arśa caused by deranged blood, (CD, 5, 114).

Diet:

1. Soup of masūra is useful in bleeding piles, (CS).
2. The following food articles are beneficial: Kulattha, yava, godhūma, rakta-śāli, punarnava, sūraṇa, takra, āmalaki, kapittha, navanīta, vāstuka, paṭola, maricha, kānji, and vṛntāka, (BR).
3. These are injurious: Fish and other sea food, curds, pinyāka, starchy food, māsha, karīra, nishpāva, bilva, tumbi and food which is constipating and hard to digest, (BR).

Ref.: SS, chikitsā, 6; CS, chikitsā, 14; AHṛ, chikitsā, 8; CD, 5; RRS.

Classical Prescriptions: Abhayārishṭa; Avipattikara-chūrṇa; Ayaskrti; Bṛhat-nṛpa-vallabha-rasa; Chandraprabha-vaṭi; Chandanādi-chūrṇa; Chāngerighṛta; Chitraka-harītaki; Dadhika-ghṛta; Dadimādi-ghṛta; Dantyādyarishṭa; Danti-harītaki; Daśamūlarishṭa; Dhānvantara-ghṛta; Haratāla-bhasma; Hutabhugādi-chūrna; Kalyāṇaka-guḍa; Kalyāṇa-kshāra; Kankāyan-guṭika; Kānta-vallabha-rasa; Kāsīsadi-taila; Kumaryāsava; Laghu-mālini-vasanta-rasa; Lodhrāsava; Lohāsava; Mahā-tiktaka-ghṛta; Maṇḍūra-vaṭaka; Mṛdvikārishṭa; Nāga-bhasma; Panchamṛta-parpaṭi; Panchasama-chūrṇa; Pippalyādi-taila; Pippalyādyāsava; Prāṇadā-gutika; Punarnavādi-maṇḍūra; Rasa-parpaṭi; Sapta-vimśatika-guggulu; Śiva-guṭika; Sukumāra-ghṛta; Sūraṇavaleha; Sūraṇa-vaṭaka; Triphala-guggulu; Vaikranta-bhasma; Viḍanga-lauha; Yogendra-rasa.

Arūmshi

Synonyms: Lomataskari (kaiyadeva, 8, 251)

Western Nosology: Furunculosis

Causative Factors: Intrinsic: Kapha

Constituents Affected: Blood

Symptomatology: Boils and abscesses on the scalp with many outlets, which are attended with copious discharge.

Prognosis: Curable.

Ref.: SS, nidāna, 13, 16.

Treatment:

1. After extracting the vitiated blood the boils are washed with a decoction of nimba. A paste of haritāla, haridra and nimba is then applied over the affected area. The oil, which is efficacious in Indralupta is to be used for massage, (SS).
2. The root of kushṭha, powdered and fried is to be applied with til oil.

Til oil medicated with haridra, dāru-haridra, triphala, nimba and chandana is efficacious if used for massage, (CD).

Ref.: SS, chikitsā, 20, 27-28; CD, 55, 82-83.

Ashṭhīla

Synonyms: Vātāshṭhīla

Western Nosology: Enlarged prostate

Causative Factors:

Extrinsic: All factors which aggravates vāta

Intrinsic: Vāta.

Symptomatology: A knotty growth which is stone-like, solid, elevated and spread upwards (from below the umbilicus) and obstructs the urine, faeces and flatus is known as asthṭhīla.

If the growth is situated side ways in the abdomen, and is painful, it is known as pratyashṭhīla, (SS). Such a growth also causes painful distension of the abdomen, (AHṛ).

Ref.: SS, nidāna, 1, 90-91; AHṛ, nidāna, 9, 24.

Treatment: See treatment of vāta roga.

Classical Prescription: Rohitakārishṭa.

Aśmari

Western Nosology: Urinary calculi, gravel, seminal concretions.

Causative Factors:

Extrinsic: 1. Sleeping during the daytime, intake of beneficial and harmful food articles in one meal, eating before the digestion of heavy and sweet food. These are especially involved in the causation of the disease in children, (SS).

2. The causative factors responsible for bringing about mūtra-krcchra (dysuria), over-exertion, intake of powerful and active (tīkshṇa) drugs and food which is dry, over indulgence in alcoholic drinks, seafood, and regular riding on fast moving animals. (CS).

Intrinsic: The vitiated kapha, (SS).

Classification: The disease can be of four kinds viz. that caused by kapha, vāta, pitta or śukra, (SS).

Pathogenesis:

1. The formation of calculi can be likened to two processes: The deposition at the bottom of a new earthern vessel of sediments from clear water and the formation of hail-stones, (SS).

Premonitory Symptoms: Pain in the urinary bladder, tastelessness, fever, dysuria, pain in the testicles, penis and supra-pubic region, body ache. The urine would have the odour of goat's urine. The colour of the urine, nature of the pain, etc. depends upon the dosha involved, (SS).

General Symptoms:

1. Pain in the umbilical region, urinary bladder, the median raphe of the perineum and penis during urination, intermittent flow of

urine, flow of urine mixed with blood, forked stream of urine, formation of turbid sediment which resembles gomeda, and is sandy and aggravation of pain while running, jumping, swimming, exposure to the sun, riding on horseback, etc., (SS).

2. Pain in the urinary bladder, the median raphe of the perineum and penis during urination, forked stream of urine, and frequent urging to urinate and defecate. During the paroxysms of pain, the patient clutches at his penis. Due to injury from passing of the calculi, there will be flow of urine mixed with blood. Relief from pain is experienced after passing the calculi, (CS).

3. Pain in the supra-pubic region is an additional symptom mentioned in AHṛ.

Symptoms of Vāta Aśmari:

1. Severe pain which makes the patient grind his teeth, press the umbilical region, rub the penis and finger his rectum. There will also be loud emission of flatus from the rectum, burning in the urethra (penis), and difficult and painful elimination of flatus, urine and stools. The calculi will be dusky in colour, rough, uneven in shape, hard and indented, (SS).

2. There will also be frequent and scanty urination, (AHṛ).

Symptoms of Pitta Aśmari:

There will be burning and sucking pain and pain as from an inflammation in the urinary bladder, and symptoms of ushṇa- vāta. The calculi will be blood-streaked, yellowish or black in colour or the colour of honey. The calculi will bear a resemblance to the seed of bhallātaka, (SS).

Symptoms of Kapha Aśmari:

There will be breaking, bursting or pricking pain in the urinary bladder and the bladder appears heavy and cold. The calculi will be white, unctuous, big in size, of the colour of flowers of madhuka and bear a resemblance to an egg, (SS).

Symptoms of Śukra Aśmari (Seminal Concretions):

A sudden cessation of sexual intercourse or excessive coition dislodges the semen from its natural receptacle. This semen dries up and is deposited at the junction of the penis and scrotum by the action of the deranged vāta. This gives rise to dysuria, pain in the urinary bladder, and swelling of the scrotum and groins. The stone sometimes vanishes when subjected to pressure, (SS).

Prognosis: A recent case can be cured by medicines, while that which is chronic needs surgery, (SS).

Ref.: SS, nidāna, 3; chikitsā, 7, 3; CS, chikitsā, 26, 36-37; AHṛ, nidāna, 9.

Treatment:

1. A patient suffering from urinary calculi should be administered the powder of or ghee prepared from pāshāṇa-bheda, vāsā, gokshura, paṭha, harītaki, trikaṭu, śaṭi, nikumbha, himsra, ajamoda, śitivāra, seeds of ervaruka and trapusha, black jeeraka, hingu, amlavetasa, bṛhati, kaṇṭakāri, hapusha, vacha and four parts of cow's urine, which is useful in dissolving the calculi.

A paste of gokshura roots, ikshuraka roots, eraṇḍa roots, bṛhati, kaṇṭakāri, and milk is mixed with sweet curds and taken for seven days, in order to dissolve the calculus. A paste of punarnavā, purified iron, haridrā, gokshura, phalgu, udumbara, pravāla, flowers of darbha, milk, water, urine and sugar-cane juice are useful in this disease. The powders of equal quantities of elā, devadāru, the five salts, yava-kshāra, kunduru, pāshāṇa-bheda, kampillaka, gokshura seeds, ervāru seeds, trapusha seeds, chitraka, hingu, jaṭāmāmsi and ajamoda and twice the quantity of triphala can be administered with any sour substances except śukta (vinegar), or meat juices, wine or gruel. This is also useful in gulma.

The gruel (yūsha) of a paste of the root of śigru, is prepared after seasoning it with ghee and oil, and after cooling, is administered with dadhi-maṇḍa (the upper layer of curd) and salt. A paste of śigru and cold water is also very useful in aśmari.

The patient should avoid exertion (exercise), suppression of natural urges, (excessive) intake of dry, unctuous food, kharjura, sāluka, kapittha, jambu, lotus stalk, and astringent food, sexual intercourse and exposure to the wind and sun, (CS).

2. An acute (recent) case of aśmari can be cured by medicines while a chronic case requires surgery.

If remedial measures such as snehana (oleation) etc. are employed when only the prodromal symptoms are present, the disease can be aborted.

In a case of vātaja-aśmari, ghee medicated with pāshāṇa-bheda, vāsuka (flowers of baka), vasira, aśmantaka, śatāvari, gokshura, bṛhati, kaṇṭakāri, kapota-vanka, ārtagala, kacchaka, uśira, gunjā, vṛkshādani, śyonāka, varuṇa, fruits of śāka, fruits of kola and kataka, barley, kulattha and drugs of the ūshakādi group, is administered internally. The patient can also partake of kshāras (caustics such as yava-kshāra), and gruels, decoctions, milk and food prepared from drugs that alleviate vāta.

In a case of pittaja-aśmari, ghee prepared from a decoction of kuśa, kaśā, śara, gundra, itkaṭa, the root of ikshu, pāshāṇa-bheda, vidāri, vārāhi, satāvari, sāli-mūla, gokshura, bhalluka, paṭola, pāṭhā, pattura, kuranṭika, punarnavā and sirisha, and a paste of śilājatu, yashṭi-madhu, seeds of indi-vara, trapusha and ervāru is to be administered. The patient can also partake of kshāras, gruels, decoctions, milk and food prepared from drugs that alleviate pitta.

In a case of kaphaja aśmari, ghee extracted from goat's milk and medicated with drugs of varuṇādi, bhadrādi and ūshakādi group, elā, guggulu, hareṇu, kushṭha, maricha, chitraka and surāhvā is to be administered. The patient should also partake of kshāras, gruels, decoctions, milk and food prepared from drugs that alleviate kapha.

The following formulations are very useful in the disintegration and expulsion of calculi: the powders of the fruits of pichuka (karīra), aṅkola, kataka and indīvara with jaggery followed by hot water; the powders of ajamoda, kadamba root, nāgara, and of bones of the camel, ass and krauncha bird, with surā (wine) or hot water; the powders of gokshura seeds made into a paste with honey, and taken with goat's milk for seven days; the kshāras of tila, apāmārga, kadali, palāśa and yava with goat's wine; the kshāras of pāṭalā and karavīra (with sweet drugs, milk, etc. in kaphaja or vātaja asmari, NiS); a paste of gokshura, madhu-yashṭi and brāhmi (with goat's urine, NiS); a paste of śigru, bhṛngarāja and eḍaka (with goat's urine, NiS); a paste of kapotavanka roots with sour gruel, wine etc, or milk medicated with the roots of kapotavanka; milk medicated with triphala (in pittaja-aśmari, NiS), and with the roots of punarnavā (in kaphaja or vātaja aśmari, NiS); and all kinds of preparations medicated with drugs of the vīrataradi group.

However, if the administration of medicated ghee, decoctions, alkalies and uttara-basti (urethral douche) do not bring about any improvement, a surgical operation has to be carried out; however, it is a very dangerous operation.

The patient should first be administered some unctuous substances, after which he should be subjected to emesis and purgation. After his weight has been slightly reduced, he should be massaged with oil, fomented, and asked to take his meal. Prayers should be offered, and the surgical instruments should be arranged in the correct order. The patient should then be reassured. A strong and well built person should be the attendant, and should sit on a couch that is as high as the knee. The patient should recline on the couch, resting the upper part of his body on the attendant's lap, with his waist being supported on a cushion. The elbows and knee should be fastened, and the umbilical region should be massaged with oil or ghee. The left side of the umbilical region should be pressed with a closed fist, in order that the calculus may be palpated. The second and third fingers of the surgeon's left hand should be introduced into the rectum. The fingers should be carried upwards, towards the middle of the perineum, so that the calculus can be brought in between the rectum and penis, where it appears like an elevated knotty growth. However, if the patient faints when the stone is handled with drooping head and fixed eyes, the operation should not be continued. If this does not happen, an incision should be made on the left side of the raphe of the perineum at the distance of a barley-corn, and big enough for the removal of the calculus. Some authorities recommend that the incision be made on the right side of the raphe, for the sake of convenience. The stone should be fully removed, without leaving any remnant behind. It should be extracted by making use of agravaktra yantra (a kind of forceps).

In women, the incision should be made in an oblique and upward direction, as the uterus is adjacent to the urinary bladder (for more details refer SS).

After the operation the patient should sit in a tub of warm water. The will prevent the accumulation of blood in the bladder. If blood accumulates there in spite of this, a decoction of kshīri trees should be injected into the urethra. For cleansing the urinary passage, jaggery solution should be administered internally. The incidental ulcer should be lubricated with honey and ghee. The patient should partake of warm gruels prepared from drugs that cleanse the urine such as gokshura, kūshmāṇḍa, pāshāṇa-bheda and drugs of tṛṇa-pancha-mūla group, for three days along with ghee. Later, for the subsequent ten days, rice well boiled and mixed with jaggery should be given, in small quantities. This acts as a diuretic, purifies blood and establishes secretion in the ulcer (wound). After ten days sour fruits and meat juices of desert animals can be partaken. The patient should then be fomented for ten days with any warm medicinal fluids or warm oils. The wound should be washed with a decoction of kshīri-trees. A paste of lodhra, yashṭi-madhu, manjishṭha and prapouṇḍarika can be applied over it. Ghee or oil medicated with the above drugs and haridrā can also be applied. The blood clots can be removed by urethral douches. If urine does not flow even after seven days, the wound should be cauterized. After normal urination, uttara-basti, āsthāpana and anuvāsana enemas can be given with a decoction of sweet drugs. If a calculus or śukra aśmari spontaneously comes down the urethral passage, the urethra can be cut open and the stone extracted by a badiśa (hook).

The patient should avoid sexual intercourse, riding on animals, swimming, strenous exertions such as climbing trees, etc. and eating heavy and indigestible food for one year after the operation.

During the operation, the mūtra-vahā srotas (vessels that carry urine); śukra-vahā (channels that convey seminal fluid), the spermatic cord, urethra, the perineal raphe, the uterus, vagina, etc., rectum and urinary bladder should be carefully protected. If the ureters (mūtra-vahā-srotas) are injured, the patient dies due to accumulation of urine in the bladder. If the śukra-vahā-srotas are injured, the patient either expires, or becomes impotent. If the spermatic cord is injured, it causes dhvaja-bhanja. Injury to the urethra causes dribbling of urine. Injury to the raphe or female generative organs engenders pain, (SS).

3. When the premonitary symptoms appear, snehana (oleation) is to be carried out.

A paste of the roots of eraṇḍa, bṛhati, kaṇṭakāri, gokshura, and sugarcane is administered with sweet curds for dissolving the calculi.

The seeds of tumbari (or gokshura, or kataka) are administed with honey and goat's milk for a week.

The kshāra of tila, apāmārga, kadali, palāśa, yava, etc. is to be administered with goat's milk.

Milk medicated with the kernel of harītaki or with punarnava is also useful. The root of mayūra-śikha can also be administered with rice water. In these cases, the diet has to consist only of milk and rice, (AHṛ).

4. A decoction of the bark of varuṇa, ginger, gokshura, and yava-kshāra, is very efficacious in vāta aśmari. A decoction of the bark of varuṇa, if partaken of with old jaggery, is useful in calculi and in relieving the pain in the bladder.

The juice of kūshmaṇḍa, yava-kshāra and jaggery is also efficacious in dissolving the calculi.

A decoction of gokshura, leaves of eraṇḍa, ginger and bark of varuṇa should also be administered early in the morning.

The juice of ripe ikshvāku is given with yava-kshāra and sugarcandy for dissolving calculi. Wine with souvarchala salt, and the ash of tila nāla (stalks of tila) with honey and milk are also beneficial in this disease. The seeds of gokshura can also be administered for a week with honey and goat's milk.

Śukra aśmari can be treated with the same drugs used for calculi, (CD).

5. The regular use of yava-kshāra with honey, and of haridra with old jaggery and kānji is useful in dissolving calculi. The stalk of vandhyā-karkoṭaki is dried, powdered and administered with honey, in this disease, (RRS).

Diet: The following food articles are beneficial: Kulattha, mudga, godhūma, old rice, yava, taṇḍulīya, ripe kūshmāṇḍa and fresh ginger, (BR).

These are contraindicated: Suppression of natural urges, food which is sour, constipative, dry and hard to digest, (BR).

Ref.: SS, chikitsā, 7; CS, chikitsā, 26, 59-72; AHṛ, chikitsā, 11, 17-33; CD, 34; RRS, 17, 18, 25, 26; BR.

Classical Prescriptions: Bṛhat-saindhavādya-taila; Chandraprabha-vaṭi; Gokshurādi-guggulu; Kumāryasava; Mūlaka-kshāra; Palāśa-kshāra; Svarṇa-bhūpati-rasa; Traikaṇṭaka-ghṛta; Vastyāmayāntaka-ghṛta; Viḍangārishṭa.

Asṛgdhara

Synonyms: Rakta-yoni, Pradara (CS).

Western Nosology: Uterine bleeding; menorrhagia, metrorrhagia.

Causative Factors:

Extrinsic:

1. Excessive intake of meat of domesticated and aquatic or wet-land (oudaka) animals, alcoholic drinks, kṛśāra, pāyasa, curds, śaktu, mastu and food that is salty, sour, hard to digest, pungent, irritant (vidāhi) and unctuous, (CS).

2. Intake of incompatible food, overeating, indigestion, abortion, excessive sexual intercourse, excessive travelling and riding on animals, grief, emaciation, lifting heavy weights, injuries, sleeping during the daytime, etc., (CSS, MN).

Classification:

1. There are three kinds of asṛgdara, i.e. that which is caused by vāta, pitta or kapha, (SS).
2. CS also includes asṛgdara that is caused by the aggravation of all three doshas.

Pathogenesis: The aggravated vāta increases the quantity of blood that circulates through the blood vessels leading to the uterus, and as a result, there is an excessive flow of blood from the uterus, (CS).

General Symptomatology:

1. Excessive bleeding during or in between the menstrual periods. Pain in the limbs, debility, vertigo, unconsciousness, thirst, burning pains, incoherent speech, anaemia, lethargy and diseases of deranged vāta, (SS).

2. Excessive uterine bleeding, (CS).

Vātaja Ashgdara:

1. The blood is frothy, thin, non-unctuous, blackish or brown in colour, or resembling the colour of the juice of the palāśa flower. Bleeding may or may not be painful. There is also severe pain in the waist, groin, chest, sides of the chest, back and pelvis, (CS).

2. The blood will be thin, frothy, brownish or black in colour, and devoid of its slimy nature. There will be rapid bleeding, (SS).

Pittaja Asṛgdara:

1. There is excessive and frequent bleeding with blood (mixed with fluid) that is bluish yellow, or black, and very hot. There is also burning pain, redness, thirst, clouded mind, fever and vertigo.

2. The blood will be blue, yellow, green, or brown in colour, foul smelling, thin, and is shunned by ants and flies, (SS).

Kaphaja Asṛgdara:

1. The blood is slimy, thick, yellowish-white, heavy, unctuous, and cold. The bleeding is only slightly painful, and is accompanied by vomiting, anorexia, nausea, dyspnoea and cough, (CS).

2. The blood will be cold, oily, thick, slimy and resembles flesh in colour. There will be slow oozing of blood. (SS)

Prognosis:

1. This disease is easily curable in young women who follow a healthy regimen, and where there are no complications, (SS).

2. If a woman who is weakened and anaemic (due to the disease) still indulges in factors that are responsible for causing this disease, the vāta is excessively vitiated, and along with the heat of pitta causes the discharge of offensive, slimy, yellowish kapha (mucous), mixed with vasā (fat of the superficial fascia) and medas (adipose tissue). The discharge will resemble ghee or bone-marrow or vasā, and will be constant, with other symptoms like thirst, fever, and burning pain. Such a patient is incurable, (CS).

3. It is incurable where there is excessive and constant bleeding, and where there are symptoms such as thirst, burning pains, fever and debility, (CSS).

Related Diseases: Yoni-roga

Ref.: SS, śārīra, 2, 18-20; sūtra, 14, 21; CS, chikitsā, 30, 16; 30, 204-224; CSS, page. 775; MN, 61.

Treatment:

1. This disease is to be treated on the same lines as Rakta-pitta, (SS).

2. Styptic (haemostatic) drugs are to be used according to the dosha involved.

The juice of varāha is administered with the soup of kulattha in cases where the vāta is involved. Patients in whom pitta is aggravated are to be administered yashṭi and nāgara with curds, honey and sugar. The root of taṇḍulīya is to be administered with honey and rice water in cases where both vāta and pitta are involved. Rasānjana can also be administered with lākshā (lac) and goat's milk in such cases. A paste of the leaves of rāḍādāna and kapittha is to be fried with ghee and administered in cases of asṛgdara. Kaphaja asṛgdara is to be treated with nimba and guḍūchi.

A decoction of kāśmari and kutaja can be used as a douche.

In cases of asṛgdara where the blood is pāṇḍura (whitish) in colour, the patient can be administered a paste of rohitaka root, or a paste of āmalaki seeds, water, honey and sugar or the powder of āmalaki with honey, or the paste of lodhra with a decoction of the bark of nyagrodha (banyan tree). A silk cloth soaked in a decoction of the bark of nyagrodha can be kept in the vagina, or a lump prepared from the bark of plaksha and honey may be inserted within the vagina. The vagina may be lubricated with oil after which a plug prepared from lodhra, priyangu, yashṭi-madhu and honey or from astringent drugs may be inserted within the vagina. The remedial measures useful in raktātisāra and rakta-arśas are also useful, (CS).

3. Immediately after the manifestation of bleeding, the patient is made to lie down on a couch with her lower limbs elevated, and covered with a soft cool bed-sheet. A cotton swab is dipped in cold water and then in ghee medicated with yashṭi-madhu and placed over the vagina. The body below the umbilicus is smeared with śata-dhouta ghṛta (ghee washed one hundred times), or sahasra-dhouta ghṛta (ghee washed a thousand time) and sprinkled with cold cow's milk, a decoction of yashṭi-madhu and nyagrodha. Cotton swabs dipped in the juice or a decoction of milk medicated with drugs having an astringent taste, such as buds of nyagrodha (banyan tree), etc. or ghee medicated with the buds of nyagrodha is administered internally. A paste of the pollen of padma, utpala, and kumuda honey and sugar can be given. Milk and ghee are also to be given. Milk medicated with priyangu, blue variety of utpala, cut and dried pieces of tender fruits of fig (udumbara), buds of nyagrodha, etc. is also beneficial.

The patient should refrain from anger, grief, sexual intercourse, and exertion, (CS, vimāna, 8, 24).

4. Asṛgdara is a life-threatening disease and should therefore be treated very seriously.

All measures employed in garbha-srāva (abortion) are useful in this condition. Emetics can be administered with sugar-cane juice or grape juice. Vaginal suppositories medicated with oil boiled with mudgaparṇi are useful.

Curds medicated with souvarchala, ajāji, madhuka, blue variety of utpala and honey are useful in vātaja asṛgdara.

The juice of vāsaka or of guḍūchi is useful in pitta-asṛgdara. A decoction of the bark of aśoka with milk is to be administered in the morning in this disease. The fruit-juice of kākodumbara is also beneficial when administered with honey.

The root of rohitaka is useful in kaphaja asṛgdara. A paste of the seeds of āmalaki, sugar candy, honey and water is also beneficial. The roots of kākajangha or kārpāsa can also be administered with benefit.

The roots of taṇḍulīyaka, if administered with tārkshya, honey and rice water relieves almost all cases of pradara. The root of kuśa if administered for three days with rice water is also very useful in asṛgdara. The seeds of bhūmyāmalaki, the buds of kāśmari and vaṭa are also extremely efficacious. Ghee medicated with flowers and gum-resin of śālmali, priśniparṇi, kāśmari, and chandana is very effective in asṛgdara. Similarly, ghee medicated with kāśmari, badara, sāriva, guḍūchi and yashṭi-madhu is useful in asṛgdara, (CSS).

5. The regular use of the root of tuvari (āḍhaki) along with cow's milk and rice water is extremely beneficial in asṛgdara, (RRS).

Diet: The diet should mainly consist of milk, rice and sugar, (CSS).

Ref.: SS, śārīra, 2, 20; CS, chikitsā, 30, 86-100; 116-119; 221; CSS; RRS, 17, 40.

Classical Prescription: Aśokārishṭa; Chandana-balā-lākshādi-taila; Dhātryadi-ghṛta; Guḍūchyādi-modaka; Pushyānuga-churṇa; Śatāvari -ghṛta; Chandrakala - rasa ; Bolabaddha-rasa.

Atattvābhiniveśa

Causative Factors: Extrinsic: Intake of food which is harmful to health, and which is too cold, too hot, too oily and too dry, and suppression of the natural urges.

Pathogenesis: The nerve channels which carry the mental processes and awareness (mano-buddhi-vatha-sirah) localise in the heart, are covered over by the rajas and tamas and vitiate the three doshas. The mind and awareness are then disturbed by the aggravated rajas and tamas.

Symptomatology: The patient is devoid of intelligence and awareness, and is incapable of discrimination.

Treatment: The patient is to be administered oleation and sudation followed by purificatory therapy such as emesis etc.

He is then to be administered food and medicines which enhance intelligence (medhya-rasayanas), such as juice of brāhmi, powder of yashṭi-madhu with milk, juice of root and flowers of gudūchi, paste of śankhapushpi, etc.

Oil medicated with laśuna; milk medicated with śatāvari, juice of kushṭha, (powder of) vachā with honey, etc. are also useful.

The patient must also have friends who are dear to him and who are his well-wishers and who are capable of teaching him virtuous living and honest ways of earning. They should equip him with wisdom, fortitude, mindfulness and concentration.

Ref.: CS, chikitsā, 10, 59-64; 1, 3, 30.

Atisāra

Western Nosology: Diarrhoea, Enteritis.

Causative Factors: Extrinsic: Intake of food which is difficult to digest, oily, too dry, excessively cold or hot, and incompatible, drinking impure water, or excess of alcoholic drinks, emotions such as fear and grief, suppression of natural urges, worm infestation, and as a complication in worms, tuberculosis, haemorrhoids, etc., (SS, CS, and AHr).

Doshas Involved: Atisāra can be caused by the vitiation of vāta, pitta and kapha.

Pathogenesis: The digestive power is weakened by the watery elements of the body which are later eliminated by the deranged vāta, (SS).

Premonitory Symptoms: Pricking pain in the chest, umbilicus, rectum, and abdomen, general weakness, incarceration of flatus, constipation, flatulent distension of abdomen, and indigestion, (SS).

Symptoms: Vātaja atisāra: Pain in the abdomen, suppression of urine, rumbling sound in the abdomen, anal prolapse, weakness in the waist, thighs and legs, and scanty stools which are frothy, dry and brown-coloured and are accompanied by flatus, (SS).

Diarrhoea caused by vitiated vāta and āma has the following symptoms: movement of flatus and rumblings within the abdomen, abdominal pain, incarceration of flatus, and painful defecation and of stools which are watery, non-slimy and have a foul odour. There will be suppression of urine.

In diarrhoea causes by vitiated vāta alone (without the involvement of āma), there will be dryness of the mouth, pain in the waist, thighs, sacral region, back, sides and knees, anal prolapse, and defecation of stools which are scanty, frothy and in hard lumps. The defecation will be attended with a rumbling sound and cutting pain, (CS).

Pittaja-atisāra: There will be thirst, unconsciousness, burning pains, perspiration, fever, and inflammation of the affected organs and gushing stools which are hot, fetid, yellow, blue or slightly red in colour, (SS).

The patient will suffer from thirst, burning, perspiration, unconsciousness, and heat and inflammation in the anal region. The stools will be yellow, green, blue or blackish in colour and will emit a foul odour, (CS).

Kaphaja atisāra: The patient suffers from lethargy, drowsiness, heaviness of the body, nausea, loss of appetite and horripilation. There will be constant urging to pass stools. Stools will be white, slimy, mixed with mucus and will be expelled without sound, (SS).

Drowsiness, lethargy, weakness, loss of appetite, horripilations, heaviness of the abdomen, anus, urinary bladder and groin, and defecation with tenesmus of stools which are slimy, white, oily, undigested, bad smelling and in the form of threads. There will also be urging which is not relieved by defecation, (CS).

Tridoshaja atisāra: Diarrhoea where all the three doshas are involved presents these symptoms - drowsiness, syncope, weakness, dryness of mouth, thirst and varied colour of stools, (SS).

Atisāra can also be engendered by emotions such as fear and grief which vitiate vāta. Such cases exhibit symptoms similar to vāta atisāra, (CS).

A case of atisāra is said to be in the āma (acute) state if the stools are found to sink in water, are slimy and emit a bad odour, (SS).

Complications: Raktātisāra (CS, SS).

Prognosis:

1. A patient suffering from atisāra is said to be incurable if he is very weak, has inflammation around the anus, if the anus is wide open and if there is distension of the abdomen, (SS).

2. Patients who are not excessively emaciated and weak and whose stools are yellow, blue, green, red, black or white in colour or like water in which meat has been washed, and who have weak digestion and loss of appetite are difficult to treat.

Patients who are afflicted with thirst, delirium, burning pains, fever, vertigo, restlessness, dyspnoea, hiccoughs and syncope, prolapse and inflammation of the anus, protrusion of rectal mucosa, excessive emaciation, anemia and weakness, pain in all the joints, and where the stools resemble slices of liver, fat, flesh, rice water, curds, ghee, marrow, oil, milk and water and are extremely blue, blood red, black, oily, putrid, slimy, etc. are to be considered as being incurable. (CS)

Ref.: SS, uttara, 40; CS, chikitsā, 19; AHr, nidāna, 8.

Treatment:

1. It is improper to suppress the first (āma) stage of atisāra by astringent drugs, as it may lead to daṇḍakālasa, grahaṇi, haemorrhoids, swelling, anaemia, enlargement of the spleen, flatulent distension of the abdomen, skin disease, gulma, ascites, fever, urinary disorders, chest pain, etc., (CS, chikitsā, 19, 15-16; SS, uttara, 40, 29-30).

However, even āma-atisāra is to be suppressed by astringents in the case of children, elderly, weak and emaciated persons and in persons of vāta and pitta constitutions, (CSS, page. 77).

2. In every case of atisāra, the physician should determine whether it is in the āma or pakva stage. Patients suffering from āma atisāra should be made to fast and are later administered drugs which are appetizing and digestive.

Patients of āma-atisāra who are troubled with griping and flatulent distension of the abdomen (and salivation, AHṛ) are made to vomit by administering a decoction of pippali and rock salt. They are then prescribed fasting, hot water for drinking, etc. They are then administered liquid food which is easily digested, such as khaḍa-yūsha, and gruel prepared from pippali. etc.

The following recipes are useful in āma-atisāra: chitraka, root of pippali, vachā and kaṭuka-rohiṇi; pāṭha, seeds of kuṭaja, harītaki and ginger; vachā, seeds of kuṭaja, rock-salt and kaṭurohiṇi; ati-vishā, musta and nāgara; the decoction of musta with milk; nāgara and guḍūchi with hot water; the stems of guḍūchi with vachā etc. If a patient has weak digestion, and scanty and frequent stools with pain, he is to be administered ghee medicated with rock-salt and yava-kshāra. The recipes given above are very useful in atisāra caused by deranged vāta and kapha, and can be used even in atisāra engendered by pitta after omitting drugs which are tīkshṇa (sharp) and hot.

A patient suffering from pakva-atisāra should be administered yashṭi-madhu, ginger and bark of śyonāka with honey and rice water (tanḍulāmbu). A decoction of musta can be administered with honey.

If the patient suffers from griping pain and dryness even after fasting, etc. he should be given ghee with sugar, ajamoda, kaṭvanga and yashti-madhu. A patient suffering from chronic, painless diarrhoea, but with good digestion is to be administered the following recipe: the barks of syonāka and pollen (keśara) of lotus (or the aerial roots of vaṭa alone) are wrapped in leaves of kāśmari or lotus, and the whole thing plastered with clay and burnt. The juice is then extracted after breaking open the outer covering, and administered with honey.

Chronic cases of atisāra with bloody, mucous stools are cured by administering a decoction of kuṭaja. The decoction is to be heated until it acquires the consistency of treacle (phāṇita).

These recipes are very useful in cases of pakva-atisāra: yashṭi-madhu and the pulp of bilva fruit with sugar and honey; and roots of badara with honey.

If a patient of atisāra suffers from thirst, he may be administered a cold infusion of the stems of śālmali (the stems are powdered or pounded and kept overnight in a vessel containing an equal quantity of water) with honey and yashṭi-madhu; or water boiled with drugs useful in atisāra. Milk is useful in cases marked by suppression of stools and urine, griping pain, tenesmus, bloody scanty stools and thirst. In chronic atisāra, milk should be given after boiling it with thrice as much water, (SS).

3. If in a case of atisāra, there is only slight imbalance in the doshas, fasting is indicated. If the doshas are moderately vitiated, the patient is to be administered decoctions of drugs which are appetizing and digestive. If the doshas are excessively vitiated, if the stools are scanty and defecation painful, harītaki is to be administered.

Decoctions of pippali, nāgara, dhānyaka, bhutika (?), harītaki and vachā (in kapha involvement, Chkp); of hrīvera, musta, bilva, dhānyaka and nāgara (in pitta involvement, ibid) and of priśṇiparṇi, gokshura, manjishṭa and kaṇṭakāri (in vāta involvement, ibid) are useful. Water boiled with vachā and prativisha, musta and parpaṭaka or hrīvera and nāgara is also beneficial in atisāra.

If the patient has a good appetite, he should partake of food which is easily digestible such as buttermilk with kānji, and thick gruel (yavāgu), khaḍa-yūsha, etc. medicated with drugs that are digestive and appetizing. The following drugs alleviate kapha and vāta, are appetizing, digestive, strength giving and are particularly useful in atisāra: śālaparṇi, prśniparṇi, bṛhati, kaṇṭakāri, balā, gokshura, bilva, pāṭha, nāgara, dhānyaka, śaṭi, palāśa, hapushā, vachā, jīraka, pippali, vrakshāmla, roots of pippali, chitraka, yavāni, hasti-pippali, dāḍima, hingu, viḍa salt and rock salt. These drugs may be used to medicate soup, etc.

Patients suffering from anal prolapse may be administered ghee medicated with chāngeri, kola, dadhyāmla, nāgara and yava-kshāra. They may also be given unctuous enemata (anuvāsana) employing ghee medicated with śaṭi, śatāvari and bilva, or vachā and chitraka. The prolapsed part is to be smeared with oil, given milk fomentation, and then gently pushed back and held in position with a suppository.

Patients suffering from pittaja-atisāra should be made to fast or given drugs which are digestive, depending on the patient's strength. If they are thirsty, they may be given water which is medicated with musta, parpaṭa, uśīra, sārivā, chandana, kirātatikta or udīchya. They are then to be administered gruel medicated with balā, atibalā, śatāvari, bṛhati, kaṇṭakāri, śālaparṇi, pṛśniparṇi, gokshura, etc. The gruel could be prepared from mudga, masūra, ādhaki or makushtha, or with the meat juices of lāvaka, kapinjala, hariṇa, eṇa, etc. The fruit and bark of kuṭaja can be administered with ativishā, honey and rice water. A paste of utpala, dhātakipushpa, the bark of dāḍima and nāgara can be administered with honey and rice water. Goat's milk is also very useful in pittaja atisāra.

Patients suffering from kaphaja atisāra should be advised to fast and are later administered drugs which are digestive and appetizing. Decoctions of the following drugs are useful in this condition: vacha, viḍanga, bhūtika, dhānyaka and devadāru; kushṭha, ativisha, pāṭha, chavya and kaṭurohiṇi; and pippali, root of pippali, chitraka and hastipippali. The patient can also be administered pippali with honey, along with buttermilk medicated with chitraka. The tender fruits of bilva are also useful, (CS).

4. Patients of pittaja atisāra are benefited by partaking of the decoctions of kuṭaja seeds or of musta or of stalks of śālmali with honey, while being on a diet of meat juices.

Patients suffering from chronic diarrhoea can also be administered decoctions of haridrā, seeds of kuṭaja and lodhra. Those who pass stools of faeces and blood alternately should be administered decoctions of the fruits of palāśa followed by warm milk. The bark of śyonāka is to be smeared with ghee, and immersed in hot water; the juice is then extracted and given with honey in cases of severe atisāra, (AHṛ).

5. A person who exhibits the premonitory symptoms of atisāra should be made to fast, and later given liquid food which is easy to digest. Water medicated with nāgara and udīchya is to be administered. These measures are sufficient to prevent or abort the disease.

The gruel named khaḍa-yūsha which is very useful in atisāra, pravāhika, jvara and arochaka is prepared from mudga, takra (buttermilk), dhānya, jiraka and rock salt.

The powders of harītaki, ativishā, hingu, souvarchala salt, rock salt and vachā are administered with hot water in āma-atisāra. A decoction of nāgara, ativishā and musta or of nāgara and dhānyaka is very useful in āma-atisāra. The leaf-juice of hijjala with honey or a decoction of the bark of kuṭaja is also useful in this condition.

A decoction of musta if administered with honey is very useful in pakva-atisāra: A paste of the root of ankoṭa with honey and rice water is very efficacious in severe atisāra. A circular ridge of āmalaki paste is constructed around the umbilical region and the juice of fresh ginger is poured into it. This immediately brings relief in severe atisāra. The gruel prepared from lājā is also very useful in atisāra. A paste of the sprouts of vaṭa, rice-water and buttermilk is extremely useful in kaphaja-atisāra. Salt is contraindicated in all cases of atisāra, (CSS).

6. Equal parts of tīksṇa loha bhasma and pārada bhasma are made into a paste with the juice of kānchanāra. This paste is very efficacious in all cases of atisāra.

Pārada bhasma can be administered with a decoction of the bark and tender leaves of trees which give off a milky exudation, (RRS).

Ref.: SS, uttara, 40; CS, chikitsā, 19; AHṛ, chikitsā, 9; CSS; RRS, 16, 5; 30, 33.

Classical Prescription: Ahiphenāsava; Ashṭākshari-guṭika; Bāla-chaturbhadrika-chūrna; Bṛhat-gangādhara-chūrṇa; Grahaṇi-mihira-taila; Jātiphalādi-chūrṇa; Jīrakarishta; Karpūrāsava; Kuṭajāvaleha; Laśunādi-vaṭi; Loha-bhasma; Kumāra-kalyāṇa-rasa; Mustā-karanjādi-kvātha-chūrṇa; Nāga-bhasma; Panchāmṛta-parpati; Piyuśavalli-rasa; Rasa-parpaṭi; Rasa-karpūra; Rajanyādi-chūrṇa; Soubhāgya-śuṇṭhi, Śūla-haraṇa-yoga; Yavanyādi-chūrṇa.

Āmatisāra: Bṛhat-kastūri-bhairava-rasa

Pakvātisara: Karpūra-rasa

Rakta-atisāra: Jīrakadi-modaka; Kutajarishṭa; Muktā-pishṭi; Ṭṛṇa-kāntamaṇi- pishṭi.

Aupasargika-meha

Synonyms: Pūya-meha, Āgantuja-meha, Vraṇa-meha.

Western Nosology: Gonorrhoea

Causative Factors: Extrinsic: This disease usually afflicts a lustful person who has sexual intercourse with prostitutes, an unclean women or a women who is menstruating.

Symptoms: The symptoms usually make their appearance about a week after the episode. Initially there is itching at the tip of the penis, and later severe pain at the time of urination. There will then be severe constant burning pain in the affected area, swelling of the genital organs, redness of the glans, pain in the testicles, and flow of pus from the urethra. There will be in some cases, constant oozing of pus from the urethra. This disease can be transmitted from person to person.

Complications: The symptoms become less severe in the course of time, but the disease causes complications such as rheumatism and certain eye diseases.

Treatment: The diseased person should strictly refrain from sexual intercourse with prostitutes. The patient should be administered drugs, diet, etc. which lessen the swelling, alleviate the pain, hasten the healing of the ulcers, are diuretic and laxative. The affected area should be washed with a decoction of the leaves of jāti.

The patient is to be administered a decoction of the gum resin of babbula with yava-kshāra, or a decoction of sārivā with navasāgara and yava-kshāra.

The patient can also be administered uttarabasti (urethral douche) with a decoction of triphala, pippali and babbula.

Ref.: BR, page. 475-476.

Avabāhuka

Causative Factors:

Extrinsic: The factors which aggravate vāta.

Intrinsic: Vāta and kapha.

Pathogenesis and Symptomatology: Vitiated vāta dries up the kapha present in the shoulder region, and contracts the blood vessels in that region, (SS).

Ref.: SS, nidāna, 1, 82.

Treatment:

1. The general remedial measures useful in vāta roga.
2. A decoction of the daśamula drugs, bola and māsha is administered with oil and ghee after the evening meal, (CD).

Ref.: CD, 22, 25.

Classical Prescriptions: Bṛhat-māsha-taila; Ekānga-vīra-rasa; Kārpasasthyādi-taila; Pariṇata-keri-kshīradi-taila.

Avapāṭika

Western Nosology: Paraphimosis

Causative Factors: Sexual intercourse with a young girl with a narrow vagina, masturbation or any trauma to the penis, forcibly folding back the prepuce, or voluntary suppression of the semen, (SS).

Symptomatology: Retraction of the inflamed foreskin, (CS, SS, AHṛ).

Ref.: SS, nidāna, 13, 48; AHṛ, uttara, 33, 17.

Treatment:

1. The foreskin should be smeared with ghee

and given mild fomentation. Poultices (upanāha) should be applied for three or five days. The glans should then be lubricated with ghee, and gently pressed, while the foreskin is drawn over it. It should then be fomented again with poultices, (SS).

Diet: Unctuous food is beneficial.

Ref.: SS, chikitsā, 20, 39; AHṛ, uttara, 34, 14-16.

Bāhyāyāma

Western Nosology: Opisthotonus

Causative Factors:

Extrinsic: Factors which aggravate vāta.

Intrinsic: Vāta

Constituents Affected: Snāyu (hard fibrous structures) (CS).

Symptomatology: The aggravated vāta affects the posterior parts (paschima-bhāga) of the fibrous structures of the ankle, calf, loin, back and neck and as a result, the body is bent outwards, like an arc. In an advanced stage, the bones of the chest, loins and thighs are broken.

Prognosis: This is incurable.

Ref.: SS, nidāna, 1, 57; CS, chikitsā, 28, 35.

Bāla roga

Western Nosology: Diseases of children.

Causative Factors:

1. The intake by a lactating mother of incompatible food, that is hard to digest, etc. causes vitiation of the doshas, which in turn adversely affects the quality of breast milk. Infants who are nourished on this milk are susceptible to various diseases.

The infant should not be breast fed when the mother (or wet-nurse) is hungry, sorrowful, fatigued, pregnant, emaciated, obese, diseased, and suffers from acid eructations after meals, (SS).

2. The health of an infant depends mostly on the quality of the breast-milk. The factors which adversely affect the quality of breast milk are : indigestion, intake of food which is incompatible and unsuitable, food articles which are salty, sour, pungent and alkaline (kshāra), pastries, sweets prepared from jaggery, kṛśara, curds, food which is abhishyandi (causes a coating within the blood vessels) and flesh of aquatic and domesticated animals, mental and physical stress, loss of sleep, anxiety, forcibly inducing or suppressing natural urges, sleeping during the daytime after a heavy meal, excessive intake of alcoholic drinks, and a too sedentary life style.

If these factors aggravate the vāta, the breast milk will acquire an abnormal taste (infants fed on this milk are emaciated, slow in development and are averse to taking feeds), will be frothy (infants suffer from hoarseness, constipation, suppression of urine, wind colic, frequent colds and śīrsha roga), or dry (this causes weakness in the infant).

If pitta is vitiated the milk will be bluish, yellow, black, etc. in colour (infants will suffer from aversion to food, discolouration of the skin, excessive perspiration and thirst, diarrhoea, and a feeling of heat) or will possess a bad odour (infants will be anaemic or jaundiced).

If kapha is vitiated, the breast milk will be oily (the infant will suffer from vomiting, salivation, dyspnoea, cough and will be peevish and drowsy), slimy (the infant will have salivation, swelling of the face, and will be dull) or heavy (the infant will suffer from heart disease). (CS).

3. The period of dentition is the time when children suffer from many diseases. The diseases especially prevalent during this period are fever, diarrhoea, cough, vomiting,

headache, inflammation of the eyes, swelling, visarpa, etc.

Infants fed on milk which has been vitiated by vāta are emaciated, and are subject to hoarseness (feeble voice), constipation, retention of urine and flatulence. Those fed on milk vitiated by pitta are subject to profuse perspiration, diarrhoea, thirst, jaundice and other such pitta diseases. Infants fed on milk vitiated by kapha are dull, drowsy, lethargic and are subject to salivation, vomiting, colic, white discolouration (paleness of skin and mucous membranes) and kapha diseases, (CSS, page 811).

The Diagnosis of Ailments: As children are unable to express themselves, the wise physician should intently observe the actions and behaviour of the sick child. The child normally weeps if the affected parts are touched or handled. A child suffering from any disease pertaining to the head is unable to open the eyes or hold up its head. A child suffering from diseases pertaining to the urinary bladder has retention of urine, intense thirst, pain and loss of consciousness. A child suffering from diseases of the alimentary tract will have constipation, retention of urine, discolouration of the skin, vomiting and flatulent distension and rumbling in the abdomen. Constant crying is an indication of a generalised disease, (SS, śārīra, 10, 34-36).

A child suffering from diseases of the head will be moaning and visibly moving the head from side to side, will lie with eye closed, and will have restless sleep.

A child suffering from ear-ache will repeatedly touch the ears, roll the head from side to side, will reject food and suffer from restlessness and sleeplessness.

In diseases of the mouth, the a child will have salivation, restlessness, irritability, aversion to breast-feeding, regurgitation of milk and loud breathing.

A child suffering from adhijihvika will have salivation, loss of appetite, lassitude, and pain and swelling of the cheek. The mouth will be open.

A child with galagraha will have fever, loss of appetite, salivation and difficulty in breathing.

In the prodromal stage of fever, the child will have restless limbs, frequent yawning and cough, aversion to breast-milk, salivation, discolouration and external heat of the body, a hot forehead and coldness of the feet, and a desire to be carried about.

In the prodromal stages of diarrhoea, there will be discolouration of the skin, restlessness, sleeplessness, flatulence and a fatigued appearance.

A child suffering from colic has an aversion to breast-milk, constantly cries while lying on its back, and has distension or rigidity of the abdomen, cold limbs and perspiration on the face.

In the prodromal stage of vomiting, there will be continuous eructations, sleepiness and yawning. A thirsty infant will not be satisfied after breast-feeding, but will continue to cry, and will have dry lips and palate.

An infant with wide open (or dilated pupils) and fixed eyes, pain in the joints, restlessness, lassitude, and retention of urine, stools and flatus is understood to be suffering from ānāha.

Sudden loud laughter (without any cause) is a prodromal symptom of apasmāra.

A child suffering from dysuria has horripilation of the skin, pain while urinating, grinding of the teeth and frequently fingers the region of the urinary bladder.

In prameha, the child feels heavy and tired, is constipated, urinates suddenly, while the urine is whitish, thick and attracts ants.

A child with haemorrhoids suffers from constipated and hard stools, flow of blood during defaecation, emaciation, and itching and pain at the anus.

A child with urinary calculi passes copious urine mixed with sediment, has painful urination, cries constantly and has an emaciated appearance.

A child with visarpa suffers from red and circular eruptions (or discolouration) on the skin, thirst, burning pain, fever, restlessness, severe pain and a desire for sweets and cold things.

A child with visūchika suffers from burning and pricking and breaking pain in the limbs, chest pain and nishṭana, while one suffering from alasaka is unable to hold up his head, has breaking pain in the limbs, yawns frequently, suffers from loss of appetite, vomiting of lumps, depression and flatulent distension of the abdomen.

A child with any eye disease suffers from restless eyes, pricking pain, swelling and redness of the eyes, lacrimation and agglutination of the eylids during sleep.

A child heading towards āma dosha suffers from lassitude, loss of appetite, drowsiness, white (pale) discolouration of the body, restlessness, aversion to play, food and sleep, and appears unclean even after a bath.

A child with anaemia has swelling in the orbital region and around the umbilicus, white discolouration of the eyes, nails and face, and loss of appetite, while a child with jaundice has yellow discolouration of the eyes, nails, face, stools and urine. Both these diseases cause lassitude and weak digestion.

A child with pīnasa (catarrh) has to frequently let go of the nipple while nursing in order to breathe, has nasal discharge, a hot forehead, constantly rubs its nose, sneezes and coughs. In uroghāta, the child has, in addition to the above symptoms, hard and rapid breathing, (KS).

Enumeration of Diseases: The diseases which usually afflict children are :

1. Ajagallika
2. Aṇāa-vṛddhi
3. Apasmāra
4. Aśmari
5. Bāla-grahas
6. Bāla-śosha
7. Choraka
8. Danta-śabda
9. Dantodbheda
10. Guāa-kuṭṭa
11. Karṇa-śūla
12. Kshirṅlasaka
13. Kukūṇaka
14. Mātulunga-kshya
15. Mṛd-bhakshaṇa-roga
16. Mukha-pāka
17. Mukha-srāva
18. Pāri-garbhika
19. Paschāttaka
20. Phakka
21. Rīti-karna
22. Rodana
23. Śayyā-mūtra
24. Sidhma
25. Sītala
26. Tālu-kaṇṭaka
27. Tuṇḍi
28. Upa-śīrshaka
29. Visarpa and
30. Utphalla

General Line of Treatment:

1. For purposes of treatment, children are classified īnto three groups :

a) Kshīrapa - An infant who is being breast-fed. In the case of diseases in such infants, drugs which are mild are to be administered with ghee and milk to the mother only.

b) Kshīrānnāda - Children who live on milk and rice (or supplements). Drugs which are mild are to be administered both to the sick child and the mother.

c) Annāda - Children who are on solids. In such cases, the child is administered a decoction, etc. of the indicated drugs.

In some diseases of nurslings, the breasts of the mother or wet-nurse are to be plastered with the paste of the indicated drugs. Theapeutic measures such as purgation, emesis, enemata etc. are contraindicated in diseases of children.

There are some drugs which are to be administered to children in order to enhance their strength, growth and intelligence. Infants who are being only breast-fed are to be given ghee medicated with siddhaārta, vachā, jaṭā-māmsi, arka-pushpi, apāmārga, sāriva, śatāvari, brāhmi, pippali, haridra, kushtha and rock salt. Children who are on milk and supplements (rice, etc.) are to be administered ghee medicated with yasthṭi, vachā, pippali, chitraka, and triphala, while children who are on solids are given ghee medicated with daśamūlas, tagara, bhadra-dāru, maricha, yashṭi, viḍanga and drāksha.

A child should not be handled roughly or in a way that causes it discomfort. It should not be scolded or suddenly woken up, abruptly lifted up or laid down. It should not be made to sit before it is capable of sitting steadily. It should be fondled and kept amused and happy with toys and play-things. It should not be exposed to the sun, rains or lightning, dust, and smoke. In the absence of sufficient breast-milk, it should be given the milk of a cow or goat.

The child should be fed on light and wholesome boiled rice in addition to milk, from its sixth month onwards, (SS, śārīra, 10).

2. If the breast-milk is found to be vitiated, the mother is given proper oleation and sudation, and is then made to vomit by administering a decoction of nimba, paṭola and salt.

After she regains some strength (after the samsarjana therapy) she is administered purgatives such as trivṛt and harītaki or harītaki alone with honey. She is then given nourishing gruels and food prepared from rice, śyāmāka, priyangu, yava, koradūsha, veṇu-yava, vamśa, mudga, masūra, nimba, vārtāka, āmalaki, trikaṭu, rock-salt, etc. Decoctions of rohiṇi, or of guḍuchi, sapta parṇa, and nāgara, or of kirāta-tikta or of śarngeshṭa, bark of sapta-parṇa and aśwagandha, etc. are administered, (CS, chikitsā, 30, 251-262).

3. CS contains a detailed description of remedial measures useful in the cases where the breast-milk is vitiated by vāta, pitta or kapha, (chikitsā, 30, 263-281).

4. The drugs which are used in diseases of children have to be sweet and astringent. They are usually administered in milk. Drugs and food articles which are too oily, dry, hot, sour, pungent, and hard to digest are to be avoided, (CS, chikitsā, 30, 285-286).

Ref.: SS, śārira, 10; CS, chikitsā, 30; KS, sūtra, 25; CSS, bāla-rogādhikāra.

Classical Prescriptions: Dhānvantara-taila (Balā-taila); Kumāra-kalyāṇa-rasa; Phala-ghṛta.

Bāla-śosha

Sanskrit: Bāla-kshaya

Western Nosology: Infantile marasmus

Causative Factors:

Extrinsic: Factors which aggravate kapha, such as excessive sleep, excessive intake of cold water, being fed on milk which is vitiated by kapha.

Intrinsic: Kapha.

Pathogenesis: The body channels (receptors) are obstructed by the deranged kapha, and as a result the child emaciates.

Symptomatology: Emaciation, loss of appetite, catarrh, fever, cough and greasiness and white discolouration of the face and eyes.

Treatment:

1. The child is to be administered the powders of panchakola along with aśoka and kaṭu-rohiṇi (or with kaṭu-rohiṇi alone).

The child can also be administered the powders of badari, dhātaki and āmalaki made into a paste with ghee.

Ghee medicated with the small variety of bṛhati, aśvagangda, surasā and pippali is also efficacious.

The child is to be massaged with lāksha taila, or oil medicated with vacha, āmalaki, harītaki, tagara, choraka, goat's urine and wine.

Ativisha alone or with śṛngi and pippali can be administered with honey in cough, fever, and vomiting, (AHṛ).

2. The child should administered the powders of the vidāri-root, wheat and yava, made into

a paste with ghee, followed by milk mixed with honey and sugar. Ghee boiled with aśvagandha and milk is also useful, (YR).

3. The paste of kushṭha, vachā, harītaki, brāhmi and suvarṇa-bhasma is given-with honey and ghee (CD).

Ref.: AHṛ, uttara, 2, 44 - 57; YR, bala-roga; CD, 64, 1.

Classical Presciptions: Aravindāsava; Aśvagandhādi -lehya; Bāla-chaturbhadrika-chūrṇa; Rasa - sindūra.

Bhagandara

Western Nosology: Fistula-in-ano.

Definition: It is so called because it effects the perinium, anal region and supra-pubic region.

Classification: This disease is of five kinds, that which is brought about by the derangement of vāta, pitta, kapha, all three combined or by extraneous causes (trauma, etc.).

Prodromal Symptoms: Pain in the hip bone, and swelling, burning pain and itching in the anal region.

Pathogenesis and Symptomatology:

Vātaja Bhagandara: The vāta is disturbed by improper food, etc. vitiates the blood and flesh of the area one or two angulas around the anus. As a result, a pustule attended with pricking pain, etc. will be formed in that area. If neglected, it suppurates, and owing to its vicinity to the bladder, exudes a slimy secretion and becomes covered over with hundreds of small sieve-like holes, through which a frothy discharge is constantly secreted in large quantities. There will be breaking, pricking, splitting and cutting pain in the ulcer. The anal region is covered over with cracks, and if the disease is neglected, jets of urine, faecal matter and semen are emitted through the holes. This kind of bhagandara is termed Śātaponaka.

Pittaja Bhagandara: If pitta is deranged, it affects the same area, and engenders a small, raised pustule resembling the neck of a camel, which is attended with sucking, burning pain. If neglected, the pustule suppurates, and the patient feels as if the ulcer is being burnt with fire. There will be a hot, foul-smelling discharge. If the disease is further neglected, jets of urine, faecal matter, etc flow out from the ulcer. This kind of bhagandhara is known as Ushṭra-grīva.

Kaphaja Bhagandara: The deranged kapha engenders in the same area, a white, hard, itching pustule. This, if neglected suppurates, and the ulcer thus formed is hard and swollen, attended with itching and a constant flow of a slimy secretion. If this is further neglected, jets of urine, faecal matter, etc. exudes through the ulcer. This kind of bhagandara is called Pari-srāvi.

Bhagandara Engendered by Vāta, Pitta and Kapha: The three deranged doshas affect the same area and cause the formation of a pustule, the size of the big toe and characterized by pricking and piercing pain, burning, itching, etc. This, if neglected suppurates, and the ulcer exudes secretions of varying, diverse colours and is attended by a kind of whirling pain. This kind of bhagandara is termed Śambūkāvarta.

Bhagandara of Traumatic Origin: Particles of bones, or other foreign bodies eaten along with meat by thoughtless persons may be carried down with hard stools by the apāna vāta, causing an abrasion or injury to the walls of the anus. This abrasion is soon transformed into a fetid and putrid ulcer infected with minute parasites. These burrow into or eat away the region of the anus and jets of urine, faecal matter etc. are emitted from these holes. This kind of bhagandara is known as Unmārgi.

Prognosis: The first three kinds of bhagandara are difficult to cure, and require prolonged treatment. The last two kinds are incurable.

Ref.: SS, nidāna, 4.

Treatment:

1. In cases where the pustule has not yet suppurated, the following eleven measures are to be employed - fasting (or intake of food that is easily digestible), application of medicinal plasters, irrigating the affected part, massaging the body (or the affected part) with oil, fomentation (measures to induce sweat), rubbing the affected area, application of a poultice, inducing suppuration, draining the pus, internal use of medicated oils, ghee, etc, inducing emesis and later, purgation.

In cases where the pustule is suppurating or has already suppurated, the patient is administered snehana and later, fomentation by a tub bath (avagāha). The physician should later examine the patient carefully to discover the situation of the ulcer and whether the mouth of the fistula is directed outward or inward. The cavity is then scraped with an Eshaṇi. If the fistula is directed inwards, the patient is asked to strain down, and it is then scraped. Cauterization with fire or alkali is generally indicated in bhagandara.

In cases like the śataponaka, the surgeon should first attend to the ulcers found in between the fistula, and later to the fistulae.

The connected abscesses should be lanced on the external side while the unconnected ones should not be incised at the same time, in order to avoid complications. The following types of incisions are indicated in the śataponaka type of bhagandhara: an incision that is equal in its two sides; an incision with one arm longer than the other; and an incision made in the region of the anus in the shape of a cross but a little removed from the raphe of the perineum. Fomentations with krśara or pāyasa prepared from drugs that are diaphoretics can be applied in the form of nāḍi-sveda. The paste of tila, castor-seeds, linseed, māsha, yava, wheat, mustard-seds, the salts and drugs of amla varga can be applied. Internally, the patient can be given the paste of kushṭha, the five salts, vachā, hingu and ajamoda mixed with ghee, wine, kānji or surā. The area should be washed with madhuka taila and other oils medicated with drugs that alleviate vāta.

3. In the ushṭra-grīva type, the ulcer should be investigated with a probe and after incision, smeared over with kshāra. A paste of tila seeds and ghee should be applied. Ghee can be also regularly used locally. Later, purificatory (śodhana) drugs should be applied followed by healing (ropana) measures.

4. In the parisrāvi type, the cavities of pus should be first removed and the sinus cauterised with fire or with an alkali. The anal region should be kept moist by sprinkling aṇu-taila. Tepid plasters mixed with yava-kshāra and cow's urine can be applied. A decoction of emetic drugs such as madana can be used locally. After the ulcer has been softened and is almost painless. it should be searched with a probe, and later operated upon and cauterised. The incision can be in the shape of a half-moon, date-palm leaf, needle's mouth, etc. The ulcer should later be purified. A plug prepared from aśvagandha, haridra, kālā, honey and ghee should be kept within the ulcer for purifying it.

If there is severe pain after the surgical measures, luke-warm aṇu-taila can be applied externally; or drugs of the bhadra-dārvādi or eranḍādi group which alleviate vāta can be used to give fomentation in the shape of nāḍi-sveda. A hot (tub) bath is also useful. The sālvaṇa type of poultice also assists in removing pain. Drugs such as trikaṭu, vacha, hingu, salts, dīpyaka (śatapushpa) can be administered with urine, kānji or a soup of kulattha.

A paste of trivrt, tila, nāgadanti, manjishṭha, rock salt, honey and milk is used in facilitating healing of the ulcers. A paste of rasānjana,, haridra, dāru-haridra, manjishṭha, nimba leaves, trivrt, tejovati and danti is useful in curing sinus. Drugs such as kushṭha, trivṛt, tila, danti, pippali, rock salt, honey, haridra, triphala and copper sulphate are useful in purifying an ulcer.

Oil boiled slowly with pippali, yashṭi-madhu, lodhra, kushṭha, ela, hareṇu, samanga, dhātaki flower, sāriva, haridra, dāru-haridra, priyangu, sarja-rasa, sudha, padmaka, padmakesara, vachā, ingalika, rock salt and bee's wax is useful in healing the ulcer and bhagandara. Drugs of the nyagrodhādi group are useful in disinfecting and healing of ulcers. An oil medicated with the roots of trivṛt, danti, haridra, arka, viḍanga, triphala, milky exudation of arka and snuhi, honey and wax is very useful in bhagandara. The oil known as syandana taila is useful in purifying and healing the bhagandara, and in removing the scar tissue after the surgical measures.

The patient should refrain from sexual intercourse, exertion, anger, and intake of heavy and indigestible food for one year after the healing of bhagandara. (SS, chikitsā, 8).

Classical Presciptions: Chitrakādi-taila; Eladi-ghṛta; Haratāla-bhasma; Kalyāṇakaguḍa; Kānta-vallabha-rasa; Kānchanāra-guggulu; Madhusnuhi-rasāyana; Mahā-pancha-gavya-ghṛta; Mahā-yogarāja-guggulu; Sapta - vimśatika - guggulu; Sārivādyāsava; Śiva-guṭika; Sūraṇa- vaṭaka; Triphala- guggulu; Viḍangarishṭa; Yogendra-rasa.

Bhagna

Western Nosology: Fractures and dislocations.

Causative Factors: Extrinsic: Various forms of trauma such as a fall, pressure, blow, violent jerking, bites of ferocious animals,etc.

Classification: There are two main sub-divisions, sandhi-mukta (dislocation) and kāṇḍa-bhagna (fracture). The former are of six kinds and the latter of twelve kinds.

Symptomatology:

I. Sandhi-mukta: The characteristic symptoms are: loss of power of extension, flexion, movement, circumduction and rotation (of the affected limbs), pain and tenderness.

1. Utpishṭa: Swelling of both sides of the articulation, and various kinds of pain, aggravated at night.

2. Viślishṭa: Slight swelling, continuous pain, and disordered functioning of the joints.

3. Vivartita (lateral displacement): Displacement of the involved bones, pain and deformity of the joints.

4. Avakshipta: Dislodged bone hangs down from the joints, looseness of the joint and severe pain.

5. Ati-kshipta: Dislocated bones are far removed from the joint, severe pain.

6. Tiryak-kshipta (oblique dislocation): Displacement of one of the bones and severe pain.

II. Kāṇḍa-bhagna: The general symptoms are: intense swelling with throbbing pain, abnormality in the position, great tenderness, presence of crepitation on palpating, looseness or dropping of the limbs, various types of pain, and a sense of discomfort in any position.

1. Karkoṭaka (shaped like a crab): Fractured bone is bent or flattened at its extremities and bulges out in the middle in the shape of a knotty growth.

2. Aśva-karṇa: The fractured bone projects upwards like the ear of a horse.

3. Chūrṇita: The fractured bone is shattered into fragments. This can be known by palpation and by crepitation.

4. Picchitam: The fractured bone is smashed (flattened out) and is marked by widespread or intense swelling.

5. Ashthi-cchallita: The fracture is characterized by splintering of the covering of the bone (periosteum).

6. Kāṇḍa-bhagna: The fractured bones are found to move about when the limb is shaken.

7. Majjānugatam: Fractures where a fragment of the fractured bone pierces into the bone and brings out the marrow.

8. Atipāṭitam (complete fracture): The fractured bone hanges down in an unnatural position.

9. Vakram: The bone is not fractured, but is bent (green-stick fracture).

10. Pāṭitam: Fractures with many perforations in the bones, and severe pain.

11. Cchinnam: Fractures occuring at only one end of the bone.

12. Sphuṭitam: Cases where there are large cracks, swelling and pain as if stuffed by bristles.

Prognosis:

These types of fractures are difficult to cure - chūrṇita, cchinna, atipāṭita and majjānugata. Both dislocations and fractures are difficult to cure in emaciated persons, old people, infants and persons suffering from kshata-kshīṇa, kushṭha and śvāsa.

These cases are considered to be incurable - fractures of the flat bones and pelvic bone ; (all kinds of) dislocations of the pelvic joints; the utpishṭa kind of dislocation of the hip, compound fracture of the flat bones, fracture into small pieces of the frontal bones, fractures of the breast bone (sternum), back bone, and temporal and cranial bones, dislocations and fractures which are improperly treated at the time of the incident, and if the union of the joints or fractured bones are disturbed in any manner.

Fractures and dislocations are also difficult to cure in a person who eats very little food, who has no self control (self control over sense organs), who belongs to the vāta constitution and where there are complications (such as fever, flatulent distension of abdomen, retention of urine, constipation, etc, NiS).

Ref.: SS, nidāna, 15; chikitsā, 3, 3.

Treatment:

General Principles:

The patient is advised to avoid intake of salty, pungent, sour, dry and alkaline (kshāra) food, sexual intercourse, exposure to the sun, and exertion. These are beneficial: old rice, meat juices, milk, ghee, gruels (yūsha) prepared from satīna and nourishing food.

The fractured bone or dislocations can be bound with splints prepared from the bark of madhūka, udumbara, aśvattha, palāśa, vaṭa, vamśa and sarja. The bandage should be neither too loose not too tight. If it is too tight, there are chances of swelling, pain and inflammation of the affected limb. The affected parts should be plastered with manjishṭha, madhūka, red sandal and rice flour mixed with ghee washed one hundred times. Fractures should be dressed and bandaged once a week in cold weather, once in five days in a moderate climate and once in three days in hot weather. The intervals can also be determined depending on the intensity of the aggravated doshas. The parts should be washed with a cold decoction of the drugs of the nyagrodhādi group, and if there is pain, with milk medicated with drugs of the laghu-pancha-mūla or tepid chakra-taila. Cold or hot lotions or plasters should be prescribed with due regard to the season and the doshas involved.

In the early morning the patient is administered cold milk from a cow with only one calf, medicated with drugs of the kākolyādi group, and lākshā and ghee. If there are ulcers they should be plastered with drugs of the nyagrodhādi group possessing an astringent taste and which are mixed with honey and ghee.

Fractures will completely heal in a month in a youth, in two months in a middle aged person, and in three months in aged persons.

The fractured or dislocated parts are brought back to the normal position by pulling up, pressing, shortening or bandaging the parts.

Treatment in Particular:

The utpishṭa and viślishṭa kinds of dislocations should not be moved or shaken. Cold lotions and pradehas (plasters) are to be employed. The affected part is first covered with a cloth soaked in ghee, and then bandaged with proper splints.

In a case of crushed (samutpishṭa) nail joint, the impure (clotted) blood is let out with the aid of an ārā (awl), and the part is plastered with rice-flour.

In a case of fractured or dislocated finger joint, the joint is brought back to its normal position, bandaged with a thin cloth, and sprinkled with ghee.

In a case of fracture of the foot, the part is (gently) massaged with ghee, carefully straightened out and bandaged after applying splints of bark of trees, (such as nyagrodha, etc. NiS).

In a case of fracture of the thigh where the fractured bone projects out, the bone is (gently reset and) bandaged with a ciruclar splint. The sphuṭita and picchita types of fractures of the thigh should also be treated in a similar manner.

In a case of fractures of the hip-bone (kaṭi) the fracture is reduced by the bone being raised up or pressed down. The patient is then administered oily enemata.

In fractures of the rib, the part should be gently massaged with ghee. The patient is then made to stand, the ribs of the left or right side are again gently massaged and the fractured rib bound with a pad (of strips of bamboo etc. NiS) (kavalika). The patient is then made to recline in a tank, full of oil.

In a case of (viślishṭa kind of, NiS), dislocation of the shoulder joint, the axilla is lifted up by means of an iron rod, and when the dislocation has been reduced, the part is bound by a svastika type of bandage.

In a case of dislocation of the elbow joint, the joint is gently rubbed with the thumb, and pressed into position after flexing and extending (the arm). The joint is then sprinkled with oil or ghee. The same procedure should be carried out in dislocations of the wrist, ankle and knee joint.

In a case of fracture of the bones and the palm, the two palms are evenly opposed to each other, and bandaged together. The parts are sprinkled with āma taila (unmedicated oil). The patient is then made to grasp a ball of clay, and later of salt and as the strength increases, a piece of stone.

In fractures of the clavicle, the bone is given fomentation, and either raised up or pressed down as the case may be, by an iron rod. It should then be firmly bandaged.

A fracture of the arm should be treated as in the case of fracture of the thigh bone.

In a case of twisting or downward displacement of the neck, the head should be straightened up by manipulating the hollow at the nape of the neck and the jaw (joint). The neck is then supported by evenly placed splints and bandaged. The patient is advised to rest on his back for a week.

In dislocation (viślishṭa, NIS) of the jaw, the parts are fomented, the portion of the jaw is corrected and the jaw is bound with a panchāngi kind of bandage. Ghee medicated with sweet drugs and drugs which alleviate vāta is used as errhines (nasya).

In cases of young people suffering from loose but not fractured teeth, the blood is pressed out, and a cold plaster is applied externally. The teeth are washed with cold water and plastered with honey, ghee, drugs of the nyagrodhādi group and substances having sandhāniya properties. The patient is advised to drink milk with the aid of a straw (lotus stem). In the case of aged person, teeth which are loose should be extracted.

In cases where the bridge of the nose is twisted, sunken or depressed as a result of trauma, a śalāka (rod) is used to straighten and correct the deformity. Two tubes, open at both ends, are inserted into the nostrils; the affected part is bandaged and sprinkled with ghee.

In cases of damage of the ear, the part is washed or plastered with ghee, straightened out to the correct position and bandaged. It is then treated as in a sadyo-vraṇa (open wound).

In fractures of the cranial bones, where there is no oozing of brain matter (mastulunga), the injured parts are rubbed with honey and ghee, and bandaged. The patient is then administered (pure) ghee for seven days.

In injuries attended with only swelling and no open wound or ulcer, cold plasters and sprinkling of cold (cooling) liquids are useful.

In cases of fractures of the leg and thigh, the patient is made to lie down on a plank (kapāta-śayana) and is bound to five pegs, in order to prevent any movement of the fractured limb. There should be two pegs on either side of the limb and one at the sole. A similar kind of plank and pegs are used in fractures and dislocations of the waist, pelvic joint, back, chest and shoulders.

Chronic dislocations are treated by anointing with oil (oleation) and fomentation, by means of which the joints are softened. The dislocations are reduced by employing measures which are most suitable.

In cases where the fractured limb has been wrongly set, the bone is to be fractured again, and correctly set and treated as in any other fracture.

Fractures and dislocations of the upper part of the body should be treated with śiro-vasti, pouring of oil into the ears, external use of ghee, and errhines (nasya); and those of the upper extremities are treated with oily enemata (anuvāsana).

Oil should be medicated with trapuśa, vibhītaka, priyāla, drugs of the kākolyādi group (i.e. possessing sweet taste) with fat (if available) and then ten times the quantity of milk. This oil if used internally, for massage, washing, for purposes of enema or as nasal drops assists in the healing of fractures and dislocations.

The fractured limb should first be sprinkled with cold water, plastered with mud, and bandaged with splints.

The powders of asthi-samhāra, lākshā, wheat and arjuna should be administered with milk, in order to promote the healing of fractures and dislocations. A paste of rasona, honey, lākshā, ghee and sugar-candy; the powder (2-3 gunja) of yellow varāṭika with unboiled milk; a paste of guggulu with babbūla, triphala, trikaṭu and ghee; milk medicated with ghee, lākshā, yashṭi-madhu, and drugs of the jīvaniya groups; a powder of the bark of arjuna with milk; and a powder of wheat with ghee are also useful in fractures.

Ref.: SS, chikitsā, 3; CD, 49, 1-16.

Classical Prescriptions: Lāksha-guggulu; Ābhā-guggulu.

Bhasmaka

Synonyms:

Sanskrit: Atyagni (CS), Tivragni (SaS)

Western Nosology: Thyrotoxicosis.

Causative Factors:

Extrinsic: Factors which aggravate vāta and pitta.

Intrinsic: Vāta and pitta.

Pathogenesis and Symptomatology:

The pitta gets aggravated in a person who has diminution of kapha, and conjoined with vāta this increases the digestive fire. As a result of the increased digestive fire, the food that is partaken of is rapidly digested, and the person begins to emaciate. There is only transient relief after eating. The patient also suffers from debility, excessive thirst, dyspnoea, burning pains, loss of consciousness, etc.

Prognosis: If the disease is left untreated, it is fatal.

Treatment: The patient is administered food that is hard to digest, oily, cold, sweet and slimy. Food is to be given at frequent intervals, even if the food previously partaken of is undigested.

The physician should prescribe medicines, food and a regimen which increases kapha, decreases vāta and pitta and restores normalcy of the digestive fire. The following food articles are beneficial: pāyasa, kṛśara, dishes prepared from flour and jaggery and jaggery and its products, flesh of sheep and aquatic animals, fish found mainly in placid waters, gruel prepared from ghee and bee wax, milk medicated with jīvanīya drugs, sugar and ghee, meat-juices with ghee and oil, cold water with ghee and bee wax, wheat powder with ghee and milk, meat-juices of aquatic animals with ghee, fat or bone-marrow, paste of bark of udumbara (fig) with breast-milk, etc.

The patient can also be purged with milk medicated with śyāma and trivrt.

The patient is also advised to sleep after meals.

Ref.: CS, chikitsā, 15, 217-234; SaS, I, 7, 16; MK on MN, 6, 4; RRS, 25, 56.

Bradhna

Western Nosology: Hernia; Hydrocele

Causative Factors: Intrinsic: Vāta and other doshas. (CS)

Pathogenesis and Symptomatology: Due to aggravated vāta, etc, there is swelling of the scrotum into which the intestines frequently enter and recede. If the swelling is filled with urine (liquid), it is soft. If the swelling is caused by the accumulation of fatty tissue, it is unctuous and hard, (CS).

Note: Bradhna is one of the complications of vātaja - gulma, (CS, nidāna, 3, 7).

Ref.: CS, chikitsā, 12, 94.

Treatment:

1. The treatment in cases where suppuration has not taken place should consist of purgation, massage with oil or ghee, nirūha-enema and external applications (or plasters, etc.,). If the swelling suppurates, it should be treated as in the case of vraṇa, (CS).

2. A paste of wheat-flour or kunduru with goat's milk can be applied when warm. A paste of ajāji, hapusha, kushṭha, wheat, wheat-flour, badara and kānji can also be applied. Medicated ghee known as śata-pushpādya-ghṛta can be administered internally. Medicated oil known as bṛhat-saindhavādya-taila can be used as anuvāsaṇa-enema, (CD).

Ref.: CS, chikitsā, 12, 95; CD, 40, 23-35.

Bhrama

Western Nosology: Giddiness, vertigo

Causative Factors:

Extrinsic: All factors which aggravate vāta.

Intrinsic: Vāta, pitta and rajas (SS), Vāta alone (CS).

Constituents Affected: Majja (bone-narrow) (CS).

Treatment: Treatment as in vāta disorders.

Ref.: CS, sūtra, 20, 11; 28, 17; SS, śārīra, 4, 56.

Classical Prescription: Bṛhat-vāta-chintāmaṇi-rasa; Chintāmaṇi-chaturmukha-rasa; Elādi-guṭika; Laghvānanda-rasa; Manjishṭhādi-taila; Tiktaka-ghṛta.

Chardi

Synonyms: Vami, Vamana

Western Nosology: Vomiting; emesis.

Causative Factors: Extrinisic: Excessive intake of liquid, oily, unpleasant and salty food, eating at untimely hours, overeating, fatigue, emotions, indigestion, worm infestation, extremely rapid eating and unpleasant or disgusting thoughts, etc. It is also common in pregnancy, (SS).

Classification: Vomiting can be engendered by disturbed vāta, pitta, or kapha, or all three doshas combined or by extraneous causes such as intake of food for which one has an aversion, or which is unclean, etc. infestation with worms, pregnancy, etc., (CS,SS).

Prodromata: Salivation, nausea and tastelessness (CS,SS); salty taste in the mouth (AS).

Aetiology and Symptomatology of Vātaja Chardi : Excessive exertion, intake of powerful drugs, grief, fear, fasting, emaciation due to other diseases, etc.

The aggravated vāta causes vomiting of frothy, astringent, blackish, scanty and thin substances with great straining and loud eructations. The patient will also suffer from pain in the chest and sides, dryness of the mouth, headache, pain around the umbilicus, cough, hoarseness and pricking pain, (CS).

There will also be back pain, exhausation and aggravation after digestion of food, (SS).

Aetiology and Symptomatology of Pittaja Chardi: Indigestion, intake of pungent, sour, vidāhi and hot food. The vomitus is hot, yellow, green., or gray, and bitter. The patient will also experience burning in the chest, syncope, thirst, dryness of the mouth, burning and heat in the head, palate and eyes, giddiness and tama, (CS).

The vomitus will be sour, very hot, yellow, green or blood streaked. The patient will also experience a pungent or bitter taste in the mouth, fever, burning pains, dryness of mouth and syncope, (SS).

Aetiology and Symptomatology of Kaphaja Chardi: Excessive sleep and intake of oily, vidāhi, unripe or uncooked food, etc.

The vomitus will be oily, thick, sweetish and filled with mucus. The patient will suffer from lethargy, a sweet taste in the mouth, increased and thick saliva, loss of appetite, drowsiness, heaviness of the body and horripilation (while vomiting). The vomiting will be easy and devoid of pain, (CS).

The vomitus is white, sweetish, thick, cold, excessive in quantity and filled with mucus. The patient will be lethargic and will suffer from horripilation, loss of appetite, and heaviness of the body, (SS).

Aetiology and Symptomatology of Tridoshaja Chardi: Intake of incompatible food, production of āma in the body, and irregular or unusual seasons.

The vomitus will be blue, thick, hot, and bloody. The patient also suffers from a sour or salty taste in the mouth, abdominal pain, indigestion, loss of appetite, burning pain, thirst, dyspnoea, and giddiness, (CS).

Aetiology and Symptomatology of the Fifth Kind of Chardi: Intake of disagreeable, unclean, spoilt and unpleasant food, food for which one has an aversion, disgusting odours, horrible sights, etc., (CS).

The sense organs coming into contact with disgusting sense objects, pregnancy, production of āma in the body, intake of food which is harmful and worms, (SS).

These causative factors aggravate one or another of the doshas. The doshas affected in each case are to be identified by the symptoms. Vomiting due to the presence of worms is accompanied by severe cramps, nausea and symptoms of Krimija Hṛdroga, (SS).

Complicaṭions: Cough, dyspnoea, fever, hiccoughs, thirst, mental disturbances, heart diseases and tamaka (darkness before the eyes) (MN).

Prognosis: A patient of chardi is deemed to be incurable when the vomiting resembles the stools and urine in smell and colour and is variegated in colour, and where there are symptoms such as thirst, dyspnoea, incessant hiccoughs and excessive vomiting. The vomiting of blood and pus is incurable in an emaciated individual, (CS, SS).

Ref.: CS, chikitsā, 20; SS, uttara, 49; AS, nidāna, 5; MN, 15.

Treatment:

1. Since the disease arises from disturbances in the āmāśaya (stomach), fasting is beneficial in all cases, except vātaja chardi. In chardi caused by pitta and kaphā, the patient may be purged by administering harītaki with honey. Debilitated patients however should not be given purgatives.

Patients suffering from vātaja chardi may be administered meat juice of tittiri, lāva or barhi or gruel prepared from kola, kulattha, dhānya, sour yava and bṛhat-panchamūlas. Patients having chest pain or palpitation may be administered ghee medicated with rock salt or with dhānya and nāgara. The juice of dāḍima with curds is also effective. Food which is unctuous and a heart tonic is also to be given along with gruel of sour substances, dāḍima and curds.

Patients suffering from pittaja chardi are to be given laxatives such as drāksha, vidāri, sugar cane juice, and trivṛt. If the pitta is excessively vitiated, sweet emetics are to be administered. The patient can be given, at the regular meal time, mantha prepared from lāja, honey and sugar, or mudga or rice or meat juice of animals residing in the desert. Cold grape juice or water cooled by lumps of parched mud, or decoctions of tender leaves of jambu and āmra taken cold with honey are useful. The powders of mudga and pippali or uśīra and dhānya or chaṇaka are to be soaked in water overnight and then administered. The cold infusions of the root of gavedhuka or guḍuchi and a paste of āmalaki and chandana are useful. Gairika and rice powder can be given with cold water.

Patients suffering from kaphaja chardi have to be first administered emetics such as a decoction of nimba, sarshapa, pippali, madana and rock salt. They should be administered gruel (yūsha) prepared from paṭola, guḍūchi and chitrāka or trikaṭu, nimba, butter-milk, and sour fruits. They can also be given old wheat, old rice, old barley, meat juice of animals living in desert areas, old honey, old sīdhu, fried mudga, masūra, chaṇaka and kalāya with honey and ginger. A paste of triphala. viḍanga and honey, or durālabha and honey, or of the juice of kapittha, powder of pippali, maricha and honey, or of the juice of kapittha, powder of pippali, maricha and honey, or of powder of manahśila, juice of bījapūra, maricha and honey is useful in this condition.

A patient suffering from tridoshaja chardi has to be treated after due considerations to the strength of the vitiated doshas of the patient and the disease.

A patient afflicted with the fifth kind of chardi has to be reassured with encouraging and pleasant words, well known anecdotes and tales, company of friends, by pleasing ornaments and decorations, pleasant sports, fragrant and variegated substances, etc., (CS).

2. Patients suffering from vātaja chardi are to be administered soup of mudga and āmalaki with ghee and rock salt or ghee prepared from milk or gruels medicated with panchamūla drugs and honey. Lukewarm oily purgatives mixed with salt are also useful.

In pittaja chardi, cool drinks, decoctions of drugs which alleviate pitta, and emetics or purgatives composed of drugs which are sweet to the taste can be administered with grape juice.

A cold infusion of gudūchi mixed with honey is extremely useful in most cases of chardi. Chardi engendered by the use of disgusting subtances, etc., can be relieved by drugs and a regimen which are agreeable to the patient. Fasting and later, the use of congenial food or the food that one is accustomed to are useful in chardi due to the use of incongenial food. Chardi due to worms is to be treated with the measures applicable in Krimija Hṛdroga.

These recipes are useful in most cases of vomiting: paste of pippali, juice of kapittha fruit and honey; powdered seeds of ātmagupta with yashṭi-madhu, honey and rice-water; gruels medicated with karanja leaves; kapittha with trikaṭu and rice water; powdered fried paddy with honey, and ghee; paste of āmalaki and sandal; powdered pippali with honey, sugar and ghee; decoction of leaves of mudga; etc., (SS).

3. Patients of vātaja chardi may be administered ghee with rock salt or ghee medicated with the juice of dāḍima, ginger, dhānya and curds. The pastes of kola, harītaki or drāksha can be given with honey in pittaja chardi. The juice of āmalaki can be administered with decoctions of the leaves of mudga in pittaja chardi. Kaphaja chardi can be relieved by giving durālabha with honey or kapittha with trikaṭu, (AHṛ).

Diet: Food that is dry, liked by the patient, agreeable, easy to digest, leafy vegetables, fruits, preparations such as kāmbalika, khalā, rāga-shādava, pānaka, etc., gargling with cold water immediately after eating and aromatic substances are beneficial.

Bathing and rubbing the body (with powders) and use of fragrant flowers, etc. are also beneficial, (AHṛ).

Ref.: CS, chikitsā, 20; SS, uttara, 49; AHṛ, chikitsā, 6, 1-24.

Classical Prescriptions: Āragvadhādi-kvātha-chūrṇa; Bāla -chaturbhadrika -chūrṇa; Balā-tailā; Bilvādi-taila; Daśamūlarishta; Drākshadi-chūrṇa; Drākshādi-kvātha-chūrṇa; Elādi-modaka; Eladi-guṭika; Nārikela-khaṇḍa; Panchāmṛta-parpati; Paṭolādi-kvātha-chūrṇa; Pippālyādi-ghṛta; Pippālyādi-lauha; Pūga-khaṇḍa; Saptāmṛta-lauha; Sīva-gutīka; Sūtasekhara-rasa; Tālīsadi-churna; Trāyantyādi-kvātha-chūrṇa, Śankha-bhasma.

Charmakīlaka

Western Nosology: Warts, condylomata.

Causative Factors: Intrinsic: Vyāna vāta and kapha.

Pathogenesis and Symptomatology: The vitiated vyāna vāta and the deranged kapha engender the production of pin like excrescences on the skin (around the anus, according to NiS).

If these are brought about by the vitiated vāta, they are attended with pricking pain. If kapha is mainly involved, they are knotty and of the same colour as the surrounding skin. If the pitta and blood are vitiated, they are dry, blackish, smooth and extremely hard.

Treatment: These excrescences are to be surgically removed or cauterized with fire.

Ref.: SS, nidāna, 2, 18-20; sūtra, 12, 10; 25, 3-5.

Chippa

Synonyms: Sanskrit: Upanakha, Akshata (SS)

Western Nosology: Felon, whitlow

Causative Factors: Intrinsic: Vāta and pitta, (SS, AS).

Constituents Affected: Blood and flesh, (CS).

Pathogenesis and Symptomatology: The vitiated vāta and pitta bring about inflammation and burning pain in the flesh surrounding the nail-bed, (SS).

The patient will also suffer from fever and pain, (AS).

There will be swelling in between the nail and the skin, with intense inflammation, which suppurates rapidly, (CS).

Treatment:

1. The patient is administered medicines which alleviate the specific dosha involved. Local treatment such as draining the pus (visrāvaṇa), hot fomentation, application of poultice and after suppuration, the treatment as given for ulcers (vraṇa-chikitsā) is advisable, (CS).

2. The affected area is sprinkled (or washed) with hot water, and drained after excision. It should be smeared with chakra-taila, dusted over with the powder of sarja and bandaged. If this treatment is not effective, the affected area is to be cauterised with fire and smeared over with an oil medicated with drugs of the madhura (kākolyadi) group, (SS).

Ref.: CS, chikitsā, 12, 88-90; SS, nidāna, 13, 21; chikitsā, 20, 9-10; AS, uttara, 36.

Choraka

Symptomatology: This is a grave condition where the child suffers from both diarrhoea and vomiting, and also has distension of the abdomen with pain.

Treatment: The child's head, palms and soles are to be smeared with the white of an egg. A warm decoction of bhadra-musta, harītaki, nimba, paṭola and āmalaki is also to be administered, (YR, KBT).

Ref.: YR, bāla-roga, KBT, 6, page, 964; PSK, page. 367.

Dāha

Western Nosology: Burning sensation; dehydration

Causative Factors:

Extrinsic: Excessive intake of alcoholic drinks, and factors which aggravate pitta.

Intrinsic: Pitta (CS)

Classification: Dāha can be brought about by abuse of alcoholic drinks, disturbances of the blood, by excessive thirst, by vitiation of pitta, by internal haemorrhage, wasting of the tissues and by trauma to vital organs (marmas), (SS).

Pathogenesis: The blood coursing through the body when vitiated becomes heated and causes coppery discolouration in the skin and eyes; and a bloody smell in the mouth and body. The patient feels as if he is surrounded by fire (or by burning coals, NiS).

Symptomatology: If thirst is not appeased, the watery elements of the body dry up, and the patient experiences dryness of the lips, palate and throat, burning sensation both within the body and on the skin, trembling of the body and protrusion of the tongue.

A patient with wasting of the body-tissues suffers from burning pain attended with syncope, thirst, feebleness of voice, and mental and physical prostration.

If the blood is vitiated by intake of improper food, grief, or any depressing emotions, the patient suffers from intense burning sensation within the body with thirst, syncope and delirium, (SS).

Prognosis: All cases of burning sensation with external coldness and which are the results of trauma are considered incurable, (SS).

Treatment:

1. The patient should be smeared with sandal paste, recline on a bed of lotus leaves, and be sprinkled with cool water. Youthful damsels decked with ornaments of lotus stems should keep him company. He should be asked to stroll about on the banks of a river with a soft, cool and sweet breeze blowing over him. Water medicated with uśīra, bālaka and chandana should be sprinkled over his body. He should take a bath with young, gay and beautiful

damsels skilled in aquatic sports refreshing him with the lotus-like touch of their cold hands, thighs, and mouth and firm breasts and with sweet words. He should lie down when tired in a cool chamber with fountains and with the floor sprinkled over with scented water and flowers and the walls smeared with a paste of sandal, teja-patra and bālaka. These measures are especially beneficial in dāha caused by abuse of alcoholic drinks.

Dāha engendered by vitiated pitta would show symptoms of pittaja jvara, and the treatment would therefore be the same.

In the dāha brought about by suppression of thirst, the main therapeutic measure would be to correct the depletion of the watery elements of the body. The patient is advised to drink large amounts of cold water, cold milk with sugar, sugar cane juice or mantha.

Dāha caused by internal haemorrhage should be treated as in a case of Sadyo-vraṇa.

Dāha produced by wasting of the tissues should be treated with drugs which are oily and which relieve vāta. The remedial measures indicated in Rakta-pitta would be also beneficial.

A patient suffering from dāha brought about by grief or depressing emotions should have his desires fulfilled, and should partake of milk, meat juices, etc. in the company of friends and well wishers.

Daha engendered by disturbances of the blood is to be treated by fasting and drugs and foods which alleviate the dosha involved. Food prepared from the meat of jāngala animals is beneficial. Venesection of veins in the extremities would be useful as a last resort, (SS).

Ref.: SS, uttara, 47, 54, 67-78; CS, sūtra, 20, 14.

Classical Prescriptions: Amṛta-prāśa-ghṛta; Chandana-balā-lākshādi-taila; Chandanādi-taila; Drākshādi-kvātha-chūrṇa; Jvarāryabhra; Laghu-chinchādi-lehya; Lākshādi-taila; Nyagrodhādhi-kvātha-chūrṇa; Tiktaka-ghṛta; Trayantyādi-kvātha-chūrṇa; Tiktaka-ghṛta; Vraṇa rāksha-taila.

Daṇḍakālasaka

Western Nosology: Spastic neuralgia.

Causative Factors:

Extrinsic: Those factors responsible for the production of āma.

Intrinsic: The three doshas.

Pathogenesis and Symptomatology: The doshas which are excessively vitiated in a person whose body channels (srotāmsi) are obstructed by āma, move in a oblique direction and render the body stiff and rigid like a rod.

Prognosis: This is a rapidly progressive and fatal disease.

Related Subjects: Alasa, Visūchika

Ref.: CS, vimāna, 2,12; AHṛ, sutra, 8,12-13.

Daṇḍāpatānaka

Causative Factors: Intrinsic: Vāta and kapha (SS); Vāta (CS).

Symptomatology: The aggravated vāta and kapha affects all the nerves of the body and deprives the body of its flexibility, rendering it stiff like a rod (SS).

The vitiated vāta causes stiffness of the extremities, head, back and pelvic region. The body is thus made as stiff as a rod, (CS).

Prognosis: This disease is difficult to cure according to SS, while CS considers it to be incurable.

Treatment: Refer to treatment of Apatānaka.

Ref.: SS, nidāna, 1, 53; CS, chikitsā, 28, 51-52.

Classical Prescription: Mahā-vishagarbha - taila.

Danta-śabda

Symptomatology: The vāta aggravated by eating very dry food, affects the siras (vessels) located at the hanu (jaws or chin) and as a result, the child grinds its teeth when asleep, (AHṛ).

Treatment:

1. The paste of karkatānghri (karkaṭa-srngi) is applied over the teeth, gums and jaws or the ghee extracted from milk that has been boiled with the same drug is rubbed externally, (CD).

2. The soles of the feet should be rubbed with milk boiled with karkaṭa-śāka, (CSS).

Ref.: AHṛ, uttara, 2, 62; CD, 56, 3, 6; CSS, bāla-roga, 150.

Dāruṇaka

Synonyms: Vernacular: Pahā, Aupahā (NiS)

Western Nosology: Tinea capitis.

Causative Factors: Intrinsic: Kapha and vāta (SS, AHṛ); Kapha, vāta & pitta (NiS).

Constituents Affected: Blood (NiS).

Symptomatology: The scalp becomes hard, dry and cracked, and itches, (SS).

Falling of hair, dryness, itching, numbness, presence of minute cracks on the scalp, (AHṛ).

The scalp is rough, resembles layers of abhra (mica) and is devoid of dandruff. There will be pricking pain if vāta is involved, itching and heaviness if pitta and the blood are vitiated. (Nyāya-chandrika on SS).

Ref.: SS, nidāna, 13, 35; AHṛ, uttara, 23, 23.

Treatment:

1. The scalp is oiled and fomented, after which venesection may be done. Abhyanga (massaging the part and the body with oil) and avapīḍa type of errhine are useful. The affected area should be washed with a solution of kshāra (ash) of burnt kodrava grass, (SS).

2. Venesection may be performed on the veins present in the forehead. Errhine therapy and śiro-basti can be done after washing the scalp. A paste of priyāla seeds, yashṭi-madhu, kushṭha, sarshapa and māsha with honey can be applied over the affected area, (AHṛ).

3. Oil medicated with the juice of bhṛngarāja and fruits of gunja is useful (when applied externally), (CD).

Ref.: SS, chikitsā, 20, 29-30; AHṛ, 24, 25-27; CD, 55, 90.

Ekānga-roga

Causative Factors:

Extrinsic: Factors which vitiate vāta.

Intrinsic: Vāta alone.

Symptomatology: This refers to a disease which is confined to one part or organ of the body. The chill or heat confined to only one part of the body as seen in certain kinds of fever are examples of this disease.

Treatment: Treatment is similar to that prescribed for vāta-rogas.

Notes: According to AS (nidāna, 15, 42) the term ekānga-roga is used as a synonym for Paksha-vadha.

Ref.: CS, sūtra, 20, 11; Chkp. on ibid.

Gadodvega

Synonyms: Sanskrit: Apadārtha-gada

Western Nosology: Hypochondriasis.

Causative Factors: Extrinsic: Mental prostration, excessive excitement, overindulgence in sex, and the disease Dhvaja-bhanga (one of the Guhya-rogas).

Symptomatology: The person imagines that

he is suffering from various diseases.

Treatment: The patient is to be reassured by conciliatory, pleasant and affectionate words which also induce confidence and enthusiasm.

The patient is also advised drugs and diet which are digestive, appetizing, laxative, which alleviate vāta and pitta and do not excessively aggravate kapha. Tonics, rejuvenative medicines and drugs which are employed in vāta rogas are also efficacious in this disease. The food is to be oily, well-cooked, clean, desirable, nourishing and easy to digest.

The physician should not tell the patient that his complaints are imaginary, but should listen to him carefully and reassure him. .

Ref.: BR, page.317.

Galagaṇḍa

Western Nosology: Goitre.

Causative Factors:

Extrinsic: Excessive use of sweet foods, (SS, sūtra, 42, 10).

Intrinsic: Kapha (CS, śutra, 20, 17); Vāta and kapha (SS).

Constituents Affected: Flesh (CS, sūtra, 28, 14); Medas (fat) (SS)

Pathogenesis: The aggravated vāta and kapha vitiate the medas (fatty tissues), and these localise in the region of the throat and neck, involving the rohiṇi (the sixth layer of skin), causing the formation of a tumour (gaṇḍa). (SS; ibid, śārīra, 4, 4).

Classification: There are three types of gala-gaṇḍa, that caused by aggravated vāta, by aggravated kapha, and by the vitiated medas, (SS).

Symptomatology: A tumour (gaṇḍa) is present on one side of the throat, (CS).

1. Vātaja gala-gaṇḍa: The tumour is blackish or brown in colour, covered over by black veins; rough, slow in growth, and rarely or never suppurates. The fatty tissues also get involved in course of time, and the tumour becomes very unctuous and painless. The patient suffers from pricking pain in the affected part, bad taste in the mouth, and dryness of the palate and throat.

2. Kaphaja gala-gaṇḍa: The tumour is large, firm, not discoloured, cold to touch and is attended by a dull pain and severe itching. It grows slowly and takes a long time to suppurate. The patient suffers from a sweet taste in the mouth, and feels as if the palate and throat is coated (with slime or mucous).

3. Medoja gala-gaṇḍa: The tumour is unctuous, soft, pale white in colour, painless, has a short neck and hangs down like a pumpkin (alābu). It has a foul odour, increases or decreases in size depending upon the growth or emaciation of the body and is attended by severe itching. The face of the patient is greasy, and a rumbling sound is constantly produced in the throat, (SS).

Prognosis:

1. The patient is considered incurable if he has dyspnoea, flabbiness of the whole body, if the growth has been present for more than a year, and if the patient is emaciated, and is suffering from tastelessness and hoarseness, (SS).

2. The patient is incurable if there are symptoms such as cararrh (pīnasa), pain in the sides, cough, fever and vomiting, (CS).

Ref.: SS, nidāna, 11, 22-28; CS, chikitsā, 12, 79.

Treatment:

1. A patient suffering from vātaja gala-gaṇḍa is to be regularly administered oil medicated with guḍūchi, nimba, hamsapādi, vṛkshaka and pippali for internal use.

The tumour has to be exposed to fomentation or nāḍi-sveda by vapours of decoctions prepared from fresh leaves of drugs which alleviate vāta, kānjika, various kinds of urine, milk, oil and meat. The vitiated blood has to be drained out (by employing leeches, NiS). The purified ulcer is then plastered with the following drugs made into a paste with surā and kānji. The paste is to be applied hot. The drugs used are: sāṇa, atasi, mūlaka, śigru, kiṇva, pulp of priyāla and tila; or ambashṭha (or trivrt), kuṭaja and tilvaka, or himsra, guḍūchi, śigru, punarnava, arka, hasti-pippali, kushṭha and madana-phala.

A patient suffering from kaphaja gala-gaṇḍa is to be internally administered oil medicated with five salts and drugs of the pippalyādi group. Emetics, errhines and inhalation of vairechanika-dhūma are beneficial.

The tumour is to be fomented (dry sveda, NiS), plastered with appropriate drugs (such as kshāras, gomūtra, etc. NiS) and drained. It is then to be plastered with a compound of ajagandha, ativisha, viśalya, vishaṇika, kushṭha, śukahvaya, alkaline water of palāsā bhasma and gunja. The plasters should be applied hot.

In the case of vātaja and kaphaja gala-gaṇḍa, which are partially suppurated, the physician should try to hasten suppuration. The diet should consist of rice, barley, gruels of mudga, honey, cow's urine, trikaṭu, śṛngavera (fresh ginger), paṭola and nimba.

A person suffering from medoja gala-gaṇḍa can be administered the sāra (essence) of drugs of the sālasāradi group, along with cow's urine every morning. The person should be oleated, and then venesection should be resorted to. A hot plaster (pradeha) of trivrt, sudhā, maṇḍūra, danti and rasanjana should be applied over the affected part.

The tumour can also be surgically opened, the fatty contents removed, and the wound sutured. It can also be cauterized by hot majja (bone-marrow), ghee, medas (lard) or honey. The cauterized part is plastered with honey and ghee, and later with a paste of kāsīsa, tuttha and go-rochana. The cauterized area can also be lubricated with oil, and the patient administered the sāra (essence) of drugs of the sālasārādi group or the bhasma of cow-dung.

Regular use of a decoction of triphala, a diet of yava (barley) and tight bandaging (gāḍha-bandha) are useful, (SS).

2. The following measures are useful in gala-gaṇḍa: venesection, purgation, use of errhines, fumigation (dhūma), fasting and internal use of old ghee, (CS).

3. The application of a warm paste of nichula and seeds of śigru or of the drugs of the daśamūla group is useful in vātaja gala-gaṇḍa. The application of a paste of devadāru and viśāla is beneficial in kaphaja gala-gaṇḍa. A paste of the roots of hasti-karṇa and palāśa and rice-water is also useful in gala-gaṇḍa.

The following recipes are efficacious in this disease : the root of white aparājita with ghee (for internal use); the fruits of tiktālābu with wine (madya); and the preparation known as kānchanāra guggulu, (CSS).

Ref.: SS, chikitsā, 18, 43-55; CS, chikitsā, 12, 80; CSS, page.533.

Classical Prescription: Sarshapādi - pralepa.

Gaṇḍālaji

Approx. Western Nosology: Swelling of the salivary glands.

Symptomatology: A stable or firm swelling in the region of the cheek, attended by burning pain and fever, (AHṛ).

Treatment: The disease is treated along the same lines as śopha, (AHṛ).

Ref.: AHṛ, uttara, 21, 10; 22, 10.

Gaṇḍa - māla

Western. Nosology: Lymphadenosis; Adenitis

Causative Factors: Intrinsic: Kapha (CSS)

Constituents Affected: Flesh (SS, sūtra, 24, 9;CS, sūtra, 28, 14); medas (CSS).

Symptomatology: Many tumours or swellings around the neck, (CS).

Tumours are found in the region of the neck, chest, and mandibular joint, in the shape of a garland. The difference between Apachi and Gaṇḍa-māla lies only in the regions affected. (Bhoja, NC and NiS on SS, nidāna, 11, 10-12).

Tumours which are slow to suppurate, are of the size of karkaṇḍa, kola or āmalaka, or are situated in axillae, neck, throat and groin, (CSS).

Prognosis: The disease is considered to be incurable if the following symptoms are present: catarrh (pīnasa), pain in the sides, cough, fever and vomiting, (CS).

Treatment:

1. See treatment for Apachi.

2. The measures useful in this disease are: venesection, purgation, errhines, fumigation (dhūma), internal administration of old ghee, fasting (langhana), rubbing the affected part (with medicated powders, etc.) and kavala-graha, (CS).

3. The following prescriptions are useful in this disease: the leaf-juice of alambusha; the decoction of the root of varuṇa with honey; a paste of bark of kānchanāra and a decoction of triphala, with ginger; a paste of bark of kānchanāra with rice water; oil medicated with juice of nirguṇḍi and a paste of the root of lāngali used as nasya (nasal drops); oil medicated with the root and fruits of gunja used as nasya and for application; oil medicated with the bark of śākhoṭaka used as nasal drops; oil medicated with bilva, karavīra and nirguṇḍi used as nasal drops; and oil medicated with chuchundaru, used for external application.

The diet has to consist of yava, mudga, gruel of kulattha and food which is not abhishyandi. Nasya, purgation and emesis are also beneficial, (CSS).

4. The following formulae are beneficial in gaṇḍa-māla: a paste of kānchani (kānchanāra), chitraka, vatsanābha and water applied externally for a week causes suppuration of the tumours. These tumours have to be plastered with the paste of muṇḍi juice and root paste. The juice is to be administered internally; the paste of purified sulphur, mercury, rock salt and milky exudation of arka is applied along with a paste of the root of kānchanāra (kānchani). The tumours will soon start to suppurate. They are then to be plastered with a paste of muṇḍi juice and root paste for a period of three weeks; the paste of the leaves of jayapāla and its (leaf) juice applied externally, (RRS).

Ref.: SS, nidāna, 11, 10-12; CS, chikitsā, 12, 79; CSS, pages. 435-438; RRS, 24, 60-65.

Classical Prescriptions: Kānchanāra-guggulu; Lāngali-taila (Nirgu-ṇḍī-taila); Madhu-snuhi-rasāyana; Sarshapādi-pralepa; Viḍangārishṭa.

Grahaṇi

Western Nosology: Malabsorption syndrome

Causative Factors: Extrinsic:

1. Factors which weaken the digestion, (SS).

2. Intake of harmful or undesirable food by a person with weak digestion who has just recovered from atisāra (diarrhoea), (SS).

3. The intake (in excess) of food which is pungent, bitter, astringent, very dry and cold, eating in too limited a quantity, excessive travelling, suppression of natural urges and excessive sexual indulgence are responsible for causing vātaja grahaṇi. The intake of food before the digestion of the food previously taken, of food which is pungent, vidāhi, sour, alkaline (kshāra), etc. are responsible for causing pittaja grahaṇi. Kaphaja grahaṇi is

engendered by intake of food which is hard to digest, very oily, and cold, overeating, sleeping immediately after a meal, etc., (CS).

Classification: There are four types of grahaṇi-roga, i.e. they are engendered by the vitiation of the three doshas individually or all three combined, (CS).

Pathogenesis: As the grahaṇi is the seat of agni (or the digestive fire), any disturbance in the agni will lead to grahaṇi roga, (SS, CS).

Prodromal Symptoms:

1. Thirst, lethargy, debility, sourness or burning sensation, slow digestion of food and heaviness of body, (CS).

2. Fermentation or vidāha of food, debility, lethargy, thirst, fatigue even without exertion, tastelessness, cough, tinnitus (sounds in the ear) and rumbling in the abdomen, (SS).

3. Salivation, bad taste in the mouth, vomiting, vertigo, and a sense of constriction in the abdomen, (AHr̥).

Symptomatology: General:

1. The food that is partaken gets converted into āma (or will be indigested or improperly digested) for many days. If this is digested, the patient suffers alternately from constipation and diarrhoea with abdominal pain and foul flatus.

The patient also suffers from emaciation, swelling of the hands and feet, pain in the sides, craving for food, thirst, vomiting, fever, loss of taste, burning pains, eructations which are sour, bitter, acid and have the smell of iron or smoke or blood, salivation, bad taste in the mouth and dyspnoea, (SS).

2. Vidāha (fermentation) of food, and downward elimination of digested or undigested food, alternate constipation or diarrhoea, thirst, loss of taste, bad taste in the mouth, salivation, dyspnoea, swelling of the hands and feet, pain in the bones and joints, vomiting, fever and eructations which are bitter, sour and smelling of iron or flesh, (CS).

3. Emaciation, headache, unconsciousness and constipation, (AHr̥).

Vātaja grahaṇi:

1. Difficult digestion of food, sourness or acidity, roughness of skin, dryness of throat and mouth, (excessive) hunger and thirst, darkness before the eyes, tinnitus, constant pain in the sides, thigh, groins and neck, visūchika, pain around the heart (precordial region), emaciation, debility, bad taste in the mouth, cutting pain (in the abdomen), craving for various kinds of food, mental prostration, distension of abdomen after or during digestion, presence of symptoms resembling those seen in vātaja gulma, vātaja hr̥droga and plīha (enlargement of spleen), cough, dyspnoea, frequent and difficult defecation of dry, watery, thin, undigested or frothy stools with emission of flatus and amelioration (of distension) after eating, (CS).

2. Dark or brown discolouration of nails, face, eyes, urine and stools, excessive pain in the anus, heart, sides, abdomen and head, (SS).

3. There are symptoms similar to those observed in vātaja arśa and pāṇḍu. (AHr̥)

Pittaja grahaṇi:

1. Indigestion, green or yellow discolouration (of body, etc.), diarrhoea with watery and yellowish stools, foul and sour eructations, burning in the chest, and throat, loss of taste, and (excessive) thirst, (CS).

2. Burning pains (in various parts of the body), and green yellow, reddish or black discolouration (of nails, face, eyes, urine and stools), (SS).

Kaphaja grahaṇi:

1. Difficult or slow digestion of food, nausea, vomiting, loss of taste, sliminess and sweet taste in the mouth, cough, spitting, cartarrh, heaviness and tightness of the abdomen, sweetish eructations, debility, aversion to sex, weakness in plump persons, lethargy, a feeling

as if the heart had congealed, and defecation of watery, loose, indigested and heavy stools which are mixed with mucus, (CS).

2. Heaviness of the body, (SS).

Note: Before beginning the treatment, the physician should ascertain whether there is presence of āma or not. The stools will sink in water due to heaviness in case of āma involvement. However, the physician should know that watery stools will float even if there is presence of āma and hard stools will sink even if there is no āma involvement, (CS).

Ref.: SS, uttara, 40, 171-177; CS, chikitsā, 15, 51-72; AHr, nidāna, 8,19-26.

Treatment:

1. The patient is to be administered purificatory measures in accordance with the dosha involved (nirūha enema, purgation and emesis, in vātaja, pittaja and kaphaja grahaṇi respectively, NiS). The patient is then given peya (gruels) which are medicated with drugs that are appetizing and digestive (such as panchakola, NiS). Drugs which are digestive (i.e.of the haridrādi group, NiS), constipative (of the ambasṭhādi group, NiS) and appetizing (of the pippalyādi group, NiS) are administered with butter milk, sura (wine), tepid water, oil or ghee, cow's urine, etc. Buttermilk even if taken alone is very useful. Ghee medicated with the paste of pippali, etc., juice of changeri and curd is very efficacious. Measures which are indicated in krimi, gulma, udara and arśa are also useful in this disease, (SS).

2. The general remedial measures in grahaṇi are oleation, sudation, purificatory measures (such as emesis), fasting, use of buttermilk and substances that are appetizing (dīpana).

If the patient suffers from constipation, salivation, pain, burning sensation, loss of taste and heaviness of the body he must be made to vomit by using warm water or a decoction of madana with pippali and sarshapa. If the doshas are located in the large intestines, he is given purgatives along with drugs that are appetizing. If the āma is mixed with the rasa dhātu, the patient is advised to fast, and is administered drugs that are digestive. He is later given a decoction of panchakola drugs, gruels (peya) etc. food that is easy to digest and medicines which are appetizing. He can then partake of small quantities of ghee medicated with drugs that appetizing. Once the agni (digestive fire) has improved, the patient can be given snehana (oleation) twice or thrice a day, subjected to massage and fomentation (sudation) and nirūha type of enema. He can also be purged with castor oil, tilvaka ghṛta, etc. In cases of constipation and dryness of the alimentary tract, anuvāsana type of enema can be given with oil medicated with drugs which are sour, appetizing and alleviate vāta. The diet can consist of food that is easy to digest, and regular use of ghee is recommended.

The following formulations are useful in grahaṇi: ghee medicated with trikaṭu, triphala, bilva and jaggery; a decoction of nāgara, ativisha and musta-which digests the āma; a paste of nāgara with hot water or nāgara, ativisha, musta and haritaki with hot water- these also assist in the digestion of ama; devadāru, vachā, musta, nāgara, ativisha and harītaki with vāruṇi, āsuta or tepid water; a decoction of dāḍima with biḍa, salt, bilva, chitraka and nāgara- in cases of undigested stools with colic; kalinga, hingu, ativisha, vachā, souvarchala salt and harītaki - in cases of abdominal colic with involvement of āma, kapha and vāta; powder with warm water of ativisha, trikaṭu, rock salt, yava-kshāra and hingu; powders of bhūnimba, kaṭuka, trikaṭu, musta, chitraka, seeds and bark of kuṭaja with jaggery and cold water; the fermented juice of flowers of madhūka which is reduced to half by boiling, is cooled and stored in a pot smeared with ela, mṛṇalā, agaru and chandana for a month; the kshāra (ash) of bhūnimba, rohiṇi, tikṭa, paṭola, and nimba with buffalo's urine; and the kshāra of stems of sudha, saindhava, souvarchala and biḍa salts, vārtāki, arka and chitraka which is made into pills with juice of vārtaka - these pills have to be taken after meals.

The powders of sour drugs, trikaṭu, sugar and the salts are to be taken with soup (sūpa), rice, rāga, etc. The gruels (yūsha) of mūlaka, panchakola, maricha, etc. with oil or ghee, medicated meat-juices, butter-milk, urine etc. are to be taken as one's diet. Butter-milk is considered to be very useful in grahaṇi.

In a case of pittaja grahaṇi, purgation or emesis, food that is easy to digest, cooling and bitter, meat-juices of animals residing in desert areas (jāngala), gruels (yūsha) and khaḍa of mudga, etc., drugs such as dāḍima, sour drugs, drugs that are appetizing and constipative (grāhi) with ghee, etc. are benefical.

A patient of kaphaja grahaṇi is made to vomit, and is later administered drugs that are pungent, sour, salty, alkaline (kshāra) and bitter. The diet has to consist of yūsha (gruel) of dry mūlaka or kulattha, buttermilk, alcoholic drinks, food that is easy to digest, etc., (CS).

3. The disease should be treated with measures indicated in ajīrṇa. A person suffering from āma should be treated with measures useful in atisāra.

Ghee medicated with bījapūra juice is useful in vātaja grahaṇi and can be used for massage also. Snehana (oleation) is extremely efficacious in enhancing the digestion and digestive fire. A patient suffering from hard stools and painful or difficult defection should be administered ghee medicated with the salts (the five kinds of salts). A person who has recovered from grahaṇi but still suffers from weak digestion should be given ghee medicated with drugs that are appetizing, (AHṛ).

4. A paste of musta, ativisha, bilva, kuṭaja and honey is very useful in all types of grahaṇi.

In vātaja grahaṇi, these recipes are useful: the gruel (yavāgu) of kapittha, bilva, chāngeri, butter-milk and dāḍima; a decoction of nāgara, musta, ativisha and guḍūchi; ghee medicated with paste of nāgara.

In pittaja grahaṇi, these formulae are used: the hot decoction of pāṭha, seeds of kuṭaja, chitraka and nāgara (this is useful in kaphaja grahaṇi also); rice water prepared by mixing thoroughly one part of rice with eight parts of water; and ghee medicated with a decoction of nāgara and bilva-garbha.

Formulae useful in kaphaja grahaṇi are: powders of nāgara, musta and viḍanga with urine, buttermilk or hot water; the powder of trikaṭu, bark of āmra and kuṭaja with rice-water; and ghee medicated with kshāras of bṛhati and chitraka.

There is a detailed procedure for partaking of buttermilk in all cases of grahaṇi, (CSS).

References: SS, uttara, 40, 178-182; CS, chikitsā, 15, 73-197; AHr, chikitsā, 10; CSS, grahaṇi-adhikāra.

Classical Prescriptions: Abhraka-bhasma; Ashṭākshari-guṭika; Bhāskar-lavaṇa-churṇa; Bṛhat-gangādhara-chūrṇa; Bṛhat-kastūri-bhairava-rasa; Bṛhat-nṛpa-vallabha-rasa; Chāngeri-ghṛta; Chitrakādi-chūrṇa; Chitrakādi- guṭika; Dadhika-ghṛta; Danti-haritaki; Dantyādyarishṭa; Daśamūlarishṭa; Grahaṇi-mihira-taila; Hingvādi-chūrṇa; Jātiphalādi-chūrṇa; Jīrakādi-modaka; Jīrakarishṭa; Kānta-vallabha-rasa; Kapardika-bhasma; Kuṭajārishṭa; Kutajāvaleha; Lodhrāsava; Loha-parpaṭi; Madhūkāsava; Mṛdvīkarishṭa; Mṛgānka-rasa; Mustakarishṭa; Nāga-bhasma; Nava-ratna-rāja-rasa; Nyagrodhādi-kvātha-churṇa; Panchamṛta-parpaṭi; Paṭola-mūladi-kvātha-churṇa; Pippalyādyāsava; Punarnavādi-maṇḍūra; Puṭapakva-vishama-jvarāntaka-lauha; Rohitakārishta; Rajanyādi-chūṛna; Rasa-parpati; Śankha-vati; Śankha-bhasma; Śatphala-ghṛta; Siddha-praneśvara-rasa; Sūla-haraṇa-yoga; Sūrana-vaṭaka; Soubhāgya-śuṇṭhi; Suvarṇa-bhūpati-rasa; Sūta-śekhara-rasa; Svarṇa-bhasma; Svarṇa-parpaṭi; Vaikrānta-bhasma; Vāri-soshana-rasa; Yaśada-bhasma; Yavanyādi-chūrṇa; Yavāni-shāḍava.

Granthi

Western Nosology: Inflammatory swellings of glands, and sebaceous cysts.

Constituents Affected: Blood, fat and flesh (SS)

Classification:

1. According to SS, there are five kinds of granthi: those engendered by vāta, pitta and kapha, that which mainly involves the fat (medas) and that which affects the blood vessels or nerves.

2. According to CS, the five kinds are: those which are brought about by vāta, pitta and kapha, that which mainly involves the flesh (māmsa) and that kind which affects the fat (medas).

3. According to AHr, there are nine kinds of granthi: those engendered by vāta, pitta and kapha, those which involve the fat (medas), blood vessels or nerves (sirā), blood (rakta), flesh (māmsa), bones (asthi) and that which is ulcerated (vraṇa-granthi).

Symptomatology:

1. Vāta granthi: The knotty growth is blackish in colour, rough and elongated like the urinary bladder. When it bursts, it exudes clear blood. The swelling feels as if it is drawn asunder, or pricked with a needle, or severed or cleft into two or elevated, (SS).

The knotty growth changes its position or becomes smaller or bigger from time to time, (AHr).

2. Pitta granthi: The knotty growth is reddish or yellow in colour, inflamed, hot and on bursting exudes extremely hot blood. There will be severe burning pain, (SS). The knotty growth rapidly suppurates, (AHṛ).

3. Kapha granthi: The knotty growth is hard like stone, very slightly painful, cold to touch, only slightly discoloured, is compact and very slow in growth. It itches internally intensely and on bursting exudes thick, white pus, (SS).

4. Medo-granthi: The knotty growth is unctuous (glossy), large, slightly painful, and increases or decreases in size with gain or loss of flesh of the patient. It is marked by intense itching, and on bursting, exudes pus which resembles (thick) ghee or pinyāka (paste of tila), (SS).

The knotty growth is painless, glossy and mobile, (CS). It is very soft, mobile, and exudes pus which is coppery coloured, black or white in colour, (AHr).

5. Sirā-granthi: This variety of knotty growth is caused by vāta which is aggravated by over-exertion in the case of weak, enfeebled persons.

The plexuses of blood-vessesls or nerves are drawn up into knotty tumours which are rounded, (SS).

The knotty tumour is painless and nishphuram, (AHṛ).

6. Māmsa-granthi: The knotty growth is large and pulsating (CS); the flesh is vitiated by the intake of meat, and causes a knotty growth that is glossy, large, hard, and covered over with blood vessels (sirānaddham), (AHr).

7. Rakta-granthi: The blood is vitiated by the aggravated doshas, and so brings about a knotty growth which is numb or insensible, and where the flesh and blood vessels are full of maggots. There will be other symptoms of aggravated pitta, (AHr).

8. Asthi-granthi: A depression or swelling of the bone due to fracture or any trauma to the bone is known as asthi-granthi, (AHṛ).

9. Vraṇa-granthi: The vāta is aggravated in a rūḍha or ārūdha kind of ulcer which exudes a liquid or is free from attachment to any organ, or due to trauma, and vitiates the blood. As a result, there will be a knotty outgrowth in the ulcer, with burning pain and itching, (AHṛ).

Prognosis: Those tumours which are painless, immobile, and large and which affect the vital organs (marma) are incurable. The sirā granthi is difficult to cure even when it is painful and mobile, (SS).

Knotty growths engendered by vāta, pitta and kapha, and those which affect the blood and medas are curable. However, those tumours which are big, hard and mobile, and which are located near vital organs or on the throat and abdomen are incurable, (AHr̥).

It is difficult to cure in children, old people and debilitated persons, (CS).

Ref.: SS, nidāna, 11, 3-9; CS, chikitsā, 12, 81, 86; AHr̥, uttara, 29, 1-14.

Treatment:

1. All care should be taken to preserve the strength of the patient, as the disease will be weakened when strength increases.

The following measures are indicated in a case of acute granthi (i.e.before it has started suppurating): fasting (or light diet), application of plasters, irrigation or spraying of medicines, massaging or anointing (with medicated oils), fomentation or measures to induce perspiration, rubbing (the affected part), application of poultices, inducing suppuration, draining the pus, internal use of oil or ghee medicated with prasāraṇi and drugs of the daśamūla group, and administering emetics and purgatives.

In vāta granthi, a plaster of himsrā, kaṭuka, rohiṇi, guḍūchi, bhārngi, śyonāka, bilva, agaru, kr̥shna-gandha, and goji should be applied. Various kinds of fomentation and poultices can be employed. When it has begun to suppurate, the pus should be drained, and the ulcer washed with a decoction of bilva, arka and āragvadha and purified by applying a paste of tila, leaves of castor and rock-salt. The ulcer should then be anointed with oil medicated with milk, viḍanga, yashṭi-madhu and guḍūchi.

In a case of pitta-granthi, the vitiated blood should be eliminated by applying leeches. The part is then washed with milk and water. The patient should be administered a cold decoction of drugs of the kākolyādi group with sugar or powder of harītaki with grape juice or sugar-cane juice. Hot plasters (pradeha) of the bark of jambu, madhūka, arjuna and vetasa, or of roots of ketaki or muchukunda with sugar are to be applied. After the granthi has suppurated, and the pus evacuated, the ulcer is washed with a decoction of (the bark of) vaṭa, plaksha, pippala and udumbara, and purified by applying a plaster of tila, and yashṭi-madhu. Ghee medicated in drugs of the kākolyādi group is then used to fecilitate healing.

In case of kapha-granthi, the doshas should be eliminated from the system (by oleation, fomentation, emetics, etc. NiS). The granthi should then be fomented and firmly rubbed with the thumb or an iron rod or a stone. A plaster of the roots of vikanṭaka, āragvadha, gunja, kākādani and ingudi is to be applied. The granthi should then be opened with an incision as soon as it starts suppurating. The ulcer should be purified by applying yava-kshāra with honey and jaggery. Oil medicated with viḍanga, haridra, and pāṭha assists in the healing of the ulcer.

In medoja-granthi, a plaster of tila paste enclosed within the folds of a linen cloth is applied to the affected part. The part should then be fomented with hot iron rods. The part can also be fomented with a ladle pasted over with heated lāksha.The granthi is then opened, and the fat removed. The ulcer is then cauterized. If the granthi suppurates, it should be washed with cow's urine. The ulcer is then purified by applying a paste of tila, suvarchika, rock-salt, haritāla, honey, ghee and yava-kshāra. Oil medicated with karanja, gunja, the scrapings (bark) of bamboo, ingudi and cow's urine is useful in promoting the healing process, (SS).

2. In a case of granthi which has not suppurated, the patient is to be administered purificatory procedure (śodhana). The affected area is then fomented and firmly rubbed with the fingers or with a rod. It is excised together with the covering (kośa) and cauterized. If it is improperly cauterized or if not fully excised,

the growth gradually grows and expands. All knotty tumours are therefore to be fully excised, after paying due regard to the area affected. The resulting ulcer is treated as a vraṇa, (CS).

3. A patient suffering from granthi is administered ghee medicated with bṛhati, chitraka, kaṇṭakari, and pippali. (He is then administered purificatory procedures such as emesis and purgation). The tumours have to be plastered with drugs which are sharp (tīkshṇa).

The vāta and kapha granthis have to be fomented and repeatedly kneaded or massaged. In pitta granthi, leeches are used, along with cold plasters. A patient suffering from sirā granthi is administered sahachara taila. Poultices composed of drugs which alleviate vāta, enemata and venesection are also useful. The māmsa and vraṇa granthis are to be totally excised and the area cauterized with fire, (AHṛ).

4. The application of a paste of pārada bhasma, triphala, root of paṭola, trikaṭu, guḍūchi, seeds of viḍanga and guggulu is very efficacious in granthi. The application and rubbing of ash (bhasma) of arimeda and palāśa is useful in medo-granthi. A paste of equal quantities of guḍūchi and sūraṇa with hot water is to be applied in medo-granthi. The pulp of putranjīva is to be made into a paste with water and applied over granthis. It is also useful in knotty growths located on the abdomen, throat and waist. The paster of vishṇu-krānta, peṭāri and kānjika or of punarnava, arka, harītaki, śigru, kupīlu, karanja, rock salt and ginger are also of use in granthi, (RRS).

Ref.: SS, chikitsā, 1, 8; 18, 3-19; CS, chikitsā, 12, 82-83; AHṛ, uttara, 30, 1-7; RRS, 24, 125-133; 30, 71.

Classical Prescriptions: Chandraprabha -vaṭi; Kānchanāra-guggulu; Khadirārishṭa; Sarshāpadi-pralepa.

Gṛdhrasi

Synonyms: Vernacular - Ranghiṇi (NiS), Ringaṇi (CSS).

Western Nosology: Sciatica

Causative Factors:

Extrinsic: All factors which aggravate vāta.

Intrinsic: Vāta (CS, sūtra, 20,11); Vāta and kapha (CS, sūtra, 19, 3, 4; chikitsā, 28, 57).

Pathogenesis: The nerves of the heels and toes are affected by the deranged vāta, (SS).

Symptomatology: Pain and inability to move the lower limbs, (SS).

In vātaja gṛdhrasi, the patient experiences frequent (attacks of) stiffness, numbness, pulsating pain and pricking pain first in the buttock and later along the loins, back, thigh, knee and leg.

In gṛdhrasi engendered by vāta and kapha, these symptoms will be accompanied by heaviness, tastelessness and lethargy (tandrā), (CS).

The symptoms present in vātaja gṛdhrasi are pricking pain, deformity of the limb, pulsation and rigidity of joints of knee, pelvis and thigh, and in gṛdhrasi caused by vāta and kapha are loss of appetite, feeble digestion, tastelessness, lethargy and salivation, (MN).

Ref.: SS, nidāna, 1, 74; CS, chikitsā, 28, 56, 57; MN, 22, 55, 56.

Treatment:

1. The treatment is given along the same lines as for other vāta diseases (see vāta roga).

Venesection is also of use in gṛdhrasi, (SS).

2. The general treatment should be on the same lines as for vāta rogas. Blood letting from the vein situated in between the ankle (joint) and the affected nerve, enemata and cauterization are also useful, (CS).

3. A decoction of leaves of śephālika or of bṛhat-pancha-mūla drugs with trivṛt; the oil of tila or ghee with the juice of ārdraka (fresh ginger) and mātulunga or with jaggery; the use of castor oil with cow's urine for a month; a fine powder of kṛshṇa (pippali) with castor oil and cow's urine; a pāyasa prepared from castor seeds, milk and ginger; and small pills of rāsna guggulu and ghee; all these are useful in gṛdhrasi, (CD).

4. The patient is advised drugs and a diet which are dry and digestive. The affected limbs are fomented by means of heated bricks, hot oil, etc. It may also be massaged and covered with plasters. The patient has then to undergo purgation and emesis; and when the digestion has improved, enemata.

When the pain and suffering is intense, venesection can be carried out at two or three sites and these are covered with a paste of gunja.

A pāyasa of purified castor seeds and milk is extremely efficacious. A yavāgu prepared along with castor seeds is also useful. Even severe cases can be cured by administering a paste of the root of mahā-nimba and water. The following recipes are also very useful: a paste of the root of tagara and buttermilk; a pāyasa prepared from (purified) castor seeds and ginger; a ghee medicated with laśuna, ginger, hingu, chavya, chitraka, kṛshṇa, amla-vetasa and rock-salt; oil medicated with gokshura, milk, fresh ginger and jaggery. This oil can also be used for purposes of enema, (CSS).

5. Pārada bhasma can be administered with śuṇthi, (root-bark of) eraṇḍa (castor) and milk, (RRS).

Ref.: SS, chikitsā, 5, 23; CS, chikitsā, 28, 101; CD, 22, 40-53; CSS, pages. 368-370; RRS, 30, 56.

Classical Prescriptions: Ajamodādi-chūrṇa; Bṛhat-māsha-taila; Mahā-vishagarbha-taila; Prasāraṇi-taila; Rāsnādi-kvātha-chūrṇa; Trayodaśānga-guggulu; Vātāri-guggulu.

Guda-bhramśa

Western Nosology: Prolapsus - ani.

Causative Factors:

Extrinsic: It is caused by the diseases pravāhika and atisāra occuring in debilitated persons with dryness of the body, (SS).

Intrinsic: Vāta, (CS).

Symptoms: Prolapse of the anus, (SS).

Treatment:

1. The prolapsed part is fomented and lubricated, and is then gently pressed back to its original (normal) position. The anal region is then bandaged, with the bandage being in the form of a gophana, with an opening for the passage of flatus. The affected part is repeatedly subjected to fomentation, (SS).

2. See treatment of atisāra according to CS.

3. Unctous enemata (anuvāsana) of ghee or oil medicated with sweet and sour drugs is useful, (SS).

Related Subject: Atisāra, Pravāhika.

Ref.: SS, nidāna, 13, 61; chikitsā, 20, 61-62; uttara, 40, 108; CS, sūtra, 20, 11; 11, 49.

Classical Prescriptions: Chāngeri-ghṛta; Pippalyadi - taila.

Guda-pāka

Western Nosology: Proctitis.

Causative Factors:

Extrinsic: 1. Factors which aggravate pitta, (CS).

2.Intake of undesirable and unhealthy food by a person suffering from atisāra, (SS, uttara, 40, 109).

Intrinsic: Pitta, (CS, sūtra, 20, 14).

Constituents Affected: Blood (CS, sūtra, 28, 12).

Symptomatology: Inflammation of the anus.

Treatment:

1. Treatment as described under pitta-roga.

2. Washing the affected area and use of oily enemata (anuvāsana) with decoctions, etc. of drugs which alleviate pitta, (SS, uttara, 40, 109).

3. The affected area is washed with a cold decoction of paṭola, yashṭi-madhu, śarkara and honey or a decoction of panchavalkala drugs, yashti-madhu, śarkara and honey or sugarcane juice, ghee, sugar and honey or goat's milk with sugar and honey.

The area can be plastered with a paste of the above drugs, and ghee. A paste of dhātaki and lodhra (with ghee) is also useful. Oil medicated with chandana, etc, śata-dhouta ghṛta can also be employed in such cases, (CS, chikitsā, 19, 89-92).

Gulma

Causative Factors:

Extrinsic: Factors which cause vātaja gulma: intake of food which aggravates vāta or use of extremely cold substances (or cold bathing, etc.), by a person of vāta constitution who is emaciated due to fever, emesis, purgation, diarrhoea, etc., administering emesis or purgation without prior oleation (snehana); forcibly inducing vomiting; suppression of natural urges; drinking too much fresh water immediately after a heavy meal; travelling over very uneven ground; excessive indulgence in sexual intercourse, exercise, alcohol and grief; trauma (of any sort); irregular posture, lying and walking on an uneven surface; etc., (CS).

Factors which engender pittaja gulma: intake of the following substances by a person who is emaciated due to fever, etc.: food which is sour, salty, pungent, alkaline (kshāra), hot, active (tīkshṇa), fermented, green and sour fruits, substances which are heat producing (vidāhi), leafy vegetables (śāka), meat, grains (dhānya), etc., partaking food before the digestion of food previously taken; indigestion (ajīrṇa), administering emesis to a person who has partaken of dry food; suppression of natural urges; excessive exposure to wind and sun; etc., (CS).

Factors which cause kaphaja gulma - intake of these substances by a person who is emaciated by fever, etc.: food which is excessive in quantity, too oily, hard to digest, sweet and cold, flour preparations, sugarcane juice, milk, tila, māsha, jaggery, and its products, excessive alcohol, maṇḍaka (unmature curd), haritaka (salads), the meat of aquatic and domesticated animals; suppressing natural urges; drinking excessive water when fasting; trauma (of any kind), etc., (CS).

Factors responsible for rakta gulma: suppression of natural urges; abortion; intake of food which aggravates vāta during menstruation or soon after parturition, (CS).

Improper diet soon after parturiton, or during menstruation; and abortion, (SS).

Intrinsic: Mainly vāta (CS, SS).

Constituents Affected: Blood (CS, sūtra, 28, 12).

Classification:

1. There are five types of gulma: those caused by vāta, pitta and kapha, that type engendered by all three doshas together (nichaya-gulma, CS) and that caused by vitiated blood (rakta-gulma), (SS, CS).

2. According to AS, there are eight types, those caused by the three doshas aggravated singly, by two aggravated doshas, by all three combined, and by the vitiated blood.

Location: Gulmas can be located either externally or internally, (AS).

The areas commonly affected are the urinary bladder, umbilical region, heart and sides, (CS, SS, AS).

Pathogenesis:

1. The doshas aggravated by the causative factors accumulate in the koshṭha (comprising stomach, small intestines, large intestine, urinary bladder, heart, lungs, colon or caecum and reservoirs of blood such as liver and spleen) and engender gulma, (SS).

2. The aggravated vāta affects the pitta and kapha, which may also be aggravated by their respective factors and when obstructed, it generates pain in the chest, umbilical region, sides, abdomen and urinary bladder. It then engenders the formation of a round and palpable tumour which is named gulma, (CS).

Prodromal Symptoms: Debility, feeble digestion, rumbling sound in the abdomen, distension of the abdomen, obstruction (or retention) of urine, faeces and flatus, constant eructations, aversion to food and inability to eat to one's satisfaction, (SS).

Aversion to food, tastelessness, indigestion, feeble digestion, burning pains after eating, vomiting and eructation without any specific reason during digestion, loss of the urge to urinate, defecate or pass flatus, obstruction or scanty elimination even if the urge is present, colicky pain in the abdomen, rumbling in the abdomen, flatulence, horripilation, udāvarta, loss of appetite, debility and intolerance to heavy food, (CS).

Symptomatology: If the gulma is located internally, the patient suffers from pain in the urinary bladder, abdomen, heart, and spleen, debility, feebleness of digestion, loss of complexion and retention of faeces, urine, flatus, etc. If the gulma is situated externally, it does not cause severe pain. The patient suffers from discolouration (of the affected area), and excessive protrusion, (AS).

A rounded knotty tumour which is either mobile or immobile, and which increases and decreases in size is situated between the heart and the urinary bladder. This is known as gulma, (SS).

Vātaja gulma - Sharp pain in the heart (chest), and abdomen, dryness of the mouth and thirst, incarceration of flatus, irregular digestion (vishamāgni) and other symptoms of deranged vāta, (SS).

Fluctuation in the area affected, size of the tumour and pain, retention of faeces and flatus, dryness of the mouth and throat, dark-brown discolouration (of skin, etc.), fever with chills, pain in the precordial region, abdomen, sides, shoulder and head, aggravation (of pain, etc.) after digestion, and by intake of dry, astringent, bitter and pungent food, and amelioration after eating. The patient also suffers from formication, various kinds of sensations such as pricking pain, breaking pain, pulsation, extension, difficult respiration, horripilation during the pains, and dryness of skin, nails, etc., (CS).

Pittaja gulma - Excessive perspiration, fever, sourness and burning after meals, thirst, redness (of the body or affected area), pungent or bitter taste in the mouth and other symptoms of vitiated pitta (such as vertigo, unconsciousness, etc.,) (SS).

Burning pain in the abdomen, heart, chest and throat, sour and burning eructations, and burning, pain, sensation of heat, perspiration, oozing, tenderness, looseness and slight horripilation around the area affected. The patient also suffers from yellow or green discolouration of the skin, nails, eyes, face, urine and faeces, redness of face and limbs, and aggravation of pain during digestion, (CS).

Kaphaja gulma - A sensation of moistness, aversion to food, debility, vomiting, salivation, sweet taste in the mouth and other symptoms of aggravated kapha, (SS).

The patient suffers from fever with chills, tastelessness, indigestion, body pain, horripilation, heart diseases (hṛdroga), vomiting, drowsines, lethargy, sensation of moistness, heaviness of the body, burning pain in the head, white discolouration of skin, nails, eyes, face, urine and faeces, nausea, and cough. The tumour will be hard, elevated, stable, heavy and numb. There will only be slight pain, (CS).

Rakta-gulma - The woman has all the symptoms of pregnancy, but does not feel the movement, nor is there any enlargement of abdomen. There are symptoms which are seen in pittaja gulma, along with pain and burning sensation, (SS).

The aggravated vāta localises in the vaginal orifice and causes amenorrhoea. Due to the suppression of the menses month after month, the abdomen enlarges. The patient also suffers from colicky pain, cough, diarrhoea, vomiting, tastelessness, indigestion, body pain, drowsiness, lethargy, sensation of moistness, salivation, appearance of milk in the breasts, dark discolouration of the lips and mammary areola, excessive sense of fatigue in the eyes, spells of unconciousness, nauses, craving for certain objects, swelling of the feet, appearance of a faint linea nigra, dilatation of the vaginal orifice, and discharge of foul smelling fluid from the uterus, (CS).

The disease rakta-gulma is observed only in women, (CS, SS).

Complications: The complications of vātaja gulma are: enlargement of the spleen, incarcerated flatus, rumbling sound in the abdomen, indigestion, udāvarta, body pain, pain in the neck, head and temples and bradhna.

The complications of pittaja gulma are fever, vertigo, burning pain, thirst, dryness of the throat, mouth and palate, spells of unconsciousness and diarrhoea.

The complications of kaphaja gulma are cough, dyspnoea, catarrh and tuberculosis, (CS).

The usual complication is śūla, (SS).

Prognosis: The gulma engendered by the vitiation of all three doshas is incurable. Where the tumour is hard like stone, elevated, extremely painful, attended with burning pain, debility, feeble digestion and prostration of body and mind is to be regarded as being incurable, (CS).

The gulma engendered by the vitiation of all three doshas is incurable, (SS).

Ref.: SS, uttara, 42, 3-15, 66; CS, nidāna, 3; chikitsā, 5, 4-19; AS, nidāna, 11, 46-47.

Treatment:

1. The following recipes are usually useful in cases of gulma: trivṛt and nāgara or jaggery and harītaki or guggulu; trivṛt, danti, dravanti, rock and vachā with cow's urine, wine, milk or grape juice depending on the strength (of the patient and disease); a paste of pīlu with rock salt; and wine medicated or given with pippali; root of pippali, chavya, chitraka and rock salt.

A patient suffering from vātaja gulma is oleated properly, given an oily (unctuous) purgative and nirūha and anuvāsana types of enema. Ghee medicated with the juice of āmalaka, pippali, roots of pippali, chavya, chitraka, nāgara, yava-kshāra, rock salt and sugar; or prepared from curd, souvīraka, decoctions of mudga and kulattha, souvarchala, sarjika kshāra, devādaru and rock salt is very useful in this condition. The patient can be given anuvāsana enema by means of bone marrow of aquatic animals, oil, ghee, curd etc. A compound of yava-kshāra, svarjika, kushṭha, and oil or of ketaki-kshāra and oil is also useful (for external use).

A patient of pittaja gulma is oleated by administering ghee medicated with drugs of the kākolyādi group. He is then purged by giving sweet drugs, and is given a nirūha type of enema. The patient can also be administered an anuvāsana enema composed of fat or ghee medicated with the flesh of jāngala and eka-śapha animals. Ghee medicated with a decoction of drugs of tṛṇa-mūla and jīvanīya group or with drugs of the nyagrodhādi group or utpalādi group is useful (when given internally).

A patient suffering from kaphaja gulma is first oleated with ghee medicated with drugs of the pippalyādi group and purged with strong purgatives (such as danti, dravanti, etc. NiS). A nirūha enema composed of the same drugs (and a decoction of drugs of āragvadhādi group, NiS) is administered. An anuvāsana enema of oil medicated with marrow of jāngala animals is benefical. The patient can also be administered (internally) ghee medicated with drugs which are appetizing, and which belong to the āragvadhādi group, or with drugs of the kshāra group or with various kinds of urines.

A person suffering from rakta gulma should be treated only after the lapse of the usual period of gestation (nine months). The remedial measures indicated in pittaja gulma prove to be beneficial. Ghee medicated with an alkaline solution of (ashes) of palāśa is to be administered internally. An uttara basti (douche) of ghee medicated with drugs of the pippalyādi group can be administered. As an alternative, the tumours can be made to open up and discharge by 'hot' drugs (such as drugs of the pippalyādi group). The measures indicated in treatment of asṛgdara should be adopted.

If a patient (of any type of gulma) is suffering from retention of faeces and flatus, plugs (vastis) medicated with (or composed of) sāmudra, ārdraka (fresh ginger), sarshapa and maricha are introduced into the rectum.

The diet should consist of warm meat juice of jāngala animals mixed with rock salt, ghee, pippali, nāgara and maricha; peyas (gruels) of drugs which alleviate vāta; soup of kulattha; phalas (of kapittha, dāḍima, takra, etc., NiS), of drugs of the panchamūla group; and milk medicated with fresh ginger in cases of constipation and milk with barley or kulmāsha with plenty of ghee or oil and rock salt in cases of retention of flatus and faeces.

Svedana (fomentation) of kumbhi, piṇḍa or ishṭika types is also efficacious, (SS).

2. No gulma of whatever type can exist without the vitiation or involvement of vāta. So a patient of gulma is treated with measures and medicines which alleviate vāta, such as oleation (snehana), fomentation or sudation (svedana), mild unctuous purgatives, enemata, and drugs and food articles possessing sweet, sour and salty tastes. Once the vāta is brought under control, gulma of any type can be cured with a slight effort. Gulma caused by any one dosha should be treated according to the dosha involved. If two doshas are involved, the general line of treatment (as indicated above) is to be adopted.

If a patient suffers from vātaja gulma which has been aggravated or caused by dry food, and excessive exertion, and if there is severe pain and retention of urine, faeces and flatus, he is to be given oily or unctuous food and drink, oil massage, potions of ghee, etc., and later administered nirūha and anuvāsana types of enema. Fomentation (snedana), is also useful. Oleation (snehana) is particularly indicated in gulma which is situated above the umbilical region. If it is located in the intestines or stomach, nirūha and anuvāsana enemas are useful. If a patient of vātaja gulma has good digestion, but retention of flatus and faeces, nourishing, hot and unctuous food and drink are sufficient. Generally in vāta gulma frequent sneha-pāna (potions of ghee, oil, etc.), nirūha and anuvāsana anemas are beneficial, but care should be taken to see that kapha and pitta do not get aggravated. Emesis is indicated in a case of vāta gulma, if kapha is aggravated and causes feeble digestion, tastelessness, nausea, heaviness of the body and lethargy. In a case of vāta-kaphaja gulma, if there are symptoms like flatulence, constipation and abdominal pain, suppositories, pills and powders composed of drugs which alleviate vāta are useful. If in a case of vāta gulma, pitta is aggravated and causes fever, etc., mild oily purgatives are employed. If these measures are not efficacious, blood letting (near the affected area) is to be done. Sudation of nāḍī, prastara and sankara types is useful if there is colic, constipation and flatulence.

If a person suffers from pittaja gulma which is aggravated by oily and hot substances, purgation is useful. If it is however aggravated by dry and hot substances, potions of ghee are beneficial. If the tumour is located in the intestines, the patient is given an enema of milk medicated with bitter drugs, or is purged with warm milk medicated with bitter drugs. If there are symptoms like fever, thirst, abdominal pains, sweating, feeble digestion and tastelessness, bloodletting is to be done. For the debility after bloodletting, ghee medicated with meat juices of jāngala animals is administered. If it is not possible to carry out bloodletting surgery is the only resort. If the tumour begins to suppurate, and there are symptoms like burning pain, abdominal pain, agitation, sleeplessness, restlessness, and fever, poultices (upanāha) are applied. If the tumour has suppurated, and the contents are being eliminated upwards or downwards, the patient is kept on a strict diet for ten or twelve days, without administering any medicines, and only preventing any complications. Later, the patient is given potions of ghee, and subjected to a purificatory procedure (śodhana). After śodhana, the patient is given ghee medicated with bitter drugs and honey.

If a person suffers from kaphaja gulma which has been engendered or aggravated by substances that are cold, heavy and unctuous, and if the digestive power is weak, the patient is advised to fast (langhana). If the digestion is weak, the pain mild, and there are symptoms like nausea, tastelessness, and constipation, etc., emesis is useful. After fasting or emesis, the patient is made to subsist on articles which are hot, pungent and bitter. If the gulma is hard and elevated, and the patient suffers from flatulence and constipation, sudation (svedana), fasting (langhana), ullekhana are indicated. When the digestion begins to improve, ghee medicated with pungent drugs and kshāras (alkalies) is administered to the patient. If the tumour has shifted its position, measures such as purgation or oily enemas composed of drugs of daśamūla group are adopted. If there are symptoms like feeble digestion and incarcerated flatus, pills, powders and decoctions mixed with ghee, oil, etc. are to be administered. Alkalies (kshāras) can be made use of in hemanta or śiśira (i.e. cold) seasons, if the tumour is stable (rigid), after examining the strength of the patient. The kshāras should be employed at intervals, and not regularly. During the kshāra therapy, the patient should partake of food which is sweet and unctuous, meat (juices), milk, ghee, etc. Arishṭas (fermented medicated drinks) are useful for cleansing the channels of the body. If all the above mentioned measures fail, the patient should be cauterized by an expert.

The following formulations are beneficial in vāta gulma: Ghee medicated with triphala, trikaṭu, dhānya, viḍanga, chavya, chitraka and milk (or wine, juice of dāḍima or curd); ghee medicated with pippali, dhānya, dāḍima, nāgara and milk; the powders or decoctions of the same drugs with anupāna of juice of mātulunga, kola, dāḍima, sour gruel, juice of bījapūra, etc.; a paste of dehusked tila, nāgara and jaggery with hot milk; castor oil with milk or vāruṇīmaṇḍa; a decoction of one part of dried laśuna with four parts of milk and four parts of water, heated until only the milk remains; śilājitu administered with yava kshāra and decoction of laghu-pancha-mūla drugs; vāṭya (a dish prepared from honey) with gruel of pippali, ghee or oil and juice of mūlaka; internal use, massage or anuvāsana enema of oil medicated with drugs that alleviate vāta.

Pittaja gulma is regarded as being dangerous. The following recipes are useful in this condition: ghee medicated with purgative or bitter drugs or with sugarcane juice, juice of āmalaki and harītaki or with vāsa roots, leaves etc., and a paste of vāsa flowers with honey; the warm decoction of trāyamāṇa is mixed with milk and administered to the patient, followed by hot milk (it should not however cause excessive purgation); the juices of drāksha and harītaki with jaggery; a paste of kampillaka and madhu drava (madhu-śigru) for causing purgation; massage with oil medicated with yashṭi-madhu; and kshīra-basti (enema of milk) medicated with drugs that are bitter, and which alleviate pitta-jvara. The diet should consist of old rice, meat of jāngala animals, milk and ghee of cow or goat; kharjūra, āmalaki, drāksha, dāḍima, parūshaka and water boiled with bola or vidāri-gandha.

The following measures are useful in kaphaja gulma: ghee medicated with drugs of the pancha-kola group, yava-kshāra and milk; purgation by administering powder of trivṛt with exudation of snuhi, honey and ghee; the pills and powders useful in vāta gulma; the kshāras used in grahaṇi; a decoction of pancha-mūla drugs with an equal quantity of vāruṇi; a decoction of pancha-mūla drugs with equal quantity of vāruṇi; and buttermilk medicated with powders of yavāni, and biḍā-lavaṇa. The diet should consist of old rice, flesh of jāngala animals and birds, gruels of kulattha or mudga or dry mūlaka, pippali and nāgara or of bilva, varuṇa or tender sprouts of chira-bilva, yavāni and chitraka; and buttermilk medicted with dāḍima, bījapūra, hingu, and amla-vetasa, yava-kshāra, and ghee.

A woman suffering from rakta-gulma has to be treated after nine months (i.e., on the tenth month). She has to be oleated, subjected to fomentation and given an oily (unctuous) purgative. She is then administered a solution of palāśa kshāra (ash) boiled with oil and ghee. If the gulma is not affected by this, she is subjected to viśodhana by employing palala (paste of tila) with palāśa-kshāra. She can be administered pastes of kshāras used in rakta-pitta, with honey and ghee, laśuna, madira, and fish having sharp (tīkshṇa) properties. She can also be given an enema of cow's urine, milk, kshāra (yava-kshāra) and drugs of daśamūla. If there is no discharge of blood (from the uterus), efforts are made to cause the disintegration of the tumour. When there is discharge, the patient is given meat-juices, massages with ghee and oil, and internally, fresh wine. If the discharge is excessive, measures useful in rakta-pitta are adopted, along with anuvāsana enema of bitter drugs, (CS).

3. The internal administration of purified vatsanābha with power of triphala and svarjika-kshāra is efficacious in gulma, (RRS).

4. The powders of equal quantities of pippali, maricha and nāgara or those of maricha, chitraka and souvarchala given with buttermilk are useful in gulma, (SaS).

Ref.: SS, uttara, 42, 16-65; chikitsā, 5, 20-182; RRS, 29, 67; SaS, II, 6,12, 53.

Classical Prescriptions: Abhayā-lavaṇa; Apāmārga-kshāra; Arka-lavaṇa; Balā-taila; Chitrakādi-chūrṇa; Chitraka-harītaki; Dāḍimādi-ghṛta; Dantī-harītaki; Dantyārishṭa; Daśamūlarishṭa; Daśamūla-harītaki; Daśamūla - shaṭ - pala-ghṛta; Dhānvantara - ghṛta; Elādi-ghṛta; Gandharva-hastādi-taila; Guḍa-pippali; Hingu-triguṇa-taila; Hingvāsṭaka-chūrṇa; Hingvādi-chūrṇa; Indu-kānta-ghṛta; Jvarāryabhra; Kalyāna-guda; Kalyāṇaka-kshāra; Kānchanāra-guggulu; Kānkāyana-guṭika; Kadali-kshāra; Kānta-vallabha-rasa; Khadirārishṭa; Kumāryāsava; Laśunadi-ghṛta; Lohāsava; Lokanātha-rasa; Mahā-yogarāja-guggulu; Miśraka-sneha; Mṛdvīkarishṭa; Nāgabhasma; Palāsa-kshāra; Pippalyādyāsava; Plihari-vaṭika; Prāṇada-guṭika; Punarnavāsava; Puṭapakva-vishma-jvarāntaka-lauha; Rasa-parpaṭi; Rohitakarishṭa; Sahacharādi-taila; Samudryādi-chūrṇa; Sapta-rasa-kvatha-churna; Sanjīvani-vaṭi; Saṭphala-ghṛta; Śiva-guṭika; Sukumāra-ghṛta; Sūtaśekhara-rasa; Trayantyadi-kvātha-chūrṇa; Vaiśvānara-chūrṇa; Vajraka-kshāra; Vāsa-kshāra; Vidāryādi-kvatha-chūrṇa; Yakrdāri-lauha; Yava-kshāra.

Halīmaka

Synonyms: Lāghava, Alasa (Chkp)

Western Nosology: Jaundice

Causative Factors:

Extrinsic: Factors which aggravate vāta and pitta.

Intrinsic: Vāta and pitta (CS, SS, KS).

Pathogenesis: This is an (advanced) stage of pāṇḍu, (CS, SS).

Symptomatology: Fever, body pain, vertigo, debility, drowsiness, emaciation and dark greenish-yellow discolouration, (of the skin, etc.,) (SS).

Dark greenish-yellow discolouration (of the skin, eyes, etc.), debility, emaciation, drowsiness, feeble digestion, mild fever, disinterest in sex, body pain, dyspnoea, thirst, tastelessness and vertigo, (CS).

Diarrhoea, yellow discolouration both internally and externally, and paleness of the eyes, (CSS).

Treatment:

1. Ghee medicated with juices of drāksha, guḍūchi and āmalaki is useful in lāgharaka, (SS).

2. The patient is first administered buffalo's ghee medicated with milk and juice of guḍūchi. He is then purged by administering trivṛt with juice of āmalaki. Drugs and diet which are sweet, drākshā-leha, agastya-harītaki, ghee medicated with sweet drugs, arishtas prepared from drāksha, yāpana-kshīra basti (a type of enema), and anuvāsana kind of enema are beneficial. The patient is also to be given pippali, madhūka or balā with milk, depending on the dosha involved, (CS).

3. Measures which alleviate vāta and pitta are beneficial in this disease, (KS).

4. The following formulae are beneficial in halīmaka: wine with maṇḍura and a decoction of khadira; a paste of sugar candy, tikta, balā, yashṭi-madhu, triphala, haridra and dāru-haridra with honey; drugs which are sweet and sour; and measures which are indicated in kāmala and paṇḍu, (CSS).

Ref.: SS, uttara, 44, 12, 36; chikitsā, 16, 132-137; KS, plīha-halīmaka chikitsā; CSS, page. 198.

Classical Prescriptions: Drākshāvaleha; Nava-ratnarāja-mrgānka-rasa; Paṭola-mūlādi-kvātha-chūrṇa; Śatāvari-guḍa.

Hanu-graha

Synonyms: Hanu-sangraha, Hanu-sramsa, Hanu-stambha

Western Nosology: Mandibular dislocation

Causative Factors:

Extrinsic:

1. Factors which aggravate vāta, (CS).

2. Eating dry and hard substances, cleaning the tongue too vigorously and harshly, and trauma of any sort, (AS).

Intrinsic: Vāta.

Pathogenesis and Symptomatology: The vāta located at the hanu-mūla (the root of the lower jaw, the condyloid process of the mandible) dislocates the jaw, and causes either a painless stiff condition where the mouth is rigidly open and cannot be closed or another condition where the mouth is firmly closed and cannot be opened, (CS).

Due to these conditions, the patient experiences great difficulty in chewing or talking, (AS).

References: CS, chikitsā, 28, 49; AS, nidāna, 15, 32; MN, 22, 49.

Treatment:

1. In the condition where the mouth is rigidly open, the jaw has to be subjected to proper sudation, and then it should be pressed downwards by the thumbs (inside the mouth), and pushed upwards by exerting pressure on the chin by the index fingers. In the condition where the jaw is firmly closed, the jaw has to be subjected to sudation and opened, (CS).

2. These conditions respond to svedana (sudation) with appropriate vāta-alleviating drugs, (AHṛ).

References: CS, chikitsā, 28, 102-103; AHṛ, sūtra, 17, 23.

Classical Prescriptions: Laghu-vishagarbha-taila; Mahā-nārāyaṇa-taila; Nārāyaṇa-taila; Prasāriṇi-taila; Trayodaśānga-guggulu.

Hikkā

Western Nosology: Hiccoughs
Caustive Factors:

Extrinsic: Excessive intake of food articles which are heat producing (vidāhi, such as maricha, sarshapa, alcohol, etc., NiS), hard to digest, constipating (such as karīra, NiS), dry (such as chaṇaka, etc., NiS), abhishyandi (such as fish, māsha, phāṇita, etc., NiS), and cold, eating too often, in too less a quantity, at untimely hours or before the digestion of food previously eaten, exposure to sun, wind, dust, smoke or cold climate, suppression of the natural urges, under-nourishment, excessive exertion, carrying heavy loads, excess of sexual intercourse, or injury, or accumulation of āma or tuberculosis, (SS).

Exposure to dust, smoke, wind, and cold climate, excessive exertion, or sexual intercourse, intake of food which is dry, heat-producing, constipating, hard to digest, abhishyandi, and aggravates kapha, excessive use of nishpāva, māsha, piṇyāka, tila oil, flour, śāluka, meat of aquatic animals, curd, and immature (or unboiled, āma), milk, obstruction or injury to the throat and chest. Hikka may also be caused by under-nourishment, debility, excessive use of eliminatory procedures (śodhana), injury to vital organs, or during the course of āma dosha, ānāha, rakta-pitta, udāvarta, visūchika, alasaka, paṇḍu or poisoning, (CS).

Intrinsic: Kapha and vāta. (CS, SS). The vitiation occurs in the āmāsaya, (CS).

Constituents Affected: All the seven dhātus, (CS).

Pathogenesis: The aggravated vāta enters the channels of the prāna vāta and vitiates the kapha present in the chest, (CS).

Classification: There are five types of hikka-mahā, gambhīra, vyapeta (yamala according to SS, NiS), kshudra and annaja, (CS, sutra, 19,4).

Prodromal Symptoms: Astringent taste in the mouth, restlessness, flatulence with rumbling in the abdomen, and heaviness of the throat and chest, (SS).

Astringent taste in the mouth, heaviness of throat and chest, and flatulence with rumbling in abdomen, (CS).

Symptomatology:

1. **Mahā hikkā:** The patient hiccoughs loudly and constantly, with discomfort in the marmas or vital centres (such as the urinary bladder, heart and head, NiS) and trembling of the whole body. The body straightens or stretches out with every bout; the patient also suffers from severe thirst, (SS).

The patient suffers from loud, violent, deepseated and constant hiccoughs which may occur in bouts of one, two or three. The patient also suffers from emaciation, debility, loss of enthusiasm (or zest for life) and lustre, loss of body heat, obstruction to the channels of prāna vāta and the vital centres (marma), unconsciousness, stiffness of the body, loss of memory, excessive lachrymation and distorted eyebrows. The patient will be irrelevantly muttering to himself, (CS).

2. **Gambhīra hikka:** The patient suffers from deep sounding hiccoughs which seem as if they appear from the navel, dryness of the lips, throat, tongue and mouth, dyspnoea and pain in the sides. There are numerous complications (such as fever, dyspnoea, thirst, etc. NiS), (SS).

The patient suffers from difficult and deep sounding hiccoughs which appear to come from the navel or intestines along with depression, emaciation, moaning, stiffness and pain in the sunken chest, obstruction of the respiratory tract, debility, unconsciousness, and yawning. The patient holds his chest with both hands, and stretches or contracts his limbs during the spasms of hiccoughs which agitates the whole body, (CS).

3. **Kshudra hikka:** The patient suffers from infrequent and mild hiccoughs, which arise from the region of the clavicles, (SS).

The vāta is slightly aggravated by exertion, and localises in the region of the kloma, heart, palate and throat. The patient suffers from mild hiccoughs which are aggravated on exertion and ameliorated on eating. It does not induce much suffering nor does it affect the marmas (vital centres) such as the heart and head. Neither does it affect the respiration or swallowing of food, (CS).

4. **Yamala hikka:** The patient suffers from hiccoughs at long intervals, and bouts of two. The hiccoughs cause trembling or jerking of the head and neck, (SS).

5. **Vyapeta hikka:** The patient suffers from hiccoughs which arise from the region of the supra-sternum, and are not continuous. They commence after eating and are aggravated at the end of digestion. The hiccoughs are accompanied by symptoms such as irrelevant speech (pralāpa), vomiting, diarrhoea, thirst, confusion of mind, dryness of the mouth, thirst, lachrymation, bending of the body, and distention (of abdomen), (CS).

6. **Annaja hikka:** This variety of hiccoughs are brought about if a person eats food too heartily or partakes of food which is heavy (hard to digest) and bitter, (SS).

This type of hiccoughs is caused by eating food too fast, or overeating, or partaking of alcoholic drinks or by extreme anger, talking too much, walking for long distances, carrying heavy loads or laughing in excess. The patient suffers from infrequent and mild hiccoughs, which do not disturb the vital organs or sense-faculties, and which are ameliorated by eating or drinking, (CS).

Prognosis: The types, mahā hikka and gambhīra hikka are incurable by nature. Cases where the patient straightens his body during the hiccough, turns the eyes upwards, where the limbs contract excessively, and where the patient is emaciated, suffers from cough and aversion to food are considered incurable, (SS).

Hikka is considered incurable in patients in whom the doshas are excessively vitiated, who are emaciated through lack of food or due to disease, in old people and those accustomed to excessive sexual intercourse. The yamaka type is incurable if the patient suffers from irrelevant speech (pralāpa), pain, thirst and unconsciousness. It is however curable in persons who are not emaciated or depressed, who have stable or firm tissues (dhātu) and sense faculties, (CS).

Patients suffering from mahā, gambhīra and vyapeta hikka where the symptoms are not fully manifested are curable. The kshudra and annaja hikka are curable even if all the symptoms are present, (Chkp. on CS).

Ref.: SS, uttara, 50, 3-15; CS, chikitsā, 17, 8-44.

Treatment:

1. The measures generally beneficial in hikka are: prāṇāyāma (breathing exercises) (especially kumbhaka, NiS); harsh words, inducing fear (in a timid person, NiS), pricking with needles, etc.

The following formulae are useful: a paste of

yashṭi-madhu with honey; or of pippali with sugar should be used for avapīḍa-nasya, (a kind of errhine therapy).

A patient who is not emaciated can be made to vomit by administering warm ghee with milk or sugarcane juice. The following errhines are also efficacious: a paste of red sandal wood with breast-milk, a paste of warm ghee with rock-salt, or a paste of powdered rock salt with water.

The region between the throat and the breasts should be fomented. The patient can be made to inhale the smoke caused by burning gum-resin of śāla, manahśila, cow's horn, etc.

The following recipes can be administered internally: a paste of svarṇa-gairaka with honey; a paste of ash of feather of barhi (mayūra); or ash of udumbara or tilvaka with honey and ghee; a paste of svarji-kshāra with juice of bīja-pūra and honey; gruels (yavāgu) mixed with ghee and warm pāyasa; goat's milk medicated with sugar, ginger and water (or a decoction of ginger); a paste of nāga-keśara, sugar and honey taken with sugarcane juice and the juice of madhūka; a paste of one part of rock salt and two parts of ghee; harītaki with the anupāna of warm water; warm ghee mixed with milk and honey; a paste of pippali, honey or of āmalaka, fresh ginger and honey; a paste of the seeds of badara, anjana (souvirānjana, NiS), lājā and honey; and a paste (or decoction) of fruits and flowers of pāṭala with honey, or of kharjūra with pippali and honey or of kāsīsa, kapittha and honey.

A strong patient can be administered purgatives. Potions of warm ghee mixed with rock salt and sugar candy are very useful in hikkā. Some authorities consider anuvāsana basti (enema) to be very useful, (SS).

2. The general line of treatment in hikkā is similar to that in śvāsa: A few formulae especially useful in hikkā are: the powder of āmalaka, and roots of śaṭi and pushkara are made into a paste with honey and administered to the patient. A paste of loha (bhasma) and honey is also efficacious. The following drugs can be used as errhines (nāvana): the roots of laśuna, palāṇḍu, or gṛnjanaka rubbed with breast-milk; chandana with breast-milk; the upper layer of warm ghee (ghṛta-maṇḍa), with powdered rock-salt; ghee medicated with drugs of the jīvanīya group can be given internally, as errhines or even sprinkled; milk alternately hot and cold, can be drunk or used as nasal drops; milk can also be used with sugar and honey.

Ghee medicated with purgative drugs; the juices of āmalaki and kapittha with pippali and honey; and a paste of kola, honey, drāksha, pippali and nāgara can also be used internally, (CS).

3. The following formulae are useful in hikka: pills prepared from the pastes of purified mercury, purified sulphur and tāmra bhasma; a decoction of rāsna, bṛhati, chitraka, balā and milk; the inhalation of smoke from burning leaves of chitraka and haridra, (RRS).

Ref.: SS, uttara, 50, 16-50; CS, chikitsā, 18, 129-136; RRS, 13, 68, 71-72.

Classical Prescriptions: Agastya-harītaki-rasāyana; Elādi-guṭika; Grahaṇi-mihira-taila; Kaṇṭakāryāvaleha; Kāsisa-bhasma; Mṛgamadāsava; Nāyopāyam-kvātha-chūrṇa; Pippalyādi-lauha; Rasa-pushpa; Sṛnga-bhasma; Svarṇa-bhasma.

Hṛdroga

Western Nosology: Heart - disease; Cardiac ailments.

Causative Factors:

Extrinsic:

1. Suppression of the natural urges, trauma, excessive use of hot and dry food, intake of food before the digestion of the food previously taken, intake of incompatible food, intake of food which disagrees with and is disliked by the person and overeating, (SS).

2. Grief, (prolonged) fasting, (excessive)

exertion, and eating food which is dry, and devoid of oilyness and too limited in quantity, will provoke vātaja hṛdroga. Anger, (over) exposure to the sun, intake of food before the digestion of the food previously taken, and intake of alcoholic drinks and food which is hot, sour, salty, pungent and kshāra engender pittaja hṛdroga. Atyādāna, lack of physical and mental activity, leading a luxurious life, excessive sleep and intake of food which is hard to digest and oily are responsible for kaphaja hṛdroga, (CS, sūtra, 17, 30, 32, 34).

Excessive exertion, trauma (of all kinds), suppression of the natural urges, (excessive) vomiting, production of āma in the body, factors which cause emaciation, excessive care, anxiety, fear and stress, excessive purging, too frequent use of enemas, and improper treatment of diseases, (CS, chikitsā, 26, 77).

A child fed continously on breast-milk vitiated by kapha has a tendency to suffer from hṛdroga, (CS, chikitsā, 30, 250).

Constituents Affected: Rasa dhātu, (SS, CS).

Classification:

1. There are four kinds of hṛdroga - those brought about by the vitiated vāta, pitta or kapha and that type which is engendered by all the three doshas (tridoshaja). The krimija hṛdroga is an advanced stage of the tridoshaja hṛdroga, (SS, NiS).

2. There are five types of hṛdroga - those caused by the vitiated vāta, pitta or kapha, or by the aggravation of all three doshas combined or that type attended with the production of organisms (krimi), (CS, sūtra, 19, 4).

Symptomatology:

1. Vātaja hṛdroga - The patient feels as if his heart is being pulled apart, or experiences pricking, piercing, bursting, or splitting pain in the (region of the) heart, (SS).

The patient suffers from palpitation, a sense of emptiness of the heart, emaciation, breaking pain, rigidity or stiffness, (spells of) unconsciousness, a sense of anxiety around (the region of the) heart, trembling (of the limbs or heart), cramping pains (in the chest) and severe pain, all aggravated after digestion of food. (CS).

2. Pittaja hṛdroga - The patient suffers from burning or sucking pain in the heart, a sense of fatigue in (the region of) the heart, pyrosis, sweating, dryness of the mouth and (spells of) unconsciousness, (SS).

The patient experiences burning pain around (the region of) the heart, a bitter taste in the mouth, bitter and sour eructations, excessive thirst, vertigo, unconsciousness, sweating, fever, yellow discolouration (of the eyes, urine, etc.) and a sense of fatigue (klama), (CS).

3. Kaphaja hṛdroga - The patient suffers from a sweet taste in the mouth, feeble digestion, tastelessness, a feeling of heaviness, and stiffness in the region of the heart, discharges (of mucous from nose, mouth, etc.) and accumulation of phlegm (in the chest), (SS).

The patient suffers from salivation, fever, cough, lassitude, tastelessness, numbness and a sense of heaviness or weight around the region of the head. He also feels as if his head is enclosed by stones, (CS).

4. Tridoshaja hṛdroga - The symptoms present in this type are: frequent expectoration, spitting or hawing (out of sputum), pricking and sharp pain (in the region of the heart), nausea and dyspnoea or darkness before the eyes.

If this type of hṛdroga is not properly treated, there may be an occurence or proliferation of organisms (krimi) along with the symptoms of tastelessness, dark-brown discolouration of the eyes and emaciation, (SS).

The patient suffers from symptoms caused by the aggravation of all the doshas.

5. Krimija hṛdroga - If a person suffering from tridoshaja hṛdroga partakes of tila, milk, jaggery, etc. (in excess), the aggravated doshas

cause a disturbance or abnormality in the rasa dhātu. This results in the formation of a granthi (knotty growth) in any one part of the heart, which begins to ooze out a liquid. This provides a fertile ground for the production of organisms (krimayah). The patient also suffers from a sense of severe, sharp, pricking or cutting pains and itching, (CS).

Complications and Concomitant Symptoms: Vertigo, debility, emaciation, dryness of the mouth, and fatigue and breathlessness even without exertion are the usual complications, (SS).

The following symptoms may be either concomitant or may appear as complications: discolouration (of skin, eyes, etc.), unconsciousness, fever, cough, hiccoughs, dyspnoea, bad taste in the mouth, thirst, pramoha, vomiting, expectoration of mucous, tastelessness, etc., (CS).

Ref.: SS, uttara, 43; CS, sūtra, 17, 31-40; chikitsā, 26, 77-80.

Treatment:

1. A patient suffering from vātaja hṛdroga is administered oleation (by means of oily food, ghee, etc.) and is then made to vomit by giving salt with ghee or oil, with a decoction of drugs of daśamūla group. He is then administered powders of pippali, ela, vachā, hingu, yavakshāra, rock salt, souvarchala salt, ginger and ajamoda (with the anupāna of) the juices of fruits (such as mātulunga, NiS), dhānyāmla, a decoction of kulattha, curd, alcoholic drinks or any sneha (oil, ghee, fat, etc.). Enemas can also be given with oil medicated with drugs that alleviate vāta. The diet should consist of old rice and meat juices of desert animals, with ghee.

A patient of pittaja hṛdroga is made to undergo emesis by administering the juices of kāśmari, yashṭi-madhu, honey, sugarcandy and kushtha. He is then advised to take ghee medicated with drugs of the kākolyādi group, and decoctions which are useful in pittaja jvara. The diet should mainly consist of the meat juices of eṇa, etc., which have a sweet taste, cooked with ghee. An enema can be given with oil medicated with yashṭi-madhu and honey.

A patient suffering from kaphaja hṛdroga is made to vomit by administering a decoction of vachā and nimba. He is then prescribed the powders recommended in vātaja hṛdroga (pippali, etc.). This powder can be taken even along with food. The decoctions of triphala or musta, etc., or madana phala, etc., are also useful. The patient may also be purged with ghee medicated with śyāma (vrddhadāraka, NiS) and trivṛt paste, or given enema with bala taila.

In a case of krimija hṛdroga the patient is made to partake of unctuous food. He is then given meat with curd and fried and powdered tila, for three days. He is then purged with a compound of ajāji, sugar-candy, salt, trivrt, nāgara, harītaki, etc. and aromatic drugs. He is then administered kānji with a large amount of viḍanga. The diet should consist of barley, rice and viḍanga, (SS).

2. A patient suffering from vātaja hṛdroga is administered the following medicines: warm oil medicated with souvīraka, mastu, butter milk and rock salt; oil medicated with cow's urine, rock salt and ambu (bālaka or water); oil medicated with a decoction of punarnava, devadāru, drugs of (bṛhat) panchamūla, rāsna, yava, bilva, kulattha and kola (this oil can be used for massage also); ghee medicated with harītaki, nāgara, pushkara-mūla, āmalaki, rock salt and hingu; a paste of pushkara-mūla, root of bījapura, nāgara, śatī and harītaki, with milk, watery ghee or salt; a paste of harītaki, śaṭī, pushkara, drugs of the panchakola group and juice of mātulunga, fried with oil and ghee; this paste is to be administered with guḍa, surā (wine) and rock-salt.

The following measures are useful in a patient having pittaja hṛdroga: cold plasters; sprinking of cold water or cold decoction; a mild purgation by administering drāksha, sugar-candy, parūshaka and honey; a paste of yashṭi and kaṭu-rohiṇi with sugar water; the medicated ghee useful in kshata-kshīṇa, the juice of dhanva, with a diet of just cow's milk; ghee medicated with the drugs of the laghu-panchamūla, and milk or juice of drāksha or sugarcane juice; and cold infusions or juice of kadali (svādu-phala) and sugarcane juice.

The diet is to consist of food articles which alleviate pitta.

A patient suffering from kaphaja hṛdroga is to be given fomentation, followed by emesis. He is then advised to fast (or partake of food which is easy to digest). He is then administered drugs and a diet which alleviates vāta. The diet should consist of kulattha, yavānna, etc. The following recipes are of use: Cow's urine medicated with kaṭphala, fresh ginger, pītadāru (devadāru), harītaki, and ativisha; the powder of kṛshṇa (pippali or maricha), śaṭi, pushkara-mūla, rāsna, vachā, harītaki and nāgara with warm water; a decoction of udumbara, aśvattha, vaṭa, arjuna, palāśa, rohitaka and khadira, with the powders of trivṛt, and trikaṭu, with warm water; and the drug silājatu as described in CS (chikitsā, 1,3). The other medicines useful in this condition are chyavanaprāśa, agastya- rasāyana, brāhma-rasāyana and āmalaki-rasāyana.

A patient of tridoshaja hṛdroga is first advised to fast (langhana). He is then recommended food which does not aggravate any of the doshas. The physician should ascertain and treat primarily the dosha which is most vitiated.

When the pain is aggravated almost immediately after eating, is slightly less during digestion and subsides after it, the patient is to be given devadāru, tilvaka, the two salts (souvarchala and saindhava), ativisha and viḍanga with hot water. Unctuous purgatives are indicated if the pain is aggravated after digestion of food. If the pain is most severe during digestion, the patient is to be given (mild) purgatives such as drāksha, kāśmari fruit, etc. If the pain is severe throughout the day, the patient is administered strong purgatives such as trivrit root, etc. Langhana and drugs which are digestive (pāchana) are very useful, (CS).

3. A person suffering from vātaja hṛdroga is to be administered ghee medicated with souvarchala salt and harītaki, or a powder of yava-kshāra and yavāni with hot water. If the patient is very thirsty, he can partake of water boiled with ginger, and the drugs of the laghu-panchamūla; or dadhi-maṇḍa or vāruṇi-maṇḍa or dhānyāmla. He can also be administered balā-taila or sukumāra ghṛta. In the case of palpitation and enlargement of the heart (dravāyāme), if there is good digestion, the patient can be given ghee, curd, jaggery, milk and flesh of aquatic animals. These are however contra-indicated in all other types of hṛdroga, and even in vātaja hrḍroga if there are symptoms like heaviness, lethargy and indigestion.

The measures most useful in hrdṛoga are anulomana, langhana and pāchana (drugs which are digestive), (AHṛ).

4. The following recipes are efficacious in chest pain (caused by heart troubles) (hṛt-sūla): the juice of bījapūra with yavakshāra; a decoction of the root of eraṇḍa reduced to one-fourth, with yava-kshāra; the ash produced by incinerating powdered deer's horn within two crucibles, given with cow's ghee (SaS).

5. The following recipes are useful in all types of hṛdroga: ghee medicated with powders of wheat and arjuna with goat's urine, given with honey and sugar; ghee medicated with harītaki and souvarchala; ghee medicated with a paste of arjuna; ghee medicated with a decoction of bala, nāgabala and arjuna, and a paste of yashṭi-madhu; the powder of pushkara-mūla with honey; the powders of godhūma and arjuna with oil, ghee or guḍa and milk; and the powder or hingu, souvarchala, nāgara, dāḍima and amla-vetasa with hot water.

The following formulae are useful in pittaja hṛdroga: milk boiled with arjuna, given with sugar-candy, or honey or balā or drugs of the pancha-mūla; and the powder of arjuna administered with jaggery, water, ghee or milk, (CSS).

Ref.: SS, uttara, 43; CS, chikitsā, 26, 81-103; AHṛ, chikitsā, 6, 25-58; SaS, madhyama, 1, 14, 42; 2, 99; CSS, pages. 448-451.

Classical Prescriptions: Abhayā-lavaṇa; Arjunārishṭa; Chandanāsava; Chintāmani - chaturmukha-rasa; Chyavana-prāśa; Dantī-harītaki; Dhānvantara-guṭika; Dāḍimādi-ghṛta; Karpūrādyarka; Kānkayaṇa-guṭika; Mānikya-pishṭi; Muktā-pishṭi; Śiva-guṭika; Svarṇa-bhasma; Trāyantyādi-kvātha-chūrṇa.

Hṛd-sūla:

Bṛhat-saindhavādya-taila; Śṛnga-bhasma; Sapta-vimśatika-guggulu; Sapta-rasa-kvātha-chūrṇa.

Hṛdaya-dourbalya:

Makaradhvaja; Muktā-bhasma; Rasa-sindūra.

Hṛt-kampa: Pravāla-bhasma.

Krimija -hṛdroga: Prāṇadā - guṭika.

Indralupta

Synonyms: Sanskrit: Rujyā, Khālityā (which occurs only in men according to NiS and Nyāya-chandrika); Khalli, Ruhya (Bhoja, quoted in Nyāya-chandrika); Chācha (AHṛ).

Western Nosology: Alopecia

Causative Factors:

Extrinsic: Abuse of salt, (CS).

Intrinsic: All three doshas.

Constituents Affected: Blood

Pathogenesis and Symptomatology: The vāta and pitta affect the scalp and cause falling of hair. The kapha is later aggravated and with the vitiated blood prevents the growth of new hair.

According to Kārtika (quoted in Madhu-kośa), indralupta refers to falling hair of the beard, khālitya to falling of hair of the scalp and ruhya to loss of hair all over body, (MN).

Treatment:

1. Venesection of veins in the head after massaging and fomentation, (SS).

Plasters of manahśila, kāsīsa, tuttha and maricha or of kuṭannaṭa (tagara according to NiS) and deva-dāru are to be applied to the scalp. Alternately the scalp can be deeply scraped and covered over with a paste of gunja. An oil medicated with mālati, karavīra, chitraka and karanja is very useful when used externally.

The patient should be administered rasāyana therapy, (SS).

2. Plasters of the root of lāngali with the juice of karavīra, or of honey and small variety of vārtāku, or of leaves of dhattūra with juice of bhallātaka or of honey, ghee, leaves of tila and gokshura are to be applied (after scraping the scalp). The ash got by burning the tusks of an elephant is used when applied with oil. Shower baths are to be avoided until the growth of new hair.

The patient can be given śodhana therapy followed by errhines, śiro-abhyanga, etc, (AHṛ).

3. The application of a paste of gokshura, flowers of tila, honey, and ghee, is useful. The paste of tikta and juice of the leaves of paṭoli is to be rubbed on the scalp, (CSS).

4. The application of a paste of āmalaki and powdered stone of āmra strengthens the hair roots. The scalp is to be scraped with the rough surface of a leaf and sprinkled with pepper powder. Oil medicated with milk, yashṭi-madhu, and fruits of āmalaki is useful as an errhine, (CD).

5. The application of a paste of haridra, dāru-haridra and fresh butter, or of flowers, roots and leaves of jāti and urine of a black cow, or of the root and fruits of gunja and the juice of

the fruits of kaṇṭakāri is beneficial. The scalp is to be scraped with leaves of dhāttūra and plastered over with a paste of bhallataka, bṛhati root and the fruits of gunja and honey. This is very efficacious, (RRS).

Ref.: CS, sūtra, 26, 43, 3; SS, nidāna, 13, 33; AHṛ, uttara, 23, 25; SS, chikitsā, 20, 24-26; AHṛ, uttara, 24, 29-33; CSS, page. 663; CD, 55; RRS, 24, 82-87.

Classical Prescriptions: Nīlikādya-taila.

Indra-vṛddha

Synonyms: Sanskrit: Viddhā (AS)

Western Nosology: Herpes zoster

Causative Factors: Intrinsic: Vāta and pitta.

Symptomatology: Eruptions (on the skin) which are arranged in a circular manner similar to the distribution of seeds in a lotus flower.

Treatment:

1. Treatment is similar to that of pitta-visarpa. When the eruptions have suppurated, ghee medicated with drugs of the kākolyadi group (having a sweet taste) are to be applied for hastening the healing process, (SS).

Ref.: SS, nidāna, 13, 11; chikitsā, 20, 7-8; AS, uttara, 36.

Irivellika

Western Nosology: Abscess.

Symptomatology: Very painful, circular eruptions on the head (and neck, AS) attended with fever and other symptoms of vitiated vāta, pitta and kapha.

Treatment:

1. The patient is to be treated along the same lines as for pittaja visarpa. The eruptions which have suppurated are to be treated with ghee prepared from drugs of the kākolyadi group (i.e. possessing a sweet taste).

Ref.: SS, nidāna, 13, 15; chikitsā, 20, 7-8; AS, uttara, 36.

Jāla-gardabha

Western Nosology: Cellulitis.

Causative Factors:

Extrinsic: Factors which aggravate pitta.

Intrinsic: Pitta.

Constituents Affected: Blood.

Symptomatoloty: An intensely painful, slightly suppurating, red swelling which spreads and is accompanied by fever and thirst, (CS).

A slight, non-suppurating swelling attended with burning pain and fever which spreads in a manner similar to visarpa, (SS). The swelling is coppery in colour, (AHṛ).

Treatment:

1. The patient is made to fast and is administered cleansing (śodhana) and drying (rūkshana) therapy. Blood-letting can also be done. Āmalaki is beneficial in such cases. Cold plasters (pradeha) can be made use of, (CS).

2. The patient is treated as in a case of pittaja visarpa. After suppuration, ghee medicated with drugs of the kākolyadi group (possessing a sweet taste) can be used, (SS).

3. The roots of nīla (nīli) and paṭola are made into a paste with water and ghee. This paste is to be applied over the swelling, (SS).

Ref.: CS, chikitsā, 12, 99-100; SS, nidāna, 13, 14; chikitsā, 20, 8; AHṛ, uttara, 31, 13, CSS, page. 651.

Jatu-Maṇi

Vernacular: Jadula (NiS), Jaṭulam (NC)

Western Nosology: Neuro fibroma

Causative Factors: Intrinsic: Kapha (SS, nidaÇa, 13, 41).

Constituents Affected: Blood (SS, ibid)

Symptomatology: Painless, very slightly elevated, smooth, reddish and circular excrescences which are congenital (sahaja) (SS, ibid).

According to AS, it is similar to charma-kīlaka, but is painful, (AS, uttara, 36, 316).

Treatment: Excision (cchedana) (SS, sūtra, 25, 46; chikitsā, 20, 32). After excision, the part is to be cauterised with kshāra of sūrya-kānta or with fire, (AHr, uttara, 32, 14).

Jvara

Synonyms: Vikāra, Roga, Vyādhi, Ātanka (CS)

Western Nosology: Fever, Pyrexia,

Causative Factors:

Extrinsic: Fever can also be caused by extrinsic causes such as trauma (abhighāta), sudden misfortune (abhishanga), malevolent magical spells (abhi-chāra) or curse (abhiśāpa). These factors first cause fever and only later are the doshas affected, (CS).

Fever can also be caused by improper or over-use of oleation, sudation, emesis, purgation and other purificatory procedures, by various kinds of trauma, due to various diseases (such as vidradhi (abscesses) etc., NiS), or suppuration, due to fatigue, due to kshaya (raja-yakshma), toxicosis, ajīrṇa (indigestion), intake of unwholesome or unpalatable food, seasonal variations, due to smell of flowers or plants, grief, mental turmoil caused by spells or curses, improper measures during delivery and after, during the onset of lactation, etc, (SS).

Intrinsic: The vāta is aggravated by excessive intake of food that is dry, light, and cold, over-use of purificatory procedures (i.e. emesis, purgation, āsthāpana and śiro-virechana), excessive excitation, very frequent indulgence in coitus, excessive loss of blood, fasting, loss of sleep, suppression of natural urges, anxiety, grief, adopting improper postures and trauma.

Pitta is aggravated by excessive intake of hot, sour, salty, alkaline and pungent food, eating before the digestion of the previous meal, excessive exposure to sun, and fire, anger, fatigue, etc.

Kapha is aggravated by excessive intake of food that is unctuous, heavy, sweet, slimy, cold, sour and salty, sleep during the daytime, lack of physical exercise and adopting a carefree attitude.

All the three doshas are aggravated by improper administration of purificatory procedures such as emesis, purgation, oleation, sudation, āsthāpana and anuvāsana enema, śiro-virechana (errhines), etc., improper care after these procedures, improper parturition and care during the puerperal period, fasting, sudden change in food-habits, drinking water that has been poisoned, living in a polluted environment, improper intake of food, etc.

Classification:

1. Depending on the causes, jvara can be of two kinds, endogenous and exogenous i.e. somatic and psychic. It can also be characterized by internal heat (antar-vega) or external heat (bahir-vega). It can also be either seasonal or unseasonal. Jvara can also be of seven kinds, depending on which of the seven dhatus are affected. Jvara can also be caused by excessive heat (in which case the patient desires cold substances and has an aversion to heat) or by excessive cold (wherein the patient desires warmth). Jvara can also be classified into five kinds, depending on the strength or weakness of the aggravated dosha and time. It can be satata, santata, anyedyu, tṛtīya, or chaturthaka.

2. Jvara is of eight types, depending on the causes (i.e. vātaja, pittaja, kaphaja, vāta-

pittaja, pitta-kaphaja, kapha-vātaja, sannipātaja or tridoshaja and caused by extrinsic factors), (SS, CS).

Pathogenesis:

1. The aggravated doshas affect the rasa-dhātu (the nutrient fluid which circulates through the blood) and displaces the jātharāgni (the internal fire). The body heat is thus augmented by this displaced internal fire associated with the morbid heat of the aggavated doshas. These doshas also obstruct the body channels (thus preventing perspiration), causing fever. The channels that are usually obstructed are the rasa-vahā-srotas (nutrient vessels and lymphatics) and sweda-vahā-srotas (coiled tubular sweat glands and their ducts), (CS).

2. The doshas that are aggravated displace the agni (internal fire) outwards, obstruct the sveda-vahā-srotas (sweat glands and their ducts) and cause fever, (SS).

Prodromal Symptoms:

1. Bad taste in the mouth, heaviness of the body, anorexia (aversion to food), congestion or watering of the eyes, sleepiness, arati (languor), yawning, stretching of limbs, tremors, exhaustion, vertigo, irrelevant speech, sleeplessness, horripilation (goose-flesh), sensitiveness of teeth, alternate desire and aversion to sound, cold wind and sun's rays, indigestion, body-pain, loss of enthusiasm, tendency to procrastinate, lethargy, inability and aversion to carry on ones normal activities, disregard for words of elders and respected people, aversion to children, indifference, aversion to food, garlands and sweets, craving for sour, salty, and pungent food, loss of complexion, (CS).

2. Debility, arati (restlesness acc. to NiS), discolouration (of skin), bad taste in the mouth, watering of the eyes, alternate desire for and aversion to cold wind and sun, yawning, body pain, heaviness, of body, horripilation, anorexia, tama (spells of blindness, of blacking out) and aversion to cold. The prodromal symptoms of vātaja, pittaja and kaphaja jvara are excessive yawning, burning of the eyes and aversion to food respectively, (SS).

Symptomatology:

I. The main symptoms of jvara are an increase in body temperature (santāpa), anorexia, thirst, body pain and distress in the cardiac region. In jvara which affects the mind, the patient suffers from grief or mental distraction (vaichitya), lethargy and arati (restlessness or languor). Patients suffering from fever caused by vāta and pitta have a desire for cold, while those suffering from fever caused by vāta and kapha desire warmth.

The symptoms of internal fever (antarvega-jvara) are a feeling of internal heat, severe thirst, delirious speech, dyspnoea, vertigo, pain in the bones and joints, lack of perspiration and constipation. The symptoms of external fever are external heat, mildness of other symptoms such as thirst, and easy curability.

The fever that occurs in vasanta (spring) and śarad (autumn) is known as prākṛta (seasonal) jvara. In these cases, the kapha that is accumulated in winter flares up in spring, while the pitta that has increased in hot weather flares up in autumn (śarad). Jvara that is seasonal partakes of the nature of the corresponding dosha.

In santata-jvara, fever is continuous, and lasts for ten, twelve or seven days and either subsides or proves fatal. The doshas that are responsible for the fever are homologous to the season, the affected constituents and the patients constitution. The doshas simultaneously affect the body tissues (dhātus) and the urine and stools. The fever proves fatal if the dhatus remain impure or diseased even at the end of seven, ten or twelve days, and vice-versa. If the twelve elements (the seven dhatus, three doshas, urine and stools) are not fully free from disease, the fever may abate on the twelfth day, but will again recur and prove intractable. In satata-jvara, the aggravated doshas affect the blood and cause fever which periodically fluctuates and increases twice in twenty-four hours. In anyedyushka-jvara, the aggravated doshas being further deranged due to either the season (time), patient's constitution and the diseased constituents of the body (dūshya) obstruct the medo-vaha-srotas (channels that transport the fatty tissue), and cause fever that recurs only once in twenty-four hours. In tṛtīyaka-jvara, which is caused by the aggravated doshas affecting the bones, the fever recurs once in two days (once in forty-eight hours). In chaturthaka-jvara, the aggravated doshas affect the bone-marrow, and cause fever that recurs after an interval of two days. The aggravated doshas lie dormant in the body and flare up when there is a decrease in the resistance or immunity, just like a seed lies dormant in the ground and sprouts forth in the appropriate season. The tritīyaka-jvara is of three types. If the vāta and pitta are vitiated, the fever is attended by severe headache. If kapha and pitta, and vāta and kapha are aggravated, the fever is accompanied by pain in the sacrum and back pain respectively. The chaturthaka-jvara is of two types. If kapha is excessively aggravated there is pain which commences in the leg (and spreads all over the body). If vāta is provoked, the pain commences in the head. All these five types of fever which are known as vishama-jvara are caused by the aggravation of all the doshas. The periodicity of these fevers depends upon the season, time, and physical and mental strength of the patient.

If the aggravated doshas affect the rasa-dhātu, there is external heat, body pain, yawning, heaviness of the body, depression, anxiety, weakness, vomiting and anorexia. If the blood is affected, there is fever with thirst, frequent expectoration of bloody sputum, vertigo, delirious speech, feeling of intoxication, redness, and appearance of red and hot eruptions. If the doshas affect the flesh (māmsa), there is internal heat, thirst, stupefaction, languor, diarrhoea, offensive body odour, and tremors. If the fatty tissues are involved, the symptoms are fever, excessive sweating, thirst, delirious speech, frequent vomiting, langour, anorexia and disgust at one's own body-odour. If the bones are affected, there is both vomiting and diarrhoea, breaking pain in the bones, moaning, dyspnoea and convulsions of the limbs. If the bone marrow is involved, the symptoms are hiccoughs, dyspnoea, cough, fainting spells, external coldness, internal heat and pain in the vital organs. The fever that is caused by the provoked doshas affecting the reproductive element of the body, proves to be fatal.

The symptoms of vātaja-jvara are irregular onset and subsidence of fever, fluctuating temperature, aggravation in the evening, later part of the night, at the end of summer (in rainy season) and after the digestion of food, roughness and brownish discolouration of nails, face, eyes, urine, faeces, and skin, cracking or splitting of the nails, various types of shifting pains, numbness of feet, cramps of the calf, a sensation of looseness or dislocation of the knee joint or other joints, weakness of thighs, various kinds of pain in the waist, sides (or the chest), back, shoulders, arms, and chest, stiffness of the jaw, tinnitus, pricking pain in the temples, astringent or bad taste in the mouth, dryness of the mouth, palate and throat, thirst, chest pain or palpitation, retching, dry cough, suppression of (inability to) sneezing and eructations, salivation, anorexia and indigestion, depression, yawning, stretching of limbs, tremors, fatigue, vertigo, delirious speech, insomnia, horripilation, sensitiveness of teeth and a desire for warmth.

The symptoms of pittaja-jvara are: generalised heat all over the body, aggravation during digestion of food, during the afternoon, at midnight and in śarad (autumn), pungent taste in the mouth, inflammation of nose, mouth, throat, lips and palate, thirst, a sense of intoxication, vertigo, debility, profuse sweating, delirious spech, appearance of red urticarial patches (koṭha), yellow or greenish discolouration of nails, eyes, face, urine, stools and skin, intense heat (fever), severe burning sensation and desire for cold.

The symptoms of kaphaja-jvara are: generalised heat, aggravation after eating, in the morning (forenoon), early part of the night, and in the spring, heaviness of body, aversion to food, hawking of mucous, sweet taste in the mouth, nausea, hṛdayopalepa, a sensation as if covered over with a moist cloth, vomiting, poor appetite, sleepiness, stiffness of the body, lethargy, cough, dyspnoea, catarrh (pratisyaya), chilliness, white discolouration of the nails, eyes, face, urine, stools and skin, appearance of cold pimples all over the body, and a desire for warmth.

The symptoms of vāta-pitta-jvara are headache, joint pain, burning sensation, horripilation, dryness of the mouth and throat, vomiting, thirst, syncope, vertigo, anorexia, sleeplessness, loquacity and yawning.

The symptoms of vāta-kapha-jvara are chilliness, heaviness of the body, lethargy, a sensation as if enveloped in a moist cloth, joint pain, headache, catarrh, cough, absence of sweat and moderate temperature.

The symptoms of kapha-pitta jvara are flashes of heat alternating with chills, intermittent sweating, stupefaction, cough, anorexia, thirst, expectoration of phlegm and vomiting of bile, coated tongue, bitter taste in the mouth and lethargy.

There are thirteen kinds of doshaja jvara, depending on the degree of involvement of the three doshas. In cases where vāta and kapha are severely provoked and pitta less aggravated, the symptoms observed are chilliness, cough, anorexia, lethargy, thirst, burning sensation, body pain and uneasiness. Fever caused by severely aggravated pitta and kapha and moderately aggravated vāta is characterised by vomiting, chilliness, flashes of heat, thirst, stupefaction and bone pain. Fever wherein vāta is severely provoked and pitta and kapha are mildly provoked is characterized by headache, joint pain, pain in the bones, delirious speech, heaviness of body, vertigo, thirst and dryness of the mouth and throat. Cases of fever where pitta is aggavated much more than the other two doshas is characterized by bloody stools and urine, burning sensations, sweating, thirst, debility and syncope. Fever where kapha is provoked much more than the other two doshas is marked by lethargy, anorexia, nausea, burning pain, vomiting, vertigo, languor, cough and weariness. In cases of fever where kapha is severely aggravated, pitta is moderately provoked and vata only slightly aggravated, the symptoms observed are catarrh, vomiting, lethargy, drowsiness, anorexia and feeble digestion. Cases where the aggravation of pittta, kapha and vāta is severe, moderate and slight, respectively, are characterised by yellow discolouration of the urine and eyes, burning sensation, thirst, vertigo and anorexia. Cases where the aggravation of vāta, kapha and pitta is severe, moderate and slight are characterised by headache, tremors, dyspnoea, delirious speech, vomiting and anorexia. Cases where the aggravation of kapha, vāta and pitta is severe, moderate and slight respectively are characterised by chills, heaviness of body, lethargy, delirious speech, headache, and intense bone pains, Cases where the provocation of vāta, pitta and kapha is severe, moderate and slight is characterised by dyspnoea, cough, catarrh, dryness of the mouth and intense joint pains. Cases where the aggravation of pitta, vāta and kapha is severe, moderate and slight are marked by diarrhoea, poor digestion, thirst, burning sensation, anorexia and vertigo. Fever that is caused by severe aggravation of vāta and pitta and slight involvement of kapha is marked by vertigo, thirst, burning sensation, heaviness of the body and intense headache. The symptoms observed in a case of fever caused by severe aggravation of all three doshas are: flashes of heat followed by chilliness, headache, pain in the bones and joints, watering of the eyes, blood shot, dull and distorted eyes, tinnitus with earache, a sensation as if there is a splinter in the throat, lethargy, stupefaction, delirious speech, cough, dyspnoea, anorexia, vertigo, dry and scorched tongue, utter weariness, expectoration of blood-streaked phlegm or phlegm with bile, rolling of the head from side to side, thirst, sleeplessness, discomfort in the cardiac region, delayed and scanty elimination of sweat, urine and stools, slight emaciation, consant moaning sound, appearance of circular, greyish or red urticarial patches, feeble voice, inflammation of body channels, heaviness of abdomen and chronicity.

The exogenous kind of fever (āgantuja-jvara) is of four kinds. Traumatic fever that is caused by blows, falls, etc. is generally caused by the aggravation of vāta, and is characterised by painful swelling, discolouration of the skin (of the affected area) and pain. Sudden anxiety, fear, grief or desire will aggravate vāta, and the person suffers from fever, marked by symptoms of aggravated vāta. Pitta will be provoked by anger, and all three doshas by the contact of bhūtas. Fever can also be caused from contact with poisonous plants or polluted air. Fever caused by desire is marked by constant obsession with the desired object with frequent sighing. Fever caused by grief is marked by weeping, while fever caused by fear is characterised by dread. Fever born out of anger is marked by excessive violence or agitation. Fever caused by bhūtas is characterised by abnormal and unnatural behaviour. Fever caused by toxicosis is marked by syncope, stupefaction, a sense of intoxication and fatigue. Even if the mind has been afflicted with grief, etc. the fever is not very severe if the doshas are not provoked. Similarly the aggravated doshas do not cause very severe fever if the mind remains unperturbed.

The symptoms during the immature stage of fever (āma-jvara) are anorexia, indigestion, heaviness of the abdomen, hrdaya-aśuddhi, lethargy, drowsiness, unremitting and high fever, salivation, nausea, loss of appetite, bad taste in the mouth, polyuria, stiffness, heaviness and numbness of limbs, excretion of indigested stools, and not much of weakness. The symptoms observed during the maturing (pachyamāna) stage are greater intensity of fever, thirst, delirious speech, dyspnoea, vertigo, nausea, and proper elimination. The fully matured (nirāma) fever is characterised by good appetite, emaciation, lightness of body, mildness of fever, and proper elimination (of morbid matter). This stage usually occurs eight days after the onset of fever, (CS).

II. The symptoms of vātaja-jvara are trembling of limbs, irregular pattern of fever, dryness of lips and throat, sleeplessness, stiffness of body, and dryness of the body, body pain, headache, bad taste in the mouth, chest pain, constipation, yawning, flatulent distension of the abdomen, and colic.

The symptoms of pittaja-jvara are intense heat, diarrhoea, insufficient sleep, vomiting, inflammation of the lips, mouth, throat and nose, perspiration, delirious speech, pungent taste in the mouth, syncope, burning sensation, sense of intoxication, thirst, vertigo and yellow discolouration of stools, urine and eyes.

The symptoms of kaphaja-jvara are heaviness of body, chilliness, nausea, horripilation, sleepiness, obstruction of the body channels, slight pain, salivation, sweet taste in the mouth, moderate heat, vomiting, debility, indigestion, catarrh, anorexia, cough and discolouration of eyes.

The symptoms of tridoshaja-jvara are insomnia, vertigo, dyspnoea, drowsiness, numbness of the limbs, anorexia, thirst, stupefaction, a sensation as if intoxicated, stiffness of limbs, burning pain, chilliness, chest pain, slow digestion (of the morbid matter), insanity, black discolouration of teeth, roughness and discolouration of tongue, headache, pain in the joints and bones, unclear and distorted eyes, tinnitus and earache, delirious speech, inflammation of body channels, moaning, semi-consciousness, and scanty elimination of sweat, urine and stools.

The symptoms of the tridoshaja-jvara known as abhinyāsa or hatoujasa are: moderate heat, semi-consciousness, feeble voice, rough tongue, dryness of throat, suppression of stools, urine and sweat, visual hallucinations, watering of eyes, aversion to food, loss of lustre, dyspnoea and delirious speech. A person suffering from this fever is bed-ridden. Another kind of tridoshaja-jvara known as ojo-nirodhaja-jvara is characterised by stiffness of limbs, chilliness, spells of unconsciousness, drowsiness, delirious speech, horripilation, prostration and mild fever. This disease is caused by severely aggravated vāta and pitta. The tridoshaja kinds of jvara aggravate on the seventh, tenth or twelfth day and either decrease or proves fatal.

The symptoms of vāta-pitta-jvara are thirst, syncope, vertigo, burning sensation, sleeplessness, headache, dryness of the mouth and throat, vomiting, horripilation, anorexia, yawning and pain in the joints. The symptoms of vāta-kapha-jvara are languor, pain in the joints, sleepiness, headache, heaviness of the body, catarrh, cough, sweating and moderate fever. The sympoms of kapha-pittaja-jvara are coating of the tongue, bitter taste in the mouth, lethargy, stupefaction, cough, anorexia, thirst and alternate heat and chills.

If emaciated (and debilitated) persons indulge in unwholesome food and regimen just after recovering from fever, the doshas which will be slightly aggravated will be further vitiated by the vāta, and as a result, five types of fever known as vishama-jvara are caused. Each type of vishama-jvara has its seat in the habitats of kapha (the satata, anyedya, tṛtīyaḳa, chaturthaka, and pralepaka are localised in the stomach, chest, throat, head and joints respectively, NiS). However, nearly every case of vishama-jvara is intimately related to some extraneous factor. The tṛtīyaka and chaturthaka jvara are caused by severely provoked vāta, while vishama-jvara accompanied by syncope is caused by the aggravation of any two doshas. The pralepaka-jvara is caused more by the aggravated kapha, although vāta is also aggravated. Fever brought about by abuse of alcoholic drinks as well as fever endemic in mountainous areas are usually caused by aggravated pitta. The stage of chill is caused by the aggavated vāta and kapha while the deranged pitta causes heat. The vishama-jvaras are distinctly periodic and may occur during any one of the six periods dominated by the deranged doshas (kapha is aggravated during the morning and the first part of the night; pitta is aggravated during noon and midnight; vāta is aggravated during the afternoon and dawn). The vishama-jvara lies dormant, never has complete remission, and causes fatigue, heaviness of body and emaciation. It is like fire that is fed with an insufficient amount of fuel (and which flares up when fed with adequate fuel). The santata kind of vishama-jvara continues without remission for seven, ten or twelve days, and has its seat in the vitiated rasa (nutrient fluid in the blood). The satata kind of vishama-jvara which has its seat in the vitiated blood aggravates twice in twenty-four hours. The anyedyu type of vishama-jvara which is localised in the vitiated flesh, aggravates once in twenty-four hours. The tṛtiyaka-jvara which has its seat in the vitiated medas (fatty tissues) aggravates every third day (once in three days), while the chaturthaka-jvara which has its seat in the bones and bone-marrow aggravates once in four days.

Of the fevers caused by extraneous causes, those caused by toxicosis are characterised by blackish discolouration of the mouth, burning sensation, diarrhoea, chest pain, anorexia, thirst, pricking pain, syncope and debility. Fever caused by smelling poisonous plants is marked by syncope, headache, vomiting and sneezing. Fever caused by unfulfilled passions (desires) are characterized by mental abberrations, drowsiness, lethargy, anorexia, chest pain, and emaciation. Fever caused by fear and grief is marked by delirious speech, while fever caused by anger is characterised by trembling (of limbs). Fever caused by malevolent magical spells and curses is marked by stupefaction and thirst. Fever that has been caused by sudden misfortune or by the influence of bhūtas is characterized by agitation, laughing, trembling and weeping.

The fever known as gambhīra-jvara is

characterised by internal heat, thirst, obstruction or suppression of stools, urine, etc., dyspnoea and cough.

The symptoms of immature jvara (āma-jvara) are: crushing pain in the cardiac region, lethargy, salivation, anorexia, drowsiness, constipation, polyuria, lack of perspiration, heaviness of the abdomen, restlessness, undigested stools, numbness, stiffness and heaviness of the body, feeble digestion, coated tongue, etc. The symptoms of matured (pakva) jvara are mildness of fever, lightness of body and elimination of the doshas, (SS).

Prognosis:

1. The tridoshaja-jvara which appears with all the symptoms along with very poor digestion and retention of the morbific matter is considered to be incurable. Otherwise, it can be cured with difficulty.

Jvara which affects the rasa-dhātu (the nutrient fluids that circulate in the blood), blood, fatty tissues and flesh (muscular tissues) is curable, while jvara affecting the bones and bone-marrow is curable with difficulty. However, jvara which affects the śukla (semen or reproductive element) is incurable.

Fever that is caused by slightly aggravated doshas in persons with strong constitutions and without any complications is easily curable. Fever that is brought about by many causative factors, where the doshas are greatly provoked, where there are many symptoms and where the sense-faculties are affected proves to be fatal. The cases of high fever attended by delirium, vertigo and dyspnoea also prove to be fatal in seven, ten or twelve days. Fever that occurs in persons who are emaciated, suffer from oedema, which is very deep seated, virulent, lasts for many days and which causes the parting of hair (keśa-sīmantakrt) is also to be considered as being incurable, (CS).

2. The tridoshaja-jvara is exremely difficult to cure. The pralepaka-jvara is also difficult to cure. Cases where heat is followed by chills are also difficult to cure. The gambhīra-jvara is incurable if it causes loss of lustre, weakness of sense-faculties, emaciation, anorexia and if there is severe fever, (SS).

Ref.: CS, nidāna, 1, 16-33; chikitsā, 3, 11-137; SS, uttara, 39, 13-96.

Treatment:

1. A person suffering from acute fever should avoid sleep during the day, bathing, massage with oil, food, sexual intercourse, anger, exertion, astringent substances and exposure to wind.

The first remedial measure to be adopted is fasting (or limited food intake), except in vātaja-jvara and jvaras caused by tuberculosis, fear, anger, passions, grief and exertion. By fasting or eating less, the digesive fire is reactivated, and the morbidity of the doshas is diminished, and there is a sense of lightness, good appetite and relief from fever. However, the patient should not continue to fast for so long as to cause weakness, because strength and vitality are the basis for good health.

In acute fever, the morbific matter, (the doshas) are reduced (or digested) as a result of fasting, fomentation (sudation), due to the effect of time and intake of gruels (yavāgu) and bitter substances.

In vāta and kapha-jvaras, the patient should appease his thirst with hot water, while water boiled with bitter drugs and cooled is to be drunk in pitta-jvara and fever caused by alcoholism. Both these drinks are appetizing, digestive, antipyretic, increase sweating and cleanse the body channels. A boiled and cooled decoction of musta, parpaṭaka, uśīra, chandana, udīchya and nāgara, which is known as shaḍanga-pānīya is useful in relieving fever and thirst.

The patient can be subjected to emesis in cases of kaphaja-jvara, where the doshas are predominently located in the stomach. However, emesis is contra-indicated if the doshas have not been precipitated and localised in the stomach, as it may cause heart disease, dyspnoea, flatulence and stupefaction.

After the period of fasting and emesis (if it was indicated), the patient should be administered gruels (yavāgu) prepared from suitable drugs, for a period of six days or until the fever subsides. First thin gruels (maṇḍa) can be used, followed by thicker gruels. Gruels are nourishing, easy to digest, promote sweating, alleviate thirst, stimulate the appetite, and regulate the passage of flatus, urine and stools. However, gruels are contra-indicated in summer, in pitta-kapha-jvara, in fevers caused by alcoholism and where there is haemorrhage from the upper orifices. In such cases, the patient can be administered refreshing (demulcent, tarpaṇa) drinks prepared from roasted paddy flour (lājā-śaktu) mixed with honey, sugar and juices of fruits that are anti-pyretic (such as drākshā, dāḍima, kharjūra, priyāla, parūshaka etc.). After this has been digested, the patient can partake of thin soup (yūsha) of mudga or meat-juice of desert animals.

At meal-time, the patient can brush his teeth with twigs that have a taste that is different from the taste experienced by the patient, and which is agreeable. This produces freshness in the mouth, good appetite and improves taste. The mouth can then be gargled with whey (mastu), sugar-cane juice or wine.

After six days from the onset of fever, the patient can partake of light, easily digestible food and can be administered decoctions (of suitable drugs). However, decoctions of astringent drugs are contra-indicated in acute fever, as they may hinder the digestion of the morbific matter, and may cause vishama-jvara (intermittent fever).

The patient can be administered light food along with soup (yūsha) of substances that are or are not sour and meat juices of desert animals, for a period of ten days. Then, if kapha is not as excessively provoked as vāta and pitta, and if the morbid matters (doshas) have been digested, the patient can partake of ghee (which is especially useful in chronic fevers). But if kapha is excessively provoked, and if the patient has not fasted, he can be administered decoctions, and can partake of light food mixed with meat juices. This can be done after ten days (after the onset of jvara).

The patient can be given milk for alleviating thirst and burning sensation in vāta-pittaja-jvara and where there is alternate constipation and diarrhoea and where there is no undigested food residue.

If the fever does not subside even after all the above measures, purgatives can be administered if the patient is not weak, or emaciated and if he has good digestive powers. But if the patient is emaciated, he can be administered a course of milk or niruha enema instead of purgation or emetics. Purgatives will eliminate either pitta or kapha and pitta that has accumulated in the small intestine, while enemata will eliminate all doshas (morbid matter) that have accumulated in the large intestines. Anuvāsana-enema can be administered in cases of chronic fever, where kapha and pitta have diminished, where there is good digestion and the stools are dry and constipated. Errhines are useful in chronic fevers with symptoms of heaviness of the head, headache, and impairment of sense-faculties. Massages with oil, external applications, affusions and tub baths are also useful in chronic fevers, depending on whether they have been caused by heat or cold. In cases where the residual effects of fever are left in the skin and in exogenous fevers, the patient can be subjected to fumigation and collyrium (anjana) procedures.

Thus, the general principles of treatment have been described.

Gruels (yavāgu) can be prepared from red rice, or varieties of old rice such as shashṭikaśāli. In the early stages of fever, when there is poor digestion, thin gruel of lājā (roasted paddy) can be taken with pippali and ginger. If there is diarrhoea or if the patient has a pittala constitution, the gruel can be taken cold with honey. If there is headache, pain in the sides of the chest and hypogastric region, gruel (peya) of red rice can be prepared with gokshura and kaṇṭakāri. If there is constipation, gruel can be prepared from sour substances and pṛśniparṇi, bala, bilva, ginger (dry), nilotpala and dhānyaka. If there is cough, dyspnoea and hiccoughs, the gruel can be prepared from drugs of vidārigandhādi group and drugs that are appetizing and sweat-inducing. If there is constipation, gruel can be prepared from pippali, āmalaki, barley and ghee. If there is constipation along with abdominal pain, gruel can be prepared fom mṛdvīka, pippali-roots, chavya, āmalaki and dry ginger. If there is sleeplessness, absence of sweating and thirst, gruels can be prepared from nāgara, āmalaka, sugar and ghee. Patients who are accustomed to soup and who like it can partake of soups prepared from mudga, masūra, chaṇaka, kulattha or makushṭaka.

The leafy vegetables that are useful in jvara are paṭola leaves and fruits, kulaka, pāṭha, karkoṭaka and kaṭhilla (the red variety of punarnava). The meats of lāva, kapinjala, eṇa, chakora, upachakra, kuranga, kāla-puccha, hariṇa, pṛśata, and śaśa are beneficial in fever. The meat of kukkuṭa, mayūra, tittiri, krouncha and vartaka are not very beneficial as they are heavy and hot. If the patient is thirsty, he can drink warm water or wine if he is accustomed to it. Food-articles that are heavy, hot, unctuous, sweet and astringent should generally be avoided in acute fevers.

Cold decoctions (or cold infusions) of musta and parpaṭaka or parpaṭaka and nāgara or of parpaṭaka and durālabha or of kirāta-tikta, musta, guḍūchi and nāgara or of pāṭha, uśīra, and udīchya are all useful in fever as they are appetizing, digestive, anti-pyretic and relieve thirst, anorexia and a bad taste in the mouth.

The following five decoctions are useful in vishama-jvara (intermittent fever): a decoction of indrayava, paṭola-leaves and kaṭurohiṇi; of paṭola, sāriva, musta, pāṭha and kaṭu-rohiṇi; of nimba, paṭola, triphala, mṛdvīka, mustā and indra-yava; of kirāta-tikta, guḍūchi, chandana and nāgara; and of guḍūchi, āmalaki and musta.

The decoctions known as vatsakādi-kashāya and madhukādi-hima are also useful in jvara. The decoction of jāti, āmalaka, musta and dhanvayāsa can be taken with jaggery. The decoction of triphala, trāyamāṇa, mṛdvika and kaṭu-rohiṇi is useful in kapha-pitta-jvara. It can also be administered with sugar and trivṛt. The decoction of bṛhati, kaṇṭakari, musta, devadāru, nāgara and kola-valli is useful in tridoshaja-jvara. Drugs such as śaṭi, pushkara-mūla, kaṇṭakāri, karkaṭa-sṛngi, durālabha, guḍūchi, nāgara, pātha, kirata-tikta and kaṭu-rohiṇi are useful in tridoshaja-jvara, especially when there are concomitant symptoms of cough heart disease, pain in the sides of the chest, dyspnoea and lethargy. Drugs such as bṛhati, kaṇṭakari, pushkara, bharngi, śaṭi, durālabha, kuṭaja, seeds (indrayava), paṭola and kaṭu-rohiṇi are useful in symptoms like cough, etc.

If the fever does not subside even after fasting, intake of light food, decoctions and emesis in a dried up individual, he can be administered potions of ghee. The element of heat which is responsible for causing fever causes dryness which in turn engenders aggavation of vāta. This is the reason why ghee has a beneficial effect. The medicinal ghees known as pippalyādi-ghṛta, vāsādi-ghṛta and balādi-ghṛta are very useful in fevers (especially chronic fevers). They also stimulate digestion.

The following prescriptons are used for giving purgation: The juices of mṛdvika or āmalaka or juice of āmalaka seasoned with ghee; or a paste of trivṛt, honey and ghee; or a decoction of triphala with honey and ghee; or āragvadha with milk or grape-juice; or a paste of trivṛt and trāyamāṇa with milk; or grape-juice with harītaki; or grape-juice followed by a draught of warm-water.

Milk medicated with drugs of the pancha-mūla group is useful in chronic fevers, cough, dyspnoea and pain in the sides of the chest. Milk medicated with eraṇḍa root or with unripe bilva fruit is useful in fever accompanied with parikartika (griping pain). Milk medicated with gokshūra, balā, kaṇṭakāri, jaggery and nāgara is useful in fever, swellings, constipation and retention (or suppression of urine). Milk medicated with nāgara, mṛdvikā and kharjūra can be administered with ghee, honey and sugar in fever with thirst. Milk boiled with four times its quantity of water is also useful in fever. Milk that has just been drawn and is still warm is very useful in vāta-pitta-jvara. Milk is especially useful in chronic fevers and can be given after boiling it with suitable medicines.

The decoctions known as patolādi-kashāya, āragvadhādi-kashāya and guḍūchyādi-kashaya can be used for giving nirūha-enema. A decoction prepared from meat-juices of desert animals, paste of pippali, madana fruit-pulp, musta and yashṭi-madhu, salt, ghee and honey can also be used as nirūha-enema. The formulations known as jīvantyādi-kashāya, paṭolādi-kashāya and chandanādi-kashāya can be used as anuvāsana-enema.

The patient can be administered errhines and fumigation with anti-pyretic drugs. The patient can also be subjected to massage with oil or ghee, external applications, and affusions after determining whether the chill stage or heat stage is prominent. The oil known as chandanādi-taila, and/or ghee washed one thousand times can be used for anointing (massage) for relieving fever and burning sensation.

The following measures are useful in relieving burning sensation in fevers: affusions and immersions (in tub-bath) with honey, kānji, milk, curds, ghee and cold water (see treatment of dāha).

In cases of fever with chills, the patient can be anointed with the medicated oil known as agarvādi-taila. The decoction of drugs used in preparing the above oil can be used for giving affusions and for bathing purposes. The thirteen kinds of sudation therapy can also be applied judiciously. The patient can also be warmly embraced by young women with comely and rounded limbs. Measures that alleviate kapha and vāta are also useful.

In a case of vātaja-jvara where there are no complications, the patient can be subjected to massage, etc. or can be administered decoctions, with the diet consisting of meat-juices. In cases of āma-jvara, kaphaja-jvara and kapha-pittaja-jvara, fasting and weight reducing measures are useful. In tridosaja-jvara, the severely provoked dosha can first be subdued. In case of fever which is not relieved by heat or cold and dry or unctuous treatment, blood-letting is to be done. In chronic fevers, nourishing and strength-giving food is beneficial.

Vishama-jvaras where vāta is mainly involved are to be treated with potions of ghee, enemata, anuvāsana-enema and food which is hot and unctuous. Cases where pitta is involved are treated by purgation, milk, medicated ghee and food that is bitter and cold. Cases where kapha is prominently involved are to be treated with emesis, fasting, hot decoctions and food that is dry and digestive. The following recipes are useful in vishama-jvara: the medicated ghee known as shaṭpala-ghṛta; a course of haritaki; a decoction of triphala or guḍūchi; a decoction of nīlini, aśvagandha, trivṛt and kaṭu-rohini which is administered just when the fever is expected to recur, and after the patient has been subjected to oleation and sudation; a paste of pippali, triphala, curd, butter-milk, ghee and pancha-gavya products; intake of rasona with oil before meals; intake of meat of fatty animals, which are hot in potency; application of collyrium of a paste of rocksalt, grains of pippali, manahśila and oil; fumigation with guggulu, nimba leaves, vachā, kushṭha, harītaki, sarshapa, yava and ghee; etc. The patient can be administered emesis (not before the fever is expected to recur).

The fever that has been localised in rasa-dhātu is treated by emesis and fasting. Fever that has its seat in the vitiated blood is treated by affusions, external applications and palliative drugs. Fever that has localised in flesh and fatty tissues is treated by purgation and fasting. The nirūha and anuvāsana enema, are useful in fever that has its seat in the bone-tissue and bone-marrow.

Traumatic fever is relieved by the internal and external use of ghee, blood-letting and use of meat-juices, and food and wines that are agreeable to the patient. Fevers caused by desire, grief and fear are relieved by reassurance, satisfying his desires, by alleviating the aggravated vāta and by pleasing the patient. Fever caused by anger, desire and fear and grief are relieved by inducing desire, anger and both desire and anger respectively.

A person suffering from fever should avoid food that is hard to digest, irritant, unwholesome, unpalatable, and incompatible. He should also avoid coitus, exertion, bathing and overeating. These activities must not be indulged in by a person who has recovered from fever, but has not yet regained his strength.

The following measures are useful in relapsed fever: mild purificatory procedures, yāpana types of enema, nourishing and light gruels (yūsha), meat juices of desert animals, massage with oil, rubbing the body (without using oil), bathing, fumigation, application of collyrium, and ghee medicated with bitter drugs.

The regular use of (a decoction of) kirāta-tikta, kaṭuki, musta, parpaṭa and guḍuchi is also useful in relapsing fevers.

The subsidence of fever may be known by relief from fatigue and distress, normal temperature and normal functioning of sense-faculties and the mind.

Fevers that are chronic usually subside without prominent symptoms (lysis). However, mild and virulent fevers which are caused by severely provoked doshas usually subside very rapidly, (crisis), with the following symptoms: moaning, vomiting, restlessness, dyspnoea, discolouration, sweating, tremors, fainting spells, delirium, burning heat, or coldness of body, loss of consciousness and glaring eyes, (CS).

2. When the prodromal symptoms of jvara appear, the patient can be administered old ghee in case of vāta involvement, or mild purgation if pitta is involved and emesis if kapha is involved. However, if oleation and purificatory procedures are both not indicated, fasting, etc., are to be enjoined.

Fasting or intake of easily digestible food is the best remedial measure when the symptoms of jvara are manifested. If the doshas are localised in the stomach, (and symptoms like nausea, salivation, etc. are present), emesis is indicated. The patient is adviced to fast until the symptoms of āma subside. Later, the patient can partake of gruel, soup etc. However, fasting is contra-indicated in fevers caused by aggravated vāta, or fevers that result from tuberculosis or mental factors and in pregnant women, aged people, children and debilitated and timid persons.

Fasting is very useful in helping the digestion of morbific matter and causes digestion of food and a sense of lightness in the body and mind. The symptoms that are manifested after fasting are proper elimination of stools, urine and flatus, good appetite, thirst, lightness of body, clarity of mind and sense faculties, and bodily weakness. However, excessive fasting causes debility, thirst, emaciation, lethargy, insomnia, vertigo, fatigue, dyspnoea, cough, hoarseness, vomiting and hiccoughs.

The patient can also partake of hot water (which has been reduced to half, NiS) which is appetizing, dislodges the kapha, alleviates vāta and pitta, and softens the body channels. Hot water is especially useful in vāta and kapha-jvaras. The cold infusions of bitter drugs, of musta, nāgara, usira, parpaṭa, udīchya and chandana (which is known as shaḍanga-pāniya) is useful in fevers caused by aggravated pitta, alcoholism or toxicosis.

Gruels (peya) prepared from drugs that are digestive are also useful in jvaras and are to be partaken at regular meal times.

If the fever does not subside after a week, even after fasting, hot-water (or shaḍanga-pāniya) and gruels, and if there is poor digestion, a bad taste in the mouth, thirst and anorexia, the patient can be administered decoctions of drugs that are digestive, anti pyretic and hṛdya. The decoctions of pancha-mūla drugs, of musta, kaṭuka, indrayava and honey and drugs of the pippalyādi group are useful in vātaja, pittaja and kaphaja jvaras respectively. But these decoctions are not to be administered just after the patient has partaken of water and food, or when he is fasting, or is emaciated, or suffers from indigestion and thirst.

Medicines are to be administered when there is mild fever, lightness of the body and proper elimination. Some authorities believe that medicines can be administered after seven or ten days after the onset of fever. Purificatory drugs administered during the āma stage cause aggravation of fever, while palliative drugs cause vishama-jvara, if administered during this stage.

Diarrhoea which occurs along with fever should be left untreated. If however, there is severe diarrhoea, it can be treated as indicated in atisāra.

The patient can be subjected to purgation and other purificatory procedures even in acute fevers if the digested doshas are localised in the alimentary tract. If these digested doshas are removed from the body, they may cause vishama-jvara or may produce severe weakness. The patient can be first subjected to emesis, followed by āsthāpana enema, purgation and śiro-virechana (errhines).

Emesis can be induced in kapha-jvara occuring in strong persons; purgation is useful in pitta-jvara, especially if there is a tendency to diarrhoea. Nirūha enema is useful in vāta-jvara if there is udāvarta and body pain. Anuvāsana enema is beneficial in cases of stiffness of the back and waist and good digestion.

Śiro-virechana is useful in cases where the kapha has localised in the head, and where there is heaviness of the head, headache and weakness of sense-faculties.

If the debilitated person suffering from jvara also suffers from flatulent distension of the abdomen with colic, a paste of devadāru, vachā, kushṭha, śatapushpa, hingu, rock-salt and kānji can be applied lukewarm over the abdomen. A suppository composed of the same drugs can be introduced into the rectum in case of obstruction of stools and urine, and upward displacement of vāta. The yavāgu (gruel) prepared from pippali, pippali root, yavāni, and chavya can also be partaken.

Ghee can be administered internally in cases where fever continues even after the purificatory procedures, and where there is dryness.

Debilitated persons and persons in whom morbidity is not severe are to be treated by palliatives (śamana), while fasting (or the ten kinds of langhana) is indicated in fevers caused by over-eating in strong persons. Such patients can drink watery gruels (yavāgu) when they are thirsty.

Persons suffering from fever caused by intoxication and other symptoms like thirst, vomiting, burning sensation and heat can be administered lājā with honey and water, which should be followed by meat, soup and meat juices. Meals consisting of meat-juices are useful in fevers caused by fasting, fatigue, tuberculosis and aggravated vāta, provided the patient possesses good digestive power. The gruel (yūsha) prepared from mudga is useful in kapha-jvara, while it can be eaten along with sugar in pitta-jvara. The gruel prepared from mudga, dāḍima and āmalaka is useful in vāta-pittaja-jvara, while gruel prepared from laghu-pancha-mūla drugs is useful in vāta-kapha-jvara. Gruel prepared from paṭola and nimba is useful in kapha-pitta-jvara. Lājā mixed with sugar and honey should be the only diet in cases of fever marked by vomiting, burning pains, weakness and thirst. Yavāgu are not useful as diet in summer, in kapha-pitta-jvara, in bleeding from internal organs and in persons who are accustomed to alcoholic drinks. In such cases, yūsha prepared from meat-juices of desert animals are to be preferred.

Alcoholic drinks can be administered along with a meal of barley in fever characterised by poor digestion. Butter-milk medicated with trikaṭu drugs is useful in kapha-jvara and where there is anorexia. Milk is useful as diet in emaciated persons, where there is less morbidity, where the person is depressed, dried-up and suffers from thirst and burning pains, and in cases of chronic fever and vāta-pitta-jvara. However, milk acts like a poison when taken in cases of acute fever.

In all fevers, the food should be easy to digest and should be taken in the proper quantity.

A person suffering from chronic fever should partake of beneficial food at regular meal times, even if there is loss of appetite, since fasting or inadequate food will weaken the body.

Food that is beneficial, palatable and easy to digest is to be partaken in santata-jvara and other vishama-jvaras.

A gruel (yūsha) prepared from mudga, masūra, chaṇaka, kulattha and makushṭhaka is useful as diet in all fevers. The leafy vegetables that are beneficial are patola leaves, vārtāka, kathilla (punarnava), pāṭha, karkoṭaka, parpaṭaka, gojihva, tender radish, guḍūchi leaves etc. The meat of lāva, ena, kapinjala, pṛshta, śarabha, śaśa, kāla-puccha, kuranga and mṛga-mātṛka can be partaken by persons accustomed to meat.

Persons suffering from acute jvara should avoid affusions, external applications, oleation, purificatory procedures, bathing, massage with oil, sleep during daytime, exposure to cold wind, exertion, coitus, emotions such as anger, fresh cereal, and food articles that are unctuous, abhishyandi, dry, astringent and hard to digest. A person who is debilitated by fever should not bathe until he has recovered his strength.

The following formulations are useful in vāta-jvara: the decoction of pippali, sāriva, drāksha, śata-pushpa, and hareṇu with jaggery; the cold infusion of guḍūchi; the decoction of balā, darbha and gokshura, with sugar and ghee; the decoction of śatapushpa, vachā, kushṭha, devadāru, and hareṇu; the decoction of kustumbara, uśira, and musta with sugar and honey; the decoction of drākshā, guḍūchi, kāśmari, trāyamāṇa and sāriva with jaggery and the expressed juices of guḍuchi and śatāvari with jaggery.

The following prescription are useful in pitta-jvara: the decoction of śriparṇi (fruits of gambhāri), chandana, uśīra, parūshaka, madhuka fruits with sugar; the decoction of drugs of the sārivādi group with sugar; the cold infusion of drugs of utpalādi group; the decoction of guḍūchi, lodhra, padmaka, sāriva and utpala with sugar; the decoction of drāksha and āragvadha (fruits) or kāśmari (fruits) or of drugs that are sweet, bitter and astringent can be administered with sugar in order to relieve thirst and heat; milk boiled with kshīri trees is also useful in relieving internal heat; the paste of padmaka, yashṭi-madhu, drākshā, puṇḍarika, utpala, fried barley, uśīra, lajjālu, and kaśmari fruit is soaked overnight in water and is administered with honey; the pastes of nāgakeśara, mātulunga, honey and rock salt or of drāksha, kharjūra, sugar and dāḍima can be kept in the mouth in order to relieve a bad taste in the mouth.

These prescriptions are useful in kapha-jvara; the decoction of saptaparṇa, guḍūchi, nimba and sphūrjaka; the decoction of trikaṭu, nāga-pushpa (naga-keśara), haridra, kaṭu-rohiṇi and kuṭaja fruits; the decoction of haridra, chitraka, nimba, uśīra, ativisha, vachā, kushṭha, indrayava, murva and paṭola with honey and maricha; the decoction of sāriva, ativisha, kushṭha, durālabha, musta and guggulu; and the decoction of musta, indrayava, triphala, kaṭu-rohiṇi and parūshaka.

A decoction of drugs of the āragvadhādhi group can be administered with honey in vāta-kapha-jvara. The decoction of nāgara, dhānyaka, bhārngi, harītaki, devadāru, vachā, parpaṭaka, musta, bhūtika, and kaṭphala can be given with honey and hingu in vāta-kapha-jvara and cough, dyspnoea, hawking of phlegm, hiccoughs, chest pain etc.

The following decoctions are useful in kapha-pitta-jvara: the decoction of balā, paṭola, triphala, yashti-madhu and vāsā, with honey; of kaṭuka, harītaki, drāksha, musta, and parpaṭa; of bhārngi, vachā, parpaṭaka, dhānya, hingu, harītaki, musta, nāgara, and kāśmari with honey; and of trikaṭu and sugar which should be drunk hot.

The decoction of guḍūchi, kirāta-tikta, drāksha, āmalaka, śaṭi with jaggery or of rāsna, vāsa, triphala, and āragvadha fruits is useful in vāta-pitta-jvara.

The following formulations are useful in all fevers: vṛśchīra (white punarnava), bilva and red punarnava are boiled with milk and water until the water has evaporated. This medicated milk can be administered. The heart wood of śimshipa is boiled with one part of milk and three parts of water until only milk remains. This is also very useful. A decoction of nala-vetasa root, mūrva root, and devadāru can also be administered. A cold infusion of ananta, bālaka, musta, nāgara and kaṭu-rohiṇi can be administered in the early morning.

The decoction of haridra, musta, triphala, kaṭu-rohini, nimba, paṭola, devadāru and kaṇṭakāri, or of triphala and ghee is useful in tridoshaja-jvara.

The treatment of vishama-jvara is as follows: the patient can be subjected to emesis and purgation. He can then be administered shaṭpala-ghṛta; a paste of triphala and jaggery; or a decoction of guḍūchi, nimba, and āmalaki wih honey; or rasona with ghee every morning; or a decoction of yashṭi-madhu, paṭola and rohiṇi, or of yashṭi-madhu, paṭola, rohiṇi and musta or yashṭi-madhu, paṭola, rohiṇi, musta and harītaki; or a paste of ghee, milk, sugar, honey and pippali; or pippali with a decoction of a daśamūla drugs; or vardhamāna-pippali with a diet of milk and meat juices; or good wine with the flesh of tāmrachūḍa (kukkuṭa); or ghee boiled with a decoction of kola, agni-mantha, and triphala and a paste of curds and tilvaka.

Medicated ghee preparations known as pippalyādi-ghṛta, guḍūchyādi-ghṛta, kalaśyādi-ghṛta, paṭolādi-ghṛta, kalyāṇaka-ghṛta, mahā-kalyāṇaka-ghṛta, pancha-gavya-ghṛta and triphala-ghṛta, are useful in fevers, particularly chronic fevers.

Boiled milk, sugar, pippali, honey and ghee should be mixed and churned with the hand. This can then be administered in vishama-jvara, tuberculosis, kshata-kshīṇa, dyspnoea and heart diseases.

Oil boiled with eight palas of paste of lāksha, nāgara, haridra, mura, manjishṭha,svarjika-kshāra and kushtha, and thirty-two palas of oil and butter-milk which is six times the quantity of oil is useful (when used externally) in fevers. Oil medicated with the milky trees (kshīri-vṛksha), asana, nimba, jambu, saptaparṇa, arjuna, sirīsha, khadira, asphoṭa (sāriva or arka, NiS), guḍūchi, vāsā, kaṭuka, parpaṭa, uśīra, vacha, tejovati (kākamarda) and musta can be used for massaging the body in chronic fevers.

When the time for the paroxysm of fever approaches, the patient of vishama-jvara should be frightened by non-venomous snakes, tamed elephants, etc. and made to fast for the day. Or he can be made to vomit repeatedly after partaking of food that is abhishyandi and hard to digest. Or he can be administered strong wine or old ghee, or ghee that has been medicated with anti-pyretic drugs (such as shaṭpala-ghṛta, NiS), or drastic purgatives or he can be fomented and subjected to nirūha-enema. The patient can also be fumigated by burning hair, and hairs of a goat, vachā, kushṭha, dāru-haridra, nimba leaves and honey. A paste of pippali, rock-salt, oil and nepati (manah-śila) can be applied as collyrium.

Fevers that are of psychic origin can be treated by inculcating vijnana (wisdom) etc. Fever caused by fatigue and tuberculosis should be treated by massage with ghee and a diet of meat-juices and boiled rice. Fevers that are caused by abhishāpa and abhichāra can be managed by performing homa (sacrifices), etc. The remedial measures useful in traumatic fever consist of drugs that are astringent, sweet and unctuous. However, all drugs that are hot are to be avoided. Fevers caused by poisons and odours of poisonous plants are treated by administering a decoction of sarvagandha drugs (aromatic drugs such as ela) or nimba and devadāru or of jāti flowers and by measures useful in toxicosis.

During the chill stage of (chronic) kapha-vāta-jvara, a paste of the drugs of bhadra-dārvādi group, surasādi group or elādi group can be applied externally. The body can be affused with warm kānji, śukta, cow's urine and whey. A paste of the leaves of surasa, arjaka and śigru can be applied. The body can be massaged with kshāra-taila mixed with śukta. A decoction of drugs of the āragvadhādi group can be administered internally. The patient can have a bath in a tub with a warm decoction of drugs that alleviate vāta. The patient is to be wrapped up in warm clothes.

In cases marked by severe heat, the measures useful in dāha can be employed. Emesis can be induced by a decoction of bimba leaves, honey and phāṇita. The body can be massaged with śata-dhouta-ghṛta and plastered with the cold paste of yava-śaktu, kola, āmalaka, vinegar, kānji, or of tender leaves of phenila (upodika), and sour drugs or of palaśa leaves and kānji, or of the froth obtained from the tender leaves of badara or arishṭa (nimba). The medicated oil known as prahladana-taila is also useful. A paste of drugs of the nyagrodhādi group, kākolyādi group and utpalādi group can also be applied. The patient can also be immersed in a tub filled with a cold infusion of these drugs.

In jvara caused by two or all three doshas, the aggravated pitta should first be subdued.

A paste of madhūka, hrīvera, utpala, madhūlika, honey and ghee is useful in fevers accompanied by salivation, haemorrhages, hiccoughs, dyspnoea and vomiting. The paste of triphala, pippali, honey and ghee is useful in cough and dyspnoea, The paste of vidāri, dādima, lodhra, kapittha and bījapūraka can be applied to the scalp in fever accompanied by thirst and heat. The paste of dāḍima, sugar, drāksha and āmalaka can be retained in the mouth in cases of tastelesness. Milk, sugarcane juice, honey, ghee and warm oil can also be used for the same purpose. A person suffering from pitta-jvara with tremors and nose-bleed can be purged by using the paste of triphala, śyāma (vṛddha-dāru), trivṛt, pippali, honey and sugar. Vertigo can be relieved by administering the paste of harītaki, honey and sugar. In vāta-jvara, nirūha-enema with drugs of bhadra-dārvādi and kākolyādi groups is useful. Anuvāsana-enema can also be employed with the same drugs.

Ghee can be administered in all fevers after the twelfth day (of fever). The symptoms which mark the subsidence of fever are: sweating, a sense of lightness in the head, slight yellowish discolouration of face, sneezing and good appetite, (SS).

A few of the rasa-preparations that are useful in jvara are trailokya-sundara-rasa, trailokya-damba-rasa, meghanāda-rasa, jvara-gajahāri-rasa, dīpika-rasa, śīta-bhanji-rasa, mṛta-sanjivani-rasa, vṛddha-jvarānkuśa-rasa, mahā-jvarānkuśa-rasa, mṛtyunjaya-rasa, sarva-jvarāri-rasa, chakra-sūrya-rasa, umā-prasādana-rasa (in intermittent fever), jvarānkuśa-rasa, etc.

Rasa-sindūra can be administered with the decoction of musta and parpaṭa for relieving all fevers. It can also be administered with pippali and a decoction of daśamūla drugs in tridoshaja-jvara, (RRS).

Ref.: CS, chikitsā, 3; SS, uttara, 39, 97 -322; RRS, 12; 30, 22-23.

Classical Prescriptions: Abhraka-bhasma; Amṛtāristạ; Āmalakyādi-chūṛna; Amṛta-prāśa-ghṛta; Āragvadhādi-kvātha-chūrṇa; Ārogyavardhini-guṭika; Balā-taila; Bālachaturbhadrika-chūrṇa; Balā-aśvagandhā-lākshadi-taila; Bilvādi-guṭika; Bṛhat-kastūri-bhairava-rasa; Chandana-balā-lākshādi-taila; Chandrāmṛta-rasa; Dāru-nāgarādi-kvātha-chūrṇa; Daśamūla-kvātha-chūrṇa; Daśamūla-shaṭpalaka-ghṛta; Daśānga-lepa; Grahaṇi-mihira-taila; Jvarāryabhra; Kacchūradi-chūrṇa; Kuṭajarishṭa; Gorochanādi-vaṭi; Kutajārishta; Kumāra-kalyāṇa-rasa; Laghu-mālini-vasanta-rasa;Lākshādi-taila; Laghvānanda-rasa; Lakshmi-nārāyaṇa-rasa; Madhu-yashṭyadi-lola; Mahā-pancha-gavya-ghṛta; Mṛtyunjaya-rasa; Pancha-gavya-ghṛta; Panchamṛta-parpaṭi; Pancha-tikta-kvātha-chūrṇa; Paṭoladi-kvātha-chūrṇa, Pippalyādi-ghṛta; Rajanyādi-chūrṇa; Rajata-bhasma; Rasa-parpati; Saptāmṛta-rasa; Shaḍanga-kvātha-chūrṇa; Shaṭpala-ghṛta; Siddha-prāneśvara-rasa; Sitopalādi-chūrṇa; Śiva-guṭika; Soubhāgya-vaṭi; Sṛngyādi-chūrṇa; Sudarśana-chūrṇa; Svarṇa-bhasma; Tarunārka-rasa; Tālisādi-chūrṇa; Trāyantyādi-kvātha-chūrṇa; Vajraka-ghṛta; Vāsavaleha; Vāsa-chandānādi-taila; Vātagni-ghṛta; Vāsavaleha; Vāsa-chandanādi-taila; Vātāgni-kumāra-rasa.

Nava-jvara: Ratna-giri-rasa

Jīrṇa-jvara: Bhārngadi-kvātha-chūrṇa; Chandanādi-chūrṇa; Chandanādi-lauha; Godanti-bhasma; Guḍa-pippali; Kadali-kshāra; Muktā-bhasma; Muktā-panchāmṛta-rasa; Nāgarādi-kvātha-chūrṇa; Puṭa-pakva-vishama-jvarāntaka-lauha; Sarva-jvarahara-lauha; Sudarśana-chūrṇa; Svarṇa-mākshika-bhasma; Vasanta-mālati-rasa; Yakṛdari lauha

Dantodbhava-jvara: Mukta-bhasma

Abhinyāsa-javara: Mukkamukkatvadi-guṭika

Āmajvara: Agni-tuṇḍi-vaṭi; Pāchanamṛta-kvātha-chūrṇa

Pitta-jvara: Godanti-bhasma; Muktā-bhasma; Muktā-śukti-bhasma.

Purāṇa-jvara: Kūshmāṇḍaka-rasāyana

Manda-jvara: Pippalyādi-lauha

Vāta-kapha-jvara: Drākshadi-kvātha-chūrṇa

Svasanaka-jvara: Gorochanādi-vati

Sūtika-jvara: Lauha parpaṭi.

Sannipāta-jvara: Bṛhat-kastūri-bhairai-rasa; Chinnodbhavādi-kvatha-chūrṇa; Chukkum-tippalyādi-guṭika; Dāru-nāgaradi -kvātha-chūrṇa; Mṛta-sanjīvani-guṭika; Mṛta-sanjīvani-sura; Soubhāgya-vati; Prabhākara-rasa; Sūtikā-bharaṇa-rasa.

Vishama-jvara: Agastya-harītaki-rasāyana; Amṛtārishṭa; Bhārngadi-kvātha-chūrṇa; Chandānadi-lauha; Dantī-harītaki; Indu-kānta-ghṛta; Mahā pancha-gavya-ghṛta; Paṭola-mūlādi-kvātha-chūrṇa; Prameha-mihira-taila; Prāṇada-guṭika; Punarnavādi-maṇḍura; Puṭa-pakva-vishama-jvarāntaka-lauha; Soubhāgya-vaṭi; Sudarśana-chūrṇa; Vasanta-mālati-rasa.

Jvarātisara: Ānanda-bhairava-rasa; Gagana-sundara-rasa; Karpūra-rasa; Siddha-prāneśvara-rasa.

Kacchapika (See Prameha piḍaka)

Causative Factors: Intrinsic: Kapha and vāta (SS), Kapha in children (KS).

Symptomatology: Five or six hard knotty eruptions shaped like the shell of a tortoise, (SS).

Treatment: The affected area is fomented, and then plastered with a paste of manahśila, haratāla, kushṭha and devadāru. If these eruptions suppurate, they are to be treated along the same lines as vraṇa, (SS).

Ref.: SS, nidāna, 13, 8; chikitsā, 20, 5; KS, chikitsā, dvivraṇīya.

Kadara

Western Nosology: Corn; Callosity

Causative Factors:

Extrinsic: Trauma to the soles of the foot caused by stepping on a stone, thorn, pieces of gravel, etc.

Intrinsic: Kapha and vāta (acc. to bhoja, NC on SS).

Constituents Affected: Fat and blood, (SS).

Symptomatology: A hard, knotty, painful growth raised or depressed in the middle which exudes a secretion. The growth is wedge shaped, about as big as a kola (fruit) and appears on the soles. According to bhoja, it may appear on the palms also, (SS; NC on SS).

Treatment: The growth is surgically removed (excised), and cauterised with hot oil or any fat, (SS).

Ref.: SS, nidāna, 13, 30-31; NC on ibid; chikitsā, 20, 23.

Kakshā

Western Nosology: Herpes Zoster

Causative Factors: Intrinsic: Pitta (SS; CS, sūtra, 20, 14), Pitta and vāta (AHṛ; CS, chikitsā, 12, 91).

Symptomatology: Painful, black eruptions in the regions of axillae, arm, sides of the thorax and shoulder, (SS).

Eruptions which are distributed crosswise across the chest like the sacred thread. (yajnopavīta), (CS). The eruptions are small, compact and resemble lāja (parched grain), (AHṛ).

Treatment: This disease is first treated along the same lines as pittaja visarpa. When the eruptions have suppurated, ghee medicated with drugs of the kākolyadi group (possessing a sweet taste) is employed.

Chakra taila is useful in this disease, (SS).

Treatment given in cases of visarpa will be found useful in this disease also, (CS).

Related Subjects: Gandha-nāma (SS), Gardabhi (AHṛ).

Ref.: SS, nidāna, 13, 16; sūtra, 44, 48; chikitsā, 20,7- 8; CS, chikitsā,13, 91-93; AHṛ, uttara, 31, 10-11.

Kālaya-khanja

Causative Factors: Intrinsic: Vāta

Pathogenesis and Symptomatology: (The aggravated vāta affects the nerves of the hip joints, and lower limbs). The diseased person suffers from loose joints, trembles before beginning to walk, and starts limping, (SS).

Treatment:

1. The patient is treated along the same lines as the other vāta rogas. Venesection is also useful, (SS).

2. The patient is to be treated as in khanja and pangu. However, snehana (oleation) is particularly useful in this condition, (BP, BR).

Ref.: SS, nidāna, 1, 78; chikitsā, 5, 22; BP; BR, page. 327, 51.

Kāmala

Western Nosology: Jaundice

Causative Factors:

Extrinsic: Excessive intake of food which aggravates pitta by a person suffering from pāṇḍu, (CS).

Excessive intake of food which aggravates pitta by a person in whom pitta is already provoked (or by a person who has the pitta constitution), (AS).

Excessive intake of alcohol, sour and harmful

food by a person who is convalescing (from the disease pāṇḍu), (SS).

Intrinsic: Pitta (CS, sūtra, 20, 14; SS).

Constituents Affected: Blood (CS, sūtra, 28, 12). Blood and flesh, (CS).

Classification:

1. A patient of kāmala who has symptoms of pain in the joints and excessive swelling (oedema) is said to be suffering from kumbhasa or kumbha-kāmala. If the condition of the patient further deteriorates with the appearance of symptoms like fever, body pain, vertigo, debility, lassitude, yawning, heaviness of the body and emaciation, the disease is called lāgharaka, (SS).

2. The disease is usually caused by aggravation of pitta in the koshṭha (alimentary tract) and śākha (the limbs). But due to intake of dry, cold, sweet and indigestible good, excessive exertion, and suppression of the natural urges, the kapha and vāta are vitiated and the disturbed vāta causes displacement of pitta from its seat in the alimentary tract. This kind of kāmala is known as śākhaśrita kāmala, and is characterised by white coloured stools (CS, chikitsā, 16, 36, 124). An advanced stage of kāmala is known as kumbha-kāmala, (CS).

Symptomatology:

1. Pale (whitish) appearance of the skin, etc., dullness of sense faculties, yawning, heaviness of body, easy fatigue, unconsciousness, emaciation, debility, confusion of mind, irrelevant and unconnected speech and even death, (SS).

2. Yellowish discolouration of the eyes, skin, nails and face, reddish-yellow discolouration of faeces and urine, greyish discolouration of the body (bheka-varṇa), weakness of sense-faculties, burning pains, indigestion, debility, anorexia and lethargy.

The śākhāśrita kind is characterized by white discolouration of faeces, yellowish discolouration of the eyes, urine and skin, flatulence, constipation, heaviness of the chest, debility, loss of appetitte, pain in the sides, hiccoughs, dyspnoea, feeble digestion and fever.

The symptoms in kumbha-kāmala are: yellowish-black discolouration of faeces and urine, excessive oedema, reddish discolouration of the eyes, face, vomitus, faeces and urine, vertigo, burning pains, tastelessness, thirst, flatulence, lassitude and confusion of the mind, (CS).

3. A child afflicted with kāmala suffers from yellow discolouration of the eyes, nails, face, urine and faeces, lethargy, indigestion and craving for blood, (KS).

Ref.: SS, uttara, 44, 10-11; śārira, 4, 49; sūtra, 15, 24; CS, chikitsā, 16, 34 -38; KS, sūtra, 25, 35; AS, nidāna, 13, 19.

Treatment:

1. The patient is to be administered trivṛt with sugar or indra-vāruṇi with jaggery or ginger with jaggery.

A patient suffering from kumbha-kāmala can be administered svarṇa-mākshika or śilajatu with cow's urine or maṇḍūra which has been immersed in cow's urine for a month with rock-salt. Maṇḍūra which is heated in a fire fed by wood from the vibhītaka trees is cooled in cow's urine. This process is repeated eight times. The maṇḍūra is to be administered with honey.

Ghee medicated with the juices of drāksha, guḍūchi and āmalaki is beneficial in lāgharaka, (SS).

2. The patient is to be first administered a purgative, and is advised to partake of the following foods: old rice, old wheat and old barley, gruel prepared from mudga, āḍhaki, masūra and meat juices of animals living in desert areas. The drugs are selected according to the dosha(s) involved.

The patient is to be administered ghee medicated with drāksha or with buffalo's milk, haridra, triphala, nimba, balā and yashṭi; powder of iron with harītaki, haridrā, milk and honey or harītaki with honey and jaggery. The cold juices of triphala or guḍūchi or nimba or dāru-haridra are to be given with honey, in the morning.

The diet can consist of mṛdvīka and juice of āmalaki. Drugs such as pancha-gavya ghṛta, mahā-tiktaka ghṛta and kalyāṇaka ghṛta can also be administered.

A patient in whom the pitta is displaced to the periphery (śākhaśrita) is to be administered the meat of barhi, tittiri and drāksha, food which is pungent, sour and dry, dry mūlaka, gruel prepared from kulattha and juice of mātulunga with pippali, maricha, nāgara and honey.

Drugs and food articles which are pungent, hot, sharp, salty and extremely sour alleviate the aggravated vāta and help in bringing back the pitta to its normal position in the alimentary tract. When the stools regain their usual colour, the patient is to be treated along the same lines as for kāmala, (CS).

3. The treatment of kāmala should consist of measures which alleviate pitta and which are not contra-indicated in pāṇḍu.

Ghee prepared with a hundred harītaki leaves and half the number of stalks is useful. Āragvadha can be administered with śuṇṭhi, pippali and maricha, and sugar-cane juice or juice of vidāri or juice of āmalaki. A paste of nikumbha given with cold water or the powder of nikumbha with honey and a decoction of triphala is also beneficial. An anjana (collyrium) of haridra, gairika and āmalaki is also useful, (AHṛ).

4. A collyrium of the juice of droṇa-pushpi is beneficial. The paste of guḍūchi leaves followed by buttermilk is also useful when administered internally. Ghee medicated with guḍūchi and buffalo's milk can also be administered, (CSS).

5. The paste of apāmārga, root of śami and buttermilk is useful. The paste of hingu with water can be applied as a collyrium. The decoction of balā, vāsa, pṛthakparṇi and guḍūchi is useful in kāmala occuring in pregnant women, (RRS).

Ref.: SS, uttara, 44, 30-36; CS, chikitsā, 16, 40-43, 52-53, 64, 98, 114, 130-131; AHṛ, chikitsā, 16, 40-2; CSS, pages. 196-197; RRS, 19, 23; 24, 23; 22, 100.

Classical Prescriptions: Arogya-vardhiṇi-rasa; Chandana-balā-lākshādi-taila; Chandraprabhā-vaṭi; Dantī-harītaki; Dhātri-lauha; Drākshāvaleha; Dugdha-vaṭi; Grahaṇi-mihira-taila; Jvarāryabhra; Kalyāṇaka-guḍa; Kumāra-kalyāṇa-rasa; Laghu-chinchyādi-lehya; Loha-bhasma; Navāyasa-chūrṇa; Maṇḍūra-bhasma; Pancha-gavya-ghṛta; Paṭolādi-kvātha-chūrṇa; Puṭa-pakva-vishama-jvarāntaka-lauha; Rajanyādi-chūrṇa; Sarva-jvarahara-lauha; Sudarśana-chūrṇa; Sūla-vajriṇi-vaṭika; Triphala-ghṛta; Vajraka-ghṛta; Vāsa-chandanādi-taila; Vāsa-guḍūchyādi-kvātha-chūrṇa; Viḍangādi-lauha; Yakṛdāri-lauha; Yakṛt-śūla-vināśini vaṭika.

Kapha-rogas

Causative Factors: Factors which aggravate kapha.

Sleeping during the day-time, lack of exercise, lethargy, intake of food before the digestion of the food previously eaten, partaking of beneficial and harmful food at the same time, intake of sweet, sour, salty, cold, oily, slimy and abhishyandi food and food that is hard to digest, intake of hayānaka (a kind of grain, NiS), yavaka (a variety of sūka-dhānya, ibid) naiṣhadhaka (a variety of grain NiS), itkaṭa (khaggali, NiS), māsha, mahā-māsha, wheat, tila, flour (of rice, NiS) and its products, curds, milk kṛśara (a yavāgu prepared with tila, rice and masha, NiS), pāyasa (a dish prepared from milk and rice, NiS), sugar cane and its products, meat and fat of aquatic animals, bisa (lotus root, NiS), mṛṇāla (lotus stalks, NiS), kaśeruka, śṛngāṭaka, fruits of nārikela, tāla, etc., and valli-phala (alābu, kūshmaṇḍa, etc. NiS), (SS, sūtra, 21, 23).

Time of Aggravation: Kapha is usually vitiated in cold seasons, vasanta-ṛtu (spring), early morning, the first part of night, soon after eating, and by all cold things. It is also aggravated in childhood, (SS, sūtra, 21, 24; AHṛ, sūtra, 1, 8).

Enumeration of Diseases Caused by Vitiated Kapha:

1. Ālasya - lack of enthusiasm.
2. Apakti - indigestion.
3. Ati-sthoulya - obesity.
4. Balāsaka - debility or milk fever (chkp.).
5. Dhamani-pratichaya-distension of blood vessels (Gangadhara, Yogindranath Sen).
6. Gala-gaṇḍa - See Gala-ganda.
7. Guru-gātrata - heaviness of the body.
8. Hṛdayopalepa - obstruction in the heart.
9. Kaṇthopaleya - obstruction in the throat or larynx.
10. Malādhikya - excessive elimination.
11. Mukha-srāva - excessive salivation.
12. Mukha-mādhurya - sweet taste in the mouth.
13. Nidrādhikya - excessive sleep.
14. Śītāgnita - poor digestion.
15. Sleshmodgiraṇa - expectoration of phlegm.
16. Staimitya - rigidity or stiffness of the body.
17. Svetāvabhāsata - white discolouration and Sveta-mūtra-netra-varcha-white discolouration of eyes, stools (and urine).
18. Tandra - uneasiness in the heart, heaviness in speech, behaviour and sensory activities, and agitation of mind and consciousness. (CS, siddhi, 9, 23).
19. Tṛpti - a feeling of satiation; a constant feeling as if one had just eaten a heavy meal (Chkp.).
20. Udarda - see udarda (CS, sūtra, 20, 17).

According to AHṛ, diseases caused by kapha are characterized by the following symptoms: oilyness, hardness, itching, coldness, heaviness, obstruction, rigidity (of joints, etc.), dullness, swelling, indigestion, excessive sleep, white discolouration, sweat and salty taste (in the mouth) and slowness (chronicity), (AHṛ, sūtra, 12, 53).

SaS mentions a few other disorders which are caused by vitiated kapha: coldness of the body, desire for warmth and bitter food, lack of intelligence and alertness, (SaS, prathama, 7,122-124).

General Line of Treatment:

1. The intake of food and drugs that are pungent, bitter, astringent, sharp (tīkshṇa), hot, and dry, including sweating (sudation therapy), emesis, errhines (śiro-virechana) and adequate exercise. These measures are useful in alleviating kapha, (CS, sūtra, 20, 19).

2. Strong emesis and purgation in strict accordance to the texts, food which is limited, dry, sharp, hot, pungent, bitter and astringent in taste, old wine, sensual pleasures or sexual intercourse, keeping awake at night, various kinds of exercise, anxiety or care, massaging of the body (without any oil), honey, yūsha prepared from drugs which reduce fat, exposure to smoke (fumigation), fasting, gaṇḍūsha and hardship, these are all useful in alleviating kapha, (AHṛ, sūtra, 13, 10-12).

Classical Prescriptions: Abhraka-bhasma; Chandana-balā-lākshadi-taila; Chaturjāta-chūrṇa; Kapha-ketu-rasa; Rasa-sindūra; Vanga-bhasma; Vāta-vidhvamsana-rasa; Vyoshādi-guggulu.

Karṇa-roga

Western Nosology: Diseases of the ear

Classification:

I. According to SS, there are twenty eight diseases of the ear.

II. According to CS, the diseases of the ear are classified into four main divisions, i.e. diseases caused by vitiated vāta, pitta, kapha or all three combined.

III. AHṛ enumerates and describes twenty-five diseases of the ear.

IV. SaS has enumerated eighteen diseases of the ear.

Symptomatology:

I. Karṇa-śūla (otalgia): The (vitiated) vāta located in the ear or displaced from its original site or obstructed by the other doshas causes severe pain around and within the ear.

2. **Karṇa-nāda (tinnitus):** If the aggravated vāta remains localised in the auditory apparatus, the patient hears various kinds of sounds in the ear.

3. **Bādhirya (deafness):** If the aggravated vāta remains localised in the auditory apparatus, and if the kapha is also deranged, the patient suffers from deafness.

4. **Karṇa-kshveḍa (tinnitus):** The vāta gets aggravated by exertion, emaciation, intake of dry, cold and astringent food, exposure to cold or śiro-virechana (errhine therapy) and engenders a humming sound in the ears (sound similar to that produced by the bamboo, NiS).

According to NiS, karṇa-kshveda is brought about by the vitiation of vāta along with the other doshas, whereas karṇa-nāda is engendered by vāta alone.

5. **Karṇa-srāva (discharges from the ear):** Due to any head injury, or immersion in water or suppuration of an abscess, there is discharge of pus from the ear which is filled by the (deranged) vāta.

6. **Karṇa-kaṇḍu (itching in the ear):** If the aggravated kapha localises in the ear-channel, the patient suffers from intense itching (within the ear).

7. **Karna-gūtha (increased ear-wax or cerumen):** If the localised kapha is dried up by the heat of the pitta, there is (excessive) accumulation of ear-wax.

8. **Karṇa-pratināha:** If the excessive ear-wax gets liquified and starts flowing out of the nose, the condition is known as karṇa-pratināha. This condition can be a precursor to various diseases of the head.

9. **Kḥmi-karṇa (vermin in the ears):** This condition is characterized by the growth or presence of parasites within the ears.

10 & 11. **Karṇa-vidhradhi (boils and abscesses in the ear):** These are of two kinds i.e. eruptions caused by any injury or trauma, and those caused by the aggravation of the doshas. This condition is marked by a discharge of reddish, brownish or bloody fluids, and pricking, burning and sucking pain.

12. **Karṇa-pāka (suppuration of the boils):** If the pitta gets deranged, it causes suppuration (of those boils) with discharges from the ear, and putridity (kotha).

13. **Pūti-karṇa (purulent discharge from the ear):** The kapha accumulated in the ear-channels is liquified by the heat of the (vitiated) pitta, and as a result, there is discharge of thick pus from the ear, with or without pain.

The ears may also be the seat for the four types of arśa, the four types of śopha or the seven kinds of arbuda, (SS).

II. Diseases of the ear which are brought about by aggravated vāta manifest the following symptoms: sounds in the ear (nāda), severe pain, dryness of ear-wax and discharge of a thin liquid. Diseases caused by vitiated pitta are characterized by swelling, inflammation, cracking (of the skin?, dāraṇa), burning pain and foul, yellow discharge from the ear. Diseases engendered by deranged kapha are marked by hardness of hearing (vai-śrutya), itching, hard (firm) swelling, slight pain and discharge of oily and white fluid. Diseases caused by all the doshas will have symptoms of all these doshas, (CS).

III. The twenty-five diseases of the ear, according to AHṛ, are:

1-5. **Karṇa-śūla (otalgia):** This can be of five

types depending on the causative factors. i.e. the deranged vāta, pitta, kapha, blood or all three doshas combined.

If the vāta is aggravated by catarrh, playing (or immersion) in water, itching in the ears, exposure to excessive noise, etc. or other aggravating factors, it localises in the ear-channels, generating pain, aversion to cold, pain confined to one part of the head (ardhāvabhedaka), (sense of) obstruction in the ears, slow suppuration, sudden feeling of emptiness (śūnya), and a feeling as if the ear was opening and closing.

If the pitta is aggravated, the patient suffers from burning pain, ear-ache, local heat, desire for cold, swelling, fever, rapid suppuration and discharge of yellow serous fluid after suppuration. The serous fluid sets up inflammation on all parts over which it flows.

If kapha is vitiated, there will be slight (dull) pain, heaviness of the head, neck and jaw; itching, swelling, desire for wamth, and discharge of white and thick matter after suppuration.

If the blood is vitiated following any injury, the pain and other symptoms will be similar to those seen in pittaja-karṇa-śūla, or the symptoms may be more intense.

If all three doshas are vitiated, there will be severe pain, swelling, fever, alternate desire for heat and cold, hardness of hearing and discharge of white, blackish, bloody or thick pus.

6. **Karṇa-nāda (tinnitus):** When the deranged vāta localises in the channels of the ear, the patient frequently hears various kinds of noises in the ear.

7. **Bādhirya (deafness):** If the disease karṇa-nāda is neglected, or if kapha and vāta are both deranged, there will be difficulty in hearing shrill sounds, which gradually leads to deafness.

8. **Pratināha:** The localised kapha is dried up by the deranged vāta and obstructs the ear (channels) causing pain and a sense of heaviness.

9. **Karṇa-kaṇḍu (itching in the ears) and karṇa-śopha (swelling around the ear):** Both these conditions are brought about by the aggravated kapha.

10. **Pūti-karṇa:** The kapha is dried up by the pitta, and as a result, there is discharge of profuse, thick and putrid matter from the ears, with or without pain.

11. **Kṛmi-karṇa (maggots in the ear):** The three doshas are vitiated and engender the growth of parasites in the watery portions (kleda) of flesh and blood. These parasites eat into the ear, and cause severe pain.

12. **Karṇa-vidradhi (abscess or boil in the ear):** Due to intense itching in the ear, the person scratches the affected area, and due to the injury an abscess is formed. It may also occur independently. For symptoms, see Vidradhi.

13. **Karṇa-śopha (swelling)**

14. **Karṇa-arśa (polypi)**

15. **Karṇa-arbuda (tumour):** These three diseases will progressively cause pain, pūti-karṇa and deafness.

16. **Kuchi-karṇaka:** If the vāta is vitiated in the internal ear, there will be contraction of the pinna or auricle (śashkuli).

17. **Karṇa-pippali**: There will be one or many fleshy, firm (or stable), painles growths which resemble (in size), the fruits of pippali.

18. **Vidārika:** All the three doshas get vitiated and result in the formation of a skin-coloured (non-discoloured), painful, stable (rigid) swelling. If this is neglected, there will be suppuration and discharge of a fluid similar to kaṭu-taila. If this condition progresses, it results in the contraction of the pinna.

19. **Pāli-śesha:** The aggravated vāta causes the emaciation of the lobule (pāli)

20. **Tantrika:** The aggravated vāta acts upon the lobule and makes it thin and dense like a string.

21. **Paripoṭa:** A painful, browish swelling suddenly appears on the lobule of the ears of delicate persons. This suppurates slowly. This condition is usually caused by the deranged vāta.

22. **Utpāta:** The pitta and blood get vitiated due to the wearing of heavy ornaments (on the ear), and engender a blackish swelling which is attended by pain, burning sensation, inflammation, redness and secretion. There will also be (a few) boils and pimples, around the swelling.

23. **Gallira or unmantha:** Due to the aggravation of vāta and kapha, there is a swelling all over the lobule of the ear. The swelling will be firm, painless, numb, not discoloured and will be attended by itching.

24. **Dukha-vardhana:** The three doshas get aggravated due to improper piercing of the ear, and cause a swelling with itching, burning, suppuration and sharp pain.

25. **Lehya:** The aggravated kapha, blood and parasites engender the formation of small eruptions, with itching, secretion and pain. If these are neglected, they eat away the lobule of the ear, (AHṛ).

Prognosis: The diseases pippali, tridoshaja karṇa-śūla, vidāri and kuchi-karṇaka are incurable, while tantrika can be palliated. All other conditions are curable, (AHṛ).

Bādhirya is incurable in children, old persons and when it is chronic, (AHṛ).

Ref.: SS, nidāna, 1, 84; uttara, 20; CS, sūtra, 20,11; chikitsā, 26, 127-12; AHṛ, uttara, 17.

Treatment:

I. The measures generally useful in all diseases of the ear are: internal use of (potions) of ghee, of drugs that are rejuvenative (rasāyana), avoidance of exertion, bathing over the head, and excess speech and celibacy.

The treatment in karṇa-śūla, karṇa ṇāda, bādhirya and karṇa-kshveḍa, all of which are caused by the aggravated vāta is as follows: The patient is oleated (both internally and externally or locally) and is then administered sudation (svedana), after which he is given an oily purgative. The nāḍi and piṇḍa types of sveda are also useful. The ear should be fumigated with fumes of burnt atasi cloth, ghee, agaru and guggulu. The patient is then made to drink potions of ghee and is subjected to śiro-basti. The patient can also be advised to fast for a day, and in the night is administered ghee with (warm) milk. The śata-pāka balā taila is to be used for śiro-basti, as nasal drops, for sprinkling, etc. Goat's milk if medicated with kaṇṭakāri and fat of a cock (kukkuṭa) and used as ear-drops is extremely efficacious. The expressed juice of laśuna, ārdraka (fresh ginger), madhu-śigru, sobhānjana, mūlaka or kadali is warmed up and used locally (ear drops). The warm juice of śṛngavera (ginger), with honey, rock salt and oil is also used as ear drops. Pieces of stem or roots of drugs of bṛhat-pancha-mūla, measuring about eighteen angulas are covered with a linen cloth and immersed in oil. The sticks are then set on fire. The oil which pours down is used as ear drops. The stems of bhadra-dāru, kushṭha, or sarala (or eraṇḍa, agni-mantha, NiS) can be used in a similar way. The fine powder of samudraphena can also be used locally.

In a case of pittaja karṇa-roga, the above mentioned remedial measures can be adopted. However, ghee medicated with drugs of the kākoladi group and milk or with bitter drugs and milk are especially useful. Ghee medicated with chandana, and yashṭi-madhu can be administered with sugar and honey. Ghee can also be medicated with drugs that have laxative properties.

In cases of kaphaja karṇa-roga, oil medicated with ingudi or sarshapa can be used for local use. Gruels medicated with bitter drugs and fomentation with drugs that alleviate kapha are also useful. The juices of mātulunga or śukta or laśuna or ārdraka can be used as ear drops. Oil medicated with any one of the above drugs can also be used in a similar fashion. Errhines and gargles (gaṇḍūsha) prepared from strong (tikshṇa) drugs are also useful.

Patients of raktaja karṇa-roga are to be treated with measures indicated in pittaja karṇa-roga.

In bādhirya, oil medicated with cow's urine, milk, water and bilva is used as ear drops. Oil medicated with sugar-candy, yashṭi-madhu, and bimbi and goat's milk is churned when still hot, with a decoction of bimbi. After it has cooled down, it is removed by hand, and again churned with a decoction of fruits of bilva, and heated with sugar-candy, yashṭi madhu, rakta-chandana and milk. The oil is extremely efficacious (when used locally). The remedial measures useful in pratiśyāya and vāta-roga can also be adopted in bādhirya.

The general measures to be employed in cases of karṇa-srāva, pūti-karṇa and kṛmi-karṇa are: śiro-virechana (errhines), fumigation, ear-drops, washing the ear, and cleaning the ear. The ear can be washed with a decoction of drugs of the rāja-vṛksha group or surasādi group, or filled with the powders of these drugs. In karṇa-srāva, the decoction of tinḍuka, abhaya, lodhra, samanga and āmalaka, with honey and juice of kapittha is used for pouring into the ear. The juice of fruits of kārpāsi, and the powder of the bark of sarja and honey can also be used for this purpose. The powders of lāksha, rasānjana and sarja are also useful (local use).

In puṭi-karṇa, where there is discharge, ghee medicated with rasānjana, breast milk and honey is used internally. Oil medicated with the juice of nirgunḍi, honey, rock salt, dhūma-rāja and jaggery can be used locally.

In kṛimi-karṇa, measures for destroying the parasites are to be adopted. The ear is to be exposed to the fumes of burnt dry vārtāku, and can also be filled with oil of sarshapa. The foul odour can be relieved by filling the ear with cow's urine, viḍanga and haratāla (powders), and by fumigation with guggulu. Emesis, gargles (kavala) and dhūma-pāna are also useful.

In karṇa-kshveḍa, oil of sarshapa can be used as ear-drops, The treatment for karṇa-vidradhi is the same as that mentioned in treatment of vidradhi.

In karṇa-gūtha, the ear should be moistened (internally) with oil, and is then fomented. After the ear-wax has softened, it is removed by using a śalāka (probe).

In a case of karṇa-kanḍu, the ear is fomented by nāḍi-sveda (tube). The patient is then subjected to emesis, dhuma (fumigation), errhines and all measures which alleviate kapha.

A case of pratināha should be treated with oleation, sudation, and use of errhines. Karṇa-pāka is to be treated with measures useful in pittaja visarp, (SS).

II. A case of karṇa-śula is treated with measures that alleviate vāta and which are useful in pīnasa. Pradāha (applications), ear drops and errhines are also beneficial. The diet has to be chosen according to the dosha involved. Sarshapa oil medicated with hingu, tumburu and śuṇṭhi or oil medicated with goats' urine, devādaru, vachā, suṇṭhi, satāhva, kushṭha and rock salt are used as ear drops. Varāṭika (cowries) are to be heated and reduced to ashes in a new earthern vessel. This is mixed with oil prepared from aromatic drugs, and the oil is medicated with the pastes of rasānjana and śuṇṭhi. This oil is very useful in otalgia (kshāra taila).

Diseases of the ear are to be treated in a manner similar to that in pīnasa, (CS).

III. A person suffering from kaphaja karṇa-śūla is administered ghee medicated with pippali, and is then made to vomit. The juices of bījapūra and kapittha are poured into the ear.

In cases where there is suppuration or discharge (srāva), the pus is removed by means of pichu-varti (cotton swabs). The ear is then fumigated by burning guggulu, and is filled with honey. The cotton swabs can be dipped in a decoction of drugs of the same group and can also be used locally.

Karṇa-nāda and bādhirya can be treated by the same measures adopted in karṇa-śūla.

Oil medicated with the leaf-juices of eraṇḍa, śigru, varuṇa and mūlaka, and eight parts of milk and the pastes of madhu-yashṭi and kshīra-kākoli can be used as ear-drops, errhines or for massage in cases of karṇa-nāda, bādhirya and karṇa-śūla. Oil medicated with prati-visha, hingu, mīśi, tvak, svarjaka-kshāra, maricha and śukta (a type of kānji) is used as ear-drops in otalgia, discharge from the ear, and karṇa-nāda. Oil of sarshapa is also useful when used locally in karṇa-nāda.

Patients suffering from swelling, discharge and difficulty in hearing should be administered emesis.

In pratināha, the ear is oleated, fomented and cleaned. It is then filled with oil medicated with śukta, rocksalt, honey and the juice of mātulunga. If the ear is very dry after cleaning it, the upper layer of ghee is used as ear-drops. The same treatment is also useful in excessive accumulation of ear-wax.

The local use of kaṭu-taila is very useful in kṛmi-karṇa. Pūti-karṇa and kṛmi-karṇa are treated as in karṇa-srāva. Vidradhi caused by trauma should be treated as in pittaja karṇa-śula. The unsuppurated vidārika should be treated as in a case of karṇa-vidradhi.

Pāli-śosha should be treated by applications indicated in vātaja-karṇa-śūla. It should then be fomented and smeared with oil medicated with seeds of priyāla, madhu-yashṭi, aśva-gandha and yava. The patient should be regularly massaged with strength-giving and nourishing medicated oils. Oil medicated with śatāvari, aśvagandha, oil of eraṇḍa, and milk is very useful in pāli-śosha. Oil medicated with a paste of the drugs of the jīvanīya group, milk and a decoction of meat of aquatic animals is also useful in pāli-śosha.

In utpāta, the ear is smeared with cold plasters. Blood-letting is also useful. In unmantha, the oil prepared from the fat of godha and karkaṭaka, tāla-parṇi, aśvagandha, arka, bākuchi fruits and rock-salt is used externally, Oil medicated with surasā and lāngali is used for errhine therapy (tīkshna-nāvana). In dukha-vardhana, the affected area is sprinkled with a decoction of leaves of asmantha, jambu and āmra, and smeared over with oil. The fine powders of yashṭi-madhu, manjisṭha, prapoundarīka, and haridra are used for dusting. Oil medicated with lāksha and viḍanga is used externally, (AHṛ).

IV. Filling the ears with a paste of haritāla and cow's urine or with oil of sarshapa is useful in kṛmi-karṇa. Oil prepared from the kshāra and a paste of apāmārga is useful (when applied locally) in bādhirya and karṇa-nāda (SaS).

Classical Presciptions:

Karṇa-roga: Asana-bilvādi-taila; Bhṛngarāja-taila; Paṭolādi-ghṛta; Vachā-lasunādi-taila.

Karṇa-nāda: Mahā-vishagarbha-taila

Karṇa-srāva: Kapardika-bhasma; Vachā-laśunādi-taila.

Bādhirya: Bhṛngāmalaka-taila; Bṛhat-māsha-taila; Mahā-nārayana-taila.

Ref.: SS, uttara, 21; CS, chikitsā, 26, 221-230; AHṛ, uttara, 18; SaS, uttara, 11, 145,151.

Kārśya

Western Nosology: Emaciation

Casusative Factors:

Intrinsic: Provoked vāta and abnormal rasa dhātu.

Extrinsic:

1. Intake of dry (rūksha) food and drink, fasting, eating less and at long intervals, excessive activity, grief, loss of sleep, suppression of natural urges, rubbing the body with dry substances, frequent bathing, old age, anger and continued illness. It can also be

hereditary (prakṛti), (CS).

2. Excessive intake of food that aggravates vāta, excess indulgence in coitus and exercise, total absorption in studies or thoughts (dhyāna), grief, keeping awake at nights, not satisfying the urges of thirst and hunger, eating less, and intake of kashāyas (decoctions), etc., (SS).

Symptomatology:

1. An emaciated person is incapable of withstanding (tolerating) exertion, over-eating, hunger, thirst, medicines, diseases, excessive heat or cold and sexual intercourse. He also suffers from diseases like plīha, cough, tuberculosis (kshaya), dysnoea (śvāsa), gulma, haemorrhoids, udara and grahaṇi, (CS).

2. A person suffering from kārśya is not capable of withstanding hunger, thirst, extremes of heat and cold, windy and rainy weather and exertion. He also suffers from diseases of aggravated vāta, and is generally weak. He quickly falls prey to diseases such as śvāsa, cough, śosha (tuberculosis), plīha, udara, feeble digestion, gulma, rakta-pitta, etc. Even minor diseases become magnified due to the weakness (SS).

Prognosis: Emaciation is far easier to cure than obesity (CS, SS, AHṛ).

Treatment:

1. The emaciated person is advised to partake of food that is nourishing (bṛmhaṇa) and easy to digest.

The following are very useful in this disease: sleeping in a soft and comfortable bed; contentment, absence of worries, restraining from coitus, exercise and mental activity; exposure to pleasant things; freshly harvested rice, new wine; meat juices of domesticated and aquatic (ānūpa) animals; well prepared meat; intake of ghee, milk, curds, sugar cane, śāli rice, māsha (black-gram), wheat and preparations of jaggery; enema of oil and sweet drugs, regular massage with oil, rubbing the body with oily substances; wearing white dresses, garlands and using perfumes; and use of drugs that are rejuvenative (rasāyana) and aphrodisiac (vṛshya).

Freedom from worries of any sort, good nourishing food and sound sleep makes a man as plump as a boar, (CS).

2. Care should be taken to prevent this disease by avoiding the causative actors.

The patient should be administered drugs such as payasyā, aśvagandha, vidāri-gandha, śatāvari, balā, atibala, nāga-bala and others possessing madhura rasa (sweet taste).

The diet should consist of milk,curds, ghee, meat, śāli-rice, rice grown in sixty days, yava and wheat. The patient should avoid coitus and exertion and should indulge in sleep during day. He should be given enema with nourishing drugs (bṛmhaṇa basti) (SS).

3. The following prescriptions are useful in this disease: pārada-bhasma or rasa-sindūra boiled in milk with aśvagandha and yashṭi; the powder of kushṭha taken in the same way; the powders of pippali, yashṭi and aśvagandha boiled in milk and given with rasa-sindūra; the powders of pippali, yashṭi and aśvagandha given with honey, ghee and śālmali juice (sātva); pārada-bhasma given with sugar and guggulu which has been boiled with castor oil and powders of trikaṭu, triphala and viḍanga.

The medicines; amṛtārṇava-rasa and pūrṇa-chandra-rasa are also useful, (RRS).

Ref.: CS, sūtra, 21; SS, sūtra, 15, 33; 24, 9; AHṛ, 14, 31; 4, 11; RRS, 18, 169-173; 27, 39-40, 30, 59.

Classical Prescriptions: Aravindāsava; Aśvagandhādyarishṭa; Balā-aśvagandha-lākshadi-taila; Balā-dhātryādi-taila; Pippalyādyāsava; Vidāryādi-ghṛta.

Kāsa

Western Nosology: Cough

Causative Factors:

Extrinsic: The general casuative factors are exposure to smoke and dust, (excessive) exercise, (excessive) intake of dry food, suppression of natural urges, sneezing, food going into the wrong tract, etc., (SS).

Intrinsic: The disease results when both prāṇa and udāna vāyu are aggravated.

Pathogenesis: The vāta prevented from going downwards enters the upward channels, acquires a tendency to move upwards, lodges in the throat and chest, fills up the channels in the head and engenders cough, (CS).

Classification: Diffrent types of cough are distinguished by pain and sound, due to the particular factors which have an impact, and by its speed of impact on vāta, (CS).

There are five kinds of cough: those caused by the aggravated vāta, pitta and kapha, that which is caused by emaciation (of either tuberculosis or of old age, Chkp.), and that which is the result of trauma (CS, SS).

Prodromal Symptoms:

1. Itching (tickling) in the throat, difficulty in swallowing food, a sticky sensation in the throat and palate, change in voice, tastelessness and feeble digestion, (SS).

2. A sensation of a splinter in the throat, itching in the throat, and difficulty in swallowing, (CS).

Symptomatology:

1. **Vātaja kāsa:** (sharp) pain in the heart (chest), temples, head, abdomen and sides, weak and hoarse voice, debility, loss of resistence to disease, frequent and continuous cough without expectoration (SS).

(Sharp) pain in the heart (chest), sides, chest, and head, hoarseness, dryess of chest, throat, and mouth, horripilation, darkness before the eyes, expectoration absent or scanty and difficult, rattling, hard breathing, dejection, agitation, amelioration after intake of oily, hot, sour and salty substances and aggravation after the digestion of food, (CS).

2. **Pittaja kāsa:** Burning in the chest, fever, dryness of the mouth, bitter taste in the mouth, thirst, yellow and pungent expectoration (with vomiting), pale-yellow discolouration of the body and burning sensation, (SS).

Bitter taste in the mouth, yellow discolouration

disorders, burning in the chest, tastelessness, vertigo, fainting spells and sparks before the eyes on constant coughing, (CS).

3. **Kaphaja kāsa:** A sticky sensation in the mouth (as if the mouth was coated with phlegm, NiS), headache, heaviness of the body, aversion to food, excessive accumulation of phlegm, debility, and thick expectoration, (SS).

Feeble digestion, tastelessness, vomiting, catarrh, nausea, heaviness of body, horripilation, salivation, sweet taste in the mouth, expectoration of thick, sweet, unctuous and copious sputum, sense of fullness in the chest and absence of pain when coughing, (CS).

4. **Kshataja kāsa (cough caused by trauma):** If the inner chest is severely injured by excessive exertion, carrying heavy weights, or any blow, the patient suffers from constant cough with expectoration of bloody sputum, (SS).

The cough is dry at first and later is attended with bloody expectoration, (NiS).

The cough is dry at first and is later attended with bloody sputum, severe pain in the throat, sharp piercing pain in the chest, pain in the joints, fever, difficulty in breathing, thirst and hoarseness. The patient undergoes severe suffering due to the pains, and will be moaning, (CS).

5. **Kshayaja kāsa:** Pain in the limbs, fever, burning sensation, fainting spells, emaciation, debility, and expectoration of pus and blood, (SS).

Intake of harmful or disagreeable food, or limited food at irregular hours, excessive sexual intercourse, suppression of the natural uges, disgust and grief are the precipitating factors. (CS)

Flushes of heat and cold, excessive appetite, debility, emaciation, a feeling as if the heart was displaced on coughing, oily and clear complexion of the face, bright and sparkling eyes, soft palms and soles, covetousness, fever with symptoms of all three doshas, pain in the sides, catarrh, tastelessness, unformed stools, hoarseness without any apparent cause, and expectoration that is offensive, green, red and putrid, (CS).

Complications: If neglected, cough turns into dyspnoea (śvāsa), tuberculosis, vomiting, hoarseness, etc., (AS).

Prognosis:

1. Kshaya kāsa is very difficult to cure. All cases of cough in old people can be only palliated (yāpya). If neglected, all kinds of cough develop into rāja-yakshma (tuberculosis), (SS).

2. The first three kinds of cough are curable. Kshataja and kshayaja kāsa are curable in persons who have a strong constitution, and where they have not become chronic. The success however depends on the (successful coordination of the) four limbs of treatment i.e. physician, medicines, nurse and patient. Cough caused due to old age can be palliated, (CS).

Ref.: SS, uttara, 52, 5-13; CS, chikitsā, 18, 4-31; AS, nidāna, 3, 43.

Treatment:

1. The powders of harītaki, sugar-candy, āmalaka and lājā or of śuṇṭhi and pippali can be made into a paste with ghee and honey and administered. The powder of pippali can also be administered with rock-salt and hot water.

The following recipes are also useful in cough: a paste of jaggery, nāgara and pippali; a paste of drākshā with ghee and honey; a paste of drākshā with sugarcandy and pippali; a paste of fresh ginger with vamśa-lochana, yashṭi-madhu, ghee and honey; paste of sugar candy, maricha, ghee and honey; paste of āmalaki, pippali, sunṭhi, sugar-candy and curd-cream (dadhimaṇḍa); paste of hareṇuka, pippali and curd; paste of haridra, dāru-haridra, devadāru, śuṇṭhi, khadira-sāra and goat's urine; paste of danti, dravanti, tilvaka and warm water; the leaves of badara pasted with rock salt and fried in ghee; a kola weight of hingu with kānji or juice of bījapūraka; paste of maricha with honey; maricha with sīdhu (a kind of fermented drink); a decoction of drākshā, bālaka, manjishṭha, śallaki (or guggulu, NiS), milk and honey; well-boiled mudga with kanṭakāri, nāgara, pippali and honey and ghee medicated with śatāvari and nāgabala.

Ghee medicated with vāsa or with drugs of the vidārigandha group is useful in vātaja-kāsa. The other measures useful in vātaja kāsa are: purgation with oily drugs, āsthāpana and anuvāsana types of enema, inhalation of smoke of wax, sarja-rasa, etc., potions of warm ghee, yavāgu (gruels) prepared from meat-juices, milk medicated with drugs that alleviate vāta and lehyas with ghee.

In kaphaja-kāsa, inducing emesis, errhines, purgations, inhalation, kavala (gargles), lehyas (lambatives) prepared from pungent drugs and intake of food that is dry, limited in quantity and easy to digest are useful. (In some cases, fasting or the various kinds of emaciating measures, langhana are indicated, NiS). Equal quantities of nāgara, maricha and pippali; or ghee medicated with the juice (or cold infusion, NiS) of viḍanga, or juice of the leaves of nirguṇḍi, are useful.

In pittaja, kshayaja and kshataja kāsa, decoctions of drugs of vidārigandha, utpala-sāriva and kākolyādi groups are used to prepare ghee (ghṛta) along with sugar-cane juice, water and milk. The ghee has to be administered in the morning. The paste of kharjūra, bhārngi, pippali, priyāla, madhūlika, ela, āmalaki, sugar-candy, honey and ghee is also useful.

The powder of āmalaki taken with milk and ghee is useful in kshataja and kshayaja kāsa. The fine powders of wheat, barley and drugs of kākolyādi group are administered with milk, honey and ghee in the three kinds of cough (i.e. pittaja, kshataja and kshayaja). A cold infusion of jaggery is boiled, cooled, mixed with honey and a little quantity of maricha and administered.

The inhalation of the smoke of bhārngi, vachā, and hingu, or veṇu-tvak, ela, rock-salt and ghee is useful in all kinds of cough, (SS).

2. The treatment in vātaja kasa should consist of oleation (snehana), potions of ghee, enemata, intake of gruels (peya and yūsha), milk, meat-juices, etc., medicated with drugs that alleviate vāta, inhalation, lambatives (lehyas), massage with oil, sprinkling (of oily substances, etc.) and measures for inducing perspiration (svedana). In cases where pitta is also vitiated, ghee (medicated with the indicated drugs) is administered after meals, while oily purgatives are used in cases where kapha is vitiated, (along with vāta).

Ghee medicated with kaṇṭakāri and guḍūchi; the paste of durālabha, śatī, drāksha, fresh ginger, sugar-candy, karkata-śṛngi and oil; the paste of duhsparśa, pippali, musta, bhārngi, karkaṭa-śṛngi, śaṭi, old jaggery and oil; the paste of pippali, rock-salt and ghee; and the essence of khadira (khadira-sāra) with madira, curd and mastu; are all useful.

The meat of domesticated and aquatic animals, old rice, barley, wheat, gruel prepared from māsha and atma-gupta, vāstuka, kākamāchi, mūlaka, sunishaṇṇaka, oily foods, milk, sugar-cane juice, jaggery and its products and substances which are sweet, sour and salty are all beneficial in patients suffering from vātaja kāsa.

Patients suffering from pittaja kāsa with expectoration are to be administered emetics prepared from ghee or a decoction of madana, kaśmarya and yashṭi-madhu or a paste of yashṭi-madhu, madana, and vidāri with sugar-cane juice in order to induce vomiting. After the phlegm has been expelled, cold and sweet drugs are administered. If the expectoration is watery, trivṛt is administered for purgation with sweet drugs, while it is given with bitter drugs in cases where the expectoration is thick. Drugs and food articles which are oily and cold are indicated where there is watery sputum, while those that are dry and cold are indicated in cases characterised by thick sputum.

The following recipes are useful in pittaja kāsa: the paste of kharjūra, pippali, padmaka, drāksha, juice of bṛhati fruit, honey and ghee; paste of mṛdvīka, pippali, sugarcandy, honey and milk; the decoction of pippali, āmalaki, drākshā, lāksha, lāja, sugar-candy; and milk with honey; all drugs that are sweet and cold; gruel (yūsha) prepared from milk, juice of kākoli, bṛhati, meda, mahā-meda, vāsa and nāgara; a decoction of the drugs of the tṛṇa-panchamūla group; pippali, drāksha and milk, with sugar and honey and the filtered juices of nāgara, udīchya, kaṇṭakāri and śaṭi, with sugar and ghee.

The food articles useful are: meat juices of desert animals, śyāmaka, kodrava, gruels of mudga, etc., bitter leafy vegetables, milk, and juices of drākshā and sugar-cane.

A patient suffering from kaphaja kāsa is to be first administered an emetic. The following recipes are beneficial: the paste of nāgara, ativisha, musta, karkaṭa-śṛngi, harītaki and śaṭi with hot water, hingu and rock-salt; the paste of pippali previously fried in oil with vibhītaki (or in a dose of one aksha), sugar-candy, and juice of kulattha; the juices of kāsamarda, aśvagandha, bhṛngarāja, vārtāka, and black surasa with honey; the paste of pippali, root of pippali, chitraka and hasti-pippali with honey; the paste of harītaki, pippali, tāmalaki, āmalaki and bhadra-musta with honey; the paste of devadāru, harītaki, musta, pippali and nāgara with honey; the paste of viśāla, pippali, musta and trivṛt with honey; and ghee medicated with pancha-kola (decoction) and juice of kulattha.

The food articles useful in kaphaja kāsa are barley, gruel (yūsha) prepared from kshāra of pippali, kulattha, mūlaka, etc.; food that is pungent, dry, hot, easy to digest and which alleviates kapha, meat of burrowing and desert animals, food that is cooked with til oil, sarshapa oil and oil extracted from bilva, hot water, buttermilk and (old) wine. The cold infusion of pushkara mūla, root of āragvadha and paṭola is to be administered with honey, before, during and after meals.

If in a case of kaphaja kāsa, there is dyspnoea caused by pitta, treatment for alleviation of pitta is indicated. If in a case of vātaja kāsa there are symptoms of aggravated kapha, treatment is to be given for alleviating kapha. If in cases of kaphaja and pittaja kāsa, there are symptoms of aggravated pitta, measures are to be taken for alleviating pitta. Bitter substances are useful in cases of kaphaja kāsa with slight involvement of pitta.

Cough engendered by trauma (kshataja kāsa) is dangerous, and requires immediate treatment with drugs which are sweet, jīvanīya, and which enhance strength and flesh. A lambative (lehya) prepared from equal quantities of barley, wheat, mṛdvīka, juice of āmalaki and oil, goat's milk, cow's milk, sugarcane juice, pippali, yashṭi-madhu and sugar-candy is to be administered with ghee and honey.

Such cases are to be generally treated along the same lines as indicated for pittaja kāsa. If symptoms of vāta and pitta are both present, massage with oil is useful. If there is excessive pain in the limbs, ghee is to be used (for massage), while oil medicated with drugs that alleviate vāta is used if there are symptoms of aggravated vāta. The meat juices of lāva, etc., are useful if there is emaciation. If there is severe thirst, goat's milk and a decoction of tṛna-pancha-mūla are beneficial. In cases of bleeding from the orifices, ghee and kshīrajam (curd) are useful.

Recent cases of kshayaja kāsa are treated with measures to induce corpulency and increase the digestive fire. If the doshas are excessively aggravated, the patient is administered a mild oily purgative. Ghee medicated with āragvadha, trivṛt, mṛdvīka juice, a decoction of tilvaka and juice of vidāri can be used for this purpose. If the patient is emaciated, and if pitta and kapha are diminished, ghee medicated with karkaṭa-sṛngi and the two varieties of balā is useful. If the urine is discoloured, and if there is dysuria, ghee medicated with vidāri, kadamba, milk and tāla-phala is benefcial. If the penis, anus, groins and pelvis are swollen and painful, anuvāsana is administered with honey and ghṛta-maṇḍa or with miśraka. The fruits of āmalaki are boiled in milk, made into a paste with ghee, and administered to the patient. Ghee medicated with juice of dāḍima, maricha, pippali and nāgara, or with goat's milk, pippali and jaggery or with yava-kshāra is administered after meals. It cleanses the channels of the chest and alimentary tract.

The following recipes are useful: the paste of maricha, ghee, honey and sugar; paste of badari leaves fried in ghee, with rock salt; and an utkārika of the paste of the leaves of tilvaka previously fried in ghee, with sugar. The first two recipes are also useful in hoarseness, while the latter is useful in vomiting and diarrhoea also.

The gruel (yūsha) of mudga medicated with the juice of kaṇṭakari, sour fruits such as dādima, and fresh āmalaki is useful in all kinds of cough.

The gruels prepared from substances which alleviate vāta, milk, and meat-juice of prasara, vishkira, pratuda, carnivorous and burrowing desert animals, are beneficial in kshayaja kāsa. The drugs used in kshayaja kāsa have to be appetizing, nourishing and should also cleanse the channels.

The important drugs useful in cough are: drāksha, harītaki, āmalaki, pippali, durālabha, karkaṭa-srngi, kaṇṭakari, vrśchira, punarnava and tāmalaki, (CS).

3. Equal quantities of tāmra bhasma, tīkshna (loha) bhasma and (kṛshṇa) abhraka bhasma are triturated with juices of agastya and kāsamarda, triphala decoction and the juice (or decoction) of amla-vetasa. It can then be administered in (all cases of) cough.

One part of roupya bhasma, one part of manahśila and four parts of haritāla are triturated for six hours each with juices of vāsa and gokshura. The paste is then subjected to heat in a bāluka yantra. This medicine is to be administered in (all cases of) cough with powders of trikaṭu and root of nirguṇḍi.

The leaves of bhṛngarāja are triturated with honey and made into small pills. These pills when kept in the mouth and sucked relieve cough and constipation. The juices of the leaves of arka and eraṇḍa are also useful in cough. The inhalation of fumes got by burning the root of danti or nirguṇḍi is also very useful. The fine powder of the root of indra-vāruṇi, bhārngi, maricha (or pippali) and tila is useful in cough brought out by wasting (or tuberculosis), (RRS).

Classical Prescription: Abhraka-bhasma; Agastya-harītaki-rasāyana; Amrta-prāsa-ghrta; Aśva-kanchuki-rasa; Balā-taila; Bāla-chaturbhadrika-chūrṇa; Balā-jīrakādi-kvātha-chūrṇa; Balā-aswagandha-lākshadi-taila; Chandanādi-chūrṇa; Chandrāmṛta-rasa; Chitraka-harītaki; Daśamūlarishṭa; Daśamūla -kaṭutrayādi -kvātha-chūrṇa; Daśamūla-shaṭpala-ghṛta;Dhānvantara-guṭika; Drāksharishṭha; Elādi-chūrṇa; Elādi-guṭika; Godanti- bhasma; Gorochanādi-taila; Grahaṇi-mihira-taila; Guḍa-pippali; Jātiphalādi-chūrṇa; Kalyāṇaka-ghṛta; Kanakāsava; Kānta-vallabha-rasa; Kaṇṭakāryāvaleha; Kapha-ketu-rasa; Karpūrādi-churna; Khadirādi-guṭika; Ḳumār-kalyāna-rasa; Kumāryāsava; Kūshmāṇḍa-rasāyana; Lavangādi-vaṭi; Mahā-kalyāṇaka-ghṛta; Mahā-lakshmi-vilāsa-rasa; Marichādi-guṭika; Mrdvīkadi -lehya; Muktā-bhasma; Muktā-panchāmṛta-rasa; Nāga-vallabha-rasa;Narasimha-chūrna; Pippalyādi-ghṛta; Prāṇadā-guṭika; Pravāla-bhasma; Sapta-vimśatika-guggulu; Śiva-gutika; Śhaṭpala-ghṛta; Soubhāgya-vaṭi; Śṛnga-bhasma; Śvāsa-kūṭhāṛa-rasa; Tālisādi-chūrṇa; Tāmra-bhasma; Vanga-bhasma;Vāsaka-kshāra; Vāsakāsava; Vasāvaleha; Vaikranta-bhasma; Vāsā-chandanādi-taila; Vatāgni-kumāra-rasa; Vidāryadi-ghṛta; Vidaryādi-kvātha-chūṛna; Yakṛtāri-lauha.

Kaphaja-kāsa: Daśamūla-kvātha-chūṛna; Daśamūla-ghṛta.

Kshayaja-kāsa: Drākshadi-chūṛna; Pravāla-bhasma.

Jīrna-kāsa: Svarṇa-vanga; Vasanta-mālati-rasa.

Vātaja-kāsa: Daśamūla-ghṛta.

Ref.: SS,uttara, 52; CS, chikitsā,18; sūtra,4, 8, 16; RRS,13, 24-26; 41-42, 46.

Khālitya

Synonyms: Khalvāṭatvam

Vernacular: Chaṇḍilatva (NiS on SS, sūtra, 3, 29)

Western Nosology: Baldness; Alopecia.

Causative Factors:

Extrinsic: Old age (SS, ibid)

Intrinsic: All three doshas especially pitta (CS, vimāna, 8, 98).

Pathogenesis: The increased body temperature and the aggravated doshas are responsible for falling hair (in young or middle-aged persons), (CS).

Treatment: See treatment of palita.

Ref.: CS, chikitsā, 26, 132; 263-282.

Classical Prescriptions: Bhṛngaṛāja-taila;

Bhṛngāmalaka-taila; Nīlī-bhṛngādi-taila; Shaā-bindu-taila; Triphalādi-taila; Nīlikādya-taila;

Khalli

Causative Factors:

Extrinsic: Factors which aggravate vāta.

Intrinsic: Vāta

Symptomatology: Bending inwards (curvature of) of the foot, leg, thigh and wrist, (CS).

According to AS and AHṛ, the symptoms of khalli are similar to those of viśvāchi and gṛdhrasi, the difference being the presence of severe pain in khalli.

Treatment:

1. Sudation (i.e. inducing perspiration) is very efficacious in khalli, (CS, sūtra, 14, 23-24).

The application of hot poultices, and intake of pāyasa, kṛśara and meat-juices mixed with oil and ghee is also effective, (CS).

2. The pain can be alleviated by massaging the affected parts with warm chukra-taila mixed with the paste of kushṭha and rock-salt. Massaging, poultices and fomentation with oily, sour and salty substances are useful in this disease, (CD).

Ref.: CS, chikitsā, 28, 57, 107; sūtra,14, 23-24; AS, nidāna, 15, 57; AHṛ, nidāna,15, 55; CD, 22, 65.

Khanja

Causative Factors:

Extrinsic: Factors which aggravate vāta

Intrinsic: Vāta (CS, SS)

Symptomatology: The vāta localised in the pelvic region affects the nerves of the lower limbs, causing a deformity in gait, (SS).

Treatment:

1. The treatment is to be given on the same lines as for other vāta rogas. Venesection may be useful, (SS).

2. Recent cases should be treated with purgation, āsthāpana and unctuous types of enema, sudation and administration of guggulu, (BR, BP).

Ref.: SS, nidāna, 1, 77; chikitsā, 5, 23; BP, BR, page. 327, 50.

Classical Prescriptions: Prasāriṇi-taila ; Simhanāda-guggulu; Vātāri-guggulu.

Kikkisa

Western Nosology: Linea nigra.

Casuative Factors:

Intrinsic: All three doshas, (CS).

Pathogenesis: In the eight month of pregnancy, the pressure of the growing foetus causes the three doshas to localise in the chest. The doshas then engender a burning sensation which leads to itching, and then to the formation of kikkisa, (CS).

Symptomatology: A thin stretch or line of wrinkled (or folds of) skin on the breasts, abdomen and thighs, (AD on AHr).

Treament:

1. The woman is administered fresh butter medicated with drugs having a sweet taste, along with a decoction of kola. Her breasts and abdomen should be gently massaged with pastes of chandana and mṛṇāla or with powders of sirīsha, dhātaki, sarshapa and yashṭi-madhu; a paste of kuṭaja, seed of ajaka, musta, and haridra; or a paste of nimba, kola, surasa and manjishṭha; or oil medicated with leaves of karavīra. The area should be sprinkled with a decoction of mālati and madhūka. The part should not be scratched as it may cause discolouration or injury. If the

itching is very severe, the part may be massaged or kneaded. The diet should consist of food articles which are sweet and alleviate vāta, with no salt and little amounts of oil or fat. Water should be taken in little quantity as anupana, (CS).

Ref.: CS, śārīra, 8, 32; AS, śārīra, 3, 9; AHṛ, śarīra, 1, 58.

Kilāsa

Synonyms: Sanskrit: Śvitra, Śveta-kushṭha

Western Nosology: Leucoderma, Vitiligo

Causative Factors:

Extrinsic: Evil deeds, evil done in the previous life and intake of incompatible food, (CS).

Intrinsic: Usually all three doshas, (CS).

Constituents Affected: Blood (CS, sūtra, 28, 11). The third layer of skin (CS, śārīra, 7,4). The fourth layer of skin (SS, śārīra, 4, 4).

Classification:

1. If the doshas are confined to the blood, there will be reddish discolouration of the skin. If the flesh (māmsa) is involved, the patient suffers from coppery discolouration. If the medas (fatty tissues) is affected, there will be white discolouration. The three kinds of kilāsa are dāruṇa, aruṇa and śvitra, (CS).

2. Kilāsa is but a variety of kushṭha, the difference between them being that kilāsa affects only the skin and does not exude any liquid. It is of three types, that which is engendered by vāta, by pitta and by kapha, (SS).

According to some authorities, only the skin is affected in kilāsa. When the other body elements are involved, the disease is known as śvitra. (NiS).

3. According to bhoja, śvitra is of two types, that which is caused by vitiation of the doshas and that which occurs due to mismanagement of vraṇa. The former type can be intrinsic or brought about by contact with persons suffering from śvitra, (NC).

Symptomatology:

1. If the blood is affected, there will be reddish discolouration of the skin. There will be coppery discolouration if flesh (mamsa) is affected and white discolouration if medas is involved, (CS).

2. If vāta is vitiated, the patient suffers from brownish circular patches, roughness of skin and desquamation (if rubbed). If pitta is vitiated, there will be discolouration resembling the petals of a lotus, and burning pains. In cases where the kapha is deranged, the discolouration will be white, oily (smooth), extensive and attended by itching, (SS).

3. In the pittaja type of kilāsa, there will be loss of hair (of the body), (AHṛ).

Prognosis:

1. Cases where the patches coalesce with each other, are extensive, and where the disease has lasted for more than an year are incurable. Dāruṇa is more difficult to cure than aruṇa while śvitra is easier to cure when compared to aruṇa.

Cases where the hairs are not reddish in colour, where the patches are limited and pale-white, slightly depressed at the centre and swollen, and which are recent are curable, (CS).

2. Cases where the discolouration occurs on the lips, palms, soles and anus, where they coalesce with each other and where the hairs turn reddish in colour and which arise after burns are incurable.

3. Cases where the hairs are black in colour are curable, (AS).

Ref.: CS, chikitsā, 7,173-177; SS, nidāna, 5, 17; AS, nidāna, 14; AHṛ, nidāna, 14.

Treatment:

1. The patient is first subjected to purification procedures such as emesis, etc. He is to be purged with juice of malāpu (kākodumbarika, Chkp.) with jaggery, oleated and should expose himself to the sun's rays. The purgative should be given for three days. When vesicles form on the affected area, they should be opened. The patient should then be administered for fifteen days, in the morning a decoction of asana, priyangu, śata-pushpa and kākodumbarika, or palāsa-kshāra with phāṇita. The measures indicated in kushṭha are also useful, especially the internal use of khadira.

The following plasters can be applied externally: the paste of manah-śila and bile of peacock; of kākodumbarika, avalguja, chitraka and cow's urine; of seeds of mūlaka, avalguja and cow's urine; of nilotpala, kushṭha, rock salt and horses' urine, of manahsila, viḍanga, kāsīsa, rochana, kanaka-pushpi (svarṇa-kshīri) and rock salt, etc.

Blood letting, rūkshana therapy and intake of saktu is also useful, (CS).

2. The patient is administered the tepid decoction of roots of bhadra (a variety of udumbara) and malāpu (is anointed with kaṭu-taila, NiS) and is exposed to the sun (after the digestion of the medicine, he is made to partake of gruel of dāḍima, NiS). Blisters would then form on the affected area, which after they burst, should be plastered with ash of the skin of a leopard or elephant and oil.

A cotton swab is soaked in a decoction of chūta (āmra) and harītaki, dipped in kaṭu-taila, and is made into a plug and lighted in a copper vessel being used as a lamp. The lamp black is triturated with milky exudation of vāṭa and a decoction of haritaki (seperately), and is applied over the patches of kilāsa, which should have previously been smeared over with kaṭu-taila. This procedure should be repeated many times.

The external application of peacock's bile or of hrīvera rubbed with the above bile is also useful (in śvitra), (SS).

3. According to Aruṇa-datta, the commentry on AHṛ, the term malayu (malapu according to CS and SS) refers to somarāji or bākuchi.

The patient is administered a decoction of the bark of phalgu and aksha mixed with the paste of indurāji (bākuchi) and made to stand in the sun until the formation of blisters. The diet should consist of butter-milk, without salt.

An earthern pot is smeared internally with ghee, and filled with chitraka, trikaṭu, cow's urine and honey. After a fortnight, this is administered to a patient of svitra. Bhṛgarāja is fried with oil in an iron vessel and administered to a patient followed by a decoction of milk and bījaka.

The tender sprouts of pūtika, arka, vyādhi-ghāta, and snuhi or of jāti are made into a paste with cow's urine and applied over the affected area. A paste of seeds of bakuchi and one-fourth the amount of harītala and cow's urine is also applied over the affected area, (AHṛ).

4. Purified kāsīsa, purified sulphur and purified mercury are trituarted with the juice of surasā (leaves of tulāsi). The paste that is obtained is heated in a crucible after being covered above and below with chāngeri (powder). After the crucible has cooled, the resulting product is powdered, and administered to the patient with honey and ghee, or curd and ghee or fresh butter, in doses measuring about seven or ten rice grains. The amount has to be gradually increased upto sixty-five rice grains. The patient is made to partake of juices of āmalaki, ārdaka, tinduka or fruit of kadali as adjuvants. This recipe is very useful in śvitra.

The powders of the leaves of nimba, haridra, pippali, and bākuchi are to be administered with milk in the early morning. Purified mercury, sulphur, tuttha bhasma, and tāmra bhasma are triturated with the decoction of bākuchi for twenty-four hours and are then administered to the patient with oil of bākuchi as adjuvant.

One part of mercury and two parts by weight of sulphur are triturated with lemon juice and smeared on three parts by weight of plates of purified copper. These are then subjected to heat by gaja puṭa. The mercury and sulphur (kajjali) are then again triturated with a decoction of khadira, of bākuchi and of nimba seperately and heated in gaja puṭa, each time. The drugs are then ground well, and are administered to a patient of kilāsa with a decoction of bākuchi (as adjuvant). The diet has to consist of rice and buttermilk.

The affected areas can be rubbed with the tender leaves of rakta-maṇḍala, and are then smeared with a paste of manah-śila, apāmārga and water. The pastes of kānchani and ankola-taila or of fruits of gunja, root of chitraka and kānji can also be applied externally. The oil obtained in a pātāla yantra from leaves or wood of ankola, nimba, and nirguṇḍi are also useful if applied over the affected area, (RRS).

Classical Prescriptions: Kilāsa

Madhūkāsava; Madhu-snuhi-rasāyana; Paṭola-mūlādi-kvātha-chūrṇa.

Śvitra: Avalgujādi-lepa; Ayaskṛti; Jyotishmati -taila; Kāśīsa-bhasma; Maṇi-bhadra-yoga; Rodhrāsava.

Ref.: CS, chikitsā, 7, 162-172; SS, chikitsā, 9, 15-26; AHṛ, chikitsā, 20, 1-18; RRS, 180-110.

Kotha

Synonyms: Ut-kotha (MN)

Western Nosology: Urticaria

Caustive Factors:

Extrinsic: Suppressing the urge to vomit (AHr); improper emesis (MN).

Intrinsic: Kapha and pitta (Chkp.).

Constituents Affected: Blood (CS, sūtra, 28,13)

Symptomatology: Transient reddish patches similar to those caused by the stings of a wasp. They are attended by itching, (Chkp.; Aruṇa-datta on AHṛ; MN, 50, 6).

Ref.: CS, chikitsā, 3, 108; AHr, sūtra, 4, 17.

Treatment: The patient is subjected to oleation, sudation and purificatory measures. He is administered medicine indicated in kushṭha, udarda and in amla-pitta.

Ghee medicated with leaves of nimba and āmalaki is useful, (CSS).

Ref.: CSS, Page. 622, 16-18.

See also Śīta-pitta.

Kroshṭuka-śīrsha

Synonyms: Sanskrit: Gairuva (Āḍhamalla on SaS, I, 7, 107)

Western Nosology: Arthritis of knee

Causative Factors:

Extrinsic: Factors which aggravate vāta

Intrinsic: Vāta

Constituents Affected: Blood

Symptomatology: An extremely painful swelling at the center of the knee joint, which resembles the head of a jackal.

Treatment:

1. The patient is to be treated on the same lines as in other vāta rogas. Venesection may also be carried out, (SŚ).

2. The patient may be administered guggulu with guḍūchi and triphala, or vṛddha-dāru with milk or castor oil, (CD).

Ref.: SS, nidāna, 1, 76; chikitsā, 5, 20; CD, 22, 62.

Kṛmi

Western Nosology: Worms; Helminthiasis

Causative Factors:

Extrinsic:

1. Indigestion, intake of food before the digestion of food previously taken, intake of harmful or dirty or undesirable and incompatible food, lack of exercise, sleeping during daytime, intake of food that is hard to digest, oily, cold, māsha, flour, vidāla, biśa, śālūka, parṇa-śāka (leafy vegetables), wine, supta, curds, milk, jaggery, sugarcane, paste of tila seeds, meat of aquatic animals, piṇyāka (oil cake of tila), pṛthuka and drinking of liquids that are sweet and sour, (SS).

2. Lack of cleanliness is the main cause for bāhya (external) malaja kṛmi.

The causative factors responsible for kushṭha are also responsible for kṛmi (blood-born parasites).

Intake of (excess) milk, jaggery, tila, fish,. meat of aquatic animals, flour products, paramānna (milk dishes), oil of kusumbha and food that is putrid, watery, unclean, incompatible, undsirable and disagreeable is responsible for the producion of kaphaja krimi and purīshaja krimi (parasites which occur in faeces), (CS).

Intrinsic: Kapha (CS), kapha and pitta (SS).

Constituents Affected: Parasites develop in the blood and faeces, (SS, CS).

Location: Parasites which are external (bāhya) are usually found in the regions of moustaches, hair of the head and body, eye lashes and clothing.

Blood born parasites are located within the blood vessels. Parasites which are kaphaja are found in the stomach (āmāsaya) primarily, and move in different directions later. Purīshaja krimi are usually located in the colon, (CS).

The parasites mainly originate in the stomach, colon, faeces, kapha and blood vessels, (SS).

The Form of the Parasites: Most of the purīshaja parasites (i.e. those found in the faeces) are white coloured and minute. A few are bigger and possess tails. One of them is reddish and elongated in shape. Parasites which originate in the vitiated kapha possess hairs either all over their body or only on the head, have tails and brownish circles on the body, are small, white-coloured and are shaped like fresh paddy sprouts (rūḍha-dhānyānkura). Parasites which origin ate from vitiated blood are reddish or black in colour, oily and thick, (SS).

Parasites which are found externally are minute, black or white in colour, have many legs and are similar in shape to that of tila. Blood-born parasites are minute, copper-coloured, rounded, devoid of legs and almost invisible. Parasites which originate in the vitiated kapha are white, thick and flat or rounded, white and coppery in colour and shaped like an earth-worm or white, minute, elongated and thin. Parasites which are seen in the feaces are minute, cylindrical, elongated, white-coloured and are like wool fibres, or are thick, cylindrical and grayish, blue, green or yellow in colour, (CS).

Classification:

1. There are twenty-kinds of parasites, seven of which are seen in the faeces (purīshaja kṛmi), six of them originate in the vitiated kapha and seven in the vitiated blood, (SS).

2. There are twenty kinds of pathogenic parasites, of which two are found externally (bāhya), six originate in the vitated blood, seven in the vitiated kapha and five are seen in the faeces, (CS).

Symptomatology:

1. The purīshaja kṛmi frequent the anal region, and produce pricking pain (in that region), abdominal colic, feeble digestion, anemia, flatulence, debility, salivation, tastelessness, heart disease and loose stools. One of them

causes itching of the anus, abdominal pain, rumbling in the abdomen, loose stools and weak digestion.

The kaphaja kṛmi eat into the bon--marrow, eyes, palate and ears and cause headache (śiro-soga), heart disease, vomiting, and catarrh.

Blood-born parasites cause diseases of the blood. (see Rakta-pradoshaja roga).

The general symptoms of parasite infestation are fever, discolouration, abdominal pain, heart-diseases, debility, vertigo, aversion to food, and diarrhoea, (SS).

2. External parasites (bāhya-malaja) cause itching and production of urticaria and pimples.

Blood-born parasites destroy hairs from the head, face, other parts of the body and eye-lashes, and nails. When they infect a wound or ulcer, they produce horripilation, itching, pricking pain, and formication. If they are present in large numbers, they destroy (eat away) the skin, blood-vessels, ligaments, flesh and cartilages.

Parasites which take their origin fom vitiated kapha cause nausea, salivation, tastelessness, indigestion, fever, unconsciousness, yawning, sneezing, flatuence, body pain, vomiting, emaciation and roughness (of skin).

Parasites which are seen in the faeces engender loose stools, emaciation, roughness (of skin) and horripilation. They are present in the anal region and cause itching of the anus. They also frequently come out of the anus, (CS).

3. Purīshaja krimi also cause anemia, (AHṛ).

Ref.: SS, uttara, 54; CS, vimāna, 7, 9-13; AHṛ, nidāna, 14, 42-53.

Treatment:

1. The patient should first be oleated, and then made to vomit by administering ghee medicated with drugs of the surasādi group and given a strong purgative. He is then given an āsthāpana enema with a decoction of yava, kola, kulattha, drugs of surasādi group mixed with salt, oil or ghee, and viḍanga. The patient is then washed with warm water, and administered food medicated with kṛmighna (anti-parasite) drugs.

The following formulations are useful: the juice of sirīsha and kiṇibhi (kaṭabhi, NiS) with honey; juice of kevuka with honey, a diet consisting of sharp (tikshṇa) drugs; the juice or paste of seeds of palāśa with rice water; the juice of leaves of pāribhadra with honey; the juice of pattura or of drugs of surasādi group (with honey); powder of viḍanga with honey; pūpalika (cakes) prepared with a paste of barley, and leaves of mūshika-parṇi followed by dhānyāmla (kānji, NiS); oil medicated with drugs of surasādi group (for internal use); dishes prepared with viḍanga (and paste of yava, NiS); the oil expressed from tila seeds which have been previously soaked in a decoction of viḍanga; the fine powders of iron, copper, silver, tin or lead should be soaked seven times each in decoctions of triphala and viḍanga, and are then administered with honey; paste of roots of pippali with goat's urine; and tin (bhasma) should be taken for a week with dadhi-mastu (upper layer of curds).

Patients suffering from worm-infestation in the head, heart, nose, ears, eyes, etc. should be administered errhines, collyrium and avapīḍa errhines. The powders of iron, etc., should be blown into the nostrils (pradhamana). Oil medicated with drugs of the surasādi group is left for some time in a vessel of kānsya (bell-metal). When the inner surface becomes blue, the oil is stirred well and used as an errhine. In cases where the hairs have been affected, the measures indicated in indralupta are useful. The treatment advised for mukha-rogas is useful in cases where the teeth are affected by parasites. Cases of raktaja kṛmi (blood-born parasites) are treated as in cases of kushṭha.

The drugs of the surasādi group, bitter and pungent food and soup of kulattha are useful in most cases of kṛmi. The following substances are injurious in this disease: milk, meat-dishes, ghee, curd, leafy vegetables and cold, sweet and salty food articles, (SS).

2. Parasites which are external should be extracted (removed); scrupulous cleanliness is enjoined on the patient, who has to avoid such regimen which produce parasites.

In all cases of kṛmi, these are the general lines of treatment: removal or extraction of the parasites, factors responsible for the growth and proliferation of parasites should be removed, and the casuative factors should be avoided.

Parasites (which are external) may be removed by the hands or with appropriate instruments. Those which are situated internally may be removed by errhines, emesis, purgation or āsthāpana (type of enema). Factors responsible for the growth of parasites can be counter-acted by (regular) use of drugs which are pungent, bitter, astringent, alkaline (kshāra) and hot, and which alleviate kapha.

The patient should be oleated and given sudation for six or seven days, and is later made to partake of milk, jaggery, curds, tila, fish, meat of aquatic animals, flour products, sweet dishes, oil of kusumbha, etc., both in the morning and evening for a day. This is in order to stimulate the parasites and entice them into the alimentary tract. If the patient gets good sleep that night, and after the food has been fully digested, the patient is administered āsthāpana enema, emesis and purgation, all in a day, if the patient is found to be strong enough.

The decoctions of mūlaka, sarshapa, laśuna, karanja, śigru, etc., or of arka, alarka, kuṭaja, aāhaki, kushṭha, madana-phala, etc., may be used for administering āsthāpana enema. The decoction of madana-phala and pippali and paste of trivṛt is useful for inducing both emesis and purgation. The patient is then washed with a warm decoction of viḍanga, made to reside in a room which is not exposed to draughts of air, and is given yavāgu (gruel) of pippali, root of pippali, chavya, chitraka and ginger. After the patient is well enough to partake of vilepi (a kind of gruel), he is subjected to anuvāsana enema with oil of viḍanga. A decoction of viḍanga should be used instead of water, for all purposes.

In cases where the parasites have affected the head, the patient is oleated, fomented and given errhines of dehusked seeds of apāmārga, etc.

In order to render the body resistant to the growth of parasites, the patient is given the juices of the following plants, either singly or in combination, with honey on an empty stomach in the morning: mārkava (bhringarāja), arka, sahachara, nirguṇḍi, bakula, kuṭaja, apāmārga, kirāta tikta, āmalaka, harītaki and vibhītaki.

Fresh tila collected in autumn should be cleaned, washed well, soaked in a tepid decoction of viḍanga until all the dirt is removed and then dehusked. It is then cleaned again, immersed twenty-one times in the decoction of viḍanga, dried in the sun, and rubbed in a mortar and made into a fine paste on a stone slab. This paste should be kept in a vessel, sprinkled over and over again with the decoction of viḍanga, and crushed with the hands until an oil is extracted. This oil is very useful in removing the susceptibility to worms.

Stems of bhallātaka are crushed and placed in an earthen vessel smeared with oil or ghee internally, and which has many minute holes at the bottom. The vessel is covered with a lid, wrapped all over except at the bottom, and is placed over another strong vessel which is also to be smeared with oil or ghee internally and is buried underground, upto its neck. The apparatus is then exposed to heat (by means of dried cow dung cakes). When the cakes are burnt, the oil is collected from the lower vessel. This oil is mixed with half its quantity of dehusked seeds of viḍanga and is kept exposed to the sun for one day. This oil if administered in the correct dosage causes good purgation. After a certain period of time, the patient is subjected to anuvāsana enema, (CS).

3. Yavāgu (gruel) prepared from viḍanga, taṇḍula (rice), trikaṭu, śigru, maricha,

suvarchala and butter-milk is useful. Thin rice gruel (maṇḍa) medicated with viḍanga and trikaṭu is also useful. In intestinal worms, the patient is advised to eat jaggery followed by the paste of pārasīka-yavāni and stale water which is to be taken in the morning, (CSS).

4. Pārada bhasma if administered with a paste of the tender leaves of nimba and honey is very efficacious in this disease, (RRS).

Ref.: SS, uttara, 5, 20-40; CS, vimāna, 7, 10, 11, 14-30; CSS, page. 187-188; RRS, 30, 54.

Classical Prescriptions: Dantyārishṭa; Kānkāyana-guṭika; Khadirārishṭa; Kṛmi-mudgara-rasa; Loha-bhasma; Maṇi-bhadra-yoga; Rasa-karpūra; Rasa-pushpa; Vanga-bhasma; Viḍanga-lauha.

Kshata-kshīṇa

Synonyms: Sanskrit: Urah-kshata; Urah-kshata-śosha, (SS).

Western Nosology: Suppurative lung disease: Pyothorax.

Causative Factors:

Extrinsic:

1. Lifting heavy weights, excessive exertion (such as stringing a bow), wrestling with a stronger opponent, falling from a height, forcibly restraining a speeding animal, injury by a stone or log of wood or by a blunt weapon, reciting loudly or at a high pitch, running at a fast pace, or alongside horses, swimming across big rivers, jumping from a height, dancing for long stretches of time, excessive sexual intercourse, habitual intake of dry and meagre amount of food, (CS).

2. Excessive exertion, lifting heavy weights, overstudying, excessive coitus, injury (especially to the chest) and strenuous activity mainly involving the chest, (SS).

Symptomatology:

1. The causative factors engender lesions within the chest, which leads to breaking and splitting pains in the chest, ulcerations within the chest cavity, oppression of (or narrowing) the sides of the chest, emaciation, tremors (or pulsations), gradual decline of strength, vitality, complexion and appetite, fever, pain or uneasiness, mental prostration, diarrhoea and feeble digestion. There is also cough with expectoration of blood-streaked mucous which is foul-smelling, blackish or yellow in colour, lumpy and copious. The patient emaciates excessively, and sufffers from depletion of ojas (resistance to disease) and sexual power.

The particular or distinctive symptoms are chest pain, vomiting of blood, constant cough, passing of bloody urine (haematuria) and pain in the back, waist and sides of the chest, (CS).

2. There are internal lesions in the chest, which lead to expectoration of putrid and bloody sputum, cough with vomiting of mucous that is blackish brownish, yellow or bloody, severe pain (in the chest) which may even cause fainting, burning within the chest, hoarseness, loss of complexion and bad breath, (SS).

Prognosis: A recent case, in a strong person, with good digestion and where only few symptoms are present is curable. If the disease has lasted for more than a year, it can only be palliated. It is incurable if all the symptoms are present, (CS).

Related Disease: Rāja-yakshma.

Ref.: CS, chikitsā, 11, 4-14; SS, uttara, 41, 24-26.

Treatment:

1. A person suffering from this disease has to be treated on the same lines as indicated for rāja-yakshma, (SS).

2. Immediately after the diagnosis is made, the patient should be administered milk medicated with lāksha and honey. After the

digestion of this medicine, he can partake of his meal with milk and sugar. This medicine should be taken with surā if the patient suffers from pain in the chest, the sides and hypogastric region, and feeble digestion. It can be administered along with ativisha, musta, pāṭha and kuṭaja, if the patient suffers from diarrhoea. A patient with strong digestive powers should be administered milk boiled with lāksha, ghee, bee's wax, sugar-candy, vamśa-lochana, wheat flour (samitam) and drugs of the jīvanīya group.

Milk boiled with ikshvālika, bisa (lotus stalk), pippali roots, padma-kesara, and chandana and mixed with honey, is useful in promoting the healing of the lesions.

If there is fever and burning pain, the patient can be given powder of yava boiled with milk and ghee or fried barley powder with honey and sugar or with milk.

If there is cough with pain in the bones and sides of the chest, a paste of yashṭi-madhu, madhūka, drākshā, dālchini, vamśa-lochana, pippali, balā, honey and ghee can be administered.

Pills prepared from powders of one-half tola each of ela, teja-patra and dālchini, one-half pala of pippali, one pala each of sugar-candy, yashṭi-madhu, kharjūra and mṛdvīka, and honey are to be used regularly.

A patient suffering from haemoptysis can be administered hen's egg with gruel or water; sparrow's egg; blood of goat or desert animal; powders of punarnava, red rice, sugar with grape juice, milk and ghee; or milk boiled with taṇḍulīyaka, yashṭi-madhu and madhūka.

If there is flatulence and distension, the patient can partake of goat's fat fried in surā and mixed with rock salt. A person who is emaciated can take the paste of wheat and barley powder, sugar, honey, jīvaka and ṛshabaka, followed by a draught of boiled milk. The soup of the flesh of carnivorous animals, seasoned with ghee, and mixed with pippali and honey is useful in enhancing flesh and blood. The patient can also partake of boiled rice with ghee extracted from milk that has been medicated with vaṭa, udumbara, aśvattha, plaksha, sāla, priyangu, tāla-mastaka priyāla, padmaka and aśvakarṇa. Ghee prepared from an equal amount of milk, a decoction of madhu-yashṭi, and nāgabala and paste of payasya, pippali and vamśa-lochana is also very useful. Similarly, ghee medicated with eight parts of milk, juice of balā and lāksha and paste of kaṭvanga, bark of dāru-haridra, bark and seeds of kuṭaja is also useful. One prastha of ghee is boiled with one prastha of a decoction of drāksha, eight palas of yashṭi-madhu, and eight palas of pippali. After it has cooled, it has to be mixed with eight palas each of honey and sugar. This ghee has to be administered with an equal quantity of śaktu (fried barley powder). Equal amounts of ghee, āmalaki fruit, vidāri, ikshu, drugs of jīvanīya group, goat's milk and cow's milk are boiled together. After it has cooled, an equal amount of honey and sugar are added. This medicated ghee is very useful in many diseases, including kshata-kshīṇa.

All these kinds of ghee can be rolled into boluses after mixing them with vamśalochana, sugar and lājā powder and honey. These boluses can be administered to patients of kshata-kshīṇa, followed by a draught of milk. It increases strength, nourishment and vitality.

If the patient also suffers from fever and cough, he can be administered milk boiled with pippali and sugar or a paste of pippali, sugar, honey and ghee. In cases where sexual over indulence has been the cause, a gruel prepared from sugarcane juice, juice of vidāri, ghee and sour fruits can be administered. A patient who is accustomed to barley can partake of a mantha (drink) prepared from fried and powdered barley, honey and ghee. Meat juices of desert animals can be fried in ghee, medicated with drugs of jīvanīya group and taken with sugar.

The patient can also partake of meat-juices of cow, buffalo, horse or elephant, with gruel (yūsha) seasoned with sour fruits, and ghee with meal of barley. If the patient has poor digestion, he should be given food articles that are appetizing and digestive.If he suffers from diarrhoea, substances that are grāhi (constipative) can be used.

The patient can also take daily for a month the juice of nāgabala root with milk beginning with half a tola and increasing gradually until a dose of one pala is reached. The diet should consist of only milk. He can also take similar courses of manḍūka-parni, nāgara or yashṭi-madhu.

The diet in a case of kshata-kshīṇa should consist of food that is non-irritant, light, cold and nourishing. The diet that has been prescribed for patients of rāja-yakshma, kāsa, and rakta-pitta can be prescribed in this disease also.

Formulations such as amṛta-prāśa-ghṛta, svadamśtrādi-ghṛta, five types of sarpi-guḍa, saindhavādi churṇa and a shāḍava preparation are also useful.

This disease, if neglected, will soon progress to rāja-yakshma, (CS).

Ref.: SS, uttara, 41; CS, chikitsā, 11, 15-95.

Classical Prescripions: Amṛta-prāśa-ghṛta; Chyavana-prāśa; Chagalyādi-ghṛta; Drākshārishṭa; Kūshmāṇḍa-rasāyana; Nirguṇḍi-ghṛta; Vaikrānta-bhasma; Vidāryādi-ghṛta.

Ksīrālasaka

Western Nosology: Lactose intolerance

Causative Factors:

Extrinsic: Drinking breast milk that is vitiated by all the three deranged doshas.

Type: This disease affects only breast fed infants.

Symptomatology: Such infants who feed on breast milk have painful diarrhoea with watery, undigested, offensive stools of varied colours. They also suffer from yellow-white urine, thirst, fever, vomiting, yawning, hiccoughs (dry eructation), loss of appetite, vertigo, restlessness, moaning, inflammation of eyes and mouth, rolling of eyes, etc.

Prognosis: This disease is very difficult to cure.

Ref.: AS,uttara, 2.

Kukūnaka

Western Nosology: Ophthalmia; Trachoma,

Causative Factors:

Intrinsic:

1. Aggravated kapha, vāta, pitta and vitiated blood, (SS).

2. Aggravated kapha and vitiated blood, (KS).

Extrinsic: Unhealthy breast milk, (SS, KS).

Symptomatology: This is a disease affecting the eyelids and occuring only in childen (SS, KS, AHṛ).

1. There is severe itching of the akshi-kūta (orbital margin, eye ball or super-ciliary ridge), photophobia and constant lacrimation. The child frequently rubs its eyes, nose and forehead, (SS).

2. In this disease which usually occurs at the time of dentition, the eyes of the infant will be swollen, infected and slimy (watery). There will be pain and difficulty in opening the eyes. The pain may also extend to the ears, nose and the orbital region (AHr).

Ref.: SS, uttara, 19, 9; KS, siddhi, 13, 3-8; AHṛ, uttara, 8, 19-20.

Treatment:

1. In this disease, blood-letting can be done (by using leeches), and the eyelids are to be scraped, and then anointed with the paste of trikaṭu and honey. The wet-nurse (or mother) should also be treated for unhealthy breast milk. The infant who is being only breast-fed

should be made to vomit by administering breast-milk mixed with fruits of khara-manjari (apāmārga), honey and rock-salt or mixed with pippali, rock-salt and honey. But these drugs should not be given if the infant suffers from vomiting.

The child who feeds on both breast-milk and semi-solid food should be made to vomit by giving milk medicated with vachā. While the child who feeds only on solid food (and is not breast-fed) should be given the fruits of madana (with or without milk). The eyes should be washed with a decoction of leaves of āmalaki, jambu, aśmantaka and āmra. Ghee medicated (boiled) with guḍūchi or triphala should be used in the form of eye drops. The pastes of manahśila, maricha, śankha, rasānjana, rock-salt, jaggery and honey, or of mūrva, yashṭi and āmraka or of black loha-chūrṇa, ghee, milk and honey; the powders of trikaṭu, palāṇḍu, yashṭi, rock-salt, lāksha and gairika or of leaves of nimba, copper powder, lodhra, yashṭi and dārvi can also be applied on the eyelids, (SS).

2. If the child is still being breast-fed, the mother or wet-nurse is given ghee medicated with khadira, śreshṭa and nimba leaves. Emesis should be done by administering pippali, yashṭi, sarshapa and rock-salt. She can also be purged (mildly) by using a decoction of harītaki, pippali and drāksha. The paste of mustā, haridra, dāru-haridra and pippali (kṛshṇa) should be applied on the breasts. The breasts should also be fumigated by burning ghee and sarshapa. A decoction of paṭola, musta, mṛdvika, guḍūchi and triphala is then given internally. The eyelids of the child can also be gently scraped, (AHṛ).

Ref.: SS, uttara, 19, 10-15; KS, khila, 13; AHṛ, uttara, 9, 24-33.

Ku-nakha

Synonyms: Sanskrit - Kunilam (SS)

Western Nosology: Onychomycosis

Causative Factors: Extrinsic: Trauma

Constituents Affected: Asthi (bones), (SS).

Symptomatology: Due to injury, the nails become dry, blackish and hard, (SS).

Note: Kunakha is a modified type of chippa where the doshas are only slightly vitiated, (CSS).

Treatment:

1. The patient is to be treated as indicated in the treatment of chippa, (SS).

2. The diseased nail has to be surgically removed, and the area is cauterised. An application of a paste of an equal quantity of milky exudation of snuhi and ṭankana is useful, (RRS).

3. The external application of ṭankana is almost infallible. Binding the affected finger with tender leaves of kāśmari will prove beneficial, (CSS).

Ref.: SS, nidāna, 13, 22; chikitsā, 20, 11; sūtra, 24, 9; RRS, 25, 6; CSS, page. 659.

Kushṭha

Western Nosology: Skin diseases, including leprosy; pellagra: etc.

Causative Factors:

Extrinsic:

1. Transgressing the rules of hygiene (sad-vṛtta), excessive intake of incompatible, disagreeable and harmful food, intake of food before the digestion of food previously taken, intake of food that is hard to digest, and milk regularly with meat of aquatic and domesticated animals, bathing in cold water immediately after being in the hot sun, exertion and sexual intercourse just after oleation or emesis, and suppression of the urge to vomit.

Kushṭha is a contagious disease which spreads from one person to another by contact, use of same clothing, by breath, by eating together, by sharing the same bed, etc.

A person who kills good and just persons and women, commits theft, and such other impious acts may also suffer from kushṭha, (SS).

Sudden changes from cold to hot and vice versa, and from nourishment to emaciation, excessive and frequent intake of honey, phāṇita, fish, lakucha, mūlaka and kākamāchi before the digestion of food previously taken, intake of milk with the chilichima fish, intake of food comprising of hāyānaka, yavaka, chinaka, uddālaka and koradūsha along with milk, curds, buttermilk, kola, kulattha, māsha, atasi and oil of kusumbha, excessive indulgence in sexual intercourse, excessive exertion and exposure to the sun after partaking of the above food articles in excess, contact of cold water just after experiencing fear, fatigue and anguish, intake of food that causes burning pain (vidāhi) without vomiting out the undigested food, suppresing the urge to vomit, and excessive oleation (snehana).

Intake of incompatible food articles, excessive indulgence in new rice, curds, fish, tila, salt, sour food, māsha, mūlaka, flour products, milk, jaggery and food that is oily, hard to digest and liquid, suppression of the natural urges, over-eating, improper fasting, sleeping during the daytime, and abuse of purificatory procedures (pancha-karma), (CS).

Intrinsic: All three doshas (CS). All three doshas and parasites, (SS, nidāna, 5, 6).

Constituents Affected: Blood (CS, sūtra, 28, 11); skin, flesh, blood and lymph (CS, nidāna, 5, 3).

Location:

The third and fourth layers of the skin, (CS, śārīra, 7, 4).

The sidhma type of kushṭha affects the first layer of the skin (third layer according to CS, ibid), the various kinds of kilāsa-kūshṭha affect the fourth layer, while the rest of the kushṭhas involve the fifth layer of skin, (SS, sārira, 4, 4).

Classification:

1. There are eighteen types of kusṭhas, among which seven belong to the major kushṭha, and eleven are of the minor variety (kshudra-kushṭha), (SS).

2. There is no kustha that results from the vitiation of only one dosha. However, even though all kushṭhas arise due to the vitiation of all three doshas, each varies from the other with regard to the degree of vitiation of the dosha, the location of the disease, the nature of pain, colour, shape, symptoms, etc. They can therefore be classified into seven, eighteen or innumerable types, (CS, nidāna, 5, 4).

Prodromal Symptoms:

1. Roughness of the skin, sudden horripilation, itching, excessive or total absence of sweating, numbness of any part of the body, black discoloration of blood, breaking down (of the affected part) and spreading (from one part to another), (SS).

2. Excessive or total absence of sweating, roughness or extreme oilyness (of the skin), discolouration (of skin), itching, pricking pain, numbness, burning pain, horripilation, induration, feeling of (local) heat, heaviness, frequent swelling which spreads, excessive formation of excreta in body orifices, suppuration or failure to heal of even trifling wounds, and severe pain in burns, suppurating wounds, bites (or insects, animals, etc.,), fractures or dislocations, and injuries, (CS, nidāna, 5, 7).

Appearances of koṭha, debility, fatigue without exertion, and rapid occurence of ulcers which are slow to heal, (CS, chikitsā, 7, 11-12).

Symptomatology:

1. The mahā-kushṭhas (major skin diseases) are of seven types:

(a) Aruṇa-kushṭha - There is predominance of vitiated vāta. The eruption is brownish in colour, thin, spreading in nature and is attended by pricking pain and numbness.

(b) Audumbara kushṭha - There is predominance of deranged pitta. The eruption is similar in colour and shape to the ripe fruits of udumbara.

(c) Ṛshya-jihva kushṭha - There is predominance of deranged pitta. The eruption is rough and resembles the tongue of the deer (ṛshya).

(d) Kapāla kushṭha - The eruption resembles black pieces of burnt clay (kapālika). This type is also characterised by predominance of aggravated pitta.

(e) Kākaṇaka kushṭha- This is marked by predominance of vitiated pitta. The eruption is intensely red with black markings, like the fruits of gunja.

The last four diseases have the common features of burning and sucking pain, and a feeling as if hot fumes are being emitted from them, speedy growth and suppuration and infestation with parasites.

(f) Puṇḍarīka kushṭha - The eruption is similar to the leaves of the white lotus.

(g) Dadru kushṭha - The eruption consists of pustules (piḍaka) which are spreading in nature, and are either coppery or coloured like the flowers of atasi.

Both these eruptions are elevated, circular, are marked by itching and are slow in developing. They are both caused by vitiated kapha.

The minor skin diseases are eleven in number:

(a) Sthūlārushka kushṭha - Deep seated, hard and big ulcers around the joints. These are difficult to cure.

(b) Mahā kushṭha - Contraction, bursting and numbness of the skin with general debility.

(c) Eka kushṭha - Reddish-black discolouration of skin.

(d) Charma-dala kushṭha-Itching, pain, burning and sucking pain in the palms and soles.

(e) Visarpa kushṭha - The eruptions rapidly spread all over like visarpa and affect the skin, blood, flesh, causing unconsciousness, burning pain, restlessness and pricking pain and later suppurate.

(f) Parisarpa kushṭha - A number of exuding pustules gradually spread all over the body.

(g) Sidhma kushṭha - White and small discolouration of skin (or eruptions) which are painless, are attended by itching and usually affect only the upper part of the body.

Sidhma kushṭha is of two types - one of them called pushpikā-sidhma is easily curable, and has therefore been included in the list of minor skin diseases. The other type is difficult to cure, and has been described under major skin diseases in CS, (NiS).

(h) Vicharchika kushṭha - Streaks or cracks all over the body which are dry, extremely painful and are accompanied by intense itching; and Vipādika - painful cracks on the feet (soles) which cause itching and burning sensation.

(i) Kiṭibha kushṭha-The eruptions are rounded, thick, oily, blackish in colour, and are attended by oozing and severe itching.

(j) Pāmā kushṭha - Small pustules with exudation, itching and burning pains; and Kacchū - similar kind of pustules along with burning vesicles which are mainly confined to the buttocks, hands and feet.

(k) Rakasa - Itching and dry pustules spread all over the body.

Among these eleven minor skin diseases, sthulārushka, sidhma, rakasa, mahā-kushṭha and eka-kushṭha are caused by vitiated kapha, while parisarpa is engendered by deranged vāta. The rest are caused by aggravated pitta.

Although kushṭha in the early stages is confined to the skin (rasa-dhātu), it spreads to all the other dhātus if neglected.

If the disease is confined to the skin (and rasa-dhātu), there will be numbness, sweating, slight itching, discolouration and roughness. When the blood is also affected, the patient experiences numbness, horripilation, sweating, itching and presence of pus (or foul odour, NiS). If the flesh (māmsa-dhātu) is affected, there will be thickness of the circular patches, dryness of mouth, roughness, eruption of pustules, and vesicles, pricking pain and hardness (induration); when the medas (fatty tissue) is involved, foul odour, increase in waste products, pus formation, parasites and breaking pain all over the body are present. When both bones and bone-marrow are affected, there will be sinking of the nasal bridge (nāsa-bhanga), eye diseases, hoarseness and presence of worms in the ulcers or eruptions. When the śukra (reproductive elements) is involved, the patient suffers from deformity of hands (and limbs), loss of power of locomotion, breaking pain or destruction of the body, and formation of ulcers all over the body.

A child born of parents both of whom are stricken with kushṭha, also suffers from the disease, (SS).

2. The symptoms of the seven major skin diseases are:

(a) Kapāla kushṭha - The eruptions are dry, brownish or black in colour, resemble pieces of an earthern jar, are filled with parasites, are uneven in shape with rough edges, thin and elevated in the periphery, numb, with horripilation, intense pricking pain, slight itching, pus formation, serous exudation and burning, and rapid in growth and suppuration.

(b) Audumbara kushṭha - The eruptions are thick, copper-coloured, filled with parasites and covered over wih coppery, rough hairs. There is excessive thick pus, blood and serous exudation, itching, sticky secretion, kotha, burning pain, inflammation and fever. They are rapid in growth and suppuration, and resemble the ripe fruit of udumbara in colour.

(c) Maṇḍala kushṭha - The eruptions are oily, heavy, swollen with a smooth, firm, yellow, margin, are white and red in colour, covered over with large quantities of white hairs, and exude copious, thick, slimy and white fluid. There is also sticky exudation and itching. They are infested with worms, are circular in shape and tardy in growth, development and suppuration, and are connected to one another.

(d) Ṛshyajihva kushṭha - The eruptions are rough, brownish or tawny in colour, darkish-gray at the centre and margins, and may be tinged with blue, yellow or copper colour. There is intense burning, pricking and cutting pains, a feeling as if a splinter is present within (the eruption), and less of itching, exudation and worm infestation. The eruptions are rapid in growth and development, are elevated at the centre and thin at the margins, are covered over with rough pustules, and are elongated and circular, like the tongue of a deer.

(e) Puṇḍarīka kusṭha - The eruptions are reddish white in colour, red at the periphery, are swol' ɜn, covered over with a network of red blood vessels, are rapid in growth and suppuration and resemble the petals of a lotus flower. There is excessive, thick reddish pus and serous exudation, itching, burning and inflammation. Worms may also be present.

(f) Sidhma kushṭha - The eruptions are rough, brownish in colour, fissured and thin at the margins, oily in the centre, have a tinge of white and red, and are sluggish in growth and ulceration. There is less of pain, itching, burning, pus formation, serous exudation and worms. They appear in large numbers and resemble the flowers of alābu in colour.

(g) Kākaṇa kushṭha - In the early stage the eruptions resemble the fruits of gunja and later manifest all the symptoms of the other skin diseases. There is severe pain. There are symptoms caused by all the three doshas.

The symptoms of the eleven minor skin diseases:

(a) Eka-kushṭha - Big eruptions resembling scales of a fish, absence of perspiration.

(b) Charma-kushṭha - The skin is thick, like the skin of an elephant.

(c) Kiṭimam - The eruption is gray coloured, rough and harsh, with callousities (of the skin).

(d) Vipādika - Cracking with severe pain of the skin of the soles and palms.

(e) Alasaka - The skin is covered with itching, inflamed lumps.

(f) Dadru - (Tinea circinata) Elevated circular eruptions with pustules, itching and redness.

(g) Charma-dala -(Erythroderma; Dermatitis) The skin is red, painful, tender, itches, is filled with vesicles and peels off.

(h) Pāma -(Scabies) Numerous pustules which are white, brown or grayish in colour, attended with itching.

(i) Visphoṭa - The skin is thin, and covered with white and brownish vesicles.

(j) Śatāru - There are numerous reddish or grey ulcers with burning pain.

(k) Vicharchika - (Pustular dermatitis) Grayish-black pustules with itching and copious exudation.

Of the seven major skin diseases, kapāla, maṇḍala and audumbara are engendered by vāta, kapha and pitta respectively, while ṛshyajihva, puṇḍarika and sidhma are caused by vāta-pitta, kapha-pitta and vāta-kapha respectively. Kākaṇaka is caused by vitiation of all three doshas.

Among the minor skin diseases; charma-kushṭha, eka-kushṭha, kiṭima, vipādika and alasaka are engendered by vāta and kapha, while pāma, śatāru, visphoṭa, dadru and charma-dala are caused by vitiation of pitta and kapha. The vitiated kapha is responsible for vicharchika, (CS).

Prognosis:

1. The disease that is confined to the rasa (skin), blood and flesh, and that occurs in a person with self control is curable.

The disease that involves the medas (fatty tissues) can be palliated. The other cases are regarded as being incurable, (SS).

2. The disease that occurs in a debilitated person and which exhibits all the symptoms is incurable. The kākaṇaka type is also incurable. Even the curable types are difficult to cure if the patient is wrongly treated or if the disease is ignored. The cases where there is debility, fever, thirst, burning pain, weakness of digestion, diarrhoea, and where the flesh etc. is eaten away by maggots are incurable.

The diseases engendered by vāta-pitta or kapha-pitta are difficult to cure while those caused by vāta-kapha or any one dosha are easy to cure, (CS).

Complications: If even the curable types of kushtha are neglected, maggots (worms) begin to infect the skin, flesh, blood, serous fluid, etc., and further vitiate the doshas, bringing about the following complications:

In vātaja kushṭha, blackish or brown discolouration (of skin), roughness and dryness, pain, emaciation, pricking pain, trembling, horripilation, contraction, debility, stiffness, numbness, fissures and ulceration.

In pittaja kushtha, burning, sweating, oozing, kotha, exudation, redness and suppuration.

In kaphaja kushṭha, white patches, coldness,

itching, stiffness, heaviness, swelling, oilyness and stickiness (upalepa).

The maggots eat away the skin, flesh, blood, fatty tissues, blood vessels, ligaments, bones and cartilages, (CS, nidāna, 5, 10).

Ref.: SS, nidāna, 5, 3-16, 20-34; CS, nidāna, 5 ; chikitsā, 7, 13-30; 37-38.

Treatment:

1. When the prodromal symptoms make their appearance, the patient is administered emesis and purgation (after oleation and sudation). If only the skin (rasa-dhātu) is affected, plasters (ālepa) of cleansing (śodhana) drugs are applied. If the blood is also involved, application of plasters of purifying (śodhana) drugs, decoctions (for internal use), and blood letting are useful. When the flesh is affected, application of plasters of purifying drugs, decoctions (for internal use), blood letting, and use of arishṭas, manthas and prāśa are beneficial. When the medas has been affected, purificatory procedures, blood letting and medicines prepared from bhallātaka, śilājatu, mākshika, guggulu, agaru, tuvaraka, khadira, asana and ayaskṛti are useful in palliating the disease.

In the early stages of kushṭha, a patient with aggravation of vāta should be advised ghee or oil medicated with meshaśṛngi (karkaṭa-śṛngi, NiS), gokshura, śārngeshṭa, guḍūchi and drugs of the daśamūla group for massage and internal use; a person with pittaja-kushṭha, is administered ghee medicated with dhava, aśva-karṇa, kakubha, palāśa, nimba, parpāṭaka, yashṭi-madhu, lodhra and samanga; while a patient of kaphaja kushṭha is given ghee medicated with priyāla, śāla, āragvadha, nimba, sapta parṇa, chitraka, maricha, vachā, and kushṭha or with bhallātaka, harītaki and viḍanga. The oil extracted from, or medicated with tuvaraka and bhallātaka can be used in all cases of kushṭha (for snehana).

The patient should then be subjected to (judicious) sudation (svedana). Venesection can also be carried out.

The elevated patches of kushṭha should be scraped with samudra-phena or leaves of śākha, goji or kākodumbarika, and anointed with a paste, of haritāla, manahśila, milky juice of arka, tila, śigru and maricha, etc.

In a case of dadru, a plaster of lāksha, kushṭha, sarshapa, gum-resin of sarala, haridra, trikaṭu and seeds of chakra-marda is effective. The plaster composed of rock-salt, seeds of chakra-marda, bakula, rasānjana and juice of kapittha is also efficacious.

A patient suffering from kushṭha should be administered emetics once a fortnight and a purgative once a month. Blood letting should be done twice a year (not profusely), and errhines can be used every fourth day.

The recipes (for internal use) useful in kushṭha are: paste of harītaki, trikaṭu, jaggery and oil; paste of āmalaki, harītaki, vibhītaki, pippali, viḍanga, honey and ghee; paste of haridra and cow's urine, to be taken for a month; paste of chitraka or rasānjana or pippali with cow's urine for a month (rasānjana should also be used for external application); paste of trivṛt and honey in cases of burning pain; old mudga is boiled in a docoction of nimba and is administered with oil in case of sloughing; and a decoction of nimba or of arka, alarka and saptaparṇa in patients having maggots.

If any part of the body is being eaten away by maggots (parasites), a paste of root of aśvamāra, viḍanga and cow's urine is applied over the affected area, and cow's urine is sprinkled over the body. Viḍanga should be taken regularly with food. The affected parts can be rubbed with the oil of karanja, or sarshapa, śigru or kośāmra or with oil medicated with drugs that are pungent, bitter and hot.

Khadira is extremely useful in all cases of kushṭha.

A paste of drugs of the lākshādi group, and cow's bile is boiled with cow's urine and oil, and it is then preserved within the kaṭukālābu gourd for a week. A patient of kushṭha should use the oil both externally and internally, while at the same time exposing his body to the sun. After elimination of the doshas from the system, he is bathed with a decoction of khadira, and made to partake of gruel (yavāgu) medicated with khadira decoction. Oil or ghee medicated with drugs of the śodhana group or kushṭhaghna group is used externally every morning. This procedure is extremely efficacious in all cases of kushṭha and even in parasitic forms.

The following diet and regimen are beneficial: śāli (old rice), rice that is harvested in sixty days, barley, wheat, koradūsha, śyāmāka, uddālaka, soup or gruel of mudga, āḍhaki, etc., mixed with leaves of nimba, and ārushkara; ghee or sarshapa oil medicated with flowers of maṇḍūka parṇi, arka, avalguja and vāsa, or with bitter drugs, meat of jāngala animals which is devoid of all fat, vajraka taila for massage, a decoction of drugs of āragvadhādi group for application (utsādana), decoction of khadira for drinking, bathing, sprinkling, etc., regular trimming of nails and hair, tranquility, regular use of medicines and wholesome food.

The following are to be avoided: use of wine, meat, animal fat, milk, curds, oil, kulattha, māsha, nishpāva, sugar-cane, flour products, sour food, incompatible food, over-eating, eating before the digestion of food previously taken, food that is heat producing, and abhishyandi, alcohol, sleep during daytime, and indulgence in sex, (SS).

2. Although kushṭha is caused by the vitiation of all three doshas, the physician should ascertain the degree of vitiation of the doshas, and treat the dosha which is most involved. The doshas which are aggravated to a lesser degree can be treated later.

The symptoms engendered by aggravated vāta are dryness, emaciation, pricking and sharp pain, contraction, extension (of parts, etc.) roughness, hardness, horripilation and dark-brown discolouration; by aggravated pitta, burning pain, redness, exudation, suppuration, foul (visra), smell, softness, and ulceration or gangrene (anga-patana); and by the deranged kapha are coldness, whiteness, itching, stability, swelling, heaviness, unctousness, exudation and eating away of tissues by parasites.

Generally, ghee is useful in vātaja kushṭha while emesis is indicated in kaphaja kushṭha, and blood letting and purgation is useful in pittaja kushṭha. Emesis is more effective in mild cases of kushṭha whereas venesection is done in severe cases. Patients of severe kushṭha should be repeatedly administered mild purificatory (śodhana) therapy. Excessive use of purificatory therapy causes aggravation of vāta and subsequent debility. After purification therapy and blood letting, the patient is given potions of ghee, etc., (sneha-pana).

For inducing emesis, the drugs used are fruits of kuṭaja, madana, yashṭi-madhu, paṭola, juice of nimba, honey, etc., in the form of cold infusions. Trivṛt, danti and triphala are used for purgation. The patient can also be administered asthāpana enema with dārvi, bṛhatī, sevya (uśīra), paṭola, pichu-marda, and āragvadha. Patients of vātaja kushṭha can be given anuvāsana enema with ghee or oil medicated with phala (madana-phala), yashṭi-madhu, nimba, kuṭaja and paṭola. Errhines (nasya) of rock-salt, danti, maricha, pippali and karanja-phala and vairechanika type of fumigation (dhūma) are also useful, if the upper part of the body is affected.

Skin eruptions that are circinate, hard and stable are to be given sudation by the prastara or nādi types, rubbed with the kūrcha and the blood extracted. Eruptions that are elevated are fomented with a warm poṭṭali (bundle) of flesh of aquatic animals, and excised. The blood can be removed by means of alābu, sṛgāla or leeches, plasters can then be applied over the affected areas.

In cases where surgical measures are not

indicated, kshāras (alkalies) can be applied, and blood letting done. Eruptions that are numb, rigid, which itch and where there is abence of sweating are to be scraped with the leaves of jāti, arka, nimba, danti, trivṛt, etc., of kūrcha or with any surgical instrument or with samudra-phena, and are then plastered with appropriate drugs.

In patients of pittaja kushṭha, the kapha, pitta and blood have to be eliminated and the patients can then be given bitter and astringent drugs, ghee, etc., and other measures that are indicated in rakta-pitta.

The following formulations are especially useful in kushṭha (for internal use): dārvi and rasānjana with cows urine; harītaki with trikaṭu, jaggery and oil, which is to be used for a month; a decoction of roots of paṭola and gavākshi, triphala, tvak, trāyamāṇa, nāgara and kaṭuka-rohiṇi is to be given to the patient for six days, in the early morning, the diet being restricted to meat juices of animals of jāngala desa, and old rice; lelitaka with juice of āmalaki and honey or with mākshika (bhasma) and cow's urine or with sulphur or with suvarṇa-makshika or śilājatu; the decoction of āragvadha, in kaphaja kushṭha; the decoctions of dārvi and rasānjana or nimba and paṭola or khadira-sāra, or āragvadha and vṛkshaka or triphala or sapta-parṇa or tiniśa or aśvamāra (karavīra) for internal administration as well as for washing the affected parts; the powders of the above drugs can be used for dusting over the affected area; a decoction of triphala, nimba, paṭola, manjishṭha, rohini, vachā and haridra is useful in kaphaja and pittaja kushtha; ghee medicated with the above drugs is useful in vātaja kushṭha also; and a decoction of khadira, asana, dāru,. nimba, vāsa and triphala.

Oil medicated with the juice of śveta-karavīra, cows' urine, chitraka and viḍanga or extracted from sarshapa, karanja, koshataki and ingudi or with khadira-sāra is useful in kushṭha. Oil or ghee medicated with bee's wax, sarja-rasa, jivanti, manjishṭha, dārvi, kampillaka, milk and tuttha is used as external application in vipādika, charma-kushṭha, eka-kushṭha, kiṭima and alasaka.

Ghee medicated with khadira-sāra or bark of nimba or darvi or leaves of paṭola is beneficial in pittaja and raktaja kushṭha.

The following plasters are also useful for external applications: kusumbara and kushṭha, in maṇḍala-kushṭha; edagaja, kushṭha, rock-salt, souvīra, sarshapa and viḍanga, in maṇḍala-kushṭha and dādru-kushṭha; edagaja, sarja-rasa and śeeds of mūlaka, in sidhma; vāsa and triphala; bṛhati, sevya, paṭola, sāriva, and rohiṇi; śata-dhouta-ghṛta, in kushṭha with burning pains.

Patients with discharge of serous fluid and proliferation of parasites are advised cow's urine, nimba and viḍanga or vāsa, kuṭaja, sapta parṇa, karavīra, karanja, nimba and khadira for internal use, bathing and application.

A diet that is beneficial consists of food that is easy to digest, bitter leafy vegetables, use of bhallātaka, triphala, nimba and ghee with food, old rice, meat of animals of jāngala-deśa, mudga and paṭola.

Food that is hard to digest and sour, milk, curds, fish, jaggery, tila, and meat of aquatic animals are to be avoided, (CS).

3. The following plasters or pastes are used for external application: paste of roots of kāsamarda, and souvira, in kiṭibha, sidhma and dadru; paste of leaves of āragvadha with aranāla (kānji), in dadru, kiṭibha and sidhma; paste of seeds of prapunnāṭa, āmalaki, sarja-rasa, snuhi and souvira, for rubbing in dadru; paste of seeds of chakra-marda, mūlaka, and water, in dadru; paste of root of śigru, in dadru; paste of equal quantities of jīraka and seeds of chakra-marda, and a small amount of root of sudarśana, in dadru; paste of gandhaka, yava-kshāra and kaṭu-taila, in sidhma; and paste of gandhaka, mūlaka and seeds of kāsamarda, in sidhma.

A few recipes useful when given internally are: a decoction of paṭola, khadira, arishṭa, triphala, kṛshṇa and vetraka, a diet consisting of bitter substances; powder of seeds of avalguja with hot water, a diet consisting of milk and ghee; the juice of nimba is given, and after it is digested, the patient should partake of rice with ghee and small quantities of gruel. This recipe is especially useful in emaciated people; a paste of leaves of indrāsana, honey, sugar-candy and ghee, is extremely useful in all skin diseases, (CSS).

4. The following formulations are efficacious in kushṭha: equal quantities of purified sulphur and maricha, and six parts of triphala triturated with the juice of śampāka (āragvadhā). This paste is very useful (when used internally), (RRS).

Ref.: SS, chikitsā, 9; CS, chikitsā, 7; CSS, page. 597-598; RRS, 3, 36.

Classical Prescriptions: Āragvadhādi-kvātha-chūrṇa; Ārogya-vardhini-guṭika; Ayaskrti; Brāhmi-ghṛta; Bṛhat-guḍūchyādi-taila; Bṛhat-manjishṭādi-kvātha-chūrṇa; Daśānga-lepa; Haratāla-bhasma; Kalyāṇaka-guḍa; Kānchanāra-guggulu; Kāsīsādi-ghṛta; Kushṭha-rākshasa-taila; Lakshmi-vilāsa-rasa; Lodhrāsava;Loha-bhasma; Madhūkāsava; Madhu-snuhi-rasāyana; Mahā-yogarāja-guggulu; Mahā-tiktaka-ghṛta; Maṇḍura-vaṭaka; Maṇi-bhadra-yoga; Nalpamarādi-taila; Nimbādi-churṇa; Pancha-tiktaka-ghṛta; Pāṭhadi-lepa; Paṭoladi-kvātha-chūrṇa; Paṭola-mūladi-kvātha-chūrṇa; Rasa-parpaṭi; Simhanāda-guggulu; Śiva guṭika; Somarāji-taila; Svarṇa-mākshika-bhasma; Tāmra-bhasma; Trikaṭu-chūrṇa; Vāri-śoshana-rasa; Vajraka-ghṛta; Vajraka-taila, Vraṇa-rākshasa-taila;Visha-tinduka-taila.

Kshudra-kushṭha: Tuvaraka-taila

Dadru-kushṭha: Devadārvārisṭa; Haridra-khaṇḍa; Kāsīsadi-ghṛta.

Pāma: Kāsīsadi-ghṛta; Rasottamādi-lepa-chūrṇa; Somarāji-taila; Śrīkhaṇḍāsava.

Pittaja-kushtha: Tiktaka -ghṛta

Purāna-tvag-roga: Amṛta-bhallātaka-leha

Mahā-kushtha: Khadirārishṭa; Tuvaraka-taila

Vicharchika: Kāsīsadi-ghṛta; Rasottamādi-lepa-chūrṇa; Sindūradi-lepa; Vraṇa-rākshasa-taila.

Visphoṭa: Chandana-balā-lākshādi-taila; Haridrā-khaṇḍa; Jātyādi-taila; Kapardika-bhasma; Rasa-karpūra; Vraṇa-rākshasa-taila.

Vipādika: Sindūradi-lepa

Makkalla

Western Nosology: Post-partum abscess, Puerperal sepsis

Causative Factors:

Extrinsic: Intake of sharp (tīkshṇa) drugs or suppression of lochia in a newly delivered woman whose body is dry, (SS).

Intrinsic: Vāta (SS).

Pathogenesis and Symptomatology: The aggravated vāta and the suppressed lochia engenders knotty tumours (granthi) below the umbilicus, on the sides of the pelvis around the urinary bladder or in the supra-pubic region. The woman also suffers from pain in the umbilical region, urinary bladder, and abdomen, pricking, stitching, breaking and cutting pain in the intestines, distention of the abdomen and retention of urine, (SS).

There will be pain in the supra-pubic region and abdomen soon after parturition, (AS).

Complications: Makkalla can also occur in mūḍha-garbha (SS, nidāna, 8, 6); raktaja vidradhi as a complication, (SS, nidāna, 9, 27).

Treatment:

1. The patient is administered a decoction of drugs of virātarvādi group with the powders of drugs of ūshakādi group. She can also be

given yava-kshāra powder with warm water or a decoction of drugs of the pippalyādi group. The powders of drugs of the same group can be administered with surā-maṇḍa, or a decoction of drugs of varuṇādi group with powder of panchakola and ela or a decoction of drugs of pṛthakparṇi group with maricha and bhadradāru or old jaggery with trikaṭu, chaturjāta and kustumbaru or just arishṭa, (SS).

2. The following formulae are beneficial in this condition: powder of yava-kshāra with ghee or warm water; rock-salt with a decoction of drugs of vatsakādi group; drugs of vatsakādi group with madira; decoction of the two amśumatis with paste of maricha and bhadradāru; and paste of bhārngi, nāgara, devadāru and hot water, (AS).

Ref.: SS, nidāna, 8, 6; 9, 27; śārīra,10, 22; AS, śārīra, 3, 35; KS, khila, 11, 7-14.

Manyā-stambha

Nosology: Wry neck

Causative Factors:

Extrinsic: Sleeping during the daytime, reclining with the head on an uneven pillow, gazing upwards for a considerable length of time or turning the head in a distorted manner, (SS).

This disease may also appear as a prodromal sign in antarāyāma and bahirāyāma (Chkp. on CS, sūtra, 28, 4) or in apatānaka (NiS on SS).

Intrinsic: Vāta (CS, sūtra, 20, 11; chikitsā, 28, 43). Vāta which is obstructed by kapha, (SS).

Symptomatology: Stiffness of the neck.

Treatment:

1. The treatment is on the same lines as in vāta roga and pakshāghāta.

Errhines which alleviate vāta and kapha and dry fomentation are useful, (SS).

2. Errhines (nasya) are beneficial (CS, sūtra, 5, 59; siddhi, 2, 22).

3. A decoction of drugs of the daśamūla group or bṛhat-pancha-mūla is useful, (CD).

4. The affected area is smeared, with (warm) katu-taila and plastered with the paste of aśvagandha, (BR).

Ref.: SS, nidāna, 1, 67; chikitsā, 5, 20; CS, chikitsā, 28, 43; CD, 22, 19; BR, page. 325, 17.

Classical Prescriptions: Bhṛngarāja-taila; Chatur-mukha-rasa; Laghu-vishagarbha-taila; Mahā-nārāyaṇa-taila; Nārāyaṇa-taila.

Mashaka

Western Nosology: Raised mole; Erythema multiforma

Causative Factors:

Intrinsic: Vāta (SS, nidāna, 13, 42). Kapha and vāta (NC on ibid)

Constituents Affected: Medas (fatty tissues) (ibid); the third layer of skin called śveta (SS, śārīra, 4, 4).

Symptomatology:

1. Hard, painless, elevated and black eruptions resembling māsha pulse, (SS, nidāna, 13, 42).

2. Soft, smooth eruptions which are skin-coloured, (Bhoja, quoted by NC on ibid).

3. The eruptions are similar to tila (seeds), (AS, uttara, 36).

Ref.: CS, sūtra, 11, 49.

Treatment:

1. Kshāras may be used externally (pratisāraṇīya kshāra), (SS, sūtra, 11, 7).

2. The eruptions may also be gradually cauterised by fire or by kshāras (alkalies), (SS, chikitsā, 20, 32).

Mastishka-apachaya

Synonyms: Sanskrit: Mastishka-hrāsa

Western Nosology: Hydrocephalus

Pathogenesis and Symptomatology: There will be growth or enlargement of the cranial bones while the brain matter will shrink. If this happens on only one part, there is usually no danger. If the shrinkage occurs throughout, the patient will not survive.

Treatment: This is usually fatal. The patient may be administered nourishing food and medicines. Measures which are useful in vāta-roga, as well as medicated ghees and oils mentioned in apasmāra treatment may be useful.

The food should be nourishing and easy to digest.

Ref.: BR, pages. 691-692, 17-22.

Mastishka-chaya

Synonyms: Sanskrit: Mastishka-vṛddhi

Causative Factors: Constitutional tendency.

Pathogenesis: The brain matter increases in size, along with the protrusion of the cranial bones. This occurs usually in children or young persons. If the growth of the brain matter is equal to the protrusion of the cranial bones, there is no danger. If however, there is increase in brain matter without any change in the cranial bones, many complaints arise.

Symptomatoloy: Headache, debility, vertigo, unconsciousness (mūrccha), paralysis, convulsions and even death.

Treatment: This is usually a fatal disease. However, medicines which are rasāyāna (rejuvenative), pancha-gavya ghṛta, and the juice of śatāvari with honey may be administered.

Ref.: BR, pages. 691, 11-16, 23.

Diet: The food should be nourishing and easy to digest.

Mastishka-kampa

Causative Factors:

Extrinsic: Mental stress.

Symptomatology: Unconsciousness (mūrccha), nausea, vomiting, lethargy, mental instability, debility, trembling (of limbs), tinnitus, foul mouth, unsteadiness of pupils of the eyes, slow pulse, coldness of body, stuttering speech and paralysis of limbs.

Treatment: The patient is to be first reassured. If his head is hot, it should be sprinkled with very cold water. If the limbs are very cold, the patient is to be wrapped up in a thick and warm blanket, and made to rest upon a bed which is to be heated from below.

Mṛta-sanjīvani-surā or any other strengthening (balya) medicine can be administered in order to restore the pulse to normalcy.

The patient can also be administered rasa-sindūra with a decoction of balā. A decoction of trivṛt, svarṇa-patri, musta, yashṭi-madhu, balā, haridra, dāru-haridra, nāgara, triphala and kaṭuka-rohini can also be given.

Measures which alleviate vāta and mastishka-roga (general line of treatment) are all useful (see vāta-roga).

Ref.: BR, pages. 690-691.

Mastishka-roga

General Line of Treatment: Panchāmṛta-loha-guggulu.

Equal parts of purified sulphur, mercury, rajata bhasma, abhraka bhasma and svarṇa-mākshika bhasma, two parts of loha bhasma and seven parts of purified guggulu are triturated in an iron vessel with an iron pestle, with the required quantity of kaṭu-taila, for six hours. The dosage is three gunjas.

Diet: Food which is laxative, easily digestible and sweet is beneficial. Milk, meat juice and alcohol are also indicated.

Ref.: BR, pages. 693, 52-55, 60.

Masūrika

Synonyms: Sanskit: Masūri (NC on SS, nidāna, 5, 33-34), Hemantika (Kaiyadeva, 8, 263).

Western Nosology: Impetigo

Causative Factors:

Extrinsic:

1. This is an infectious disease, (ibid).

2. Excessive intake of pungent, sour, salty and alkaline (kshāra) food, incompatible food, impure water, and unclean or polluted nishpāva, leafy vegetables, etc., polluted air, fasting and over-eating, (MN).

Intrinsic: Pitta (NC and NiS on SS). All three doshas (MN).

Constituents Affected: Blood (NC and NiS on SS; MN).

Pathogenesis: The aggravated pitta and the vitiated blood cause a pustular eruption all over the body, (NC and NiS on SS).

Classification: The masūrika may be engendered by the deranged vāta or pitta or kapha or all the three combined or by vitiated blood, (MN).

Symptomatology:

1. Copper coloured and yellowish vesicles (sphoṭa) all over the body, face and inside the mouth, with burning pain, fever, and sharp pain, (SS).

2. Pustules (piḍaka) resembling masūra, mudga and māsha (in size), and similar to kola, which are found all over the body, (NC and NiS on SS).

3. In vātaja masūrika, there will be brownish or dark-gray coloured vesicles which are dry, hard, slow to ripen and severely painful. The patient will also suffer from breaking pain in the joints and bones, cough, trembling of the limbs, restlessness, fatigue, dryness of lips, palate and tongue, thirst and tastelessness.

In pittaja masūrika, the vesicles will be reddish or yellowish, white in colour, and will be attended with burning and severe pain. They will suppurate rapidly. The patient will also suffer from watery or unformed stools, body pain, burning sensation, thirst, tastelessness, ulcers in the mouth, eye diseases and high fever.

The type that is brought about by impure blood manifests symptoms similar to those of pittaja masūrika.

In kaphaja masūrika, there will be white, unctuous looking large vesicles with dull pain and itching. They suppurate slowly. The patient will also suffer from nausea, tastelessness, drowsiness, sleepiness, lethargy and heaviness of body, and headache.

The types that are engendered by all the doshas will manifest pustules which are blue, broad and flattened with a depression in the centre, severe pain and foul discharge. They are slow to ripen. There will also be tastelessness, dificulty in swallowing, irrelevant speech, restlessness, and stiffness (of the body). The pustules are known as charma.

If the skin (rasa dhātu) is involved, the eruptions will be like water bubbles, and on breaking will ooze out a watery fluid. If the blood is affected, the eruptions will be red like blood, rapid in growth and suppuration, while blood will ooze out. When the flesh is involved, the skin will be rough, and the eruptions hard, oily and slow to ripen. There will also be body pain, thirst, itching, fever, and restlessness. When the medas is involved the eruptions will be circinate, soft, slightly elevated, large, oily, painful and attended with high fever, confusion (of sense faculties) and restlessness. When the marrow is involved, the eruptions will be small, skin coloured, dry, flattened, slightly elevated and accompanied by extreme confusion, pain and restlessness. The vital organs will be affected. If the bones are also affected, there will also be stinging pains all over the body. When the śukra is affected, the eruptions will be oily, small in size, severely painful and attended by restlessness, stiffness or rigidity of body, confusion (of mind), burning pain and insanity (unmāda), (MN).

Prognosis:

1. If eruptions resembling coral (pravāla) appear all over the body and disappear immediately (after its appearance), the condition is incurable. (CS)

2. Cases of masūrika which are caused by aggravated pitta or kapha or kapha and pitta are easily curable. Likewise cases of masūrika confined to the skin or blood are easily curable. Those which affect the flesh are difficult to cure, while cases in which medas is involved are very difficult to cure. Masūrika where the bone-marrow and śukra are involved is fatal.

Cases which are caused by aggravated vāta, vāta and pitta or kapha and vāta are difficult to cure, and those which involve all three doshas are incurable.

Cases where the patient suffers from cough, hiccough, prameha, high fever, delirium, restlessness, syncope, thirst, burning pains, spitting of blood, nose-bleed, blood shot eyes, rattling sound in the throat, difficulty in breathing, swelling in the elbow and wrist joints, thirst, and hard nasal breathing are incurable. (MN)

Ref.: SS, nidāna, 13, 38; CS, indriya, 11, 14; AHṛ, uttara, 31, 8; MN, 54.

Treatment:

1. A person suffering form masūrika is treated as in the case of kapha-pittaja visarpa. Plasters employed as external applications in kushṭha can be applied, (CS ; SS).

2. The patient has to be treated on lines similar to that in pittaja visarpa, (AHṛ).

3. At the very onset, the patient is to be exposed to fumigation of veṇu-tvak, surasa, lāksha, stone of kārpāsa, yava-pishṭa, ghee, vachā, brāhmi, etc. This may abort the disease.

In all types of masūrika, the patient is administered emesis by giving a decoction of paṭola, arishṭa, vāsaka, and paste of vachā, vatsa, yashṭimadhu and madana-phala. The juice of brāhmi and hila-mochika can also be given with honey. After emesis, the patient is to be purged. In a debilitated person, however, śamana therapy is advisable.

If the patient is subjected to emesis and purgation, there will be no complications, less pain and pus, and speedy maturation of the pustules.

The following prescriptions are beneficial in all cases of masūrika: the leaf-juice of sushavi with turmeric powder; a decoction of paṭola, kundali, musta, vāsa, dhānya, yavāsa, bhūnimba, ṇimba, bāluka and parpaṭa - this is very efficacious in relieving fever; a decoction of paṭola, musta, aruṇa, and taṇḍuliya with the paste of haridra and āmalaki; the decoction of the root of paṭola, aruṇa-taṇḍuliya, āmalaki and khadira; the decoction of the pancha-tikta drugs; the juice of nimba alone or of hilamocha with the paste of śveta-chandana- these are to be administered at the very first stage; pārada bhasma with leaf-juice of bilva, with the adjuvant being the juice of hilamocha.

In vātaja masūrika, the decoction of paṭola śariva, musta, pāṭha, kaṭu-rohini, khadira, pichu-marda, balā, āmalaki and vikankata is useful. A paste of the bark of nyagrodha, plaksha, manjishṭha, sirīsha, udumbara and ghee is to be applied. (A decoction of) guḍūchi, yashṭi-madhu, drākshā, moraṭa, dāḍima and jaggery helps in the maturation of the pustules. The powder of badara and jaggery also hastens maturation.

In pittaja masūrika, the patient is given powder of lājā with sugar. The diet has to consist of soup of bitter drugs or meat juice of animals of the pratuda group. The decoction of nimba, parpaṭa, pāṭha, paṭola, the two chandanas, vāsa, durālabha, āmalaki, trikaṭu and kaṭu-rohini is administered with honey and śugar. A paste of the bark of sirīsha, udumbara, asvattha, pīlu, nyagrodha and ghee is applied externally. A decoction of moraṭa, fruit of kāśmari, sugar-candy and the powder of lājā helps in the maturation of the eruptions. A decoction of durālabha, parpaṭaka, paṭola and kaṭu-rohini is useful (when administered internally).

In kaphaja-masūrika, a decoction of duralābha, parpaṭaka, paṭola and kaṭu-rohiṇi or of bhūnimba, mustā, vāsa, triphala, indra-yava, pichu marda and paṭola, with honey is useful. The leaf-juice of vāsa can be given with honey. A paste of the leaves of khadira and arishṭa, and bark of sīrīsha and udumbara is applied externally (also in pittaja masūri). A paste of curds and saktu helps in the maturation of the pustules.

The juice of pūti-karanja and āmalaki is given with honey and sugar for reducing the swelling in kapha-pittaja masūrika. A decoction of drugs of the amṛtadi group also relieves the swelling.

In raktaja masūrika, blood-letting will be of use.

A paste of the kesara (filament) of mātulunga and souvīra relieves burning pain and hastens maturation (when applied externally). If eruptions located on the foot cause burning pain, the affected area can be sprinkled with rice water. In ulceration of the mouth and throat, gargles (gaṇḍūsha) of a decoction of leaves of jati, manjishṭha, dārvi, fruit of pūga, śami, yashṭi-madhu and fruit of āmalaki are useful. If the eyes are affected, they can be washed with a decoction of gavedhuka and yashṭi-madhu. The paste of the bark of bahuvāra can be applied as collyrium. A decoction of bark of nimba, babbūra, aśoka, bimbi, and vetasa can be used for washing the parts.

During the time of maturation of pustules, the vāta will be aggravated, and therefore the patient has to be given nourishing food. The gruel (yūsha) of dāḍima and sour drugs is useful in anorexia.

In swelling of the elbow and wrist joints, measures indicated in vrana-śotha and dushta-vraṇa and which alleviate vāta are useful. Blood letting can also be employed, (CSS).

4. The following recipes are efficacious in masūrika: ananta mūla (sāriva) with jyeshṭhambu (decoction of triphala); kajjali prepared from one part of purified mercury and two parts of purified sulphur; tender leaves of haridra or amlika with cold water; the powder of badara with jaggery for promoting the maturation of the pustules; purified guggulu with a decoction of triphala, for relieving pain, and burning sensation and for purifying the eruptions; the powders of pippali and harītaki with honey in cases where the throat is involved; and the five bitter drugs (pancha-tikta) for internal and external administration, (CD).

5. Pārada bhasma, if administered with coconut water is extremely efficacious in masūrika, (RRS).

Ref.: CS, chikitsā, 12, 93; SS, chikitsā, 20, 31; AHṛ, uttara, 32, 5; CSS, pages. 644-650; CD, 54; RRS,30, 71.

Mūḍha-vāta

Western Nosology: Flatulence

Causative Factors:

Extrinsic: Over - nutrition (CS, sūtra, 23, 22).

Intrinsic: Vāta

Symptomatology: The apānā vāta is obstructied giving rise to flatulent distension of the abdomen, abdominal pain, and constipation.

Treatment:

1. Tālisādi chūrṇa is useful (CS, chikitsā, 8, 147).

2. Milk medicated with taṇḍulīyaka and the pastes of yashṭi-madhu and madhūka is useful. Ajamoda can be fried with surā and administered with rock-salt, (CS, chikitsā, 11, 27).

3. Tarpaṇa is useful, (AS, sūtra, 24, 61).

4. Sour food articles help in eliminating the obstructed flatus, (AHṛ, sūtra, 10, 11) .

Classical Prescriptions: Pippalyādi-taila; Sūraṇāvaleha.

Mūka

Extrinsic: Excessive or untimely smoking (dhūma) (CS, sūtra, 5, 38).

There are four body channels about the two sides of the food pipe or oesophagus (kantha-nāḍi. Any injury to these channels will cause mukatva, (SS, śarīra, 6, 27).

If the cravings of a pregnant woman are not fulfilled, there may be aggravation of vāta, which may cause dumbness in the child, (SS, śārīra, 2, 51).

Talking in a loud voice (ucchaih) may also cause dumbness, (SS, chikitsā, 39, 30).

Intrinsic: Vāta (CS, sātra, 20, 11). Vata and kapha (SS, nidāna, 1, 85).

Pathogenesis and Symptomatology: The aggravated vāta and kapha obstruct the channels responsible for transmitting sound, and cause dumbness, (SS, nidāna, 1, 85).

Treatment:

1. The patient is to be administered ghee internally and should also be given nasal drops (nāvana), collyrium and tarpaṇa, (CS, sutra, 5, 38).

2. The patient is to be treated with measures indicated in vāta roga.

Mukha-dūshika

Synonyms: Sanskrit: Yuvana-piḍaka; Varaṇḍaka, (madhukośa on MN, 55, 33).

Western Nosology: Acne

Causative Factors:

Intrinsic: Kapha and vāta

Constituents Affected: Blood

Symptomatology: Pustules (piḍakas) resembling the spikes on the śalmali tree, which appear on the face of young people (yūnam).

Ref.: SS, nidāna, 13, 39.

Treatment:

1. The patient is to be administered emesis. The pastes of vachā, lodhra, rock-salt and sarshapa or of kustumbara, vachā, lodhra and kusṭha can be applied externally, (SS).

2. The application of pastes of lodhra, dhānya and vachā, or of maricha with gorochana is useful. The paste has to be as thick as one fourth, one half or one-third of an angula. It should be removed as soon as it becomes dry, (CSS).

Ref.: SS, chikitsā, 21, 37; CSS, page. 654.

Classical Prescription: Kunkumādi-taila.

Mukha-roga

Causative Factors:

Extrinsic: Excess intake of fish, meat of buffalo and pig, immature mūlaka, soup of māsha, curds, milk, śukta, sugarcane juice and phāṇita, sleeping on the face, failure to brush the teeth, subjecting one self to fumigation, emesis and gaṇḍusha, and unnecessary venesection, (AHṛ, uttara, 21, 1-2).

Classification:

1. The diseases of the oral cavity can be broadly classified into four groups, those caused by the

vitiated vāta, pitta, kapha and all three doshas combined, (CS, sūtra, 19, 3).

2. According to physicians of the śālākya branch, there are sixty-four diseases of the oral cavity, depending on the location, the body constituents involved, symptoms present and nomenclature, (CS, chikitsā, 26, 12).

3. There are sixty-five diseases of the oral cavity of which eight affect the lips, fifteen the gums, eight the teeth, five the tongue, nine the palate, seventeen the throat and three the mouth in general, (SS, chikitsā, 16, 3).

Symptomatology:

I. Diseases of the Oral Cavity: Where vāta is aggravated symptoms are characterised by dryness, roughness, pain, looseness (of teeth, etc.), blackish or brown discolouration, cold salivation, pulsation, and pricking and breaking pain.

The diseases wherein pitta is vitiated are characterised by thirst, fever, boils or vesicles, burning of the palate, cracking (of skin, etc., avadīrṇata), unconsciousness (mūrcha),various kinds of pain, a sensation as if filled with smoke and different kinds of discolouration except white and brown.

The cases engendered by deranged kapha are characterised by itching, heaviness, whitish discolouration, oilyness, anorexia, lethargy, expectoration of phlegm, nausea (utkleśa), feeble digestion, dull pain and sliminess.

Cases engendered by all the doshas are attended with symptoms caused by all of them, (CS, chikitsā, 26, 119-122).

II. A. Diseases of the Lips:

1. If vāta is vitiated, the lips become rough, dry, rigid or stiff, blackish in colour, very painful, are cracked and wrinkled.

2. If pitta is aggravated, the lips are yellow or blue in colour, covered with pustules, resembling mustard seeds, which burn, ripen and suppurate.

3. If kapha is deranged, the lips are covered with painless, non-discoloured pustules, are heavy, cold, stony, swollen and attended by itching.

4. If all three doshas are vitiated, the lips may vary in colour, being black, yellow or white, and are covered by pustules of many colours.

5. If blood is affected, the lips are blood red in colour, are covered with eruptions coloured like the fruits of kharjūra, and ooze out blood.

6. If māmsa is involved, the lips become heavy, thick, swollen as from lumps of flesh, while the corners of the lips are infected with parasites.

7. If medas is affected, the lips begin to itch, are heavy, soft, numb, appears as if smeared with the upper layer of ghee and exude a clear, crystal-like liquid.

8. If the lips are injured, they are cracked, chapped (vidīryate), knotty and begin to itch.

III. Diseases of the Gums (Roots of the Teeth, Danta-mūla):

1. Sītāda - This is caused by kapha and blood. Occasional bleeding from the gums, the gums become soft, offensive, black in colour, and slimy. They gradually begin to wear out.

2. Danta-pupputaka - This is also engendered by deranged kapha and blood. Painful swelling occurs around the roots of two or three teeth.

3. Danta-veshṭa - This is brought about by the vitiation of blood. Teeth become loose, and there is exudation of pus and blood.

4. Soushira - This is caused by kapha and blood. Painful swelling with itching around the roots of the teeth, with excessive salivation.

5. Mahā-soushira - This is engendered by all the doshas. The teeth become loose while the gums and palate are inflamed. The gums are also fissured, and the entire oral cavity is inflammed.

6. Paridara - This is caused by deranged kapha, pitta and blood. The gums wear out and the patient spits out blood.

7. Upakuśa - This is caused by aggravated pitta and blood. There is burning and inflammation of the gums, looseness of teeth, bleeding and dull pain when the teeth are brushed or shaken; the entire mouth is swollen and offensive.

8. Vidarbha - This results from injury. There is looseness of the teeth, and great swelling around the roots of the teeth.

9. Vardhana - This is caused by deranged vatā. Painful eruption of the additional teeth (wisdom tooth). The pain subsides after the tooth emerges.

10. Adhi-māmsa - This is caused by deranged kapha. There is a very painful and big swelling of the jaw, opposite the last teeth, with excessive salivation.

11-15. There are five types of sinuses affecting the roots of the teeth. They may be caused by vāta, pitta, kapha, all three doshas or may result from trauma (see Nāḍi-vraṇa).

IV. Diseases of the Teeth:

1. Ḍālana - This is caused by aggravated vāta. Many of the teeth ache intensely as if they are being torn asunder.

2. Kṛmi-dantaka - This is also a vātaja disease. The teeth turn black, are filled with minute holes, are loose, very painful, attended with swelling and salivation. The pain appears without any apparent cause.

3. Danta-harsha - This is also engendered by vitiated vāta. The teeth are very sensitive to both heat and, cold and touch.

4. Bhanjanaka - This is caused by deranged kapha and vāta. The mouth or face is distorted, the teeth break off and there is severe pain.

5. Danta-śarkara - The teeth are covered over with impurities which become hard like gravel, and which (gradually) destroy the teeth.

6. Kapālika - The gravelly impurities (tartar) break off along with the outer covering of the teeth.

7. Śyāva-danta - Due to aggravated pitta and blood, teeth turn blue or blackish in colour.

8. Hanu-moksha - Due to the action of vitiated vāta, there is dislocation of the jaw. The symptoms are similar to those of ardita.

V. Diseases of the Tongue:

1. Vātaja kaṇṭaka - The tongue is cracked, numb, and rough.

2. Pittaja-kaṇṭaka - The tongue is yellowish, and covered with blood red pappilae, with burning pain.

3. Kaphaja-kaṇṭaka - The tongue is heavy, thick and covered with fleshy nodules resembling the spikes of the śālmali tree.

4. Alasa - this is caused by vitiated kapha and blood. This is a swelling under the tongue which increases, causes stiffness of the tongue and severe inflammation of the root (of the tongue).

5. Upa-jihvika - This is also engendered by aggravated kapha and blood. There is a swelling under the tip of the tongue which pushes the tongue upwards. There is also itching, salivation and burning pain.

VI. Diseases of the Palate:

1. Gala-śuṇḍika - This is brought about by deranged kapha and blood. There is an elongated swelling around the uvular region of the palate, which is like an inflated bladder. There is also thirst, cough and dyspnoea.

2. Tuṇḍikeri - This is also caused by the vitiation of kapha and blood. A thick swelling (near the uvular region) (resembling the fruit of vanakārpāsi, NiS) with pricking pain, burning and suppuration (pra-pāka).

3. Adhrusha - This is caused by vitiated blood. There is a numb, reddish, painful swelling of the palate, with high fever.

4. Kacchapa - This is engendered by aggravated kapha. A painless, gradually appearing, whitish swelling resembling the shell of a tortoise.

5. Arbuda - This results from a vitiated condition of the blood. A lotus (pericarp) shaped swelling appears in the middle of the palate, with symptoms similar to those of rakta-arbuda.

6. Māmsa -sanghāta - The aggravated kapha vitiates the flesh and causes a painless fleshy outgrowth around the extremity of the palate.

7. Tālu-pupputa - The deranged kapha and medas engender a painless, firm swelling as big as the kola fruit, in the region of the palate.

8. Tālu-śosha - The aggravated vāta and pitta causes severe dryness of the palate with piercing pain and dyspnoea.

9. Tālu-pāka - The deranged pitta brings about an intense inflammation of the palate.

VII. Diseases of the Throat:

1-5. Rohiṇi (Diptheritic tonsillitis) - These may be caused by vāta, pitta, kapha, all three doshas combined or by vitiated blood. The doshas vitiate the blood and flesh and so result in fleshy nodules which obstruct the throat and cause death.

In vātaja rohiṇi, extremely painful, fleshy nodules crop up all over the tongue and obstruct the throat. There will also be other symptoms of aggravated vāta.

In pittaja rohiṇi, the disease occurs rapidly, progresses quickly to suppuration, and is accompanied with high fever and burning pain.

In kaphaja rohiṇi, the nodules are heavy (big), firm, slightly painful and obstruct the throat.

The nodules, in the tridoshaja rohiṇi, are very deep seated and attended with symptoms caused by all the doshas.

In raktaja rohiṇi, the growths are covered over with vesicles (sphoṭa). There will be other symptoms caused by the aggravated pitta.

6. Kaṇṭa-śālūka - The aggravated kapha engenders the formation of a knotty tumour of the size of the stone of the kola fruit, and resembling the bulbs of utpala, which is hard and stable. The patient feels as if there is a splinter in the throat. This disease is amenable to surgical treatment.

7. Adhi-jihva - The aggravated kapha, (pitta, acording to NC and NiS) and blood bring about the formation of a swelling shaped like the tip of the tongue, which occurs above the root of the tongue. It is considered to be incurable once it starts to suppurate.

8. Valaya -Due to vitiated kapha, a circular, raised, swelling obstructs the oesophagus.

9. Balāsa - Due to the aggravation of kapha and Diptheritic tonsillitista, a painful swelling occurs in the throat along with dyspnoea.

10. Eka-vṛnda - This disease is caused by aggravated kapha and blood. There is a circular and elevated swelling which is soft, heavy, which slightly supurates, and is accompanied by burning pain and itching.

11. Vṛnda - The vitiated pitta and blood bring about the formation of an elevated, rounded swelling with high fever and severe burning pain. If vāta and blood are affected, there will be pricking pain.

12. Śataghni - This is caused by the vitiation of all three doshas. An elongated large swelling with fleshy outgrowth, which increases in size and obstructs the throat and is accompanied by various types of pain (burning, pricking, itching, etc). (It resembles a huge stone studded with iron spikes, NC, NiS).

13. Gilāyu - The aggravated kapha and blood engender a knotty growth of the size of the stone of the āmalaka fruit, which is firm and slightly painful. The patient feels as if a morsel of food is stuck in the throat.

14. Gala-vidradhi - The vitiated three doshas bring about an extensive painful swelling all along the inner throat. The symptoms are similar to those seen in tridoshaja vidradhi.

15. Galougha - An extensive swelling which obstructs the passage of solid food and even liquids and the passage of air, and which is attended by high fever. This is caused by vitiated kapha and blood.

16. Svaraghna - This is caused by the aggravated vāta. The deranged kapha obstructs the air passages (larynx) bringing about frequent fainting, stentorous breathing, hoarseness, and dryness and paralysed condition of the throat.

17. Māmsa-tāna - The three aggravated doshas bring about an extensive swelling which obstructs the throat. It gradually increases and becomes pendulous.

18. Vidāri - A reddish swelling marked by burning and pricking pains occurs within the throat. The flesh becomes putrified and sloughs off. The disease is caused by pitta, and is found more on the side on which the patient lies.

VIII. Diseases of the Oral Cavity:

1. Vātaja sarvasara - The mouth is covered over with vesicles attended with pricking pain.

2. Pittaja sarvasara - The mouth is covered over with reddish or yellowish small vesicles, with burning pain.

3. Kaphaja sarvasara - The mouth is covered with non-discoloured (same colour as the surrounding area), slightly painful vesicles which are attended by itching.

4. Raktaja sarvasara - This is only a modification of the pittaja kind. Some authorities refer to this variety as mukhapāka, (SS, nidāna, 16).

1. **Diseases of the Lips:** If the lips are split, the disease is known as khandeshṭa. It is caused by vitiated vāta.

In diseases of the lips caused by kapha, there is sensitivity to cold.

In the disease known as jālārbuda, which is engendered by vāta and kapha, the lips are covered with vesicles which resemble water bubbles.

2. **Diseases of the Teeth:** In ḍālana, the tooth pains as if it is being cleft apart. It can bear heat but is very sensitive to cold.

In danta-harsha, the teeth are very sensitive to air, sour and cold things, and when in contact with some food hurts intensely and feels as if it is loose.

In danta-bheda, there will be pricking, breaking and pulsating pain in the tooth.

In danta-chāla, the teeth (or tooth) are loose, and ache intensely while chewing.

In karāla, the teeth are unevenly placed and are very irregular.

In danta śarkara, either due to absence of cleanliness or kapha which has been dried up by the aggravated vāta, the teeth are covered over with hardened dirt which emits an offensive smell.

The description of the other diseases of the teeth are the same as described in SS.

3. **Diseases of Gums or Roots of Teeth:** The disease upakuśa is attended with itching also. The swelling in danta-pupputa resembles the stone of the badara fruit and suppurates rapidly.

In danta-vidradhi, the aggravated doshas and blood engender a heavy (big) swelling on the gums, both internally and externally. There is pain, burning sensation, and exudation of putrid blood when the swelling ripens. The disease sushira (soushira) is caused by aggravated pitta and blood. In mahā-sushira (mahā-soushira), there is pain, fever and exudation of putrid blood. The disease adhi-māmsa is characterised by a wedge shaped swelling near the last teeth, which causes pain in the jaw and ear and obstructs the swallowing of food.

4. **Diseases of the Tongue:** The disease alasa is characterised by the aggravated kapha and pitta bringing about a swelling under the tongue which renders the tongue immobile.

When it suppurates, it emits a filthy odour. It destroys the flesh.

In the disease adhi-jihva, there is a painful swelling shaped like the tip of the tongue under the root of the tongue. The swelling is covered with nodules, is rough and causes salivation, burning pain, rigidity of the tongue, and itching. It is caused by the aggravated kapha, pitta and blood and causes difficulty in talking and swallowing. The same kind of swelling located above the tongue is known as upa-jihva.

5. **Diseases of Palate:** In the disease tālu-pūtika, the flesh of the palate is disturbed by the vitiated vāta, and is covered over by rough, painful, thick, numerous eruptions (pustules) which discharge a fluid.

In gala-śuṇḍika, the swelling is soft, hanging down, causes difficulty in swallowing, thirst and vomiting.

A painless, fleshy swelling in the middle of the palate is known as tālu-samhati.

Tāla-pāka is characterised by inflammation with severe pain and discharge of pus.

Tālu-śosha (dryness of mouth) may be caused by the aggravated vāta or pitta or by fever or exertion.

6. **Diseases of the Throat:** In vātaja rohiṇi, there will be dryness of the mouth and throat, pain in the jaw and ear. Pittaja-rohiṇi is characterised by fever, a tenderness and intense redness. The rohiṇi caused by vitiated blood will be marked by pain in the ears and red discolouration. In the disease vṛnda, the śwelling is found along the sides of the throat.

In tuṇḍikeri (which according to SS is a disease of the palate), there is a hard, slightly painful unctuous swelling resembling the fruit of kārpāsi. The swelling is located in the throat near the mandibular joint (hanu-sandhi).

In the disease galougha there is a big swelling around the throat, both internally and externally (visible) with heaviness of the head, lethargy, salivation and fever.

The disease valaya is painless or only slightly painful. In gilāyu, a thick, wedge shaped, fleshy, slightly painful, swelling causes difficulty in breathing and also swallowing. There may be one or more swellings.

The disease śataghni is attended with intense thirst, fever, headache and severe pain. In gala-vidradhi, the abscess ripens rapidly, is very painful and discharges an offensive putrid secretion.

In galārbuda, a painless, non-suppurating, firm, reddish growth occurs between the root of the tongue and the beginning of the throat.

7. **Diseases of the Oral Cavity:** In vātaja mukha-pāka, the mouth is covered with ulcers which are dry, brownish in colour and spread. The lips also turn brownish and become cracked. The tongue is sensitive to cold, becomes heavy, cracked and covered with nodules.

In the disease ūrdhva-guda, the aggravated vāta is pushed upwards due to arśa, gulma, the derangement of kapha, etc., and causes offensive mouth odour.

In pittaja mukha-pāka, there is a bitter taste in the mouth and burning or pain. The mouth feels as if it is covered with alkali (kshāra).

In kaphaja mukha-pāka, there is a sweet taste in the mouth.

In mukhārbuda, there is a swelling inside the cheek which is blackish or pale-white in colour, which grows even if it is excised, (AHṛ, uttara, 21).

Prognosis: Of the mukha-rogas the following are incurable: the diseases of lips caused by three doshas, flesh and blood; mahasoushira and the disease caused by all three doshas affecting the gums; ḍālana, śyāva-danta and bhanjanaka which involve the teeth; the diseases of the tongue named alasa; the disease of the palate known as arbuda and the nine diseases of the throat, viz., svaraghna, valaya, vṛnda, vidāri, balāsa, galougha, māmsa-tāna, śataghni and rohiṇi, (SS, chikitsā, 22, 77-81).

Treatment:

I. The patient has to be subjected to dhūma (fumigation), pradhamana type of errhine, purgation, emesis, fasting and should partake of food which alleviates the doshas involved.

The following medicines are to be kept in the mouth: the powder of pippali, bark of dārvi, yava-kshāra, rasānjana, paṭhā, tejovati, and harītaki, with honey-in all mukha-rogas; the powders of gṛha–dhuma (soot), yava-kshāra, pṛtha, trikaṭu, rasānjana, tejovati, triphala, lodhra, and chitraka with honey-in mukha-rogas, especially diseases of the throat and teeth; the powders of manahśila, yava-kshāra, haritāla, rock salt, and bark of dārvi with honey and the upper layer of ghee - in all mukha-rogas, especially those affecting the throat; mṛdvīka, kataka, trikaṭu, bark of dārvi, triphala and ghana with the upper layer of ghee – in diseases of the throat; and pātha, rasānjana, mūrva and tejohva with honey – in diseases of the palate.

The decoction of kaṭuka, ativisha, pātha, dārvi, musta, kalinga and cow's urine is administered internally in diseases of the throat. The expressed juice of dārvi is boiled until it acquires a semi-solid consistency. This is given with honey in mukha-rogas especially sinuses and cases where there is vitiation of blood.

A person suffering from tālu-śosha without thirst is given pure ghee after meals. The nāvana type of errhine and drugs that are cold, sweet, and oily are also useful.

A person suffering from mukha-pāka is subjected to venesection, errhine therapy and purgation. He is also advised to gargle with cow's urine, oil, ghee, honey, milk, etc. The mouth is frequently gargled with a decoction of mṛdvīka, triphala, pāṭha, tender leaves of jāti and honey or of drugs that are astringent, bitter and cold, (CS, chikitsā, 187-205).

II. Treatment in Diseases of the Lips: In the diseases of the lips caused by vāta, the lips are smeared with oil or ghee, etc., medicated with bees' wax, and a decoction of drugs which alleviate vāta. The lips are then fomented by the nāḍī-sveda process. Then they are plastered with sālvaṇa poultice. Oil medicated with drugs that alleviate vāta are used for errhine therapy and śiro-basti. The lips are then smeared with sri-veshṭak, sarja-rasa, devadāru, guggulu and powder of yashṭi-madhu.

In diseases caused by pitta, vitiated blood and injury, blood letting with leeches is useful. All the measures indicated in pittaja vidradhi will be found useful.

In disease engendered by vitiated kapha, blood-letting is to be followed by errhines, fumigation, sudation and gargles (kavala). The lips are smeared with the paste of trikaṭu, svarjika-kshāra, yava-kshāra, biḍa (salt) and honey.

In the disease caused by medas, the lips are fomented, opened up and cauterised with fire. They are then smeared with a paste of priyangu, triphala, lodhra and honey.

Treatment in Diseases of Gums (Roots of Teeth): In śitāda, the blood should be let out, and later, the decoction of nāgara, sarshapa, triphala, musta and rāsanjana should be used for gaṇḍusha. The paste of priyangu, musta and triphala is applied externally. Ghee or oil medicated with triphala, utpala and yashṭi-madhu should be used for errhine therapy.

In acute cases of danṭa-pupputaka, blood-letting is to be done. The pastes of the 'five salts', yava-kshāra and honey is smeared over the affected area. Oily food, śiro-virechana (errhines) and nasya (medicated snuff) are also useful.

In danta-veshṭa, the vitiated blood should be let out (along with pus), and a paste of lodhra, patanga, yashṭi-madhu, lāksha and honey is applied externally. The milky exudation of trees such as vaṭa, aśvattha, audumbara, etc., is used as gaṇḍūsha along with honey, ghee and sugar. Ghee medicated with milk and drugs of the kākolyādi group is used as nasya (nasal drops).

In soushira, the blood is let out. A paste of rodhra, musta, rasānjana and honey is applied over the affected area. A decoction of the kshiri trees which have a milky-exudation is used as gaṇḍūsha. Ghee medicated with sāriva, utpala, yashṭi-madhu, savara (lodhra), agaru and chandana and milk is used as an errhine.

Cases of paridara are treated as in śītāda.

In cases of upakuśa, the patient is subjected to purgation, emesis and errhine therapy. The blood is let out by rubbing the affected part with leaves of kākodumbarika, or goji. A paste of the five salts, trikaṭu and honey is applied externally. The tepid decoctions of pippali, white sarshapa, nāgara and fruits of naichula (vetasa) is used for gargling (kavala). Ghee medicated with drugs of the kākolyādi group is used as an errhine and for gargling.

In cases of danta-vaidarbha, the region around the roots of the teeth is opened with surgical instruments and anointed with kshāra. Cooling measures are also useful.

In adhi-danta, the extra tooth should be extracted and the area cauterizd with fire. Measures indicated in kṛmi-danta are to be employed.

In adhi-māmsa, the growth (swelling) is excised, and the area plastered with the paste of vachā, tejovati, pāṭha, svarjika-kshāra, yava-kshāra and honey. A paste of pippali and honey (and water, NiS) is used for gargling. The decoction of paṭola, triphala and nimba is used for washing the part. Errhines and vairechanika type of fumigation are also useful.

The treatment in danta-nāḍi is as follows: the measures useful in nāḍi-vraṇa can all be employed. The tooth which is very close to the sinus is extracted, and the flesh excised, provided the tooth is not in the upper jaw. The area is then cleansed, and cauterised with fire or alkali (kshāra). If the tooth is not extracted, the sinus may affect the bone of the jaw. A loose or broken tooth should be fully extracted, along with the root. However a tooth of the upper jaw which is firmly implanted should not be extracted, as it might cause severe haemorrhage with all its after effects, kāṇa (eye-diseases), ardita (facial paralysis) etc. A tooth in the upper row should not be extracted even if it is loose. The decoction of jāṭi, madana, svādu-kaṇṭaka and khadira is used to wash the area. Oil medicated with jātī, madana, kaṭuka, svādu-kaṇṭaka, yashṭi-madhu, rodhra, manjishṭa and khadira is used externally.

Treatment of Diseases of the Teeth: In danta-harsha, the following measures are useful: gargling with warm oil or ghee or traivrta ghee, decoctions of drugs which alleviate vāta, the snaihika type of fumigation, errhine therapy, unctuous food, meat juices, gruels (yavāgu) prepared from meat juices, milk, santanika (milk cream), ghee, śiro-basti and other remedies useful in vāta-roga.

In danta-śarkara, the tartar (deposit) is gently removed in such a way that the roots of the teeth are not affected. A paste of the powder of lāksha and honey is applied externally. The measures useful in danta-harsha may also be employed.

The same treatment may be given in kāpālika which is very difficult to cure.

In kṛmi-danta, if the tooth is firm, it is fomented, and the accumulated blood, pus, etc., is drained. The avapīḍa type of errhine, and gaṇḍūsha of oil or ghee, plasters of punarnava and drugs of the bhadra-dārvādi group, and intake of unctuous food are useful. If the tooth is loose, however, it should be extracted, and the area cauterised. Oil medicated with vidāri, yasṭi-madhu, sṛngāṭaka, kaseruka and parts of milk is used as errhine (nasya).

A case of hanu-moksha is treated as in a case of ardita.

In diseases of the teeth, sour fruits, cold water, dry food, brushing the teeth and chewing very hard food are prohibited.

Diseases of the Tongue: The measures indicated in disease of the lips caused by vāta are useful in vātaja-kaṇṭaka. In pittaja-kaṇṭaka, the tongue is scraped (with the leaves of goji, śephalika, etc., NiS) and the vitiated blood is eliminated. Sweet drugs are used for external application, gaṇḍūsha and errhine therapy. In kaphaja kaṇṭaka, the growths are excised, and the vitiated blood let out. The drugs of pippalyādi group are made into a paste with honey and applied over the affected area. The patient is also advised to gargle with white sarshapa and rock salt. A soup (yūsha) of paṭola, nimba, vārtāka and yava-kshāra is advised as diet. In upa-jihva, the swelling is excised, and the area rubbed with an alkali (yava-kshāra). Fumigation, gaṇḍusha and errhines (śiro-virechana) are beneficial.

Diseases of the Palate: In gala-śuṇḍika, the swelling is drawn out by forceps or with the thumb and finger, and excised with a maṇḍalāgra instrument. But only three quarters of the length of the growth should be excised. If too much is excised (severed) there will be haemorrhaging which might kill the patient. If too little is severed, there will be swelling, salivation, sleepiness, vertigo and darkness before the eyes. The part is then plastered with a paste of maricha, ativisha, pāṭha, vachā, kushṭha, śyonāka, rock-salt and honey. The patient is made to gargle with a decoction of vachā, ativisha, pātha, rasona, kaṭu-rohiṇi and nimba. Twice a day, the patient is made to inhale the smoke emitted by burning sticks prepared from the five parts (panchānga) of ingudi, kaṭabhi, danti, sarala (trivṛt, acording to NiS) and devadāru, which also alleviates kapha. The diet consists of soup (yūsha) prepared from mudga treated with kshāras or yava-kshāra.

The diseases tuṇḍikeri, adhrusha, kacchapa, māmsa-sanghāta and tālu-puppuṭa are treated in a similar manner. The surgical procedure however varies.

Tālu-pāka is treated with measures which alleviate pitta (see pitta-roga).

In tālu-śosha, the patient is subjected to snehana (oleation) and svedana (sudation) and other measures which alleviate vāta, (see vāta-roga, treatment of).

Diseases of the Throat: The curable cases of rohiṇi should be treated with bloodletting, emesis, fumigation, gaṇḍūsha, and errhine therapy. In the vātaja type, the area is plastered with a paste of the salts, after bloodletting. Frequent gaṇḍūsha of warm oil or ghee is useful. In the pittaja type, a paste of patanga, sugar and honey should be applied. Gargling with a decoction of drāksha and parūshaka is also useful. In kaphaja rohiṇi, the affected area is rubbed with a paste of soot and kaṭuka oil medicated with rock salt, śveta, viḍanga and danti is used for gargling and errhine therapy. The rohiṇi engendered by the vitiated blood is treated as in the pittaja type.

In kaṇṭha-śālūka, the tumour is bled, and treated as in tuṇḍikeri. The patient is advised to partake of meals consisting of small amounts of barley rice with ghee or oil.

The treatment of adhi-jihvika should be the same as that of upa-jihvika.

In eka-vṛnda, blood-letting is resorted to, followed by śiro-virechana, fumigation, applications of kshāras (alkali) and such other purificatory measures.

A case of gilāyu is treated surgically. If the gala-vidradhi is found in a place that is not vital (marma), it should be opened up when it starts suppurating.

Diseases of the Oral Cavity: In vataja sarvasara, pastes of the salts are applied externally. Oil medicated with drugs which alleviate vāta is used as nasal drops and for gargling. The snaihika kind of fumigation is also beneficial.

In pittaja sarva-sara, the patient is subjected to purificatory therapies (such as enemas, purgation, etc., NiS). Drugs that are sweet and cold are used for external application, gaṇḍūsha, fumigation. etc.

In kaphaja sarva-sara, measures that alleviate kapha should be employed, (see kapha-roga treatment). The patient is also administered one dharana measure of ativisha, pāṭha, musta, devadāru, kaṭuka-rohiṇi, fruit of kuṭaja and cow's urine (every day).

Gargling with milk, sugarcane juice, cow's urine, curds, mastu (curd-cream), sour kanji, oil or ghee is useful in all diseases of the mouth, depending on the dosha involved, (SS, chikitsā, 22).

III. In diseases of the lips caused by vitiated vāta, the paste of madhu-yashṭi may be applied. The lips may be fomented through a nāḍi (tube) by boiling tender leaves of eraṇḍa and milk. Lips which are affected by aggravated vāta may be plastered with a paste of rodhra, sarja-rasa, yashṭi-madhu and honey. Ghee medicated with guḍūchi, yashṭi-madhu and pattanga may also be used (externally). The paste of pāṭha, yava-kshāra, yashṭi-madhu and trikaṭu is applied in diseases of the lips caused by deranged kapha (after blood letting). In the disease known as jālārbuda, the vesicles are opened up, cleaned and rubbed with the paste of pippali, marichika, etc., and honey. If the vesicles are deep seated and extensive, cauterisation with alkalies or fire is useful.

In the diseases of the teeth known as ḍālana (śīta-danta) the patient is fomented with warm water. The edge or margin of the tooth (with the gums) is scraped (with a vrīhi-mukha instrument) and cauterised with oil. The pastes of the bark of dāḍima, vara (triphala), tārkshya, kānta (loha), stone of the jambu fruit, nāgara, honey, rock-salt and ghana (musta) are applied. A decoction of drugs having milky exudation is used for gargling. Aṇu-taila can be used as nasal drops. In danta-harsha, milk boiled with tila and yashṭi-madhu is used as gaṇḍūsha. This is also useful in danta-bheda.

In looseness of the teeth (chala-danta), a decoction of drugs of the daśamūla group is used as gaṇḍūsha along with some oil or ghee. The teeth have to be rubbed with tuttha, rodhra, pippali, triphala, patanga and rock salt. Oily things, ghee, etc., can be used as part of the diet, errhine therapy, for gargling etc. In the case of adhidanta, the tooth is plastered with kshāra (alkali) until it becomes loose and infirm. It is then treated as in a case of kṛmi-danta. If the bleeding continues for a long time or if the blood is impure, it is to be given the treatment indicated in burns (dagdha-vraṇa). In danta-śarkara, a paste of yava-kshāra and honey is applied (after gently removing the deposits). The disease kāpālika is treated in a similar manner along with the measures useful in danta-harsh. In kṛmi-danta, the cavities are to be filled with jaggery, and cauterised with (hot) bee's wax. The pain of kṛmi-danta is relieved by applying the milky exudation of sapta-parṇa and arka. The pain is also relieved by applying the powders of hingu, kaṭphala, kāśīsa, svarjika-kshāra, kushṭha and valli (viḍanga) tied in a piece of cloth. The oil medicated with these drugs or with a decoction of eraṇḍa, kaṇṭakāri, bṛhati and bhu-kandanka can be used for gaṇḍūsha. If the pain persists even after all these measures, the tooth is extracted with a small samdamśa or danta-nirghatana instrument after first separating the root of the tooth from the gum. Then oil medicated with powder of yashṭi-madhu or honey with yashṭi-madhu is used for gaṇḍūsha. Teeth should not be extracted (if they are firm) in debilitated, emaciated and elderly persons and persons in whom there is aggravation of vāta. The teeth of the upper row should not be extracted. After the extraction of teeth, measures consisting of oily, sweet and cold substances should be employed.

Treatment in Diseases of the Gums: In cases of upakuśa, the gums are fomented with hot water, and are scraped with leaves or maṇḍalāgra instrument. The warm upper layer of ghee (ghṛta-maṇḍa) is useful for gaṇḍūsha. In danta-puppuṭaka, the area is fomented, excised or incised or scraped. The paste of yashṭi-madhu, svarjika-kshāra, nāgara and rock-salt is to be applied externally. In abscess (vidradhi), pungent, sharp (tīkshṇa), hot and dry drugs are used for gargling and external application. The abscess is then scraped or rubbed with kaṭuka, kushṭa, vrischikah and yava. Suppuration can be prevented by using cold drugs (both internally and externally). If it suppurates, it is to be lanced. If it is deeprooted, it may have to be cauterised.

In danta-nāḍi, after the measures explained in SS, a decoction of trees having milky exudation is used for gandusha. Oil medicated with these drugs is used for errhine therapy.

In the disease of the tongue known as adhi-jihvika, the swelling is raised up with the help of the badiśa instrument, and is excised with the mandalāgra instrument. Drugs which are hot and sharp (tīkshṇa) are used for scrubbing the area.

In the disease of the palate known as gala-śunāika, measures which alleviate kapha are to be employed. In tālu-pāka which has not ripened, the part is to be rubbed with kāsīsa, honey and rasāñjana. Cold infusions of drugs which are sweet are used for gargling. If it ripens, it is to be incised in eight places (or in a quadrupartite fashion), and anointed with drugs that are sharp and hot. Infusions, etc., of bitter drugs such as vāsa, nimba, paṭola, etc., are used for gargling.

In tālu-śosha, if the patient is not thirsty, potions of ghee are administered after meals. The decoction of pippali and nāgara is given internally. Sour substances (like kānji) are used for gaṇḍūsha. Unctuous meat-juices of animals of desert areas are to be partaken of. Ghee extracted from milk is used as nasal drops.

Treatment of Diseases of the Throat: In diseases of the throat, the patient is subjected to blood-letting, errhine therapy, etc., and is administered a decoction of bark of dāru-haridra, nimba, rasāñjana and kalinga or a decoction of harītaki with honey. The decoction of śreshta (triphala), trikaṭu, yava-kshāra, dāru-haridra, rasāñjana, chitraka, pātha, tejini, and nimba with śukla and cow's urine is used for gargling. Pills composed of the same drugs are used for external application. The paste of nichula, kaṭabhi, mustā, devadāru, nāgara, vachā, danti and mūrva is applied when warm, in order to relieve pain and swelling.

In vātaja-rohiṇi, fomentation is given both internally and externally. The nodules are excised by the anguli-śastra or with the nail smeared with rock-salt. The decoction of the (bṛhat) panchamūla drugs is used for gargling. Oil is used for gaṇḍūsha and errhine therapy.

In pittaja rohiṇi, blood-letting is done, after which the part is rubbed with priyangu, sugar and honey. A decoction of these drugs and rodhra and patanga is used for gargling. The decoction of drāksha and parūshaka is also used for gargling.

In kaphaja-rohiṇi, oil medicated with fruits or seeds of apāmārga, śveta (giri-karṇika), danti, viḍanga and rock salt is used for ganāūsha and nasya.

The same treatment is indicated in vraṇa, śāluka, tuṇḍikeri and gilāyu.

An abscess (vidradhi) is opened surgically, and the paste of triphala, gorochana, rasāñjana, gairika, rodhra, rock-salt, patanga and pippali is used for rubbing the area. A decoction of the same drugs is used for gaṇḍūsha.

In diseases of the oral cavity (mukha-pāka), a decoction of triphala, paṭha, mṛdvika, fresh leaves of jāti and honey is used for washing the mouth. The above drugs or drugs of the harītaki group are chewed and spat out.

In vāta mukha-pāka, the paste of pippali, rock salt and ela is applied externally; oil medicated with drugs that alleviate vāta is used for gargling and nasya.

In arbuda which is recent and not well developed, the growth is excised, and then plastered with the paste of svarjika-kshāra, nāgara and honey. A decoction of pastes of guḍūchi and nimba along with honey and oil is used for gaṇḍūsha. The diet has to consist of yavā-anna. Oil medicated with sharp drugs is used for massage and nasya.

In bad breath (ūrdhva-guda or pūti-mukha), the patient is subjected to emesis and fumigation and nasya of sharp drugs. The decoction of samanga, dhātaki, rodhra, phalini and padmaka is used for washing the mouth. The powders of the same drugs can be dusted inside the mouth. Nasya useful in śitāda and upakuśa are useful.

Some Recipes: One hundred pala weight of nila-sahachara is boiled with water (and reduced to one-forth quantity, and filtered). The paste of one half pala of khadira, jambu, yashṭi-madhu, sāriva, apāmarga and nilotpala is added to it along with one prastha of oil and boiled. This oil is to be kept in the mouth and retained there for a while. It is useful in all disease of the mouth, especially in looseness of teeth.

The decoction of kaṇṭakāri, guḍūchi, tender leaves of sumana (mālati), dāru-haridra, yavāsa and triphala is used as a gargle with honey in all diseases of the mouth.

The powders of soot, rasānjana, pāṭha, trịkaṭu, yava-kshāra, chitraka, loha (bhasma), triphala and tejovati is used with honey as an external application in all diseases of the mouth, teeth and throat.

The powders of the bark of dāru-haridra, rock salt, manahśila, yava-śūka, and haritāla is also applied with honey in diseases of the mouth, teeth and throat.

Harītaki is to be boiled in cow's urine and is then triturated with a decoction of miśi and kushṭha. This is given internally as a prophylactic for all diseases of the mouth.

The decoction of paṭola, nāgara, triphala, viśāla, trāyaṇti, tiktaka, haridra, dāruharidra and guḍuchi can be administered with honey internally or used as gaṇḍūsha. It relieves all diseases of the mouth.

The decoction of dāru-haridra is boiled until it becomes semi-solid. It is then mixed with gairika and honey and applied externally in mukha-pāka and fistulae (nādi-vraṇa). The decoction of khadhira, agaru or loha bhasma, triphala, arjuna, madayanti and arimeda is used as gaṇḍūsha for strengthening the teeth.

Barley, soup prepared from (yuva) trna-dhānya (such as mudga, etc.), yava-kshāra and ghee or oil is beneficial. All measures which alleviate kapha are useful in diseases of the mouth, (AHṛ, uttara, 22).

III. Equal quantities of pra-pouṇḍarīka, manjishṭha, vatsa-nābha and tinḍuka (kāraskara) are made into a paste. The oil medicated with this paste is used for the purpose of gaṇḍūsha in diseases of the mouth.

The powder of āmalaki taken with milk is useful in nodules of the throat (gala-kīlaka). Pills prepared from visha-tinḍuka, nāgara and harītaki are to be kept in the mouth and sucked (in the above diseases). The paste of rock salt and milky exudation of arka is applied externally.

The bark(?) of nirguṇḍi and stalk of nilotpala are to be chewed in upa-jihvika. The powder of harītaki is heated in a copper vessel for a little while, with honey. It is then made into pills, which when kept in the mouth cures kṛmi-danta. Pills prepared from purified kāśīsa, hingu, alum, devadāru and water are to be kept in the mouth. This relieves the pain in kṛmi-danta. The powder of fruit of indra-vāruṇi is sprinkled on a piece of heated iron. The smoke causes the parasites to fall out. Teeth which are loose become firm if one chews the leaves of jāti and koranti first thing in the morning. The seeds of mūlaka when kept in the mouth (and chewed) strengthen the teeth.

Pills composed of svarṇa-mākshika bhasma, abhraka bhasma, tuttha bhasma, purified manhaśila, rājāvarta bhasma, śilājatu, guggulu and pārada bhasma (rasa-sindūra) are useful in mukha-roga. The paste of manḍūra (bhasma) and buffalo's urine is slightly warmed up and applied in diseases of the throat.

Svarṇa-bhasma, rajata bhasma, purified pārada (rasa-sindūra) and purified haratāla are triturated with milk. The paste is then boiled in oil in a dola yantra. It is then administered with honey in looseness of the teeth, (RRS, 29, 116; 24, 30-66).

Classical Prescriptions:

Mukha-roga: Arimedādi-taila; Gomutra-harītaki; Kālaka-chūrṇa; Kanaka-taila; Kunkumādi-taila.

Mukha-pāka: Khadirādi-guṭika.

Gala roga: Gorochanādi-vaṭi; Kālaka-chūrṇa; Khadirādi-guṭika; Mṛdvīkārishṭa; Trikaṭu-chūrṇa.

Danta-chālana: Bhringāmalakādi-taila; Shaḍ--bindu-taila.

Danta-kḥmi: Khadirādi-guṭika

Danta-roga: Arimedādi-taila; Kālaka-chūrṇa; Kāyyonnyādi-taila; Khadirādi-guṭika; Nārāyaṇa-taila.

Mūrccha

Western Nosology: Fainting ; Syncope

Causative Factors:

Extrinsic:

1. Regular intake of unwholesome food by a person where mind is over powered by rajas and tamas, (CS, sūtra, 24, 26).

2. Intake of incompatible food articles, suppression of natural urges, injuries, emaciation and prostration or weakness of mind (hīna-sattva), (SS, uttara, 46, 3).

Intrinsic: All three doshas, (CS). Mainly pitta (SS, ibid, 8).

Constituents Affected:

1. Channels which transmit blood and rasa dhātu, (CS, ibid, 25).

2. Sense faculties and mind, (SS, ibid, 4).

Classification:

1. According to CS, there are four types of mūrccha, those that are engendered by vāta, pitta or kapha or all three combined, (CS, ibid).

2. According to SS, there are six types of mūrccha, those that may be caused by vitiation of the three doshas individually, by the deranged blood, by intake of alcohol and by poisoning, (SS, ibid, 7).

Prodromal Symptoms: Discomfort or pain around the pre-cordial region, yawning, lethargy, loss of consciousness and debility, (SS,ibid, 5).

Symptomatology:

1. In vātaja mūrccha, the patient loses consciousness while perceiving that the sky is blue, black or brownish in colour. He recovers consciousness immediately. He will also suffer from trembling (of limbs), body pain, pain in the region of the heart, emaciation and grayish-brown discolouration (of skin, etc.).

In pittaja mūrccha, just before losing consciousness, the patient perceives the sky to be yellow, green or reddish in colour. He sweats while recovering consciousness. He also suffers from thirst, fever, reddish-yellow tinge in the eyes, looseness of stools and yellow discolouration (of skin, etc.).

In kaphaja mūrccha, the patient feels as if the sky is dark or enveloped by thick clouds, just before losing consciousness. He recovers with a moist skin. He also suffers from salivation, nausea, and heaviness of body.

In sannipātaja mūrccha, all the symptoms may be present, and the patient looks as if he has apasmāra, but without the hideous actions seen in that disease, (CS, sūtrā, 24, 35-41).

2. The symptoms of vātaja, pittaja and kaphaja mūrccha are similar to those of vātaja, pittaja and kaphaja apasmara.

In raktaja mūrccha there is stiffness or rigidity of the limbs and eyes, and deep breathing (almost imperceptible respiration, according to NiS).

In mūrccha due to alcohol, there will be delirious speech, mindlessness, mental agitation, while the patient will convulsively jerk his limbs while lying on the ground.

In mūrccha caused by poisoning, there will be trembling, thirst, rigidity (of limbs), drowsiness and specified symptoms brought about by each poison, (SS, ibid, 9, 12-13).

Prognosis: Mūrccha is considered to be more serious than mada and not as serious as sanyāsa, (CS, sūtrā, 14, 24, 27).

Treatment:

1. The patient has to be subjected to oleation and sudation, followed by the five purificatory procedures (pancha-karma), with due regard to the dosha involved.

The patient can be administered triphala with ghee, honey and sugar or śilājatu with milk or pippali or chitraka with milk. Medicines such as kalyāṇaka ghṛta, mahā-tiktaka ghṛta, shatpala ghee or just old ghee are useful. Blood letting, study of scriptures and company of good people are also advised, (CS, ibid, 54-58).

2. The general line of treatment consists of sprinkling (of water, etc.), tub baths (avagāha), wearing of precious stones and garlands, cold applications, (plasters, pradeha), fanning the patient, a cool breeze and administering cold and fragrant decoctions, etc.

The patient is to be administered beverages containing sugar candy, priyāla and sugar-cane juice or juices of drāksha and madhūka or kharjūra and kāśmari; and ghee medicated with drugs of the jīvaniya group. He can also be given milk medicated with the drugs of the kākolyādi group, meat juices of desert animals with dāḍima, and red-rice, satīna and barley (yava).

The following prescriptions are also useful: equal quantities of nāgakeśara, maricha, uśīra, and pulp of badara with cold water; bisa (lotus fibre) and mṛnāla (lotus stalk) with cold water; pippali with honey; harītaki with sugar candy; breast-milk; ghee medicated with a decoction of harītaki or juice of āmalaki; and decoctions useful in pittaja jvara along with drāksha, sugar candy, dāḍima, lājā, padma and nīlotpala.

If there are repeated attacks of mūrccha, frequent use of errhines and inducing emesis with active drugs are useful, (SS, ibid, 14-20).

3. In mūrccha brought about by use of alcohol, the patient is administered an emetic, and allowed to sleep for as long as he desires. In mūrccha caused by poisoning, the appropriate vishagna (antidotes to poisons) drugs are administered.

A decoction of nāgara, guḍūchi, kaṇṭakāri, and pushkara with pippali is useful. The patient can also be advised to take triphala with honey at night, and jaggery with fresh ginger in the morning, with a suitable diet, for a week's time.

The person can be aroused from mūrccha by use of powerful (tīkshṇa) collyrium, avapīḍa-nasya, fumigation (dhūma), pradhamana nasya, pricking with a needle, burning the skin (with an alkali), by pressing below the finger-nails, pulling at the hairs of body and head, grinding of teeth, rubbing the body with ātma-gupta, etc., (CD, 17,1-12).

Classical Prescriptions: Aśvagandhādyarishṭa; Balā-taila; Drākshādi-kvātha-chūrṇa; Dhātryādi-ghṛta; Eladi-guṭika; Pūga-khanḍa; Soubhāgya-vaṭi; Vāta-kulāntaka-rasa.

Nāḍī-vraṇa

Symptoms: Nādi-vrana

Western Nosology: Fistulae; Sinuses; Carbuncle

Causative Factors:

Extrinsic: Neglecting (to open) a localised swelling which has ripened, improper diet and regimen when the vraṇa has been filled with pus (has fully suppurated), (SS, AHṛ).

Pathogenesis: The pus burrows inwards, in the form of a channel (from the vraṇa-sthānas, localities of the vrana, such as the skin, etc.). There will be excessive infiltration of pus, and many cavities within, (SS, AHṛ).

Types: There are five types, namely vātaja, pittaja, kaphaja, tridoshaja (caused by all three doshas) and śalyaja (caused by the presence of a imbedded foreign body), (SS, AHṛ).

Symptomatology:

The vātaja-nāḍi-vrana is very painful, foul and narrow-mouthed with a frothy discharge which increases at night.

The pittaja-nāḍi-varṇa is characterised by fever, local heat, thirst, fatigue (lethargy), pricking pain and hot and yellow discharge which is worse during the day.

The kaphaja-nādi-vraṇa is characterised by itching, hardness (induration), slight benumbing pain and nightly discharge of thick, slimy, whitish pus.

The nādi vraṇa caused by the aggravation of all the doshas presents signs and symptoms characteristic of all the doshas. In addition there will be fever, burning pain, dysnoea, syncope and dryness of the mouth.

Śalyaja-nāḍi-vraṇa: A foreign object which has been imbedded in the body and is not outwardly visible tends to pierce through the flesh, etc., and form a nādi (sinus). In such cases, there will be severe constant pain, local heat and sudden (forcible) ejection of hot, frothy, bloody, swirling discharge, (SS).

Prognosis: The tridoshaja-nāḍi-vraṇa is difficult to cure (SS).

Ref.: SS, nidāna, 10, 9-14; AHṛ, uttara, 29, 26-31.

Treatment:

1. In vāta-nāḍi-vraṇa, a poultice (upanāha) should first be applied, and then the course of the sinus should be probed and opened, and then bandaged after applying a paste of tila. apāmārga fruits, and rock-salt. The ulcer should then be regularly washed with a decoction of bṛhat-panchamūla drugs. An oil medicated with himsra, haridra, kaṭuka, balā, gojihva and bilva roots should be used for purifying the ulcer and promoting granulation and healing.

In pittaja-nāḍi-vraṇa, an utkārika type of poultice should be applied after mixing with milk and ghee. The sinus should be surgically opened, and the ulcer should be washed daily with a decoction of soma, nimba and haridra.

The ghee medicated with śyāma (vṛddha-dāru), tṛivrt, triphala, haridra, dāru-haridra, lodhra, kuṭaja and milk is very efficacious in promoting healing of an ulcer even if it is located in the koshṭha (visceral organs).

In the kapha-nāḍi-vraṇa, the area is softened by applying a poultice of kulattha, siddhārtaka (white mustard), saktu and kiṇva (surā-bija). The sinus should first be probed carefully and then opened. The paste of tila, nimba, danti, surāshtra (a kind of earth/mud) and rock-salt should be applied. The decoction of karanja, nimba, jāti, aksha and pīlu should be used for washing the ulcer. An oil medicated with suvarchika, rock-salt, chitraka, danti, tali-tala (mushali root), white arka, apāmārga fruits, and cow's urine is used for healing.

In the śalyaja-nāḍi-vraṇa, the foreign body is first extracted (as per the directions given in SS, sūtra, 27) and the ulcer is then cleansed (purified), by applying a paste of tila, and large amounts of honey and ghee. Oil medicated with a decoction of the tender fruits of kumbhika, kharjūra and kapittha and the paste of mustā, sarala, priyangu, sugandhika, mocha-rasa, ahipushpa, lodhra and dhātaki flowers is useful in healing the ulcer rapidly.

In the case of a nāḍi-vraṇa occuring in weak, debilitated and timid persons, or occuring in the vital organs, a kshāra-sūtra should be used instead of a knife.

The different kinds of varti (plugs) described in SS, chikitsā, 1, can be used in this disease also. Other kinds of varti are also described in SS, chikitsā, 17. The medicine bhallātaka-taila is very efficacious in nāḍi-vraṇa, (SŚ).

2. A paste of chanchu-fruits applied externally is very efficacious in nāḍi-vrāṇa, (AHṛ).

3. The following medicines are useful in nāḍi-vraṇa; Saptānga-guggulu; Svarjikādya-taila; Kumbhikādya-taila; Bhallatākadya-taila and Nirguṇāi-taila, (CD).

4. The following medicines can be administered in nāḍi to promote healing: the paste of khadira and exudation of white eraṇḍa, applied externally; the application of a milky exudation of asphoṭa; and the internal use of powders of viḍanga, triphala and pippali taken with honey ,(BR).

Ref.: SS, chikitsā, 17, 17-41; AHṛ, uttara, 30, 37,; CD, 45; BR, page. 562.

Classical Prescriptions: Haratāla-bhasma; Jātyadi-taila; Lakshmi-vilāsa-rasa; Panchatiktaka-guggulu-ghṛta; Somarāji-taila; Vraṇa-rākshasa-taila.

Nīlika

Synonyms: Sanskrit-Nīli

Causative Factors:

Extrinsic: Emotions such as grief and anger, (AS).

Intrinsic: Pitta (CS, sūtra, 18, 25; 20, 14). Vāta and pitta (AS).

Constituents Affected: Blood (CS, sūtra, 28, 12).

Pathogenesis and Symptomatology: The aggravated pitta engenders dryness in the blood, causing this disease, (CS, sūtra, 18, 25).

The aggravated vāta and pitta bring about the formation of circular black discolouration (and swelling, CS) on the body. If vāta is mainly involved, there will be dryness of the skin and greyish discolouration. If pitta is mainly involved, the discolouration will be bluish with copper-coloured borders. If kapha is involved, there will be itching and whitish borders. If the blood is deranged, there will also be burning and smarting pain in the affected areas, (AS).

There will be painless, isolated (SS, MN) blackish discolouration either of the body or face. According to bhoja (madhu-kośa on MN) and AS, the discolouration will be confined to the body only. The face will not be affected.

Related Diseases: Vyanga

Ref.: SS, nidāna, 13, 46; AS, uttara, 36; MN, 55, 40.

Treatment:

1. The external application of paste of jātiphala and massage of the body in the evening with kaṭu-taila will be very useful.

The decoction of yashṭi-madhu is boiled with the paste of priyangu, manjishṭha, chandana, nilotpala and nāga-keśara, and til-oil. This oil known as kanaka-taila can be used for external application.

The remedies useful in vyanga can be employed in treating this disease also, (CD).

2. The remedial measures indicated under nyaccha can be used in this disease also,(SS).

Ref.: CD, 55, 50, 58-59.

Classified Prescriptions: Kanaka-taila,; Kunkumādi-taila; Mahā-triphalādya-ghṛta; Somarāji-taila.

Niruddha-prākaśa

Western Nosology: Phimosis

Causative Factors:

Extrinsic: Factors which aggravate vāta

Intrinsic: Vāta

Symptomatology: The prepuce covers the glans penis and obstructs the flow of urine. If the glans is only partially enveloped, a thin stream of urine is emitted with slight pain. Even if the glans is completely covered, there will not be any fissure in the glans.

Treatment: A tube made of iron, wood or shellac (lāksha) which is open at both ends, is smeared with ghee and gently introduced into the urethra. The marrow or fat of śiśumāra or boar or chukra-taila medicated with drugs that alleviate vāta is sprinkled over the affected area. Every third day, slightly thicker tubes should be introduced into the urethra. The diet should consist of unctuous food preparations.

As an alternative mode of treatment, an incision should be made along the prepuce, avoiding the sevani (raphe) and this should be treated as in an open wound (sadyo-vraṇa).

Related Diseases: Parivartika, Avapāṭika.

Ref.: SS, nidāna, 13, 52-53; chikitsā, 20, 43-46.

Nyaccha

Synonyms: Sanskrit - Lānchana (in vernacular) (NiS) on (SS).

Western Nosology: Mole

Casuative Factors:

Intrinsic: Vāta and pitta (NC and NiS on SS).

Constituent Affected: The second layer of skin known as rohitā (SS, śārīra, 4, 4); blood (SS, sūtra, 2, 9).

Symptomatology: Congenital, painless, small or large whitish or blackish circular discolouration of the skin, (SS).

Treatment: The patient can be subjected to blood-letting. The affected areas can also be rubbed with saumudraphena, etc., and plastered over with the paste of the bark of kshīri trees and milk, or a paste of the bala, ati-bala, yashṭi-madhu and haridra; or a paste of arka-pushpi, agaru and black chandana or a paste of kapittha and rajadāni, (SS).

Related Diseases: Vyanga, Nīlika

Ref.: SS, nidāna, 13, 44; chikitsā, 20, 33-36.

Mūtrāghāta

Western Nosology: Obstructive uropathy

Types:

1. According to SS, there are twelve kinds of disease included under the general heading of mūtrāghāta. They are vāta-kuṇḍalika, vātashṭhila, vāta-basti, mutrātīta, mutra-jaṭhara, mūtrotsanga, mūtra-kshaya, mūtra-granthi, mūtra-śukra, ushṇa-vāta, and two kinds of mūtroukasada.

2. CS has enumerated eight kinds of mūtrāghāta; three types engendered by the vitiated vāta, pitta and kaphā, that which is caused by the provocation of all the three doshas, that which is caused by aśmari (calculi) or by śarkara (gravel), or by the śukra or vitiated blood, (CS, sūtra, 19, 4).

The following thirteen diseases have also been described: mutrotsanga, mūtra-kshāya, mutrātīta, mūtrashṭhīla, vāta-basti, ushṇa-vāta, vāta-kuṇḍalika, rakta-granthi, vit-vighāta, basti-kuṇḍa, mutra-jaṭhara, kṛcchramūtra and mutroukasāda, (CS, siddhi, 9, 15-16).

3. AS has enumerated and described twenty kinds of mutrāghāta. They are: the four types of kṛcchra engendered by vāta, pitta, kapha and all three combined; the four types of aśmari, viz. those caused by the vitiated vāta, pitta, kapha and śukra; vāta-basti, ashṭhīla, kuṇḍalika, mutrātīta, mūtra-jaṭhara, mutrotsanga, mūtra-granthi, mūtra-śukra, viḍ-vighāta, ushṇa-vāta, mūtra-kshaya and mutra-avasāda, (AŚ, nidāna, 9, 3).

4. MN has enumerated thirteen kinds of mutrāghāta, viz., the twelve types mentioned in SS and additionally basti-kuṇḍa, (MN, 31).

Pathogenesis and Symptoms of Vāta-kuṇḍalika:

1. Due to excessive intake of dry food, suppression of natural urges, etc. the vāta is aggravated, localises in the urinary bladder, and causes the urine to revolve in eddies. The urine is therefore passed in small quantities, or is passed in very small quantities with pain, (SS).

2. The aggravated vāta obstructs the normal flow of urine, and as a result, the urine is deflected (within the bladder). There is severe pain, obstruction (retention) of urine and stools, heaviness of body and difficult urination, (CS).

Pathogenesis and Symptoms of Vātashṭhīla:

1. The vāta that is aggravated and localises in the region between the urinary bladder and anus engenders the formation of a stable, raised, thick knotty growth, which causes retention of stools and urine, flatulent distension of the abdomen, and pain in the region of the urinary bladder, (SS).

2. The aggravated vāta localises in the region of the anus and urinary bladder, causes flatulent distension, and the formation of a stony tumour which is very painful. There is also obstruction of stools and urine, (CS).

3. There is also obstruction to flatus, (AS).

Pathogenesis and Symptoms of Vāta-basti:

1. In a person who foolishly suppresses the urge to urinate, the aggravated vāta obstructs the mouth of the urinary bladder, causing retention of urine and pain in the bladder and abdomen, (SS).

2. In addition to the above symptoms, there will also be itching, (CS).

3. Occasionally, the urinary bladder is displaced from its normal position due to the aggravated vāta, and is elevated, thick and swollen, resembling the swollen belly of a pregnant woman. The urine dribbles in drops and flows when the bladder is pressed. The patient also suffers from pain, burning pain, stiffness and pulsation, (AS).

Pathogenesis and Symptoms of Mūtrātīta:

1. If a person suppresses the urge to urinate, and later attempts to pass urine, it is often impossible to do so. Only after much straining, is there dribbling of urine, with mild pain, (SS).

2. If the urge to urinate is suppressed for a long time, the urine does not flow out easily. It flows in a feeble stream after much straining, (CS).

Pathogenesis and Symptoms of Mūtra-jaṭhara:

1. Suppressing the urge to urinate causes aggravation of apāna-vāta and udāvarta. The aggravated vāta fills up the abdomen, and causes flatulent distention and severe pain in the region of abdomen below the umbilicus. There is also obstruction of stools and urine, (CS, SS).

Pathogenesis and Symptoms of Mūtrotsanga:

1. The displaced (and aggravated vāta) causes feeble flow of urine and dribbling of urine, with or without pain, or flow of bloody urine with tenesmus. The urine is obstructed at the urethra or glans penis, (SS).

2. Due to aggravation of vāta and kha-vaiguṇya, a small amount of urine is retained at the region of the glans penis, and is later emitted slowly, with or without pain. The penis also becomes swollen or heavy due to the retention of urine, (CS).

Pathogenesis and Symptoms of Mūtra-kshaya:

1. The vāta and pitta are aggravated and localise in the urinary bladder, in an emaciated and dried up individual, and as a result there is scanty formation of urine. There will also be burning sensation and pain, (SS).

2. The urine (present in the bladder) dries up due to the aggravation of vāta, (CS).

Pathogenesis and Symptoms of Mūtra-granthi:

1. A stable, rounded, painful, small knotty

tumour that grows rapidly and is located within the bladder obstructs the outlet (from within). The other symptoms are similar to those found in aśmari, (SS).

2. The aggravated kapha and vāta, and the vitiated blood engender the formation of a knotty tumour at the outlet of the bladder. The urine therefore can be emitted with difficulty. The pain, will be similar to that in aśmari. This disease is also known as rakta-granthi, (CS).

Pathogenesis and Symptoms of Mūtra Śukra (Seminuria): If a person indulges in sexual intercourse after suppressing the urge to urinate there will be forcible discharge of semen either before or after the urine, while the urine will the colour of a solution of ashes (kshāras), (SS, AS). - See kṛcchra-mūtra.

Pathogenesis and Symptoms of Ushṇa-vāta:

1. As a result of excessive exertion, walking for long distances or exposure to the sun, the pitta is aggravated, and localises in the bladder along with the aggravated vāta. The patient suffers from burning pain is the urinary bladder, penis (urethra) and rectum, and painful urination of yellowish or bloody urine or discharge of only blood (through the urethra), (SS, AS).

2. The aggravated vāta and pitta dry up the urine, cause pain and burning along the urethra and urinary bladder, and difficult (painful) urination, the urine being yellowish-red, (CS).

Pathogenesis and Symptoms of Mūtroukasāda:

1. There are two kinds, one caused by the aggravated pitta and the other by the deranged kapha. In the former type, urine is non-slimy, yellow, thick, and when dry, leaves a sediment resembling the powder of cow's bile (rochana). In the latter kind, the urine is slimy, thick, whitish and when dry leaves a sediment that is white like powdered śankha (conch). The urine is emitted with difficulty, (SS).

2. The aggravated kapha and pitta and the slightly provoked vāta causes a flow of urine that is thick, yellowish, whitish or red, and dense. There is also burning micturition. All the symptoms of the aggravated doshas may also be present, (CS).

Pathogenesis and Symptoms of Kṛcchra-mūtra: If a person indulges in sexual intercourse after suppressing the urge to urinate, there is aggravation of vāta, and semen is discharged either before or after the urine, (CS).

Pathogenesis and Symptoms of Viḍ-vighāta: The vāta that is aggravated in a debilitated and dried up individual obstructs the passage of stools, and as a result the urine has the smell of faeces and may be mixed with it, (CS, AS).

Pathogenesis and Symptoms of Basti-kuṇḍala: The urinary bladder is displaced from its normal position in a person due to injury, over-exertion, or fasting, and resembles the foetus. There will be burning, pain and pulsation, along with dribbling of urine. The urine flows if the bladder is pressed. If pitta is vitiated there will be burning sensation, pain, and discolouration of urine. If kapha is aggravated, there will be a sense of heaviness, swelling, and thick and white urine, (CS), (see vāta-basti).

Prognosis:

1. The disease basti-kuṇḍala is incurable if there is complete retention of urine, or if pitta is excessively vitiated. It is very difficult to treat if vāta is aggravated. It is also incurable if there is dyspnoea, or hṛd-moha, along with the displacement of the bladder, (CS).

2. The following diseases are difficult to cure: vāta-kuṇḍalika and vāta-basti, (SS).

Ref.: SS, uttara, 58, 3-26; CS, siddhi, 89, 25-48; AS, nidāna, 9; MN, 31.

Treatment:

1. The treatment should consist of decoctions, pastes, oils, food articles, lehyas, milk, kshāras (alkalies), alcoholic drinks, etc., prepared from medicated drugs, fomentation and uttara-basti

(urethral douches). Measures that are useful in aśmari and mūtra-udāvarta are also useful.

The following prescriptions are useful: the paste of ervāru seeds, rock salt and dhānyāmla; wine preparred from pishṭa (or flour) with souvarchala salt, or wine prepared from jaggery; a paste of kumkum that is soaked overnight in a solution of honey and water; the paste of ela, jeeraka, nāgara, wine (prepared from flour), the juice of daḍima and rock salt; the paste of musta, harītaki, devadāru, yashṭi-madhu, mūrva (and honey); the paste of harītaki, āmalaki and vibhītaki (triphala) with rock salt and water; the paste of drāksha soaked overnight in the expressed juice of udumbara and taken the next morning; the expressed juice of kaṇṭakāri; the expressed juice of āmalaka with honey; the juice of āmalaki, with ela and honey; the paste of tender roots of kola with rice water; the juice of trapusha and white variety of karkaṭaka is taken with milk in the early morning; a decoction of drugs of the sweet group (kākolyādi) with milk and ghee; the ashes of burnt pāṭala wood should be strained through a cloth seven times, and taken with a little quantity of til oil; the paste of nala, pāshāṇa-bheda, darbha, sugarcane (ikshu), ervāru, trapusha and beejaka should be washed in milk, filtered and taken along with the kshārodaka (alkaline water) prepared from the ashes of pāṭala, yava-kshāra, pāribhadra and tila; a paste of the above drugs and jaggery can also be taken.

The decoction of milk, root of gokshura and drugs of vidārigandhādi group is to be taken, when cold, with honey and sugarcandy in cases of mūtra-ghāta caused by vāta or pitta.

Generally, a person suffering from mūtrāghāta should be subjected to oleation (snehana), sudation (svedana), and purgation. After these measures, he should be administered uttara-basti (urethral injections).

If a person suffers from discharge of blood through the urethra due to sexual excesses, he should be asked to avoid sexual intercourse, and should be subjected to bṛmhaṇa (nourishing) therapy. He can be administered uttara-basti with the fat (lard) of kukkuṭa and oil.

One part of ghee extracted from milk and one-half part of honey, and one-half part of sugar, drāksha, fruits of ātmagupta, ikshwāka and pippali (together) are strained well in a vessel. A person suffering from this disease should lick one paṇi-tola measure of this compound, and drink milk after it.

Equal quantities of bala, stones of kola fruits, yashṭi-madhu, gokshūra, śatāvatri, lotus stem, kaseru, ikshuraka seeds, sahasravīrya (darbha), amśumati (śālaparṇi), payasya (arkā-pushpi), kālā (a kind of sariva), pṛśniparṇi, ati-balā and drugs with a sweet taste (i.e. drugs of kākolyādi group excluding guḍūchi), should be boiled with four parts of milk (or water) and one tola of jaggery, until only one droṇa of water (or milk) is left. This is then boiled with one āḍhaka weight of ghee. This should then be mixed with some amount of honey and stored in an earthern vessel. This is very useful in all kinds of mūtrāghāta, (SS).

2. In the disease mūtra-jaṭhara, the patient should be administered diuretics. The powders of hingu, vachā, chitraka, kushṭha, suvarchika (svarjika-kshāra) and viḍanga, taken in increasing amounts are given along with warm water, (CS).

3. The patient can be administered expressed juice of dhanvayāsa or a decoction of kakubha or the paste of triphala, rock salt and water, or a decoction of kaṇṭakāri and gokshura or gruel prepared from kaṇṭakari, gokshūra and phānita or a decoction of drugs of the vīratarādi group or the powder of śilājatu with the latter decoction or gruel prepared from meat-juice of tāmra-chūḍa (kukkuṭa), (AHṛ, chikitśa, 11, 37-39).

4. The following prescriptions are useful in mutrāghāta: the expressed juice of durālabha or the decoction of vāsa; the decoction of fruits, roots and leaves of gokshura with honey and

sugar-candy; the expressed juice of kaṇṭakāri with buttermilk; the paste of the root of barhi-śikha with rice-water, a diet consisting only of curds; and the paste of bhadra, pāshāṇabheda root, śatāvari, chitraka, rohiṇi, kokilaksha, krouncha, sthūla and gokshura with wine.

A person suffering from ushṇa-vāta should take a paste of chandana, rice water and sugar. The diet should consist of rice with boiled and cooled milk. This is also useful in bleeding from the urethra, (CSS).

5. The paste of khadira seeds and water of the root of rudra-jaṭa and buttermilk is very useful in mūtrāghāta. Powder of karpūra (camphor) can be inserted into the urethra.

The juice of kūshmāṇḍa can be taken with yava-kshāra and sugar in ushṇa-vāta, (CD).

Related Diseases: Mūtra-kṛcchra

Ref.: SS, uttara, 58, 27-64; CS, siddhi, 9, 30-31; AHṛ, chikitsā, 1, 37-39; CSS, pages. 460; CD, 33, 12, 15.

Classical Priscriptions: Gokshūrādi-guggulu; Guḍuchyādi-modaka; Nyagrodādhi-chūrṇa; Svarṇa-vanga.

Mūtra-kṛcchra

Western Nosology: Painful urination; Dysuria.

Causative Factors:

Extrinsic: Excessive physical exertion, intake of powerful drugs, very dry food and excessive alcoholic drinks, continuously riding on fast moving animals, excessive intake of fish and meat of aquatic animals, over-eating and eating before the digestion of the previous meal, (CS).

Pathogenesis:

1. The three doshas being provoked either singly or together due to the respective causes localise in the urinary bladder, and cause compression (on the bladder) which results in painful urination, (CS).

2. The aggravated pitta along with kapha and vāta adversely affects the urinary bladder, and causes painful urination, (KS).

Types:

1. There are eight types of mūtra-kṛcchra namely those causd by the aggravated vāta, pitta or kapha, or all three combined, or due to vitiated blood, or due to urinary calculi (aśmari) or due to obstruction of semen or due to obstruction of faeces.

2. The eight types of mūtrakṛcchra according to SS are the same as in CS, excepting that śarkaraja-mūtra-kṛcchra is instead substituted by śukraja-mūtrakṛcchra.

Symptomatology:

Vātaja-mūtra-kṛcchra:

1. There is severe pain in the groins, supra-pubic region and urethra, and scanty and frequent urination, (CS).

2. There is pain in the scrotum, penis (urethra) and urinary bladder, bursting pain (in the above areas), and scanty, frequent and difficult urination, (SS).

Pittaja-mūtra-kṛcchra:

1. There is frequent urination with burning sensation and pain, the urine being yellowish, and mixed with blood, (CS).

2. The scrotum, urethra and urinary bladder feel as if they have been set on fire, while the urine is hot, yellowish and bloody, (SS).

Kaphaja-mūtra-kṛcchra:

1. There is swelling and a sensation of heaviness in the area of the urinary bladder and penis (urethra), while the urine is slimy, (CS).

2. There is horripilation (hairs standing on end) and a sense of heaviness in the scrotum, penis (urethra) and region of the urinary bladder, while the urine is cold, unctuous (slimy) and white, (SS).

Tridoshaja-mūtra-kṛcchra: The aggravated vāta dries up the urine along with the pitta and semen or kapha, and then as a result,there is the gradual formation of a calculi, just like the formation of the gall-stone from the bile of a cow.

The calculus is very similar to a stone and may resemble the flower of kadamba or may be smooth, soft or triangular. If this calculus enters into the urethra, it obstructs the flow of urine, and causes pain in the urinary bladder. There will also be pain in the penis, urinary bladder and sevani (the raphe), while the urine does not flow in a single stream but is scattered or is forked. Due to the pain, the patient may squeeze his penis, or may involuntarily pass stools or semen. If the calculi causes damage to the urethra, there is flow of bloody urine, while the passage of the calculi results in free and painless urination. If this calculi is broken up into small pieces known as śarkara by the vāta, it can easily be eliminated through the urethra, (CS).

Śarkaraja-mūtra-kṛcchra: The condensed kapha is digested through the action of the pitta, broken up into pieces through the action of vāta, and pebbles (śarkara) which are in the shape of small engender pain in the cardiac region, trembling, pain in the abdomen, weak digestion, syncope, and painful urination or retention of urine. If the śarkara are eliminated through the urine, there is relief from pain. If the urethra is again obstructed there is obstruction of urination or dysuria.

Śukraja-mūtra-kṛcchra: If a person suppresses the ejaculation of semen, he will suffer from pain in the groins, urinary bladder and penis, and painful swelling of the testis. The urine is passed with difficulty as if it is obstructed by the semen. This condition is also known as aṇāa-stabdha.

If the doshas localised in the urinary bladder either individually or together obstruct the flow of semen, there will be pain in the urethra (penis) and bladder, and retention of urine and semen. The bladder and testis become painful, swollen and indurated, (CS).

Rakta-mūtra-kṛcchra: If the blood that is present in the urinary bladder is vitiated either due to any injury or due to depletion of body tissues, it gets obstructed in the bladder and causes painful urination or is converted into a calculi and causes distention and a sense of heaviness in the bladder. If this is eliminated, the bladder appears light, (CS).

Related Subjects: Mūtrāghāta

Ref.: CS, chikitsā, 26, 32-44; SS, uttara, 59.

Treatment:

1. A person suffering from vātaja-mūtra-kṛcchra has to be subjected to massage (with oil), anuvāsana and nirūha types of enemata, poultices of unctuous substances, uttara-basti (urethral douche) and affusion with a decoction of drugs of the sthirādi group or drugs that alleviate vāta.

Tila oil mixed with ghee, the fat of bear and hog, and medicated with a decoction of punarnava, eraṇḍa, śatāvari, pattūra, vṛschīra, balā, pāshaṇa-bheda, drugs of daśamūla group, kulattha, kola and yava and a paste of the above drugs and five salts is efficacious in vātaja-mūtra-kṛcchra.

A paste of these and other useful drugs can be applied as poultices. Oil seeds mixed with oil or ghee and sour substances can also be used as poultices, and should be applied when lukewarm.

In a patient of pittaja-mūtra-kṛcchra, cold affusions (sprinkling, seka), cold tub-baths, application of a paste of cold drugs, the regimen and food recommended for summer, enemas, the internal use of milk, purgation, etc., are to be employed. The patient can also partake of drāksha, vidāri, sugarcane juice and ghee. A cold decoction of śatāvari, kāśa, kuśa, gokshura, vidāri, rice, ikshu (sugarcane), and kaseruka can be administered with honey and sugar. The (cold) decoction of kamala and nilotpala, or of śṛngāṭaka or of vidāri or of roots of daṇḍairaka can be admnistered. Pure cold water is also useful.

The paste of ervāru seeds, trapusha, kusumbha, kumkuma, vṛkshaka (vāsa) with grape juice is very useful (when used internally) in all types of mūtra-kṛcchra, and urinary calculi. The paste of ervaru seeds, yashṭi-madhu, devadāru and rice water is very useful (when taken internally) in pittaja-mūtra-kṛcchra. Dāruharidra can be administered with honey and juice of āmalaki in similar cases.

In a case of kaphaja-mūtra-kṛcchra, the patient can partake of drugs and food-articles that are alkaline (kshāra), hot, and sharp, barley preparation, buttermilk, and oil medicated with bitter drugs, can be subjected to sudation, emesis and nirūha type of enemata. The above mentioned oil can also be used externally for massage.

The powders of trikaṭu, gokshura, ela, and the bones of the sarasa bird can be administered with cow's urine and honey. The paste of ela can be administered with honey and juice of banana (kadali) or of kaiḍarya. The paste of sitivāra seeds and butter, or pravala chūrṇa with rice water can also be administered.

The decoction or gruel prepared from saptaparṇa, āragvadha, kevaka, ela, dhava, karanja, kuṭaja and guḍūchi can be administered with honey.

In a case of tridoshaja-mūtra-kṛcchra, enemata, purgation and emesis are to be administered if vāta, pitta, and kapha respectively are involved.

In aśmarijanya-mūtra-kṛcchra, measures which alleviate kapha and vāta are to be employed.

A patient suffering from raktaja-mūtra-kṛcchra, should be administered (a decoction, etc., of) the stalk of nilotpala, tāla, kāśa, ikshuvala, ikshu, and kaseruka with honey and sugarcandy. Sugarcane (juice), vidāri and trapusha are also useful. Ghee medicated with gokshura-juice, eight parts of milk, and drugs of laghu-pancha-mūla, drugs of katākadi group, either seperately or together, is also useful. The patient can also be subjected to (uttara ?) basti (with milk medicated with drugs of the sweet group or with oil medicated with sweet fruits (such as madhuka fruit, etc.). The drugs, etc., indicated in pittaja mūtra-kṛcchra are also useful in this disease.

In cases of mūtra-kṛcchra engendered by the obstruction of semen, the dosha involved should be ascertained after examination. Meat juices medicated with a decoction of kārpāsa roots, vāsa, pāshana-bheda, bala, gavedhuka, drugs of laghu-pancha-mūla group, vṛschīra, aindri, punarnava, śatāvari, asana, etc., is useful if vāta is aggravated. If pitta is aggravated, ghee or milk medicated with the above drugs is useful. If there is aggravation of kapha, gruels and food prepared from the above drugs are beneficial. If these do not produce any lasting benefit, the patient should be administered old wine or madhūkāsava, or meat of birds. He can be subjected to urethral douche, after which he can be comforted by young women, and administered aphrodisiac drugs, (CS).

2. The remedial measures indicated in the treatment of aśmaṛi are useful in this disease also.

In vātaja-mūtra-kṛcchra, oil, lard and ghee, or oil or ghee medicated with gokshura, kumbhi, hapusha, kaṇṭakāri, bala, śatāvari, rāsna, vaṛuna, girikarṇika and drugs of the vidāri-gandhādi group can be used both internally and for administering anuvāsana types of enema. Uttara-basti (urethral douche) is also useful. Oil medicated with milk, nāgara, jaggery, and expressed juices of gokshura can be used similarly.

In pittaja-mūra-kṛcchra, ghee or milk medicated with drugs of the tṛṇa-panchamūla, utpalādi, kākolyādi and nyagrodhādi groups is very useful (for internal use). The above ghee or milk can also be used for uttara-basti and anuvāsana and nirūha types of enema. The patient can also be purged by giving sugarcane juice, grape-juice, etc., (with purgative drugs).

In kaphaja-mūtra-kṛcchra, oil medicated with drugs of surasādi, ūshakādi, mustādi and varuṇādi groups and yavāgu (gruel) prepared from these drugs can be administered internally.

In tridoshaja-mūtra-kṛcchra, treatment can be given after due consideration of the dosha predominantly affected.

The powders of phalgu, vṛśchīra, darbha, and śilājatu can be administered with (cold) water, surā (wine), sugarcane juice or a decoction or juice of darbha (in all cases of mūtra-kṛccha).

In mūtra-kṛcchra caused by (the suppression of) faeces (purīshaja-mūtra-kṛcchra), measures that alleviate vāta such as sudation, tub baths, massage wih oil, enemata, etc., are to be employed, (SS).

3. The best diet in mūtra-kṛcchra is one of cow's milk, while the drugs of the vīratarādi group are very efficacious, (AHṛ).

4. The formulations that are useful in all types of mūtra-kṛcchra are: a decoction of roots of atibala; the expressed juice of kaṇṭakāri with honey; the powder of yava-kshāra with an equal amount of sugarcandy; the paste of loha bhasma with honey, and the decoction of brhaṭi, kaṇṭakari, pāṭha, yashṭi-madhu and indrayava; etc.

In vātaja mūtra-kṛcchra, the decoction of guḍūchi, nāgara, āmalaki, aśvagandha and gokshura is very efficacious.

The recipes that are useful in pittaja-mūtra-kṛcchra are: the decoction of kuśa, kāśa, śara, darbha, and ikshuka (tṛṇa-pancha-mūla drugs); milk boiled with the above medicated drugs, which is especially useful in bloody urination; a paste of equal quantities of jaggery and āmalaki; and a decoction of gokshura and nāgara.

The decoction of gokshura seeds and yava-kshāra is useful in purīshāja-mūtra-kṛcchra.

The paste of śilājatu and honey is efficacious in śukraja-mūtra-kṛcchra, (CD).

5. Equal quantities of purified tuttha, rasa-sindūra and tāmra bhasma are triturated with the expressed juice of śatāvari (for a day). The bolus is then boiled in kaṭu taila (for three hours). This can then be administered internally in mūtra-kṛcchra, (RRS).

Classical Prescriptions: Bṛhat-saindhavādya-taila; Chandanāsava; Chandraprabhā-vaṭi; Chāngeri-ghṛta; Chandra-kalārasa; Daśamūla-harītaki; Gokshurādi-guggulu; Guḍūchyādi-modaka; Mūlaka-kshāra; Kumarī-āsava; Nyagrodhādi-chūrṇa; Palāśa-kshara; Prāṇada-guṭika; Pravāla-bhasma; Pippalyādi-taila; Śatavari-guḍa; Śivaguṭika; Traikanṭaka-ghṛta; Vastyāmayāntaka-ghṛta; Yava-kshāra.

Mūtra-sāda: Pravāla-bhasma

Mūtra-sanga: Saptāmṛta-loha.

Related Diseases: Aśmari, Mutraghāta

Ref.: CS, chikitsā, 26 , 45-58; 69-75; SS, uttara, 59, 16-27; AHṛ, sūtra, 5, 23; 15, 25; CD, 32; RRS, 17, 8.

Nāśā-roga

Western Nosology: Catarrh, Rhinitis

Enumeration: There are thirty-one diseases of the nose, namely apīnasa, pūtinasya, nāsā-pāka, śonita-pitta, pūya-śonita, kshavathu, bhramshathu, dīpta, nāsānāha, parisrāva, nāśā-śosha, four kinds of nāsā-arśas, four kinds of swellings (nāsā-śopha), seven kinds of arbudas and five types of pratiśyāya, (SS).

According to CS, the diseases of the nose that are commonly seen are pratiśyāya, dushṭa-pratiśyāya, kshavathu, nāsa-śośa, pratināha, nāsa-srava, pūtinasya, apīnasa, ghrāṇa-pāka, nāsā-śotha, nāsā-arbuda, pūya-rakta, arūmshika and dīpta.

Causes, Pathogenesis and Symptomatology of Pratisyāya:

1. Suppression of the natural urges, indigestion, exposure to smoke, mist and dust,

excessive speech, anger, seasonal irregularities, diseases of the head, loss of sleep, or excessive sleep, intake of very cold water, excessive sexual indulgence and excessive weeping are the precipitating factors.

These factors aggravate vāta which in turn causes pratiśyāya. If only vāta is aggravated, the patient suffers from pain and pricking sensation in the nose, sneezing, watery discharge from the nose, hoarseness and headache. If pitta is also aggravated, the patient suffers from inflammation of the tip of the nose, fever, dryness of the mouth, thirst and discharge of yellow and hot fluid from the nose. If kapha is aggravated, the patient suffers from cough, anorexia, thick and profuse discharge from the nose and heaviness and itching in the nose - nasal passage. If all the three doshas are vitiated there is severe pain, discomfort and presence of all these symptoms.

If a patient suffering from any of the above mentioned types of pratiśyāya indulges in unwholesome food or ignores his disease, his condition will worsen, and progress to dusṭa-pratiśyaya which in turn may lead to sneezing, nāsā-śosha, pratināha, pari-srāva, pūti-nasya, apīnasa, nāsa-pāka, nāsā-śotha, nāsā-arbuda, pūya-rakta, arūmshi, diseases of the head, ears and eyes, baldness, greying of hair, thirst, dyspnoea, cough, fever, rakta-pitta, hoarseness and rāja-yakshma.

The symptoms of dusṭha-pratiśyāya (atrophic rhinitis) are obstruction, ulceration, discharge, dryness and inflammation of the nose, loss of sense of smell, bad odour from the mouth, and chronicity (i.e. recurrent attacks of the disease), (CS).

2. The causes for pratiśyāya are excessive sexual intercourse, disease of the head, exposure to dust, smoke, excessive cold and heat, and suppression of the natural urges.

The disease (pratiśyāya) may be caused by the aggravated vāta, pitta, kapha, all three doshas combined or by the vitiated blood.

The prodromal symptoms are heaviness of the head, sneezing, body pain, horripilation or appearance of gooseflesh on the skin etc.

If vāta is aggravated, there is a sense of distension or obstruction in the nose, discharge of thin fluid from the nose, dryness of the palate, throat and lips, a pricking pain in the region of the temples and hoarseness. If pitta is aggravated, there is a hot, yellowish discharge from the nose, emaciation, paleness of mucous membranes and skin (paṇḍu), a sensation of heat, thirst and a feeling as if smoke was issuing from the nostrils. If kapha is aggravated, there will be frequent discharge of white and cold fluid from the nose, whitish discolouration (of skin, etc.), swelling around the eyes, heaviness of the head, and intense itching in the head, throat, lips and palate. If all the doshas are provoked, the symptoms of all the doshas will be present and will frequently recur without any apparent cause. If the blood is vitiated, there will be bleeding from the nose, chest pain, reddish discolouration of eyes, loss of sense of smell, foul odour from the mouth, and presence of minute white parasites in the nostrils. The patient will also suffer from symptoms seen in krmija-śiro-roga.

If this disease is not treated properly, the patient will suffer from dushṭa-pratiśyāya where there is alternate dryness of the nose and coryza (running in the nose), alternate ānahyate (obstruction) and vivriyate (opening), bad odour from the mouth, and loss of smell.

If the disease (pratiśyāya) is further neglected, the patient will suffer from deafness, blindness, loss of sense of smell, serious eye-diseases, cough, poor digestion, swellings, etc., (SS).

Pathogenesis of Kshavathu: The deranged vāta localises in the head and its passages, and engenders sneezing, (CS).

The aggravated vāta localises in the marma (vital part) of the head, and is expelled forcibly from the nostrils along with mucus, in the form of sneezing. Sneezing is often precipitated by the smell of pungent and sharp (tīkshṇa) substances or by gazing at the sun, or by the presence of any foreign matter in the nostrils.

Pathogenesis and Symptoms of Nāsā-śosha (Ozena): The aggravated vāta dries up the kapha (localised in the nose) and causes loss of smell and atrophy of śrngāṭaka (turbinated bones), (CS).

The kapha that is present in the nose is dried up by the aggravated vāta and pitta, and as a result, there is drying up of the nose and subsequent difficulty in breathing through the nose, (SS).

Pathogenesis and Symptoms of Pratināha: The aggravated kapha and vāta engenders obstruction of the nose, (CS).

The udāna-vāyu is obstructed by the aggravated kapha, and as a result, there is blocking of the nose, (SS).

Pathogenesis and Symptoms of Nāsā-srāva (Nāsā -parisrava, SS): There is discharge of thick, yellow matter from the nostrils, (CS).

There is clear, watery, and constant discharge from the nose, which is aggravated at night, (SS).

Pathogenesis and Symptoms of Pūti-nasya (Ozena): If the above mentioned disease (i.e. nāsā-srārva) is neglected (or is improperly treated), there is swelling of the nose, foul odour, discolouraion and vertigo, (CS).

The aggravated doshas (including blood, NiS) which are localised in the throat and uvular region of the palate (tālu-mūla) will be eliminated by the action of the aggravated vāta, in the form of a foetid discharge, (SS).

Pathogenesis and Symptoms of Apīnasa: There is obstruction and sense of dryness in the nose, softening of (or discharge from) the nose, a sensation as if smoke is being let out from the nostrils, and loss of smell and taste. If vāta and kapha are both aggravated, the symptoms will be similar to those seen in pratiśyāya, (CS, SS).

Pathogenesis and Symptoms of Nāsā-pāka: In this disease, which is caused by the aggravated pitta and the deranged blood, there is an inflammatory swelling (of the nose) with redness and burning pain, (CS).

The aggravated pitta that is localised in the nose causes ulcers in the nose, and subsequent inflammation (suppuration), with discharge and kotha (foetid odour), (SS).

Pathogenesis and Symptoms of Pūya-rakta: There is discharge of blood with pitta from the nostrils, ears and mouth, (CS).

Due to the aggravation of the doshas or as a result of injury to the forehead, there is discharge of putrid blood from the nostrils, (SS).

Symptoms of Dīpta: The patient feels as if the nose was kindled or set on fire, (CS).

There is severe burning pain within the nose, a sensation as if hot smoke was coming out of the nostrils, and as if the nose has been set on fire, (SS).

Pathogenesis and Symptoms of Arūmshika: The aggravated doshas and the vitiated dhātus (like rakta, etc.,) bring about a swelling around the nose, (CS).

The four kinds of śotha have the same symptoms that are described under śotha, (SS).

Pathogenesis and Symptoms of Nāsārbuda: The aggravated doshas vitiate the flesh and blood, and result in the formation of a tumour which causes obstruction of the nose, (CS). See arbuda, (SS).

Pathogenesis and Symptoms of Bhramśathu: The kapha that accumulates in the head is liquified by the aggravated pitta and is forcibly expelled through the nose, in the form of a thick, salty discharge, (SS).

Pathogenesis and Symptoms of Nāsā-arśas (Nasal Polyp): See under Arśas.

Ref.: CS, chikitsā, 26, 104-117; SS, uttara, 22; 24, 3-17.

Treatment:

1. In a case of vātaja-pratiśyāya, where there is cough and hoarseness, the patient can be administered ghee with yava-kshāra, or meat-juices, or hot-milk, or snaihika types of fumigation (dhūma). The patient can also smoke a cigar (varti) prepared from śatapushpa, dālchini, roots of balā, eraṇḍa and bilva, bark of āragvadha, bee's wax, ghee and animal fat (vasā). The patient can inhale the smoke from burning śaktu (barley which is dehusked, fried and powdered) and ghee, in a case of recent pratiśyāya. If a person has acute pain in the temples, head and forehead, he can be gently fomented (or massaged) by the palms or a poultice can be applied. In sneezing, coryza or obstruction of nose, the patient has to be rubbed with oil and subjected to fomentation by the methods of sankara-sveda, etc. The powders of rohisha, ajāji, vachā, tarkāri, choraka, or of dālchini, teja-patra, maricha, ela and upakunchika can be used as snuff. In cases of dryness of the nasal passages, śṛngātaka and eyes, oils can be used as nāvana (nasal drops).

Tila seeds are soaked in goat's milk and subjected to mild heat. The powder of madhu-yashṭi is added and oil is expressed from this. This oil is to be boiled again with a decoction of daśamūla drugs and a paste of rāsna, rock salt and yashṭi-madhu. This oil that is known as aṇu-taila is very efficacious. A patient of vātaja pratiśyāya can be given āsthāpana type of enema after massaging him with this oil. The patient can partake of easily digestible foods with meat juices of domesticated animals, etc., and unctuous, hot and sour substances. He can bathe in hot water, and should stay in a warm room that is free from draughts. A person suffering from vātaja pratiśyāya should avoid worry, exertion, excessive speech and sexual intercourse.

A person suffering from pittaja-pratiśyāya should be administered medicated ghee and milk medicated with nāgara (ginger) in order to ripen or digest (the accumulated mucus), after which errhines can be used. The oil medicated with pāṭha, haridrā, dāru-haridra, mūrva, pippali, tender leaves of jāti, and danti can be used as nasal drops. In cases of pūya-rakta, errhines, etc., that are useful in rakta-pitta can be administered. In nāsā-pāka, burning pain and arūmshika, sweet and cold decoctions can be used as errhines, and cold plasters and affusions (sprinklings) can be employed. If pitta is only mildly aggravated, purgation can be carried out by using unctuous substances. The diet can consist of ghee, milk, barley, rice, wheat, meat-juices of desert animals, soup of mudga, leafy vegetables that are bitter, and cold and sour substances.

In a case of kaphaja-pratiśyāya, where there is heaviness of the head, anorexia, etc., the patient is advised to fast. The head has to be smeared with ghee, after which fomentations and sprinkling (of hot liquids) can be done. The patient can be asked to partake of garlic mixed with flour of mudga, trikaṭu, yava-kshāra and ghee, and is later given an emetic. In kaphaja-pratiśyāya, apīnasa, pūti-nasya, and nāsā-srāva with itching, the patient can be exposed to fumigation and errhine therapy with pungent drugs. The powder of manahśila, vachā, trikaṭu, viḍanga, hingu and guggulu can be used as snuff (or pradhamana). Mustard oil is boiled with the paste of lāksha, vachā, kaṭu-tumbi, viḍanga, kushṭha, pippali and karanja and cow's urine that has been boiled with bhārngi, madana, tarkāri and tulasi, etc. This oil is used for nasal inhalation in kaphaja-pratiśyāya and cases where the nasal discharge is thick and resembles fat (medas). When the condition of the patient has become less serious, the patient can be oleated, and subjected to emesis, with a decoction of emetic drugs and gruel (yavāgu) prepared from tila and māsha. The patient of kaphaja-pratiśyāya can partake of soup of vārtāka, kulaka, trikaṭu, kulattha, mudga, and āḍhaki. Hot water should be used (both externally and for drinking), (CS).

2. Persons suffering from apīnasa and pūti-nasya have to be subjected to oleation and sudation, and later, emesis and purgation.

After these eliminative procedures, the patient can partake of food that is sharp and easy to digest, in a limited quantity, and prepared? According to the prescribed rules; hot water can be used for drinking. The patient can also smoke medicated cigars at the proper time. The compound consisting of hingu, trikaṭu, vatsaka, sivāṭi (white variety of punarnava ?) lāksha, kaṭphala, sourabha, vachā, kushṭha, śigru and viḍanga can be used daily in the form of avapīḍa-nasya. Mustard oil medicated with cow's urine and the above drugs can be used in the form of nasal drops.

In cases of nāsā-pāka, measures which alleviate pitta are to be employed both internally and externally (as paste, affusions, etc.). The patient can also be subjected to blood-letting at the affected area, after which a paste of bark of kshīri trees and ghee can be applied.

A case of pūya-rakta has to be treated on the same lines as for nāḍi-vraṇa. The patient can be subjected to emesis, which should be followed by avapīḍa nasya and fumigation or smoking of sharp drugs or drugs that are cleansing (śodhana).

In cases of kshavathu and bhramśathu, drugs belonging to the śiro-virechana group have to powdered and inhaled through a pipe (as snuff). The head can also be fomented, and snigdha dhūma can be employed.

Persons suffering from dīpta have to be treated with drugs, regimen and food that alleviate pitta. Cold and sweet drugs and food are particularly useful in this disease.

In a case of nāsānāha, the patient can be internally administered, potions of ghee or oil, after which sneha-dhūmas and śiro-basti are used. Balā-taila or any other oil indicated in vāta-rogas may be used.

In nāsā-srāva, powders of the śiro-virechan group are used as snuff, and are introduced though a pipe into the nostrils; sharp drugs can be used as avapīda-nasya, and the affected area can be exposed to smoke by burning devadāru and chitraka. The patient can partake of goat's meat.

In a case of nāsā-śosha, ghee extracted from milk as well as oils prepared in the same way as aṇu-taila can be used in the form of nasal drops. The patient can be administered oil or ghee internally, while the diet can consist of meat of desert animals. He can also be subjected to oleation, sudation and snaihika-dhūma.

All cases of pratiśyāya, excepting recent and acute cases are treated by potions of ghee (taken internally), sudation (fomentation), and the patient should partake of sour and hot food or milk medicated with fresh ginger, or sugar-cane products (such as jaggery, etc.). After these measures have accelerated the maturing process, and the discharge has become thick and viscous, śiro-virechana drugs are used as errhines. Purgation, āsthāpana enema, dhūma-pāna and medicated gargles can also be prescribed. The patient should reside, sleep and move about in rooms that are not exposed to draughts of air, and his head should be warmly covered. Strong drugs should be used for admin istering errhines and dhūma (fumigation). Harītaki should be given internally. The diet should consist of barley and dry food. The patient should avoid cold water (for bathing, drinking, etc.), sexual intercourse, worries, suppression of natural urges, excessively dry foods, leafy vegetables, and newly prepared alcoholic drinks.

If the patient of pratiśyāya also suffers from vomiting, debility, fever, heaviness of body, anorexia, restlessness, and diarrhoea, he should be made to fast, and is administered drugs and food that are appetizing and digestive. If a young adult suffers from pratiśyāya caused by vāta and kapha, he should be made to vomit after drinking large amounts of fluids.

A patient of vātaja-pratiśyāya can be administered (internally) ghee, either by itself or medicated with drugs of vidāri-gandhādi group and the five salts. Errhines which are useful in ardita can also be used.

A person suffering from pratiśyāya caused by pitta and vitiated blood should be administered ghee medicated with sweet drugs (belonging to the kākolyādi group). Cold washes (affusions) and applications (plasters) are also useful. Gargles with śrīveshṭaka, sarja-rasa, patanga, priyanju, honey and sugar, or drākshā, madhūlika (guḍūchi), gojihva, kaśmīri, and yashṭi-madhu; and purgation with sweet drugs are also beneficial. An oil medicated with ten parts of milk, and the paste of bark of dhava, triphala, trivṛt, tilvaka, yashṭi-madhu, śrīparṇi (kaśmīri), and haridra can be used in the form of nasal drops.

In the case of kaphaja pratiśyāya, the patient has to be oleated, made to partake of gruel of tila and māsha, and is made to vomit. Later, measures which alleviate kapha are employed. An oil medicated with the two varieties of bala, bṛhati, kaṇṭakāri, viḍanga, gokshura, śveta-roots, kāśmari and punarnava is used as an errhine. Cigars prepared from trivrit, kaṭabhi, devadāru, danti and ingudi are then to be smoked, in the prescribed manner.

In a case of tridoshaja-pratiśyāya, ghee medicated with pungent and bitter drugs, dhūma of strong drugs, and pungent drugs (and food) are useful. An oil medicated with rasānjana, ativisha, musta, and bhadradāru is used as an errhine. The decoction of musta, tejovati, pāṭha, kaṭphala, kaṭuka, vachā, sarshapa, root of pippali, pippali fruits, rock salt, chitraka, tuttha, karanja seeds, salt and devadāru is used a śiro-virechana.

Milk with half the amount of water mixed with it is boiled with the meat of desert animals and birds, drugs of vidārigandhādi group, and acquatic flowers, until all the water has evaporated. Ghee extracted from this milk is again boiled with drugs of eladi group, sugar, sāriva (ananta), yashṭi-madhu, chandana, and with ten parts of milk. This ghee can be used as nasya.

In cases of pratiśyāya where there are worms, the above mentioned drugs can be taken along with cow's urine and bile of cow, and drugs that are useful in kṛmiroga, (SS).

3. The powders of equal amounts of trikaṭu, chitraka, tāliśapatra, tintiḍika, amla-vetas, chavya, and ajāji and one-fourth parts of dālchini, and teja-patra are to be administered with old jaggery in pratiśyāya. The oil medicated with kaṇṭakāri, danti, vachā, śigru, tulasi, trikaṭu and rock salt can be used as nasya for relieving pūti-nāsa. An oil prepared from cow's urine and paste of trikaṭu, viḍanga, rock salt, bṛhati-fruits, śigru, surasa (tulasi?) and danti is also useful (as nasya) in the same disease. The patient (of pūti-nāsa) can also be administered avapīḍa nasya from the compound of indrayava, hingu, maricha, lāksha, tulasi, kaṭphala, kushṭha, vachā, śigru and viḍanga. Mustard oil medicated with the above drugs and cow's urine can be also used in the form of nasal drops in the same disease.

Oil or ghee medicated with a paste and decoction of nāgara, kushṭha, pippali, bilva, and drāksha is used as an erhine in kshavathu.

Drinking a lot of cold water just before retiring to bed is very useful in relieving pratiśyāya. The juices extracted by the puṭa-pāka method from jaya leaves, and which is mixed with rock salt and til oil is very efficacious in all varieties of pratiśyāya. A paste of maricha and jaggery, and a diet of unctuous food and sour curds is useful in acute pratiśyāya.

Partaking of fermented māsha with rock salt soon after meals is efficacious in relieving all varieties of chronic pratiśyāya. An avapīḍa nasya prepared from pippali, śigru seeds, viḍanga and maricha is beneficial in pratiśyāya.

An oil medicated with flowers of red karavīra, flowers of jāti, asana and mallika (flowers) is useful in nāsā-arśas (nasal polypi). Oil medicated with chitraka, chavika, ajamoda, kaṇṭakāri, karanja, rock salt, arka and cow's urine is also useful in this disease, (CD).

4. The powders of nāgara, harītaki, pāṭha, trāyanti and vatsanābha are used (as nasya)

in pūti-nāsa. The nasya of white jīraka and sugar candy is useful in pūya-rakta. The nasya of a paste of kumkuma and ghee is useful in pīnasa, (RRS).

Classical Prescriptons: Nāsā-roga : Paṭolādi-ghṛta.

Pīnasa: Chitraka-harītaki; Kaccūrādi-chūṛna; Kapha-ketu-rasa; Mahā-lakshmi-vilāsa-rasa; Rāsnādi-chūrṇa; Sahacharādi-taila; Śiva-guṭika; Trikaṭu-chūrṇa.

Pratiśyāya: Triphalādi-taila.

Related Diseases: Arbuda, Arśas, Śotha

Ref.: CS, chikitsā, 26, 134-157; SS,uttara, 23; 24, 18-24; CD, 58; RRS, 24, 21, 22; 29, 115.

Netra-roga

Western Nosology: Disease of the eye.

Introduction: A brief description of the eye: The bulb of the eye (the eyeball) is circular, shaped like the teat of a cow, is two angulas in transverse diameter, about the breadth of one's thumb in depth and two and a half angulas all round (in circumference). It is formed by all the five mahā-bhūtas, the pṛthvī, ap, tejas, vāyu and akāśa, being responsible for the formation of the muscles, the sclera, the blood supply, the iris and the lacrimal apparatus respectively. The iris forms one-third of the extent of the while eyeball, while the pupil occupies one-seventh part of the iris. The eye consists of five maṇḍalas (different circular or circle-forming structures of the eye), six sandhi (joints) and six paṭalas (different layers or coverings of the eye or eyeball).

The five mandalas are pakshma-maṇḍala (eye-lashes, or ciliary circle), vartma-maṇḍala (the eyelids), śveta-maṇḍala (sclera), kṛshṇa-maṇḍala (iris) and dṛshṭi-maṇḍala (pupil or lens).

The six joints are pakshma-vartma-sandhi (point of junction of cilia with the lid margin), vartma-śukla-sandhi (fornix of the conjunctiva), śukla-kṛshṇa-sandhi (sclero-corneal junction), kṛshṇa-dṛshṭi-sandhi (contact of the iris with the lens), kanīnika-sandhi (medial angle of the eye) and apānga-sandhi (outer junction of eyelids).

The six paṭalas are the two eyelids, the tejojalāśrita-paṭala (the cornea), piśitāśrita-paṭala (the iris), the parts of the eye that consist of fatty tissue (medas) and the covering known as dṛshṭi (pupil). The dṛshṭi is as big as the māsura-dala, is enveloped by the (tejo-jalāśrita) paṭalas and is like an aperture.

Causative Factors:

Extrinsic: Getting drenched immediately after being exposed to the hot sun, gazing constantly at distant objects, loss of sleep, continuous weeping, anger, grief and anxiety, injury, excessive coitus, excessive intake of śukta, kānji, sour food, kulattha and māshā, suppression of the natural urges, excessive sudation, exposure to smoke, over-administration of emetics, suppression of tears and vomiting, and gazing at minute objects,. (SS).

Classification:

1. There are seventy-six kinds of eye-diseases of which ten are caused by the aggravated vāta, ten by pitta, thirteen by kapha, sixteen by the vitiated blood, twenty-five by the vitiation of all three doshas and two by external factors.

Of these seventy-six diseases, nine are confined to the sandhis, twenty-one to the eyelids, eleven to the sclera (śukla-bhāga, the white of the eye), four to the iris (kṛshṇa-bhāga, the black portion of the eye), seventeen to the entire eye and twelve to the pupil or lens (dṛshṭi). The two diseases that are of traumatic origin affect chiefly the pupil or lens (dṛshṭi), (SS).

Prodromal Symptoms: Watering of the eyes, slight inflammation, clouded vision, itching of the eyes, increase in the mucous (or agglutination of eyes), heaviness, burning and sucking sensation, and redness, (SS).

I. Diseases of the Sandhis (Joints or Junctions):

1. Pūyālasa: A suppurating swelling (affecting the inner canthus, NiS) which exudes a thick and offensive pus. It is caused by the vitiation of all three doshas, but is curable, (SS).

2. Upanāha (lacrimal cyst): A fairly big knotty growth which is painless, and is situated at the kṛshṇa-dṛshṭi-sandhi (the contact of the iris with the lens). It is attended by itching, and does not suppurate. It is caused by the provoked kapha and is curable.

3. Pūya-srāva (disease of tear gland): The aggravated doshas bring about inflammation at the inner canthus (medial angle of the eye) along with discharge of pus. This disease is incurable.

4. Śleshma-srāva: The aggravated kapha causes discharge from the inner canthus that is whitish, slimy and thick. This condition is painless.

5. Rakta-srāva: There is discharge (from the inner canthus) that is bloody, warm, slightly thick and copious. This condition is engendered by the vitiated blood and is incurable.

6. Pitta-srāva: The aggravated pitta causes the secretion of a bluish or yellowish, hot, watery fluid from the inner canthus. This is also considered to be incurable.

7. Parvaṇi: There is a small rounded copper-coloured swelling that is attended by burning and pain, which is situated at the sclero-corneal junction. This is caused by the vitiated blood and is curable.

8. Alaji: This is a bigger swelling situated at the sclero-corneal junction, that is caused by the vitiation of all the three doshas. It is considered to be incurable.

9. Kṛmi-granthi: This is a disease affecting the fornix of the conjunctiva. Minute parasites are found in the affected region which cause itching (irritation) of the eyelids. The normal functioning of the eye is also affected. This disease is caused by the aggravated kapha and is curable.

II. Diseases of the Eyelids:

1. Utsargiṇi: A small round indented swelling (piḍaka) on the inner surface of the lower eyelids, is caused by the aggravation of all the doshas. It is curable.

2. Kumbhika: A number of small piḍakas will be formed at the junction of the eyelashes with the lid margin. These pustules which resemble the seeds of kumbhika, will later burst. This disease is also caused by the vitiation of all three doshas, and is curable.

3. Pothaki: The eyelids will be covered by a number of red and large piḍakas (or small circumscribed swellings) resembling the seeds of rakta -sarshapa. There will be pain, itching and secretion. This disease is engendered by the deranged kapha and is curable.

4. Vartma-śarkara: A large and hard piḍaka (a local, circumscribed swelling) surrounded by a number of smaller and thick pidakas appears on the eyelids. This disease is engendered by all the three doshas, but is curable.

5. Arśo-vartma: Small and rough piḍakas which resemble the seeds of ervāru and are very slightly painful appear on the eyelids. This is also caused by the vitiation of all three doshas, but is curable.

6. Śushkārśa: A deep seated, large, rough and painless ankura (tumour, cyst, papilla) is seen on either of the eyelids. This disease is also engendered by all the three doshas, and is curable.

7. Anjana-nāmika: Due to vitiated blood, small, soft, slightly painful, copper-coloured piḍakas appear on the eyelids. There is also pricking and burning pain. This disease is curable.

8. Bahala-vartma: The eyelids are covered with crops of piḍakas that are of equal size and of skin colour. This is caused by the vitiation of all three doshas, and is curable.

9. Vartma-bandha: The vitiated three doshas bring about swelling of the eyelids attended with

itching, slight pricking pain and inability to fully open the eyes. This disease is also curable.

10. Klishṭa-vartma: Both the eyelids become copper-coloured, soft and slightly painful. There is at times slight oozing of blood. This disease is caused by the vitiated blood and is curable.

11. Vartma-kardama: When the pitta is aggravated along with the blood, there is exudation (secretion) from the eyelids (in addition to the other symptoms of klishṭa - vartma). This disease is also curable.

12. Śyāva-vartma: The aggravated three doshas bring about painful, dark-brown swelling of the eyelids, along with secretion, burning pain and itching. There is blackish discolouration of eyelids both internally and externally. This disease is also curable.

13. Klinna-vartma: The aggravated kapha causes secretions, itching and pricking pain within the eyelids, and a painless swelling externally. This disease is also curable.

14. Aklinna-vartma: The deranged three doshas cause the repeated agglutination of eyelids, without signs of inflammation. This disease is curable.

15. Vātāhata-vartma: The eyelids seems to be paralysed, and the patient is unable to blink. There may or may not be pain. The disease is engendered by the provoked vāta and is incurable.

16. Arbuda: A hard, painless, reddish, knotty growth of irregular shape dangles from in between the eyelids. This is caused by all the three doshas and is curable.

17. Nimesha: Due to the vitiation of aggravated vāta, there is twitching of the eyelids. This is considered to be incurable.

18. Śonitārśas: The vitiated blood causes the formation of soft polypi on the eyelids which often reappear even after excision. The polypi are attended by itching and burning pain. This is considered to be incurable.

19. Lagaṇa: A large, hard, non-suppurating, painless and slimy knotty growth of the size of a kola fruit (or seed) attended with itching appears on the eylids. This is curable, and is caused by kapha.

20. Biśa-vartma: The deranged three doshas engender swelling of the eyelids. The swelling consists of small punctures resembling the pores in the stem of a water filled lotus plant. This disease is curable.

21. Pakshma-kopa: Due to the aggravation of the three doshas, the eyelashes become rough, and point inwards. These therefore cause pain and irritation in the eyes, which are relieved when the offending hairs are plucked out. There may also be photophobia and aversion to wind. This disease can be palliated.

III. Diseases of the White of the Eye:

1. Prastāryarma: A thin and extended knotty swelling which is reddish-blue in colour appears on the śukla-bhāga. This is caused by the vitiation of all three dushas and is curable.

2. Śuklarma: The white of the eye is gradually covered over by a soft, whitish, fleshy growth which gradually increases in size. This disease is caused by the vitiated kapha and is curable.

3. Lohitārma or kshatajārma: The vitiated blood engenders the formation of a fleshy growth resembling the lotus (leaf or flower) on the white of the eye. This disease is also curable.

4. Adhimāmsa-arma: There is an extended, thick, soft, fleshy growth that is greyish or liver-coloured. This is caused by the vitiation of all three doshas, and is curable.

5. Snāyu-arma: A fleshy growth that is pale-white in colour and rough appears on the white of the eye. This is also caused by the aggravation of all three doshas, and is curable.

6. Śuktika: Small dark-brown dots resembling either oyster-shells or flesh appear on the sclera. This is caused by the aggravation of pitta, and is curable.

7. Arjuna: A single spot of the colour of the blood of a hare appears on the sclera. This is brought about by the vitiated blood and is curable.

8. Pishṭaka: An elevated circular spot which is either white like flour or transparent like water appears on the sclera. This is caused by the aggravated kapha and is curable.

9. Sirā-jāla: The sclera is covered over by extensive red patches of hardened veins which appears like a network. This is engendered by the vitiated blood and is curable.

10. Sirā-piḍaka: Small pustules (eruptions) covered over by minute veins (blood-vessels) appear on the sclera, near the iris. This disease is caused by the aggravation of all three doshas and is curable.

IV. Diseases of the Kṛshṇa-bhāga (Iris):

1. Sa-vraṇa-śukla: A small painful depression similar to that produced by a pin or needle, along with the secretion of acrid (hot) discharge is seen in the iris. This is caused by the vitiated blood and is incurable.

However, if the ulcer is far from the pupil and is not very deep seated or painful and if there is not much secretion, the condition may be cured. But, if the ulcer is covered over by flesh, or by a network of veins, or if the vision is affected, or if there is bleeding or eruption of blackish pustules, the disease is to be considered as being incurable.

2. Avraṇa-śukla (corneal opacity): A white spot from which oozes a liquid, appears on the iris, just as a cloud appears on the sky. This is neither painful not is there much lacrimation. This condition is also engendered by the vitiated blood, but is curable.

3. Pākātyaya (keratitis): There appears on the iris, a white film which gradually envelops it. This is very painful and usually develops from akshi-kopa. This disease is engendered by the aggravated three doshas and is incurable.

4. Ajaka (prolapsed iris; anterior staphyloma): A fleshy growth resmbling goat's dung (which is very dry) appears on the iris and later bursts. It will be reddish, painful, and there will be a reddish and slimy secretion. This condition is brought about by the vitiated blood and is incurable.

V. Diseases Which Affect the Entire Eye:

1. Vāta-abhishyanda (conjunctivitis): There will be a sense of dryness in the eye or flow of cold tears, headache, roughness, irritation, stiffness and pricking pain in the eyes, and horripilation. This is curable.

2. Pitta-abhishyanda: There will be yellow discolouration of the eyes, clouded vision, discharge of profuse, hot tears, burning pain and inflammation (of eyes) with desire for cold substances. This is also curable.

3. Kapha-abhishyanda: There will be swelling and heaviness of the eyes, itching, frequent flow of cold and slimy tears, white discolouration of eyes, excessive formation of waste in the eyes, and desire for warmth. This is also curable.

4. Rakta-abhishyanda: There will be red stripes on the eyes, flow of tears that are copper coloured, and red discolouration of eyes. Other symptoms of aggravated pitta will be present. This condition is curable.

Adhimantha (uveitis): If the disease abhishyanda is ignored or improperly treated, it develops into the disease known as adhimantha. This disease is characterised by excruciating pain. This patient feels as if the eyeball is being torn out. The pain usually extends upwards, involving one-half of the head.

5. Vāta-adhimantha: There is tearing, twisting, piercing and splitting pain, irritation, swelling and tremors. The pains are felt not only in the eye, but also in a major portion of the head. This condition is curable.

6. Pitta-adhimantha: There is reddish-discolouration of the eyes, flow of hot tears, swelling, sweating, inflammation, yellow discolouration of eyes, fainting fits and burning

pain in the head. The eyes resemble a slice of liver, and feel as if they have been smeared with caustics (kshāra). This condition is also curable.

7. Kapha-adhimantha: Swelling of eyes with slight congestion, lacrimation, itching, a sensation of coldness, heaviness and sliminess, clouded vision, excess accumulation of mucous, dilated nostrils and headache. This is also curable.

8. Rakta-adhimantha: There will be bright-red discolouration of the eyes, intense pain, tenderness, piercing pain, blood-streaked secretion and red canthi. The object of vision seems as if it is enveloped in flames. This is also curable. However, improper treatment and care may cause blindness, at once, or after five, six or seven days in pitta-.rakta- vāta and kapha-adhimantha, respectively.

9. Sa-śopha-pāka: An inflammatory swelling with itching, burning and pricking pain, heaviness, coppery discolouration, accumulation of waste in the eye, lacrimation and discharge of alternately hot and cold, slimy fluid.

10. A-śopha-pāka: This is characterized by the same signs and symptoms as sa-śopha-pāka, except there is absence of swelling. Both these disease are caused by the aggravation of all three doshas and are curable.

11. Hatādhimantha: If the disease vāta-adhimantha is neglected or improperly treated, the vāta is further provoked, and localises in the inner siras (blood-vessels or nerves), causing intense pain and blurring of vision. This is caused by the aggravated vāta and is considered to be incurable.

12. Vāta-paryaya: The aggravated vāta localises in the regions of the eye-lashes and eye-brows and causes pain alternately in the eye-balls and regions of eye-brows and eye-lashes. This is curable.

13. Sushkākshi-pāka: The eyelids will be hard (stiff) and dry, and will be closed. The patient will find it very painful to open his eyelids. There will also be clouded vision. This is caused by the aggravated vāta and is curable.

14. Anyato-vāta: The aggravated vāta is localised in the head, nape and sides of the neck and causes severe pain either in the eyes or eye-brows. This is also curable.

15. Amlādhyushita: The excessive intake of sour and irritant (vidāhi) food engenders swelling of the eyes, with a bluish-red tinge. This is caused by the aggravated pitta and is curable.

16. Sirotpāta: The veins present in the eye become copper-coloured, with or without pain. They, however, frequently return to normal. This disease is caused by the vitiated blood and is curable.

17. Sirāharsha: If the above disease (sirotpāta) is neglected, there will be blindness, with discharge of profuse copper-coloured clear fluid. This is also caused by the vitiated blood and is curable.

VI. Diseases of the Pupil (Drshti):

There are six diseases affecting the patalas (which envelop the pupil), and six diseases involving the pupil proper.

1. Linga-nāśa: If the vitiated doshas affect the first patala (consisting of kālakāsthi, Nis), the patient perceives only a blurred image of objects. (If vāta is mainly provoked, objects appear shaky, unsteady and brownish in colour. If pitta is involved, objects appear yellowish, etc., NiS).

If the second patala (consisting of medas, NiS) is affected, there is more disturbance in vision. The patient is unable to guage the distance of the objects, and is unable to thread a needle even with great effort. He perceives false images of insects, hairs, nets, cob-webs, etc. The objects seem enveloped in a mist, as if laid under a sheet of water, or as viewed in rain or in a mirage.

If the third patala (consisting of māmsa, NiS), is affected, the patient is able to perceive only the upper part of objects. Even large objects appear as if shrouded by a piece of cloth. People are seen as bereft of eyes, ears or nose. The aggravated doshas impart their respective colours to the objects. The doshas localising below, above and to the sides of the pupil respectively obstruct the view of objects situated near, distant or laterally. If the doshas localise all over the pupil, all objects appear dim. If the doshas are localised at the centre of the pupil, a single object is seen as if there are two. On the other hand, if the doshas are distributed over the pupil, one object is seen as many.

When the fourth patala (tejo-jalāśrita, NiS) is affected, the patient suffers from the disease known as timira (?ametropia, loss of vision). If there is complete blindness, the disease is known as linga-nāśa (? cataract). However, if this disease is not very deep-seated the patient can perceive faint images of the sun, moon, stars, a flash of lightning and such other brilliant objects.

The disease linga-nāśa has the synonyms of kācha and nīlika.

In the timira caused by aggravated vāta, objects appear hazy, flickering, crooked and brownish in colour. If pitta is mainly aggravated, objects seem to be inverted with the colours of the rainbow, glow-worm, a flash of lighting or with blue and black colours. If kapha is mainly provoked, objects appear unctuous (cloudy), white and hazy, unctuous and a thick white coat appears to intervene between the objects and the eye. If blood is vitiated, objects appear red, smoky or enveloped in darkness, and are inverted with gray or variegated colours. If all the three doshas are aggravated, objects appear variegated, confused, and appear to the trebled; the patient also perceives stars floating in his vision.

Due to vitiation of the blood by the aggravated pitta, the patient perceives the heavens as being yellow and resplendent with the light of the rising run, and trees which seem to sparkle with fireflies, such a disease is known as parimlāyi.

In the six kinds of timira explained above, the colour (of the pupil?) will be brownish, blue or bluish-yellow, reddish white, and variegated (i.e. in vātaja, pittaja, kaphaja, raktaja and tridoshaja timira respectively). In parimlāyi, a circular patch coloured bluish-yellow and resembling fire or a piece of thick grass is formed on the pupil.

In vātaja-linga-nāśa, there will be a rough, fluctuating and brownish circular patch on the pupil. In pittaja-linga-nāśa, the patch will be bluish, yellow or of the colour of bell-metal. In kaphaja-linga-nāśa, the patch will be thick, white, unctuous, resembling the conch-shell or the moon, or a white drop of water on the lotus-leaf. In raktaja-linga-nāśa, the circular patch is red, like a (red) lotus-petal or coral. In tridoshaja-linga-nasa there will be variegated colour.

Thus there are six kinds of linga-nāśa, namely:

1. Vātaja-linga-nāśa

2. Pittaja-linga-nāśa

3. Kaphaja-linga-nāśa

4. Raktaja-linga-nāśa

5. Sannipatika (tridoshaja) – linga-nāśa

6. Parimlāyi

7. Pitta-vidagdha-drshti: The aggravated pitta localises in the third patala and as a result, the patient suffers from day-blindness. All objects also appear yellow. This disease is curable.

8. Kapha-vidagdha-drshti: The aggravated kapha localises in all the three patalas, and as a result, the patient suffers from night-blindness. All objects appear white. This is also curable.

9. Dhūma-darśi: The doshas, especially pitta, are aggravated due to grief, fever, fatigue, head-injury, etc., and as a result, objects appears as if obscured by smoke. This disease is also curable.

10. Hrasva-jāḍya: The patient is able to perceive minute objects with great difficult (even) in daytime. This is caused by provoked

pitta and is considered to be incurable.

11. Nakulāndhya: In this disease, which is engendered by the derangement of all the doshas, the drshti (eyeball or pupil) becomes lustrous, like that of a mongoose, and in daytime, all objects appear to the inverted with many colours. This is also incurable.

12. Gambhīrika (glaucoma): Due to the aggravation of the deranged vāta, the drshti (pupil) is deformed, contracted and sunken, and there is also intense pain in the affected area. This is also considered to be incurable.

VII. Diseases of Traumatic Origin:

1. As a result of head-injury, the person suffers from symptoms similar to those seen in abhishyanda.

2. If a person gazes at very bright shining objects, he suffers from symptoms similar to those observed in linga-nāśa. However the eye looks lustrous, resembling vaiḍūrya (a precious stone).

Both these disease are considered to be incurable.

Treatment:

I. Of the seventy-six eye-diseases, eleven, nine, five and fifteen of them are to be treated by chedana (incision), lekhana (scarification), bhedana (excision) and vyadhana (venesection) respectively. Seven diseases can only be palliated and twelve of them should not be operated upon. Moreover, fifteen eye diseases are considered to be incurable.

The eleven diseases that are to be incised are arśo-vartma, suśkarśa, arbuda, sirā-piḍaka, sirś-jāla, the five types of arma and parvaṇika.

The diseases in which scarification is employed are utsargṇi, bahala-vartma, kardama-vartma, śyāva-vartma, baddha-vartma, klishṭa-vartma, potaki, kumbhiṇi and śarkara-vartma.

The diseases which are to be excised are sleshmopanāha, lagaṇa, biśa-vartama, kṛmigranthi and anjana.

Venesection is considered to be useful in sirotpāta. siro-harsha, aśopha-pāka, saśophapāka, anyato-vāta, puyālasa, vāta-viparyaya, the four types of adhimantha and four types of abhishyanda.

The following twelve diseases should not be operated upon: śushkākshi-pāka, kapha-vidagdha-dṛshti, pitta-vidagdha-dṛshti, amlādhyushita, śukra-roga, arjuna, pishṭaka, aklinna-vartma, dhūma-darśi, śuktika, praklinna-vartma and balāsa.

The Procedure of Lekhana (Scraping): The patient should be subjected to oleation, sudation and purificatory procedures. He should then be asked to recline in a room which is not exposed either to the sun or to wind. The eyelid should be gently turned outwards with the thumb and index finger. The part is scraped with a scraping instrument. After the bleeding stops, the part is to be fomented and gently rubbed with the powders of manhśila, kāsīsa (iron sulphate), trikaṭu, rasānjana, rock salt and mākshika. It is then washed with tepid water and lubricated with ghee. The subsequent treatment should be similar to that of vraṇa. After three days, fomentation and avapīḍa (nasya) should be carried out. The signs of proper lekhana are stoppage of bleeding, subsistence of swelling and itching, and smoothness of the affected part, (which should be like the surface of a finger nail).

Vāta-abhishyanda: The patient should first be administered old ghee. The eye should then be fomented and subjected to local venesection, followed by sneha-basti (a kind of enema). Later, measures such as aschyotana (eye-drops), nasya (errhines), etc., can be employed. The part can be washed with kānji or a decoction of drugs that alleviate vāta or which are prepared with the meat of aquatic or wetland animals. Poultices composed of milk, vesavāra, pāyasa, etc., or śalvaṇa-upanāha can be applied. The patient should also be administered ghee medicated with triphala, or old ghee, or milk medicated with drugs that alleviate vāta or with drugs of vidāri-gandhādi group. The decoction of milk diluted with an equal quantity of water, rock-salt, balā, yashti-madhu and pippali can be used for washing the eye, and as eye drops. If there is pain, goat's milk can be boiled with water, hrīvera, tagara, manjishtha and udumbara bark and used as eye drops. A thin paste of yashti-madhu, haridra, harītaki, devadāru and goat's milk is used as collyrium in acute abhishyanda. A paste of gairika, rock salt, pippali and nāgara, the quantity of each double the quantity of the preceding drug, is also useful when used as collyrium. The affected part can be washed with goats' milk boiled with leaves, roots and bark of eraṇḍa or with roots of kaṇṭakāri.

Pitta-abhishyanda: The measures useful include bloodletting, administration of purgatives, use of plasters and eye-drops, errhines, collyrium etc. The remedial measures useful in pittajavisarpa can also be used with benefit.

Ghee or goats' milk medicated with gundra, rice, saivala (dūrva, NiS), pāshaṇa-bheda, dāru-haridra, ela, utpala, lodhra, mustaka, padma leaves, sugar, darbha, sugarcane, tāla, vetasa, padmaka, drāksha, chandana, honey, yashti-madhu, breast-milk, haridra, and ananta (utpala-sāriva, NiS) can be used either internally or as nasya. Ghee extracted from milk can be used as nasya, eye-drops, etc. The juice of palāśa or sallaki can be applied as collyrium, along with honey and sugar. The rasakriya (thick liquid extract) of palindi (sariva or a variety of trivrt, NiS) or yashṭi-madhu can be used (as collyrium). The extract of musta, samudraphena, utpala, viḍanga, āmalaki and bījaka can be used similarly. A paste of talīsa, ela, gairika, uśira, śankha and breast-milk can also be used as collyrium. The powder or rasa-kriya of āmalaki and syandana can also be used as collyrium. Gold leaf rubbed with breast milk or the paste of palāśa flowers (kimśuka) and honey can also be used as collyrium. The paste of lodhra, drākshā, sugar, utpala, yashti-madhu, vachā and breast-milk can also be used as anjana. Samudra-phena can be rubbed with honey or breast-milk and applied as collyrium. The powder of yashṭi madhu, lodhra, drāksha, sugar and utpala are to be soaked in breast-milk and folded up within a cloth which should then be squeezed. The liquid can be used as eye drops. Ghee medicated with yashṭi-madhu and lodhra, or with bala, kāśmari, āmalaki, harītaki and kaṭphala can be used as eye drops.

Kapha-abhishyanda: The remedial measures include venesection, fomentation (sudation), avapīda type of errhine, application of collyrium, fumigation (dhūma), affusion (parisheka) application of plasters, gargles, eye-drops consisting of non-unctuous substances, and puṭa-pāka of similar (non unctuous) substances. The patient is advised to fast once in three days and partake of titkaka ghrṭa on the morning of the next day (after fasting). The diet should consist of articles that do not aggravate kapha. The affected area can be fomented using tender stems or leaves of tagara, asphoṭa, phaninjaka, bilva, pattūra, pilu, arka and kapittha. A paste of bālaka, nāgara, devadāru and kushṭha can also be applied. Vartis (sticks) prepared from hingu, rock-salt, triphala, madhuka, prapouṇdarīka, rasānjana, tuttha and tāmāra or from harītaki, harida, yashṭi-madhu, and anjana (rasājana), or from trikaṭu, triphala, haridra, and viḍanga or from bālaka, kushṭha, devadāru, śankha, pāṭha, anala (chitraka), trikaṭu, manahśila and flowers of jāti, karanja and śigru can be used for applying collyrium. The vartis can also be prepared from seeds of prakīrya (kaṇṭaki-karanja), rasānjana, rock-salt, chandana, manahśila, haratāla, and laśuna and used for applying collyrium.

Rakta-abhishyanda: The patient has to first be subjected to snehana with old ghee or with a copious quantity of meat juice. He can also be subjected to venesection. Later on, the patient can be administered purgatives and then subjected to śiro-virechana employing ghee medicated with sugar and śiro-virechana drugs. The remedial measures that are also useful include plasters, affusions, errhines, fumigation (dhūmapāna), medicated eye drops, massages with ghee (or oil), refreshing measures, and puṭapāka. A paste of nilotpala, uśira, dāruharidra, kaliyaka, yashṭi-madhu, musta, lodhra, padmaka and ghee can be applied. If there is severe pain, milk fomentation or blood-letting by leeches, is useful. Large draughts of ghee can also be administered, The measures useful in pitta-abhishyanda are also useful. Rain water may be medicated with powdered kaseruka and yashṭi-madhu and squeezed through a cloth, and used as eye drops. The paste of flowers of pāṭala, arjuna, kāsmari, dhātaki, āmalaki, bilva, bṛhati, kaṇṭakāri, bimbilota, manjishṭha, and honey or sugarcane juice can be used as collyrium. The paste of chandana, kumuda, tej patra, śilājat, kunkuma, loha (bhasma), tāmra (bhasma), tuttha, rasānjana, the gum-resin of nimba, trapu (bhasma), kāmsya and honey can also be used as anjana.

Diseases of Sandhis:

Puyālasa: The affected area is subjected to oleation, sudation and bloodletting. Poultices can also be applied. The remedial measures useful in akshipāka are also to be employed. A paste of fresh ginger, rock-salt, kāsīsa and iron dust, copper dust and honey can be used as collyriums.

Krmi-granthi: The affected area is fomented, incised and plastered with the rasa-kriya (semi-solid extract) of triphala, tuttha, kāsīsa and rocksalt.

Upanāha: The affected area is to be incised and rubbed with the paste of pippali, rock-salt and honey. It should then be scraped with a maṇḍalāgra instrument.

Parvaṇī: The joint should be fomented. A quarter part of the growth should be kept apart, while the remaining three quarters should be excised. One half of the remaining quarter should then be excised very carefully (care being taken to avoid creating a sinus). The area is then rubbed with a paste of rock-salt and honey. The area can then be covered over by powders of lekhana drugs.

Diseases of Vartmās (Eyelids):

Praklinna vartma: The paste of kāsīsa, samudra-phena, rasānjana, buds of jāti flowers and honey is applied as collyrium. The paste of rock-salt, śveta-maricha, and nepāla-jaṭa (manahśila), and mātulunga, if used as collyrium relieves the itching. The paste of nāgara, deva-dāru, musta, rock-salt, buds of jāti flower and cow urine can be used as collyrium for relieving the swelling and itching. The patient should also be subjected to oleation, sudation, emesis, purgation, etc., depending on the dosha involved. Eye drops prepared from musta, haridra, yashṭi-madhu, priyangu, siddhārta, lodhra, utpala and sāriva can be used. The paste of resānjana and honey can be used as collyrium. The extract of the leaves and fruits of āmalaka or of triphala and flowers of palāśa, can be applied as collyrium. The paste of kajjala (kajjali?) and tuttha should be rubbed with ghee on the surface of a copper vessel, and can be used as anjana.

Aklinna-vartma: The powders of rock-salt, śankha, mudga, samudra-phena and white maricha can be used as collyrium for relieving the itching.

The diseases known as pothaki, bahala-vartma, vartmāvabandha, and klishṭa-vartma should be scraped as described above.

The diseases known as śyāva-vartma and kbārdama-vartma should not be scraped too deeply or too superficially.

In the disease utsangini, vartma-śarkara and kumbhika, the eruptions (growths) should be excised, and the area scraped later.

Śuśkārśas: The powders of śankha, samudraphena, maṇḍuki (śukti), sphaṭika, kuruvinda (padmarāga), pravāla, asmantaka (a variety of precious stone), vaiḍūrya, pūlaka (a kind of sphaṭika), mukta, iron, copper and srota-anjana can be applied as collyrium.

Arbuda: The same powder (described above)

can be used as collyrium.

In any of the diseases affecting the inner lining of the eyelids, the following measures are useful: The affected area is fomented. The eyelid is then turned upwards, and the growth or pustule should be lifted up with a needle, and excised at its base with the help of a maṇḍalāgra instrument. The part is then rubbed with the paste of rock-salt, pippali and kāsīsa. If there is still a residue of the vitiated blood, the affected area can be cauterised. If there is a remnant of the growth remaining, it can be scraped with kshāras (caustics). The patient can also be administered decoctions of emetics and purgative drugs.

Lagana: The affected part should be incised, and the paste of rochana, yava-kshāra, tuttha, pippali and honey can be applied therein. But severe cases may require to be cauterised.

Bisa-vartma: The affected eyelid should be fomented. The puncture-like holes are then incised. The area can be dusted with the powders of rock-salt, kāsīsa, māgadhi (pippali), pushpānjana, manahśila and ela. A paste of honey and ghee can then be applied. The eyelid should then be loosely bandaged.

Anjana-nāmika: The affected area should be first fomented. If it spontaneously bursts, it should be pressed well and rubbed with the paste of manahsila, ela, tagara, rock-salt and honey. If it has not burst, it should be fomented, and incised, rubbed with rasānjana and honey and plastered with the lamp-black collected from a burning lamp flame.

Pakshma-kopa: The patient is first subjected to snehana (oleation), and is then seated in a proper position. An incision shaped like a barley corn is made in the eyelid horizontally parallel to the inner and outer canthi leaving two parts below the eyebrow and one part above the eyelashes. The two edges of the incisions should be sutured with horse's hair. A paste of ghee and honey should be applied to the incised area. It should then be treated as in the case of a vrana. A piece of cloth should be tied around the forehead and the horse's hair (used for suturing) should be attached to it. The horse's hair should be removed after the cuts have healed.

If the above described procedure fails to cure, the eyelid should be lifted up, and the diseased vali should be cauterised with fire or kshara. Or, as an alternative, all the eyelashes should be removed, and the eyelid should be rubbed with a paste of harītaki and tuvaraka (lodhra) after having previously secured the lid with three hooks (badiśa). Other measures that are likely to be useful include purgatives, eye drops, earrhines, fumigation, plasters, collyrium, etc.

Diseases of the Sukla Bhāga (White of the Eye, Sclera):

1. Śuktika: A paste of vaiḍūrya, sphaṭika, pravāla, mukta, śankha, silver, gold, sugar and honey can be used as collyrium. The paste of cooling drugs can also be applied as collyrium. The patient should also be administered triphala ghṛta, or tilvaka-ghṛta or just old ghee. All the measures useful in pitta-abhishyanda except bloodletting can be employed with benefit.

2. Balāsa-granthi: The patient has first to be subjected to oleation, sudation and cleansing procedures. Then nīla (unripe, NiS), barley grains with the bristles should be soaked in cow's milk (i.e. subjected to bhāvana) for seven days and burnt into ashes. These ashes should be mixed with the ashes of flowers of arjaka, asphoṭaka, kapittha, bilva, nirguṇḍi and jāti. These should be converted into kshārodaka (alkaline solution) to which rock-salt, tuttha and rochana should be added. The solution should then be subjected to heat. The resulting product is to be applied as collyrium.

3. Pshṭaka: The paste of śuṇṭhi, pippali, musta, rock-salt, śveta-maricha (seeds of śigru acc. to NiS) and juice of mātulunga can be applied as collyrium. Or ripe bṛhati fruits devoid of seeds should be filled with the paste of pippali and sroto-anjana. The paste can also be preserved within the fruits of vārtāku, śigru, paṭola, indravāruṇi, kirāta-tikta and āmalaka.

4. Arjuna: The paste of sugarcane juice, honey, sugar, breast milk, daru-haridra, yashṭi-madhu and rock-salt can be used as collyrium. Kānji can be used in the form of eye drops. The paste of sugar, yashṭi-madhu, kaṭvanga, mastu, kānji (or any sour liquid), honey, rock-salt, bījapura, kola and dāḍima or any other sour fruit can be used for preparing eye drops. The paste of sphaṭika, pravāla, śankha, yashṭi-madhu and honey or of śankha, honey, sugar and samudraphena or of rasānjana and honey or of rock-salt, kataka and honey, or of kāsīsa and honey can be used as collyrium.

5. Armas: The patient should be asked to partake of unctuous food, and then sit at ease. The affected eye should then be irritated by dusting it with rock-salt, and then fomented and rubbed with the hand; the patient should then be instructed to gaze at the outer canthus, and the growth should be secured by a badiśa (hook), and muchunḍi or sūchi-sutra instrument. The eyelid should not be lifted up suddenly, but the two eyelids should be firmly drawn apart. The growth should then be scraped with a sharp manḍalāgra instrument. The root of the growth should be pushed towards the inner canthus, away from the iris and sclera, and carefully excised. However one-fourth of the growth should be left intact. A lekhana anjana can then be made use of.

An arma which is in the form of a network (jāla) should be made pendent by rubbing it with rock-salt. It should then be secured with a badiśa (hook) and excised by a manḍalāgra instrument, at the junction of the eyelid and sclera. The area is then rubbed with a paste of yava-kshāra, rock-salt and trikaṭu, fomented and carefully bandaged. The patient is then subjected judiciously to oleation. The bandage is removed after three days. The affected eye should then be gently fomented with the palms. Eye drops prepared by boiling milk with Karanja seeds, āmalaki, and yashṭi-madhu and mixed with honey are useful in relieving pain. A plaster composed of yashṭi-madhu, pollen of utpala, dūrva, milk and ghee can be applied to the scalp.

6. Śirā-jāla and Sirā-piḍaka: These have to be excised as described above.

The anjaan described in the treatment of śuśkārśas (consisting of śankha, etc.,) is also used in these diseases.

Diseases of the Kṛshṇa-bhāga (Iris):

1. Avraṇa and Śa-vraṇa Śukra: A case of śukra should be treated as prescribed in the case of raktaja-abhishyandi. The affected part can be scraped with the paste of sirīsha seeds, maricha, pippali and rock-salt or with rock-salt alone. The paste of copper dust, manahśila, maricha and rock-salt can be applied as collyrium. The kshāra-anjana described in the treatment of balāsa-granthi can also be applied. The paste of fried dehusked mudga, śankha, sugar and honey, or of the pith of madhuka and honey or of the inner pulp of the stones of vibhṭtaka and honey can be applied as collyrium. Kshārodaka (caustic solutions) should be prepared from the ashes of bamboo sprouts, arushkara, tāla and nārikela. The ashes of elephant bones should be subjected to bhāvana with this solution several times. It can then be used as an anjana in order to remove the discolouration (the powder can be rubbed on the affected area, and this eye washed with a decoction of triphala).

2. Ajaka: The thin, watery matter that accumulates should be drained out by making a puncture on either side with a needle. The ulcer should then be packed with the paste of beef and ghee. If the ulcer becomes elevated, it can be scraped.

Diseases Involving the Entire Eye:

1. The diseases known as vāta-adhimantha, pitta-adhimantha, kapha-adhimantha and raktaja-adhimantha should be treated on the same lines as vāta-abhishyanda, pitta-abhishyandha, kapha-abhishyanda and rakta-abhishyanda respectively.

2. The diseases known as anyato – vāta and vāta-paryaya should be treated on the same lines as vāta-abhishyanda. The patients can

partake of draughts of ghee and milk before meals. Ghee medicated with vṛkshādaṇi, kapittha, bṛhatpanch-mūla drugs, karkata and milk can be administered internally. Ghee medicated with pattūra, ārtagala and ajamoda or with milk and mesha-śṛngi or with vīratara can also be administered.

3.Śuskākshi-pāka: The paste of rock-salt, nāgara, devadāru, the juice of mātulunga, breast-milk, water and ghee should be used as collyrium. The patient can be internally administered ghee medicated with drugs of the jivanīya group. The medicated oil known as aṇu-taila can be used in the form of nasal drops. The eye can be washed with cold milk mixed with rock-salt or medicated with haridra, devadāru and rock-salt. The paste obtained by rubbing ginger over a stone slab along with ghee and breast-milk can be used as collyrium. The paste of vasā (fat) of aquatic or wet land animals, nāgara and rock-salt can also be used as anjana.

4. Sirotpāta: The paste of honey and ghee, or of rock-salt, kāsīsa and breast-milk, or of śankha, tutha, manahśila, dāru-haridra, rock salt and honey or of svarṇa-gairika and honey or of maricha, honey, wine and juices of sirīsha flowers can be applied as collyrium.

5. Sirā-harsha: The paste of phānita and honey or of rasānjana and honey or of rock-salt, kāsīsa and honey, or of amla-vetasa, rock-salt, phāṇita and breast-milk can be used as collyrium.

6. Akshi-pāka: The affected eye can be subjected to oleation and sudation, followed by blood-letting. Eye-washes, eye drops, errhines and puṭa-pāka measures are also useful. The patient can also be subjected to cleansing procedures. Later, the paste obtained by rubbing rock-salt, ghee and curd or curd-cream on a copper vessel or of rust of bell-metal and ghee or of rock-salt and breast-milk, or of a paste of madhūka, gairika and honey or of rock-salt, copper dust, ghee and breast-milk can be applied as collyrium. The rasa-kriya of dāḍima, araveta, aśmantaka, kola, rock-salt and sour juices can also be used. Eye-drops prepared from animal flesh, rock-salt, ghee, ginger and breast-milk can be used. The paste of rock-salt, jāti flowers, nāgara, pippali, dehusked viḍanga and honey can be used as collyrium.

7. Amlādhyushita: The measures useful in pittaja-abhishyanda are to be employed in this disease also.

Diseases Affecting the Drshti (Pupil):

1. Dhūma-darsi: The patient should be administered draughts of ghee. Other remedial measures useful in pittaja-visarpa and rakta-pitta can also be employed.

2. In the diseases known as pitta-vidagdha-dṛshṭi and kapha-vidagdha-dṛshṭi, measures such as errhines, affusions, collyrium, plasters, putapāka, etc., are useful. Triphal ghṛta and traivṛta ghṛta are useful in pitta-vidagdha-dṛshṭi and kapha-vidagdha-dṛshṭi respectively. The patient can also be administered potions of old ghee. The paste of gairika, rock-salt, pippali and soot obtained by burning cow's teeth or of beef, maricha, sirīsha seeds and manah-śila, or of stalks of kapittha fruit and honey, or of ātmagupta and honey can be used as collyrium. The paste, known as pushpānjana, dravānjana and guṭikānjana can be applied in the form of collyrium. The paste of rasānjana, the juice (of jāti or āmalaki), honey, tālīśa-patra, svarṇa-gairika and cow-dung juice or the preparation known as chūrṇa-anjana can be used as collyrium. The paste of kāśmari flowers, dārvi, lodha, yashṭi-madhu, rasānjana and honey can also be used (as collyrium), in pitta-vidagdha-dṛshṭi.

A varti (plug) prepared from rock-salt, souvīranjana, pippali, reṇuka and goat's urine is useful in kapha-vidagdha-dṛshṭi (as anjana). The varti prepared from tagara, dāru-haridra and juice of cow-dung or from tagara, balā, trikaṭu, harītaki, manahśila, samudra-phena and goat's milk can be used as anjana in kapha-vidagdha-dṛshṭi. The anjana known as rasa-kriya-anjanas are also useful in this disease. The liver of a godha should be partially opened and stuffed with pippali coated over with clay and roasted. The pippali is then used as an anjana. It is considered very useful in night blindness. The liver of a goat can be used instead of godhā. The paste of rock-salt, green mudga or śankha, souvīranjana, trikaṭu, manśila, haridra, dāru-haridra and chandana is used as anjana in pitta-vidagdha-dṛshṭi.

3. The treatment of the six kinds of timira is as follows: The patient should be oleated, fomented and administered old ghee medicated with purgative drugs. If vāta is aggravated, castor-oil can be administered with milk. If pitta and kapha are involved, triphala-ghṛta can be administered. Ghee medicated with trivṛt can be administered in cases where kapha is vitiated, while oil medicated with trivṛt is useful where all the doshas are vitiated. Old ghee which has been preserved in an iron vessel is useful in all cases of timira. Ghee medicated with triphala or mesha—śṛngi is also useful. Triphala can be administered with ghee, oil and honey in pittaja, vātaja, and kaphaja timira respectively. Ghee can be used as nasya in pittaja-timira. Oil medicated with drugs of the kākolyādi group or vidārigandhādi group or aṇu-taila can be used in the form of nasal drops in timira where vāta and blood are deranged. Milk should be boiled with the meat of aquatic or wet-land animals, and ghee extracted from it. This can be used as nasya in vataja-timira. Sroto-anjana should be soaked in milk for three days, and then used as anjaan in vātaja kācha.

Ghee extracted from milk and medicated with drugs of the kākolyādi groups is to be used as nasya or tarpaṇa in pittaja-timira. The drugs of the kākolyādi group and flesh of desert animals can be used in the form of puṭa-pāka. The paste of rasānjana, sugar, honey, manahśila and yashṭi-madhu can be used as (in pittaja-timira). The powders of souvrānjana and tuttha can be used as anjana. The paste of soulvirānjana, mesha-śṛngi and sroto-anjana is used as collyrium in pittaja-kācha. The rasa-kriya prepared from the juices of pālaśa, rohitaka, madhūka, honey and the upper layer of madira is used as anjana in this disease.

Oil medicated with uśira, lodhra, triphala and priyangu can be used in the form of nasal drops in kaphaja-timira. Fumigation with viḍanga, pātha, apāmārga and ingudi bark is also useful. Ghee medicated with kshīri tree, haridra and uśira can be used for akshi-pūraṇa. The puṭa-pāka prepared from the meat of desert animals, pippali, honey and rock-salt is also useful (in kaphaja timira). The rase-kriya prepared from manahśila, trikaṭu, rock-salt honey, śankha, kāsīsa and rasānjana or from kāsīsa, rasānjana, guḍa and nāgara can be used as collyrium.

Sroto-anjana should be heated and soaked many times in a decoction of triphala prepared with eight kinds of urines, stuffed inside the hollow bones of nocturnal birds (such as vultures) and immersed in unruffled water for a month. This can be used as collyrium along with yashṭi-madhu and mesha-śṛngi in tridoshaja-kācha.

The timira known as parimlāyi shuld be treated on the same line as pittaja-timira. The measures useful in abhishyanda can be employed in timira also.

A person who regularly partakes of old ghee, triphala, śatāvari, paṭola, mudga, āmalaka, and yava will not suffer from timira. The pāyasa pepared from śatāvari or āmalaka or a meal of barley corns cooked with a decoction of triphala and copious amount of ghee is useful in timira. Articles such as sunisharṇnaka, jīvanti, taṇḍuliya, vāstuka, chilli, mūlaka (bāla-mulaka), meat of lāva, etc., and desert animals, paṭola, karkoṭaka, kāravella, vārtāku, tarkāri, kāsīsa, śigru, ārtagala etc. cooked with ghee are useful in timira.

The surgical treatment in the case of kaphaja linga-nāśa has also been described, (SS).

Ref.: SS, uttara, 1-17.

Classical Prescriptions: Aśva-bilvādi-taila; Balā-dhātryādi-taila; Bhṛungarāja-taila; Danti-varti; Kapardika-bhasma; Karpūradi-kuzambu; Kāyyonnyādi-taila; Mṛdvīkārishṭa;

Muktādi-mahānjana; Tāmra-bhasma; Tāmradi-guṭika; Triphala-chūrṇa; Tunga-drumadi-taila; Vajra-bhasma.

Netra-kaṇḍu : Vimala-varti
Netra-dāha : Balā-dhātryādi-taila
Netra-ruja : Manjishṭhādi-taila
Netra-śukra : Paṭolādi-ghṛta
Netra-adhimāmsa : Chandrodaya-varti
Netra-abhishyanda : Mahā-triphāladya-ghṛta
Naktāndhya : Mahā-triphalādya-ghṛta; Paṭoladī-ghṛta.

Pāda-dāha

Western Nosology: Burning of soles

Casuative Factors:

Extrinsic: Excessive walking, (SS).

Intrinsic: Vāta and Pitta, (SS).

Constituents Affected: Blood, (SS).

Symptomatology: The patient suffers from burning of soles, (SS).

Treatment:

1. The patient is to be treated along the same lines as indicated in vāta-roga.

2. The patient is subjected to venesection after which a paste of thorns of nāga-keśara and śata-dhouta ghṛta is applied. The soles can be washed with a decoction of daśamūla. The soles can also be smeared with butter and given fomentation, (CD).

Ref.: SS, nidāna, 1, 80; AHṛ, sūtra, 27, 16; CD, 22, 58-59.

Classical Prescriptions: Guḍūchyādi-modaka; Śatāvari-guḍa.

Pāda-dāri

Synonyms:

Sanskrit :Vipādika (NiS on SS)

Vernacular :Miśrāvāku (NiS on SS)

Western Nosology: Fissures

Causative Factors:

Extrinsic: Excessive walking

Intrinsic: Vāta

Symptomatology: Painful cracks on the soles of the feet.

Treatment:

1. The feet are smeared with oil and given fomentation. Blood letting is performed by venesection. The paste of bee's wax, vasā and majja (animal fat), powder of sarja, ghee, yava-kshāra and gairika (red ochre) is applied, (SS).

2. The paste of sarja-rasa, rock salt, honey and ghee is churned with kaṭu-taila. This paste can be applied over the soles, (CD).

Ref.: SS, nidāna, 13, 29; chikitsā, 20, 20; CD, 55, 12.

Classical Prescription: Sindūrādi – lepa

Pāda-harsha

Western Nosology: Peripheral Neuritis

Casuative Factors:

Extrinsic: Factors which aggravate vāta.

Intrinsic: Vāta and kapha, (SS).

Symptomatology: The patient suffers from a tingling sensation and numbness of the soles, (SS).

Treatment: The patient can be administered an enema of honey, ghee, meat-juice, musta and vibhītaka, (CS).

The patient can be subjected to blood letting by venesection. The remedial measures useful in vāta roga can also be employed, (SS).

Ref.: SS, nidāna 1, 81; chikitsā, 5, 23; CS, siddhi, 12, 18 (15).

Padmiṇī-kaṇṭaka

Western Nosology: Papilloma of skin

Causative Factors:

Extrinsic: Factors which aggravate kapha and vāta.

Intrinsic: Kapha and vāta.

Constituents Affected: The avabhāsini layer of skin (the stratum corneum layer of epidermis).

Symptomatology: Whitish circular patches on the skin covered over by small eruptions resembling the thorns on the lotus stem, and attended by itching.

Treatment: The patient is subjected to emesis by administering a decoction of nimba. The patient is then administered ghee medicated with nimba, along with honey. The paste of nimba and āragvadha is to be rubbed over the affected areas, (SS).

The kshāra (ash) of the lotus stem is used for external application, (CD).

Ref.: SS, nidāna, 13, 40; śārīra, 4, 4; chikitsā, 20, 38-39; AS, uttara, 36; CD, 55, 21-22.

Paksha-vadha

Synonyms: Sanskrit - Pakshāghāta (CS, sūtra, 14, 21), Ekānga-roga, (CS).

Western Nosology: Hemiplegia

Causative Factors:

Extrinsic: Factors which aggravate vāta, (CS,SS).

Intrinsic: Vāta (CS, sūtra, 11, 49; SS)

Symptomatology: The aggravated vāta causes immobility of either side of the body, with pain and inability to speak. The blood vessels and hard fibrous structures are dried up, and there is contraction (deformity) of the hand or foot, attended by pricking and sharp pain, (CS).

The aggravated vāta affects the nerves of the body, causes weakness and loss of power in the joints of one side of the body, and immobilises that part. If the part becomes entirely immobile and numb, the patient may suddenly fall down and expire, (SS).

Pricking pain, emaciation, immobility (paralysis) and coldness of the affected area, (RRS).

Prognosis: Those cases where only vāta is vitiated are difficult to cure, whereas cases in which either pitta or kapha is also involved are curable. Pakshavadha that is brought about through the depletion of the body tissues is incurable, (SS).

Ref.: CS, chikitsā, 28, 53-55; SS, nidāna, 1, 60-63; AS, nidāna, 15, 43; RRS, 21, 66.

Treatment:

1. The patient should be given the general measures indicated in vāta-roga.

The specific measures that are useful in pakshāghāta are nāḍi type of fomentation, application of poultices (upanāha) of meat of aquatic animals, oleation and purgation, (CS).

2. Only the patient who does not suffer from emaciation of the affected part, and who suffers from pain (in the affected part) should be treated. The patient should be first oleated and fomented, and then subjected to mild purificatory measures (such as emesis and purgation). Later, after the stipulated period (fifteen days after emesis or one week after purgation), āsthāpana kind of enema is administered. The remedial measures employed in ākshepaka are to be made use of.

The specific measures useful are mastishka śiro-basti with massage of aṇu-taila, the application of sālvaṇa poultice, and anuvāsana type of enema with balā-taila. These measures are to be followed continuously for about four months, (SS).

3. The patient should be administered rasa-

parpaṭi and any one of the guggulu preparations with ghee. The decoction of eraṇḍa, chitraka, nāgara and guḍūchi or a decoction of chaṇaka should be used as anupāna.

The oil extracted from sarja can be used for massage, (RRS).

Ref.: CS, chikitsā, 28, 100; SS, chikitsā, 5, 19; RRS, 21, 67-69.

Classical Presciptions: Chaturbhuja-rasa; Dhānvantara-taila; Ekāngavīra-rasa; Kārpāsāsthyādi-taila; Laghu-vishgarbha taila; Rasarāja-rasa; Rāsnādi-kvātha-chūrṇa; Yogendra-rasa.

Palita

Western Nosology: Greying of hair

Casuative Factors:

Extrinsic: Excessive exertion, emotions such as anger and grief, (SS).

Intrinsic: All three doshas, especially pitta, (CS, SS).

Constituents Affected: Rasa (CS, sūtra, 28, 10; SS, sūtra, 24, 9).

Varieties: Palita may be due to old age, or may be untimely, (AS).

Pathogenesis and Symptomatology: The aggravated doshas and the (increased) body heat affect the scalp and cause graying of hair, (SS).

If vāta is mainly affected, the hair will be rough, dry, will split in the middle and will turn grayish in colour. If pitta is mainly involved, the hairs will be yellowish and appear as if they have been singed by fire. There will also be burning pain (in the scalp). If kapha is affected, the hairs will grow well, will be thick, unctuous and whitish in colour. If graying of hair occurs due to (chronic) headache, there will be tenderness of the scalp, (AS).

Prognosis: Palita caused by all the three doshas (sannipātaja) is incurable.

Treatment:

1. Nīli-taila: The juice of bhrngarāja and a decoction of triphala is made into a paste with powders of the leaves of nīli (indigo), bark of arjuna, bhṛngarāja, piṇḍītaka (madana?), iron, flowers of bījaka and sahachara, triphala and mud which is found sticking to lotus bulbs (which weighs as much as all the other drugs mentioned above). This paste is kept inside an iron vessel, which is well covered. After a fortnight, this paste is heated with til oil along with the juice of bhṛngarāja and a decoction of triphala. For testing the quality of the oil, the feathers of a crane are dipped in it. If they turn a deep blue colour, the oil is of good quality. The oil should be preserved for a month, after which it can be used externally.

A paste is prepared of the flowers of saireyaka, jambu, arjuna and of kāsmari, seeds of tila and bhṛngarāja, stones of mango, punarnava (two varieties), kaṇṭakāri, kāsīsa, seeds of madana, triphala, powdered iron, rasānjana, yashṭi-madhu, nilotpala, sāriva, mallika, and a decoction of the essence (sāra) of bījaka (asana). This paste is mixed with the decoction of sāra of bījaka and kept for ten days in an iron vessel. This is later boiled with oil of vibhītaka and preserved in another iron-vessel for a month. This oil can be used as nasal drops and for external application. The diet has to consist of māsha and kṛśara, (SS).

2. The patient has to be subjected to snehana (oleation) and svedana (fomentation). Medicated oils such as aṇu-taila can be used as nasal drops (nasya). Medicinal plasters can be applied on the scalp. Oil medicated with drugs of the vidārigandhādi group or jīvanīya group can be used in the form of nasal drops. A medicated oil prepared in a stone vessel by boiling milk, sahachara, bhṛngarāja, juice of sourasa, and paste of yashṭi-madhu can be used in the form of nasal drops. The paste of dugdhika or karavīra with milk can be applied on the scalp after extracting the gray hairs.

The oil medicated with bhṛngarāja juice, milk, and paste of yashṭi-madhu can be used as nasal drops. Oil medicated with prapouṇḍarika, yashṭi-madhu, pippali, chandana, utpala, and āmalaki juice can be used for pratimarśa-nasya (a kind of errhine) A paste of milk, priyāla, yashṭi-madhu, taila, drugs of jīvanīya groups and kṛshna (pippali) is used for external application. The paste of āmalaki, tila, kinjalka (kesara), yashṭi-madhu and honey is very useful in graying of hair and baldness, when used externally. The hair has to be washed well and plastered with the paste of rock salt, śuktaka, powder of iron and taṇḍula (rice) which have been boiled together. The hair has to be washed, the next morning with a decoction of triphala. This is very useful in graying of hair, (CS).

3. The following formulations are useful in gray hair: the paste of yashṭi-madhu, leaves of nili, iron, bhṛngarāja and goat's milk, applied externally; a hole is bored into a half-ripe coconut which is filled with the paste of triphala powder, iron powder and juice of bhṛngarāja; the coconut is then kept covered up for a month; the person suffering from gray hair should then shave his head. The coconut is broken open, and the contents are stirred well and applied on the scalp and covered by leaves of kadali. After seven days, the scalp is washed with a decoction of triphala. The diet has to consist of milk and meat-juices. This procedure is very useful in palita; a paste of nilotpala and milk is kept in an iron-vessel which is placed for a month inside a pit dug in the ground. The paste can later be used for external application; bathing over the head regularly after applying a paste of maṇḍūra-bhasma, āmalaka and flowers of japa are also very useful; the seeds of nimba are triturated with the juices of bhṛangarāja and asana for seven days. The oil extracted from these seeds is used in the form of nasal drops, the diet should consist only of milk and rice. This will also be very effective in turning the gray hair black; oil medicated with juice of bhṛngarāja, milk and yashṭi-madhu is be used as nasal drops; (CD).

Classical Prescriptions: Amṛta-bhallatāka-leha; Aṇu-taila; Bhṛngāmalakādi-tails; Kāyonnādi-taila; Nīlibhṛngādi-taila; Nīlikādya-taila; Triphalādi-taila; Yashṭi-madhuka-taila.

Ref.: SS, chikitsā, 25, 28-31; CS, chikitsā, 26, 263-282; CD, 55, 112-134.

Pānajirṇa

Western Nosology: Sub-acute drunkenness

Casuative Factors:

Extrinsic: Abuse of alcoholic drinks.

Inrinsic: All three doshas, especially pitta.

Sytmptomatology: Flatulent distention of the abdomen, vomiting of sour fluid, and burning (along the alimentary tract).

Treatment: The patient is made to vomit by administering milk medicated with tiktalābu, dhāmārgava, fruits of kuṭaja and kakodumbara. After a few days, if there is a good appetite and stimulation of the digestive fire, the patient can partake of wine.

The patient can also be administered phalāmla (sour fermented wine prepared from dāḍima, bījapūraka, etc., along with dālchini, pippali, nāgapushpa and viḍa (salt) or with hingu, maricha and ela. The compound consisting of rock salt, viḍa, dālchini, chavya, ela, hingu, pippali, roots of pippali and nāgara can be given with hot water.

The diet can consist of appetizing khaṇḍayūsha.

Classical Prescription: Śri khaṇḍāsava

Related Diseases: Pānātyaya, Pāna-vibhrama, Para-mada.

Ref.: SS, uttara, 47, 20-21; 37-38.

Pānaki

According to some authorities, quoted by NiS, Pānaki is an advanced stage of pāṇḍu or kumbhāsa. The symptoms are: fever, unformed stools, yellowish discolouration of the eyes, skin, urine, etc., paleness and eye-disease.

Related Diseases: Kāmala, Pāṇḍu.

Ref.: NiS on SS, uttara, 44, 11.

Panasika

Western Nosology: Furuncle; Boil.

Causative Factors:

Extrinsic: Factors which aggravate kapha and vāta.

Intrinsic: Kapha and vāta.

Symptomatology: Extremely painful eruptions resembling lotus bulbs on the back or on the external ear.

According to Bhoja, there will be also burning pain, (NiS).

Treatment: The affected area is subjected to fomentation, after which a paste of manahśila, haratāla, kushṭha and devadāru is applied externally. When the eruptions come to a head, they are incised and treated as in vrana, (SS).

Ref.: SS, nidāna, 13, 12; chikitsā, 20, 5-6; AS, uttara, 36.

Pānātyaya

Synonyms: Sanskrit - Madātyaya

Western Nosology: Alcoholism

Causes

Extrinsic:

1. Excessive and improper intake of alcoholic drinks by persons who are accustomed to dry food and regular exertion. While alcoholic drinks taken in the correct dosage and at the prescribed time act as elixirs, they act as poisons when taken in excessive quantity and at improper timings. However, even excessive amounts of alcoholic drinks do not bring about adverse affects in persons who have been accustomed to alcohol, who take alcoholic drinks after food, and who have a strong body and mind. Even small amounts of alcohol cause adverse effects in persons who are debilitated, who have weak mental powers (sattvaḍurbalah), who suffer from vishṭabdha (a kind of ajirṇa), in persons who are hungry or thirsty, in persons of vāta or pitta consitution, who are used to dry and limited food, who are irritable, emaciated, exhausted; and when taken improperly, (CS).

2. Intake of alcoholic drinks on an empty stomach, in excessive quantity by ignorant persons. Intake of alcohol by persons who are angry, frightened, thirsty, grief-stricken, hungry, who have been weakened by exertion such as lifting heavy loads, walking, etc., by persons who have suppressed their natural urges, by persons who have spoiled their digestion by eating excess of sour foods, by debilitated persons, by persons who eat food before digestion of the previously taken meal, and by persons who have been exposed to the sun (for long periods), (SS).

Intrinsic: All three doshas.

Pathogenesis: The alcohol interacts with the kāyāgni (the digestive fire) and causes intoxication (mada), (SS).

Alcohol has properties which are diametrically opposed to the qualities of ojas, and it thus weakens ojas, and through it, adversely affects all the dhatus, (CS).

Symptomatology:

1. In the first stage of intoxication, the ojas is not affected, and the mind is stimulated. The person is happy, affectionate, can appreciate the taste, etc., of food and drink, is able to sing and play music, crack jokes, tell stories, etc., and is able to sleep well and wake up refreshed. The consciousness and memory are not affected.

In the second stage of intoxication, there will be episodes of forgetfulness, irrelevant speech and mumbling and occasional loss of concentration regarding the place (situation), food and conversation. The person will also be reeling about.

After the second stage, and just prior to the third stage, the intoxicated person whose mind is enveloped with rajas and tamas will be capable of commiting all unrighteous acts, and will lose control of oneself. It is as if the person is insane.

In the third stage of intoxication, the person will fall down like a log of wood. His mind will be clouded, and although living, the person is as if dead. He will lose the faculty of discrimination and enjoyment and will be in a despicable condition.

If vāta is severely provoked, the intoxicated person will suffer from hiccoughs, dyspnoea, pain in the sides of the chest, insomnia, unsteadiness of head (neck) and irrelevant speech.

If pitta is mainly aggravated, the patient will suffer from thirst, burning pain, fever, sweating, diarrhoea, syncope, vertigo and greenish discolouration (of the skin, eyes, etc.,).

If kapha is deranged, the patient suffers from vomiting, anorexia, nausea, lethargy, heaviness of the body, chilliness and a sensation as if covered with a wet cloth.

If all the doshas are provoked, the person will suffer from uneasiness in the cardiac region, loss of taste, intense thirst, fever, flashes of heat and chilliness, lightning-like pains in the head, sides of the chest and joints, constant yawning, tremors, pulsation, weakness, a sense of obstruction or constriction in the chest, cough, hiccoughs, dyspnoea, insomnia, diseases of the ears, eyes and mouth, stiffness in the sacral region, vomiting, diarrhoea, nausea, vertigo, irrelevant speech, hallucinations, delusions and nightmares, (CS).

2. Due to intoxication, there is an adverse affect on the consciousness, mind and sense-faculties, and even the innermost thoughts are revealed.

In the first stage, of intoxication, there is an enhancement in enthusiasm, pleasure, contentment and speech, laughter, etc. In the second stage, there is irrelevant speech, confusion of mind and episodes of improper behaviour. In the third stage, the person falls down unconsciousness, (SS).

3. In the first stage of intoxication, the alcoholic drink adversely effects the qualities of ojas, and disturbs the mind (cheats). In the second stage, under the influence of alcohol, the foolish person indulges in improper behaviour and forfeits his happiness. In the next stage, the intoxicated person who is enveloped by rajas and tamas behaves like an unrestrained vicious elephant, running amuck. The person then falls down unconscious.

Excessive and improper intake of alcohol is the cause for delusion (clouded mind), fear, grief, anger, unmāde, mūrccha, epilepsy (apasmāra), apatānaka and even death. The most important cause for all ailments is error of judgement and discrimination. It also destroys ones intelligence, courage and modesty.

The common symptoms of intoxication are cloudiness of mind, uneasiness in the cardiac region, diarrhoea, intense thirst, poor digestion, fever, loss of appetite, headache, joint pain, pain in the sides of the chest, tremors, stiffness of the back (trika), a sense of constriction in the chest, cataract (timira), cough, dyspnoea, insomnia, excessive sweating, flatulence (vishṭambha), swellings, mental disorders (chitta-vibhrama), irrelevant speech, vomiting, nausea, vertigo and nightmares.

If vāta is aggravated, there will be insomnisa, dyspnoea, trembling, headache, and dreams of roving about, or falling to the ground or holding conversation with ghosts. If pitta is vitiated, the symptoms seen are fever, burning pain, sweating, diarrhoea, clouded mind, thirst, vertigo, yellow or green discolouration of the skin and red discolouration of the eyes and cheeks. If kapha is disturbed, the person suffers from vomiting, nausea, sleepiness, urticaria (udarda) and heaviness of the body, (AS).

Complications: The complications are hiccoughs, fever, vomiting trembling, cough, vertigo and pain in the sides of the chest, (SS).

Prognosis: The disease is difficult to treat, (CS).

A patient exhibiting the signs and symptoms of sunken lips, excessive chilliness or sensation of severe heat, oilyness of the face, blackish or blue discolouration of the tongue, lips and teeth and yellowish or blood red appearance of the eyes is considered as being incurable, (SS).

Related Diseases: Pānājīrna, Paramada, Pānavibhrama.

Ref.: SS, uttara, 47, 9-23; CS, chikitsā, 24, 29-107; AS, nidāna, 6, 5-22.

Treatment:

1. Although all the three doshas are involved in this disease, the physician should identify the dosha that is predominantly aggravated Since the disease process originates from the locality of kapha (i.e. the ojas), treatment should be given first for the deranged kapha and later for the vāta and pitta.

The disease that arises from improper, excessive or too limited intake of alcohol will be relieved from proper and judicious intake of that alcohol itself. Likewise, the ailment caused by the digestion of āma madya will subside by the (proper) intake of alcohol. The alcoholic drink should be medicated with souvarchala, bīḍa and saindhava kinds of salts, juices of mātulunga and fresh ginger and water, and should be drunk cold.

If a person suffering from sour eructations and pyrosis partakes of an excess of hot and sharp alcoholic drinks, the food juices becomes alkaline (kshāra) and it causes fever, burning pains, thirst, clouded mind, intoxication and vertigo. In such cases, alcohol itself is to be administered. Alkaline substances (kshāras) rapidly become sweet when they are combined with sour alcoholic drinks and alcohol is the best of all sour substances.

Due to excessive intake of alcohol, the body channels are obstructed, and vāta is aggravated, and causes severe (sharp) pain in the head and joints. In such cases, alcoholic drinks are to be administered along with other medicines, as alcohol is vyavāyi, sharp and hot.

The following substances are useful in vātaja pānātyaya: paishṭika madya (i.e. alcoholic drinks prepared from rice flour, wheat flour, etc,) with bīja-pūraka, vṛkshāmala, kola, daḍima, powders of yavāni, hapusha, ajāji, nāgara and rock salt, oil or ghee and avadamśa (any pungent food that is appetizing); meat juices of lava, tittira, drāksha, and śikhī with oily and sour substances; meat juices of prasaha and bhūśaya animals with boiled rice; meat of aquatic animals, fish etc.; vesavāra (a preparation of meat) of the above mentioned kinds of meat that is tasty, and is mixed with oily, hot, salty and sour substances, along with the upper layer of vāruṇi; the dish known as māshapūpalika; alcoholic drinks along with the above mentioned kinds of meat (juices) but which is not very oily or sour, mixed with maricha and fresh ginger, or juice of dāḍima; dishes such as rāga, shādava, flour preparations, leafy vegetables, barley, wheat, rice, etc., ; drinks such as vāruṇimaṇḍa, juices of dāḍima, decoction of panchamūla drugs, water boiled with dhānya and nāgara, the upper layer of curds or of sour kānji, etc., can be used in case of thirst. The patient can be exposed to fumigation by burning agaru. He can also be subjected to massage, hot water bath, etc., and is to be warmly covered. The patient can also be embraced by young women with warm waists, thighs and breasts.

Those formulations are useful in pittaja madātyāya: the cold juices of bhavya, kharjūra, mṛdvīka, parūshaka, and dāḍima with saktu (barley that is dehusked, roasted and powdered); grape wine with sugar, which is well diluted; the meat of śaśa, lāva, kapinjala, eṇa and black-tailed deer; sour and sweet food articles and rice that is harvested in sixty days; the meat juice of chaga (goat) with soup of paṭola or soup of satīna and mudga or with dāḍima and āmalaka; refreshing gruels and meat-juices along with or prepared from juices of drākasha, āmalaka, kharjūra and parūshaka; etc.

If the patient (suffering from pittaja madātyaya) is very thirsty, he can be frequently given small amounts of diluted wine, which should appease thirst and not intoxicate. The cold juices of pīlu and parūshaka or cold infusion of śālaparṇi, pṛśniparṇi, mudgaparṇi and māshaparṇi or juice or decoction of musta, dāḍima and lāja, etc., are also useful in relieving thirst.

Cool foods and drinks, cool beds, breezes and gardens, the contact of silken gaments, precious stones and of women smeared with sandalwood paste, etc., are also recommended in pittaja madātyaya. The paste of phalini, uśīra, lodhra, musta, etc., or of the tender leaves of badara, nimba and phalini can be applied externally to alleviate burning pain. The juice of mātulunga, honey, sour curds, sura wine, etc., are also used for sprinkling and external application. Cold water can be used for administering in tub baths and as affusion.

In severe cases of alcoholism where the pa-

or of musta alone can also be given, as these will aid in the digestion (elimination) of the doshas. The above mentioned decoctions can be administered in all cases of madātyaya, as they are harmless, and alleviate fever and thirst, After the āma has been digested and the patient feels hungry, he may partake of sugar-wine or old honey or sīdhu with honey, or dry and refreshing (tarpaṇa) food mixed with yavāni and nāgara. The diet has to consist of barley, wheat, dry or ununctuous* gruels (yūsha) prepared from kulattha or dried radish. These should be easily digestible, and should be pungent, sour and mixed with a slight amount of ghee. The patient can also partake of dishes of barley along with sour soup (yūsha) of paṭola or soup of āmalaka mixed profusely with pungent substances, or sour soup (or gruel) mixed with trikaṭu or soup of amlavetasa or sour meat-juices of goat or desert animals, without much oil or ghee. Meat should be fried or roasted until it is fully dry and then mixed with sour, salty and pungent substances and partaken with honey. The patient should eat only at his regular meal time, after duly considering the state of his digestion. The food should be generously mixed with ginger. Wholesome wine can also be taken. The paste of one part of sugar and one-half part each of souvachala salt, ajāji, vṛkshāmla, amlavetasa, tvak (dālchini), ela and maricha is very useful in kaphaja madātyaya, as it stimulated the digestion, and cleaneses the body channels. The paste can be diluted with sweet and sour juices, and can be taken along with wheat and barley preparations and meat dishes.

The paste (chutney) of white grapes divested of the seeds, pungent spices, juices of mātulunga and dāḍima, souvarchala salt, ela, maricha, ajāji, dālchini and ajamoda can be taken with honey, as it is an excellent appetiser and digestive. Mṛḍvika can also be used in the same manner, instead of white grapes; and it has to be mixed in the same manner, with śukta and matsyandika. The pastes (chutneys, rāga) of mango pulp or pulp of āmalaka can be mixed with dhānya, souvarchal, ajaji, kāravi, maricha, jaggery and honey, so as to impart a sour and salty taste to them, and these may be used along with the food as they facilitate good digestion.

Dry and hot food, bathing with hot water, exercise, fasting, keeping awake at nights, massage without oil, rubbing the body, wearing heavy cloths (so as to induce sweating), application of a paste of agaru, embraces by young women, massage by women masseurs, are all useful in kaphaja madātyaya.

If all the above mentioned measures do not succeed in curing the patient suffering from madātyaya, wine (alcoholic drinks) would have to be stopped completely, and a milk-diet advised. Patients who have been weakened by excessive use of alcoholic drinks, and in whom there is aggravation of vāta and kapha are immensely benefited by using milk. After the disease has been cured by milk, and after the patient has regained his strength, milk can be gradually replaced with alcohol, (CS).

2. In a person suffering from vātaja pānātyaya alcohol (wine) mixed with chukra, maricha, ārdraka, ajamoda, kushṭha and souvarchala salt can be administered. Shāḍava (a kind of preparation) or cool juices prepared from āmalaka, mango fruits, dāḍima and mātulunga can also be given. The cooked meat of aquatic animals can be seasoned with the juices of the above fruits and partaken.

A patient of pittaja madātyaya can take alcoholic drinks, mixed with a decoction of drugs of the sweet group (i.e. kākolyadi group without guḍūchi), sugar, honey and aromatic substances. Wine (madya) mixed with large amounts of sugar cane juice can be taken, immediately followed by an emetic. Meat juices of lāva, eṇa and tittiri without any sour substances or soup of mudga with sugar and ghee can be partaken.

A person suffering from kaphaja pānātyaya is made to vomit by administering alcohol mixed with juices of bimbi and vetasa. The diet can consist of meat-juices of desert animals mixed with bitter and pungent substances or soup of mudga which should be also bitter and pungent. Barley can also be eaten.

The following preparation is useful generally in all forms of pānātyaya and relieves the delirious state of mind: the fine powder of equal amounts of dālchini, nagā-kesar, ela, pippali, madhuka, dhānya, ajāji and maricha is to be mixed with a copious amount of juices of kapittha, parūshaka and water and filtered; this is useful in all kinds of pānātyaya. The paste of hrīvera, padma, paripelava, karavīra, padmaka, drugs of the sārivādi group and aquatic flowers can be applied externally. The body can also be sprinkled over with clear and cold water. The pānaka consisting of dālchini, patra, chocha, maricha, ela, nāga pushpa and flowers of śleshmāntaka, jaggery and drāksha should be filtered and given to a person suffering from pānātyaya. The pānaka prepared from yashṭi-madhu, kaṭuka-rohiṇi, drākshā, and roots of trapusha or of kārpasa roots, nāga bala and souvarchala salt is also useful.

Objects that are pleasing to the senses, intake of mild alcoholic drinks, partaking of things that are relieving and satisfying, embrace by beautiful young women, etc., are all useful in a patient of pānātyaya.

The juice of kūshmāṇḍa mixed with sugar, madhūka, and drugs of the trijātaka group, and the powders of nāgakeśara, ajājī, pippali and maricha is to be administered.

In cases of severe thirst that is experienced by drunkards, a cold infusion of pāṭala, stalks of utpala, mudgaparṇi and pippali can be administered, (SS).

3. These prescriptions are useful in all types of pānātyaya: a mantha prepared from kharjūra, mṛdvīka, vṛkshāmla, amlika, dāḍima, purūshaka and āmalaka; ghee medicated with milk, punarnava, decoction, and paste of yashṭi-madhu; the powders of chavya, souvarchala salt, hingu, bījapūraka, nāgara and ajamoda are to be given with alcohol (wine); the pānaka of drāksha, kapittha, and dāḍima, with plenty of honey and sugar, ghee medicated with the juice of āmalaka; etc.

Refreshing drinks can be made by churning well, four parts of coarse powder of drugs mixed in sixteen parts of cold water.

In a case of vātaja pānātyaya, wine is diluted and mixed with souvarchala salt and trikaṭu and drunk. In pittaja pānātyaya, the patient can be administered soup of mudga with sugar or meat-juices medicated with sweet drugs. In kaphaja pānātyaya the patient is advised to fast, and is administered appetizing drugs, (CD).

Classical Prescriptions: Dhātryādi-ghṛta; Elādya-modaka; Rajatabhasma;

Srikhaṇḍāsava.

Ref.: CS, chikitsā, 24, 107-211; SS, uttara, 47, 24-53; CD, 18.

Pāna-vibhrama

Causative Factors:

Extrinsic: Abuse of alcoholic drinks

Intrinsic: All three doshas.

Symptomatology: Pricking pain in the praecordial region and limbs, vomiting, fever, burning sensation in the throat, syncope, hawking of mucous, headache, burning (along the alimentary tract) and aversion to food and wine.

Treatment: The patient should be administered pānaka (refreshing drink) prepared from drākhshā, kapittha and dāḍima fruits, honey and sugar-candy or from the juices of āmrātaka, and kola with honey and sugar-candy.

The cold infusion of kharjūra, vetraka, karīra, parūshaka, drāksha, trivṛt and sugar or with śrīparṇi can also be administered. The following drugs can be administered in the form of a cold infusion along with yashṭi-madhu and nīlotopala: tender sprouts of vata, etc., (kshīri-trees), biśa, (mṛṇāla, lotus stem), jīraka, nāga-pushpa, ela, śāriva, padma, amrātaka, kara-marda, kapittha, kola, vṛkshāmla, fuits of vetra, jiraka, dāḍima etc.

Related Diseases: Pānātyaya, Pānājirṇa, Paramada.

Ref.: SS, uttara, 47, 21-22; 39-41.

Pāṇḍu-roga

Western Nosology: Pallor, anaemia

Causative Factors:

Extrinsic:

1. Excesive sexual intercourse, sleep during daytime, excessive intake of alcoholic drinks, and substances that are salty, sour and sharp (tīkshṇa) and eating mud, (SS).

2. Sleep during daytime, excessive exertion and sexual inter-course, suppression of the natural urges, emotions such as lust, anxiety, fear and anger and grief, being subjected to improper and untimely emesis, purgation etc., (pancha karma), and excessive intake of- nishpāva, māsha, piṇyāka, tila-taila (sesamum or gingelly oil) and substances which are alkaline(kshāra), sour, salty, hot, unpleasant and imcompatible. Eating mud is also a causative factor, (CS).

Infants who are fed on bread and milk that is vitiated by deranged kapha are also prone to develop this disease, (CS, chikitsā, 30, 245).

Intrinsic: All three doshas, especially pitta, (CS).

Constituents Affected: Blood (SS), All the body elements (dhātus), (CS).

Prodormal Symptoms:

1. Cracks in the skin, frequent desire to spit, weakness, desire to eat mud, swelling around the eyes, yellow discolouration of urine and stools, and indigestion, (SS).

2. Pulsation in the precordial region, dryness of skin, failure to sweat and fatigue, (CS).

Types:

1. According to SS, there are four types of pāṇḍu: pāṇḍu engendered by the derangement of each of the three doshas, and that caused by the derangement of all the doshas together.

2. According to CS, pāṇḍu can be caused by the derangement of the three doshas separately and together (i.e. four types) and by eating of mud.

Symptomatology General:

1. Allthough there may be many kinds of discolouration (of skin, faces, etc.) the most frequent symptom observed is paleness (white

discolouration), (SS).

2. The three deranged doshas affect the dhātus (tissues) and cause debility and heaviness of the body. This is followed by excessive depletion of the attributes of ojas such as strength, complexion etc. The patient usually suffers from lack of blood (anaemia), emaciation, loss of lustre, weakness of sense organs, and discolouration (of skin, urine, faeces), tinnitus, loss of appetite, indigestion, vertigo, body pain, fever, dyspnoea, the limbs feel bruised, swelling around the eyes, green discolouration of skin, dryness of hair, irritability, aversion to cold, drowsiness, and cramping pain in the calves and weakness on ascending (steps, etc,), (CS).

Vātaja Pāṇḍu: Dark discolouration of eyes, stool, urine and face, darkish veins in the eyes, and other symptoms of vāta-rogas, (SS).

Blackish discolouration, dark and brownish skin, body pain, pricking pain, shivering, pain in the sides and head, dryness of stools, bad taste in the mouth, weakness, flatulence and swelling, (CS).

Pittaja Pāṇḍu: Yellowish discolouration of the eyes with prominent yellow veins, yellowness of stools, urine, nails and face, and other symptoms of aggravated pitta, (SS).

Fever, burning pain, thirst, syncope, excessive sweating, desire for cold, loss of appetite, pungent taste in the mouth, sour eructation, pyrosis, especially during digestion of food, bad odour (from the body), debility, unformed stools and yellowish or green discolouration of eyes, face etc. Hot and sour food disagrees with the person.

Kaphaja-Pāṇḍu: Whitish discolouration of eyes with prominent whitish (pale) veins, whitish stools, urine, nails and face, and other symptoms of deranged kapha, (SS).

Heaviness of body, lethargy, vomiting, vertigo, weakness even without any exertion, horripilation, salivation, weakness, dyspnoea, cough, drowsiness, loss of appetite, hoarseness, swelling, sweet taste in the mouth, whitish discolouration of urine, eyes, stools and face, and desire for pungent, dry and hot substances (CS).

Tridoshaja Pāṇḍu: Symptoms caused by all three deranged doshas will be present, (SS,CS).

Mṛd-bhakshaṇa Pāṇḍu: (Pāṇḍu caused by eating mud). Intake of mud that is astringent, alkaline (kshāra), and sweet aggravates vāta, pitta and kapha respectively. It also causes dryness in the dhātus (tissues), and as it is indigestible it obstructs the body channels. The patient suffers from loss of strength, complexion, resistance to disease and acuteness of sense faculties, loss of digestive power, swelling of feet, umbilical region (of abdomen), chest, region around the eyes and penis, worm infestations, and diarrhoea with colic and mucous stools, (CS).

The symptoms of this disease are loss of enthusiasm, feeble digestion and craving for blood, (KS).

Complications: Loss of appetite, thirst, vomiting, fever, headache, feeble digestion, swelling (oedema), weakness, vertigo, pressing pain in the chest, and dyspnoea (gasping for breath), (SS).

Prognosis: The patient who has been suffering from a severe kind of pāṇḍu roga for a long time, who suffers from swelling (oedema) and perceives everything as being yellow, who has diarrhoea with greenish, scanty and mucous stools, or constipation, who is emaciated, very pale, who suffers from vomiting, syncope, thirst, etc., is considered as being incurable, (CS).

Ref.: SS, uttara, 44; CS, chikitsā, 16, 3-33.

Treatment:

1. The patient should first be subjected of snehana (oleation) by means of ghṛta (ghee) (such as kalyāṇaka ghṛta, mahātiktaka ghṛta, etc., NiS), and then (mild) emesis and purgation. For purgation, the powder of harītaki with honey and ghee or ghee medicated

with haridra, or triphala, or tilvaka ghṛta or any purgative drugs with ghee are to be administered. The powder or paste of dantī boiled in buffalo's wine or guḍa boiled with harītaki or the decoction of drugs of the āragvadhā group can be employed for inducing purgation. However, the patient should be administered only very mild purgation for many days, as severe purgation causes swelling (oedema).

The following recipes are useful in pāṇḍu: the paste of purified iron, maricha, pippali, śunṭhi, viḍanga, ghee and honey; paste of haridra with triphala, ghee and honey; the juice of āmalaka with honey; sugarcane juice with honey; mantha with honey; māgadhika (pippali) with milk; the decoction or powder of yashṭi-madhu with honey; the paste or pulp of fruits of āmalaka, vibhītaki, and harītaki with purfied pravāla, mukta, śankha and rasānjana with cow's urine; the powder of purified svarṇa-gairika with cow's urine; the paste of purified maṇḍūra (or maṇḍura bhasma), chitraka, viḍanga, harītaki, trikaṭu and svarṇa-mäskshika with cow's urine and honey; the paste of vibhītaka, purified maṇḍura (or maṇḍura bhasma), nāgara, tila seeds and jaggery is made into small pills which can be taken with buttermilk; the powders of souvarchala salt, hingu and kirāta-tikta with tepid water, the powders of mūrva, haridra and āmalaki are soaked in cow's urine for seven days and then used; the paste of roots of balā and chitraka with tepid water or cow's urine; the fruits of śigru and rock salt can be taken with tepid water, a diet consisting of only milk; the cold decoction of drugs of nyagrodhādi group with sugar candy and honey; the power of āmalaki with honey; the drugs of sālaśrādi group with honey; etc., (SS).

2. The patient is subjected to emesis and purgation (with mild, bitter drugs) after oleation. The medicated unctuous preparations etc, can be used (for oleation).

The diet has to consist of old (red) rice, old barley, old wheat, soup or gruels of mudga, āḍhaki, meat juices of desert animals, etc. The decoction or infusion of drugs of the laghu-pancha mūla group is useful as a substitute for water.

The following formulations are useful in pāṇḍu: the (hot) infusion of fruits of kāśmari and fruits of danti with warm milk and cow's urine; the juice of drāksha; cow's or buffalo's urine and triphala with cow's urine, which is to be taken for a week; the fine powder of purified iron is triturated with cow's urine and is administered with milk for a week; the paste of purified iron powder, triphala, trikaṭu, viḍanga, bark of dārvi, honey and ghee; and arishṭa (alcoholic preparation) prepared from manjishṭha, haridrā, drāksha, root of balā, powder of purified iron and lodhra.

These yogas (formulations) have been recommended in pāṇḍu: dāḍimādya ghṛta, kaṭukādya ghṛta, pathyā ghṛta, dantī ghṛta, drāksah ghṛta, navāyasa chūrṇa, maṇḍūra vaṭaka, yogaraja, silā-jatu vaṭaka, dhātravayeha, dhātryarishṭa, punarnava maṇḍūra and bījakarishta,

In pittaja pāṇḍu, the powder of trivṛt is to be given with sugarcandy. In kaphaja pāṇḍu, the powder of harītaki is administered with cow's urine. In mṛt-bhakshaṇa pāṇḍu (i.e pāṇḍu caused by eating mud), the patient is subjected to purificatory procedures after considering the strength of the patient. The patient is then given ghṛta (ghee) medicated with strength-giving drugs. To create aversion to mud, ghee medicated with kesara, yashṭi-madhu, yava-kshāra, pippali and dūrva or with viḍanga, ela, ativisha, leaves of nimba, pāṭha, vārtāki, kaṭu-rohini, mūrva and kuṭaja is administered.

As a general rule, patients suffering from vātaja pāṇḍu, pittaja pāṇḍu and kaphaja pāṇḍu are administered unctuous preparations, cold and bitter drugs and pungent, bitter and hot drugs repectively, (CS).

3. In all cases of pāṇḍu, and its complications, pills prepared from purified iron, tāla, trikaṭu, and svarṇa-mākshika bhasma are beneficial

when administered with honey. The powder of purified maṇḍura is soaked in cow's urine, and is then administered with jaggery, in all cases of pāṇḍu. Ghee medicated with haridra or triphala, is also useful, (CSS).

4. Purified rasa-sindūra, tāmra bhasma, purified sulphur and purified vatsanābha (aconite) are triturated with a decoction of the juice of chitraka. The mass is then subjected to mild heat (for three-fourths of an hour) until all the water content evaporates. This mass is then powdered and administered in doses of 1/2 to 2 rathis in cases of pāṇḍu and swellings (oedema). The powder of the devadāli plant is administered with milk or water, daily for a month in cases of pāṇḍu. The paste of apāmārga, roots of sāmi and buttermilk is useful. Pārada bhasma can be administered with a decoction of triphala, (RRS).

Ref.: SS, Uttara, 44, 14-27; CS, chikitsā, 16, 40-123; CSS, pages 192-195; RRS, 19, 73, 91, 93; 30, 45.

Classical Prescriptions: Abhraka-bhasma; Aśoka-vaṭi; Ayaskṛti; Chandana-balā- lākshadi-taila; Chandraprabha-vaṭi; Chaturmukha-rasa; Dāḍimadi-ghṛta; Dantī-harītaki; Daśamūla-shaṭpala-ghṛta; Dhānvantara ghṛta; Dhātri-lauha; Drākshāvaleh; Dugdha-vaṭi; Elādi-ghṛta; Haratāla-bhasma; Hinguvādi-chūṛna; Hutabhugādi-chūrṇa; Kalyāṇaka-ghṛta; Kānta-vallabha-rasa; Kāsīsa-bhasma; Khadirārishṭa; Laghu-chinchādi-leha; Laghvānanda-rasa; Lohāsava; Lodhrāsava; Loha-bhasma; Loha-parpaṭi; Mahā-kalyāṇaka-ghṛta, Mahā-tiktaka-ghṛta; Maṇḍūra-bhasma; Loha-parpati; Maṇḍūra-bhasma; Maṇḍūra-vaṭaka; Mṛgānka-rāsa; Navaratna-rāja; Navāyasa-chūṛṇa; Pradarāntaka-lauha; Prāṇada-guṭika; Punarnavādi-maṇḍūra; Puṭa-pakva-vishama-jvarāntaka-rasa; Rajanyādi-chūṛna; Rasa-parpati; Śiva-guṭika; Śūla-vajrini-vaṭaka; Svarṇa-bhasma; Vāsa-chandanādi-taila; Vāsa-guḍūchyādi-kvātha-chūrṇa; Vāri-soshaṇa-rasa; Vidangādi-lauha.

Pittaja-pāṇḍu: Dhātryādi-ghṛta.

Pārada-vikārah

Western Nosology: Mercurial poisoning

Causative Factors:

Extrinsic: Intake of improperly purified mercury.

Symptomatology: The general symptoms are: pain, swelling and redness of gums, ulceration of mouth (gums), the gums become spongy, and bleed easily. The teeth become loose, there is excessive salivation, and the tongue become swollen, and fissured. The patient becomes emaciated, and suffers from gala-śuṇḍika (see mukharoga), etc., swelling of glands around the parotid region, jaw and throat, an unpleasant metallic taste in the mouth, fever, weakness, mental prostration, softening (kshāraṇa) of mandible, ulceration in the mouth, anaemia, disease of pitta and impure blood, etc. If mercury is continuously administered in large doses, it may prove fatal.

Constant inhalation of mercury causes tremors, especially in the arms and thighs, intense muscular weakness and disturbances in the sense faculties.

Acute symptoms of mercurial poisoning are swelling and pain in the stomach and intestines, vomiting, dysentery with bloody stools, syncope and death.

According to some authorities, the symptoms of mercurial poisoning are: sunken nose bridge, catarrh, falling out of teeth, headache, and fistula, visarpa (a skin disease), disease of mouth and eyes, koṭha (urticarial eruptions), itching and discolouration of skin, ulceration of nose, etc., skin diseases, symptoms of upadamśa, knotty and painful swellings, paralysis (pakshā-ghāta), rheumatism, burning pain of bones, lethargy and other mental disorders.

Ref.: BR, pārāda-vikāra, pages. 574.

Treatment:

1. If the patient suffers from eructation, he is to

partake of rice with curds, or black fish with jīraka. If there are symptoms of vāta-roga, the patient should be massged with nārāyaṇa-taila, etc. In cases of restlessness, cold water should be sprinkled on the head. In severe thirst, the patient is administered coconut water and gruel of mudga (green-gram) with sugar, (RRS).

2. The patient should be administered four ratti's of purified sulphur everyday. There is no medicine as effective as purified sulphur in antidoting the bad effects of mercury.

The decotion of triphala, kaṭuka, śatāvari, paṭola (leaves), gudūchi and parpata is also useful. The diet should be the same as that recommended in vāta-roga and kushṭa, (BR).

Ref.: RRS, 11,132-133; BR, pages, 575.

Paramada

Causative Factors:

Extrinsic: Abuse of alcoholic drinks.

Intrinsic: All three doshas.

Symptomatology: A feeling of heat and heaviness of the body, bad taste in the mouth, loss of taste, constipation, suppression of urine, excessive accumulation of phlegm (śleshma), thirst, headache and pain in the joints.

Related Diseases: Pānātyaya, Pānajīrṇa, Pānavibhrama.

Treatiment: A pānaka (refreshing drink) prepared from kāśmari, dāru (deva-dāru), biḍa salt, dāḍima, pippali and drāksha should be administered along with juice of bījapūraka. Pānaka prepared from drāksha, sugarcandy, yashṭi-madhu, jīraka, dhānyaka, pippali and trivṛt or from souvarchala salt, meat juices of desert animals and juice of sour fruits (such as dāḍima) can also be partaken of. The sprinkling of a decoction of bhārgni is also useful.

Also see treatment of pānātyaya, pānājirṇa and pāna-vibhrama.

Ref.: SS, uttara, 47, 19-20; 34-36.

Pārigarbhika

Synonyms: Paribhava

Causative Factors: This disease is seen in infants who are fed on the breast milk of pregnant women, (MN, CSS).

Symptomatology: The child suffers from cough, loss of appetite, weak digestion, vomiting, lethargy, emaciation, vertigo and enlarged abdomen.

Treatment:

1. The child is given food that is dīpana (which stimulates the apetite). Aśwagandhā-ghṛta is useful in this disease, (CD).

2. The ghee medicated with pippali, pippali-root, kaṭuki, devadāru, yava-kshāra, svarjika-kshāra, viḍanga, ajāji, bilva, chitraka, curd, souvīra and surā-maṇda is useful, (GN).

3. The ghee boiled with yava-kshāra, sarjika-kshāra, devadāru, śuṇṭhi, chitraka, pippali, granthika and tiktaka, souvīra, curd and surā is very effective in pārigarbhika, (CSS).

Ref.: MN,68, 101-1; CD, 64, 66; GN, bāla-roga, 11, 128-131; CSS, bāla-roga, 190-191; KBT,6.

Pariṇāma-śūla

Synonyms: Sanskrit: Pakti-śūla (Madhukośa)

Causes:

Extrinsic: Similar to those responsible for śūla.

Intrinsic: All three doshas, (MN). Predominantly pitta (Madhukośa).

Constituents Affected: Channels which carry rasa (nutrient fluid) (Madhukośa)

Symptomatology: The common symptom is pain in the abdomen during digestion of food, (MN).

According to some authorities, the pain is felt in the abdomen, stomach, sides of the chest, umbilical region, around the urinary bladder, and around the sternum. It may also be felt in the lower back. The pain subsides soon after eating or after eating rice, (Madhukośa).

If vāta is predominantly aggravated, the patient suffers from flatulent distension of abdomen, constipation, retention of urine, restlessness, tremors and amelioration by unctuous and hot substances.

If pitta is mainly vitiated, the paitent suffers from thirst, burning pain, restlessness, sweating, aggravation from food that is pungent, sour, and salty, and amelioration from cold.

If kapha is vitiated, the symptoms are vomiting, nausea, slight pain, chronicity (of complaints), syncope, and amelioration from pungent and bitter food, (MN).

Prognosis: If all the three doshas are vitiated, and if there is depletion of strength, muscular tissue and digestive power , the patient cannot be cured, (MN).

Related Diseases: Anna-drava-śūla, Śūla, Gulma.

Ref.: MN, 26, 15-20; Madhukośa on MN, ibid.

Treatment:

1. The measures beneficial in this disease are: emesis, purgation, intake of bitter and sweet drugs and enemas.

The following formulae are very useful: Semi-solid pills prepared from viḍanga, trikaṭu, trivṛt, dantī, chitraka, and jaggery, followed by hot water, milk boiled with jaggery, nāgara, and tila seed; śankha bhasma with hot water; the paste of triphala, pippali and honey; the gruel of kalāya with śaktu, which is to be taken for a week; the paste of triphala, loha bhasma, honey and ghee; the paste of jaggery, pippali harītaki, and loha bhasma; the paste of harītaki, purified manḍūra, nāgara, honey and ghee; a coconut full of water is filled with rock-salt and subjected to heat. The pulp is then administered; the paste of triphala, yashṭi-madhu, loha-bhasma, honey and ghee, followed by a glass of milk; ghee medicated with milk, jaggery and pippali; ghee medicated with pippali, taken with honey; and followed by milk; one prastha of cow's milk is boiled with 8 palas of purified manḍūra and 1/2 āḍhaka of cow's urine, this milk is very useful; paste of purified manḍūra or loha bhasma and jaggery; the decoction of triphala is boiled with loha bhasma. This can be taken with jaggery.

The pastes of tila, nāgara, harītaki, śambhuka bhasma and jaggery are triturated and made into boluses. These have to be taken in the morning with cold water. The diet has to consist of milk and meat-juices in the evening, (CD).

Ref.: CD, 27, 1-58.

Classical Prescriptions: Dāḍimadi-ghṛta; Kapardika-bhasma; Kumāryāsaya; Nārikela-lavana; Samudrādya-chūrṇa; Śankha-bhasma; Vaiśvānara-chūrṇa.

Partivartaka

Sanskrit: Nivṛtta-charma (AS, uttara, 38).

Causative Factors:

Extrinsic: Excessive handling of the organ, rubbing and pressing it, injury, etc.

Intrinsic: Vāta and kapha: Vyāna vata and kapha, (Bhoja, in NC).

Symptomatology: Due to the disturbance of the vāta, the prepuce retracts behind the glans penis, becomes contracted and swollen and hangs down like a knotty growth. It is painful, attended by burning pain, and in some cases gets inflamed.

In some patients, there is aggravation of kapha also and in these cases the prepuce becomes hard and there is itching, (but there is only slight pain, Bhoja in NC).

Related Diseases: Avapāṭika, Niruddha-prakāśa.

Treatment: The same treatement as in Avapāṭika.

Ref.: SS, nidāna, 13, 47-49; chikitsā, 20, 40-42.

Paschāttaka

Synonyms: Pascha-rujam(BR)

Causative Factors:

Intrinsic: The aggravated pitta.

Extrinsic: Drinking unhealthy breast milk.

Type: This disease occurs in infants.

Symptomatology: The rectum is the seat of an inflamed ulcer (vraṇa) that bears a resemblance to the belly of a leech (jalouka). The infant also suffers from high fever, cough, and yellowish stools, (greenish-yellow stools according to BR).

Treatment: Blood letting can be done by using leeches. The area should be washed with a warm decoction of the kshīri trees. The paste of mandhuraka is to be applied. The paste of chandana, the two types of śariva and śankha-nabhi can be applied locally and also administered internally with honey. The fine powder of asana flowers is also useful in this disease. Many other prescriptions are given in CSS.

Ref.: CSS, bāla-roga, 114-125; BR, bāla-roga, 76-79.

Pāshāṇa-gardabha

Causative Factors:

Extrinsic: Factors which aggravate kapha and vāta.

Intrinsic: Kapha and vāta

Symptomatology: A slightly painful, firm, swelling in the mandibular joint (hanu-sandhi).

Treatment: The swelling is to be fomented and plastered with the paste of manahśila, haratāla, kushṭha and devadāru. After it ripens, it is to be incised and treated as a vraṇa.

Ref.: SS, nidāna, 13, 13; chikitsā, 20, 5-6; AS, uttara, 36.

Phakka

Western Nosology: Rickets

Definition: A child is said to be suffering from phakka if it does not walk about even after it is one year old.

Types and Causative Factors:

1. If the child is breast fed on milk which has been vitiated by aggravated kapha.

2. If the mother has become pregnant and stops breast feeding, the child either suffers from this disease or expires.

3. Phakka may be caused by disease, usually grhaṇi.

Symptomatology: The child suffers from loss of strength, flesh and lustre, emaciation especially of arms, thighs and buttocks, swelling of the abdomen and face, yellowish discolouration of skin, horripilation, frequent urination and defaecation, weakness, especially of lower limbs, bad odour of body, excessive secretion of waste products of eyes, etc., and loud, rattling breathing. The child has an emaciated body, large head, crawls about on all fours, has long nails, is irritable and is infected with worms and insects.

Treatment: As the children suffering from phakka usually have an improperly functioning grahaṇi, they are unable to digest and assimilate food. Due to feeble digestive power, the stools are watery and diarrhoeic. Therefore, the main aim of treatment should be to improve digestion (stimulate the agni).

The child has to be administered kalyāṇaka ghṛta or shatpala ghṛta which act as elixirs in this disease. After seven days, the child is given the decoction of trivṛt and milk which acts as a laxative.

The child is also to be given milk medicated with punarnava, ekaparṇi, eraṇda, śatapatra, pīlu, drāksha and trivṛt. Along with this, the diet has to consist of boiled rice. These measures build up strength. The child is then to be massaged with oil medicated with the above mentioned drugs. The child can also be given rāsna ghṛta, rāsna taila, milk, gruel (yūsha), meat-juices, etc.

In phakka caused by intake of breast milk vitiated by kapha, the child should be given milk mixed with a small quantity of cow's urine.

An expert carpenter should be asked to prepare a three legged vehicle which the child can push and thus learn to walk.

If the child is also suffering from any vāta roga, it should be subjected to enema therapy, fomentation and udvartana (a kind of massage). It should be administered gruels, etc., mixed with ghee or oil.

Ref.: KS, phakka-chikkitsā.

Classical Prescriptions: Aravidāsava; Aśvagandhādi-lehya; Rasa-sindūra.

Phiranga-roga

A disease common in phiranga-deśa (Europe)

Synonyms: Sanskrit -Gandha-roga

Western Nosology: Syphilis

Causative Factors:

Extrinsic: Sexual intercourse with a person suffering from phiranga.

Type: This disease manifests in three forms: external, internal and both external and internal.

External phiranga: slightly painful, vesicular, eruptions which later suppurate.

Internal phiranga: Rheumatic pains in the joints followed by swelling (of joints). The symptoms are similar to those in āma-vāta.

The third type of phiranga is characterised by symptoms of both the external and internal varieties.

Complications: Emaciation, debility, depression of the nasal bridge, loss of appetite, asthi-śosha (necrosis of bone), bone deformities, etc.

Prognosis: The disease of recent onset and where there are no complications is easily curable. The external kind of phiranga is also easily curable while the internal kind is curable with difficulty.

The patient who suffers from symptoms of both exernal and internal phiranga, and in whom complications arise cannot be cured.

Ref.: BP; MN, 71.

Treatment:

1. The powder of chopachini is to be administered in a dosage of one śāna with honey. Salt has to be strictly avoided. If the patient cannot do without salt, however, rock salt can be used in small quantities. Drugs and food articles having sweet taste are beneficial.

Kajjalyādi-modaka: Equal quantities of purified mercury, purified sulphur and powder of khadira are triturated together well. Later, the powder of haridra, nāgakeśara, small variety of ela, the two kinds of jīraka, yavāni, chandana, pippali, vamśalochana, jāṭā-māmsi and teja-patra are added and the mixure is again triturated. Honey and ghee are added; and small pills are prepared. This is very useful in phiranga. This preparation does not cause any adverse effects either. However, salt should be avoided while taking this formulation.

According to some authorities (BR, pariśishṭa), the patient is first given a purgative. Later, he can be administered rasa-karpūra. The powders of āmalaki, harītaki and (leaves of) nimba are also useful.

Ref.: BR, pages. 573-574; 786-787.

Classcial Prescriptions: Rasa-karpūra, Svarṇa bhasma: Rasa-pushpa.

Plīhā-vṛddhi

Synonyms: Plīha

Western Nosology: Enlarged spleen

Causative Factors:

Extrinsic: Factors which vitiate vāta and blood.

Intrinsic: All three doshas.

Constituents Affected: Blood (CS, Ahṛ.)

Types: There are five types, namely plīha caused by vāta, pitta, kapha, all three doshas and vitiated blood (CS).

Pathogenesis and Symptomatology: The provoked vāta causes a gradually progressive enlargement of the spleen, (CS).

Complications: This disease, if left untreated, causes udara (ascites) which in turn leads to generalised dropsy (CS).

Ref.: CS, sūtra, 18, 28; 19, 3-4; 11, 49.; 28, 12; nidāna, 8, 18; Ahṛ, sūtra, 11, 8.

Treatement:

1. Buttermilk is particularly useful. (Ahṛ.)

2. The following prescriptions are efficacious the powders of detoxified vatsanābha, dravanti, madhūka, drāksha, rāsna, śaṭhi, and pippali; of detoxified vatsanābha, viḍanga, śatapushpa and yava-kshāra; or pārada bhasma triturated with cow's urine and laśuna, given with a decoction of drugs of the nyagrodhādi group or asanādi group. The vein at the back (lumber region?) can be opened, and later smeared with a paste of rock-salt and milky exudation of arka, (RRS).

3. The following prescriptions can be usefully employed for curing plīha; the powders of ajamoda, chitraka, yava-kshāra, root of pippali and danti, and pippali can be administered with hot water or an aśava; the decoction of śigru can be administered with the powders of rock-salt, pippali and maricha and juice of amlavetasa; the juice of ripe mango with honey; the decoction of śarngeshṭha can be given with rock salt and tintiḍika; the powders of equal quantities of pippali, śuṇṭhi and root of danti, of double the quantity of harītaki and one-fourth amount of bīda-lavana can be administered with hot water; the kshāra of flowers of tāla can be given with jaggery; the powder of pippali can be used after triturating it with palāśa-kshāra; the bhasma of śankha-nābhi can be administered with lemon-juice; or the decoction of harītaki and rohitaka-bark can be given with yava-kshāra and pippali, (BR).

Ref.: Ahṛ, sūtra, 5, 34; RRS, 29, 69; 30, 40; 18, 59; BR.

Classical Prescriptions: Dantī-harītaki; Dantyārishta; Dāḍimādi-ghṛta; Daśamūla-harītaki; Gandharva-hasta-taila; Jvarāryabhra; Kāsīsa-bhasma; Loha-bhasma; Maṇḍūra-bhasma; Maṇi-bhadra-yoga; Palāśa-kshāra; Pīlhāri-vaṭaka; Punarnavādi-maṇḍura; Puṭapakva-vishama-jvarāntaka-lauha; Rajata-bhasma; Rohitakārishṭa; Rohitaka-lauha; Śankha-bhasma; Sapta-rasa-kvātha-chūrṇa; Sarva-jvara-hara-lauha; Shatpala-ghṛta; Sudarśana-chūrṇa; Sukumāra-ghṛta; Sūraṇa-vaṭaka; Yakṛadāri-lauha; Yava-kshāra.

Chitraka-vaṭaja (BR); Arka-lavaṇa (BR); Kadalyādi-kshāra-taila (CSS); Pūitika-kshāra (CD).

Prameha

Synonyms: Sanskrit: Meha, Mūtra-dosha (RN, 20,19)

Western Nosology: Urinary disorders including diabetes.

Causative Factors:

Extrinsic:

1. Pandering to the pleasures of the palate, comfort in sleep, (excessive) intake of curds, milk, new rice, dishes prepared from jaggery and meat of aquatic and domesticated animals and all factors which aggravate kapha, (CS, chikitsā, 6, 4).

Absence of mental exertion is also responsible for provoking prameha, (CS, Sūtra, 17, 79).

The frequent and excessive intake of new (fresh) grains such as hayānaka, yava (barley), chīnāka, uddālaka, etc., gruels prepared form ghee and new hareṇu and māsha, meat of aquatic and domesticated animals, excessive intake of tila, leafy vegetables, flour, pāyasa, kṛśara, vilepi and products of sugarcane juice, milk, new wine, manḍaka (immature curds), curds, and sweet and liquid food, lack of exercise, infrequent bathing, indolence, excessive sleep, and other factors which aggravate kapha and meadas and engender polyuria; those are responsible for kaphaja prameha.

The excessive intake of hot, sour, salty, alkaline (kshāra), incompatible, pungent, and sharp food, over-exposure to sun, and fire, fatigue, and anger; these factors engender pittaja prameha.

Excessive intake of astringent, pungent, bitter, dry, cold food, and food easy to digest, suppression of natural urges, over-use of purgatives, emetics, errhines and enemata (āsthāpana), excessive indulgence in sex, too much exercise, frequent fasting, trauma, over-exposure to sun, severe loss of blood, grief, loss of sleep, and irregular posture; these are responsible for bringing about vātaja prameha, (CS, nidāna, 4, 5, 24, 36).

People who are lethargic, obese and gluttons are prone to develop prameha, (CS, nidāna, 4, 51).

2. Those persons are prone to develop prameha who are accustomed to sweet, cold, oily, liquid and fattening food, sleeping during daytime, lack of exercise and an indolent life style, (SS, nidāna, 6, 3).

Intrinsic: All three doshas are involved in the disease (CS, nidāna, 4, 3; SS, nidāna, 6, 7).

Constituents Affected: The fatty, fleshy, watery and reproductive tissues, blood, bone-marrow, lymph, resistance to disease (ojas) and the nutrient fluid that circulates throughout the body, (CS, nidāna, 4, 7; chikitsā, 6, 8).

The fatty tissues are mainly affected. However, blood is also affected in pittaja prameha and bone-marrow in vātaja prameha, (SS, nidāna, 6, 4, 9).

Pathogenesis: The mere presence of the causative factors is not sufficient to engender prameha. The presence or absence of immunity to disease depends on the relation between the aetiology, the doshas concerned and the constituents affected. If these three factors are disimilar or only slightly similar, the disease will either be unmanifest or will manifest itself slowly or in a mild form. If the three factors (the aetiology, dosha and constituents affected) are very similar, the disease will be manifested quickly and with all symptoms, (CS, nidāna, 4, 4).

Classification: There are twenty kinds of prameha, ten of which are predominantly caused by kapha, six by pitta and four by vāta, (SS, CS, AHṛ).

Prodromal Symptoms:

1. Matting of hair, sweet taste in the mouth, burning and numbness of palms and soles, dryness of mouth, palate and throat, thirst, apathy, excessive formation of waste in the body and orifices (such as eyes, nose, etc.), numbness and burning of the limbs, attraction of insects to the urine, excessive sleep, abnormalities of urine, foul smell of the body, a continuous feeling of lethargy and drowsiness, perspiration, debility, desire for ease, luxury and sleep, rapid growth of hair and nails, and craving for cold (substances).

(CS, nidāna, 4, 47; chikitsā, 6,14).

2. Burning of palms and soles, heaviness, sliminess and oilyness of the body, sweet taste and whiteness of urine, drowsiness and lethargy, debility, thirst, bad breath, coating (of slime or mucus) of palate, throat, tongue and teeth, rapid growth of nails and matting of hair, (SS, nidāna, 6, 5).

Symptomatology: General and characteristic symptoms: Profuse urination and turbidity of urine, (SS, nidāna, 6, 6).

Symptoms of kaphaha prameha:

I.

1. Udaka-meha: the urine is watery, clear, profuse, whitish, cold and devoid of smell.

2. Ikshu-vālika-rasa-meha: the urine resembles sugarcane juice, is extremely sweet, cold, turbid and slightly slimy.

3. Sāndra-meha: the urine becomes thick and dense when kept overnight in a vessel.

4. Sāndra-prasāda-meha: the urine when kept overnight is dense below and clear near the surface.

5. Śukla-meha: frequent urination, the urine being white in colour, resembling flour.

6. Śukra-meha: frequent urination, the urine resembles or is actually mixed with semen.

7. Śita-meha: the urine is copious, cold and extremely sweet.

8. Sikatā-meha: the urine contains small hard gravel.

9. Śannair-meha: dribbling of urine with very little force.

10. Ālāla-meha: the urine is slimy and appers full of threads, (CS, nidāna, 4, 12-23; chikitsā, 6, 9).

II.

1. Udaka-meha: the urine is white and resembles water. Urination is painless.

2. Ikshu-vālikā-meha: the urine resembles sugarcane-juice.

3. Surā-meha: the urine resembles surā (wine).

4. Sikatā-meha: the urine is mixed with gravel, and urination is painful.

5. Śanair-meha: the urine is slimy, mixed with mucous and is emitted slowly (without force).

6. Lavaṇa-meha: the urine resembles salt-water and is clear (non-slimy).

7. Pishṭa-meha: the urine resembles water mixed with flour, the patient also suffers from horripilation.

8. Sāndra-meha: the urine is thick and (externally) dirty (turbid).

9. Śukra-meha: the urine resembles semen.

10. Phena-meha: the urine is clear, frothy and is emitted in small quantities, frequently, (SS, nidāna, 6, 10).

AHṛ mentions the same symptoms and classification as described in CS and SS, with a few differences:

1. Surā-meha: the urine resembles surā, is dense below and clear towards the surface.

2. Pishṭa-meha: the urine is thick like flour; the patient also suffers from horripilation. (AHr, nidāna, 10,8-13).

Symptoms of pittaja prameha:

I.

1. Kshāra-meha: the urine resembles kshāra (alkalies) in smell, appearance, taste and touch.

2. Kāla-meha: the urine is hot, profuse and black in colour.

3. Nīla-meha: the urine is sour and blue like the feathers of the chāshā bird.

4. Rakta-meha: the urine is salty, hot, bloody

and has an odour like that of raw flesh.

5. Manjishṭha-meha: the urine has the colour of the decoction (or juice) of manjishṭha and has a strong smell of raw flesh.

6. Haridrā-meha: the urine is pungent and has the colour of the decoction of haridra (turmeric).

(CS, nidāna, 4, 28-35; chikitsā, 6, 10)

II

1. Nīla-meha: the urine is clear, frothy and blue in colour.

2. Haridra-meha: the urine resembles (the decoction of) haridra (turmeric); the patient also suffers from burning micturition.

3. Amla-meha: the urine is sour in smell and taste.

4. Kshāra-meha: the urine resembles a filtered alkaline solution.

5. Manjishṭha-meha: the urine is coloured (red) like the decoction of manjishṭha.

6. Śonita-meha: the urine is similar to blood.

(SS, nidāna, 6, 11).

Symptoms of vātaja prameha:

1. Vasā-meha: the urine either resembles vasā (muscle fat) or is mixed with it.

2. Majjā-meha: the urine is mixed with marrow.

3. Hasti-meha: the patient passes large quantities of urine like an elephant in rut. The urine is mixed with lymph, (lasīka).

4. Madhu-meha: the urine is astringent, sweet, dry and pale-white in colour. The urine is mixed with ojas (the factors responsible for strength or resistance to disease).

(CS, nidāna, 4, 37-45; chikitsā, 6, 11).

1. Sarpir-meha: the urine has the appearance of (cow's) ghee.

2. Vasā-meha: the urine resembles vasā (muscle fat).

3. Madhu-meha: the urine has the taste and appearance of honey.

4. Hasti-meha: the urine flows continuously like that of an elephant in rut. (SS, nidāna, 6, 12).

Sarpir-meha is the same disease named in CS as majjameha, while hasti-meha is synonymous with lasika-meha, (NC on SS, ibid).

Complications:

1. Thirst, diarrhoea, fever, burning pains, debility, tastelessness, indigestion, and formation of carbuncles and abscesses, (CS, nidāna, 4, 48).

2. The complication in kaphaja prameha are: Attraction of flies (to the urine, body, etc,), an inordinate love of pleasure, aversion to discomfort, disinclination to work without any debility; increase in muscular (fleshy) growth; catarrh, debility, loss of taste, indigestion, salivation, vomiting, sleepiness, cough and dyspnoea.

The complications in pittaja prameha are: Cracks of the scrotum (or tearing pain in the testicles), breaking pain in the urinary bladder, pricking pain in the penis, chest pain, pyrosis (sour eructations, NiS), fever, diarrhoea, tastelessness, vomiting, feeling of heat all over the body, burning pains, unconsciousness, thirst, loss of sleep, the disease pāṇḍu (anaemia), and yellow discolouration of stools, urine and eyes.

The complications in vātaja prameha: Oppression (tightness) of the chest, ravenous appetite, sleeplessness, stiffness of the body, tremor, piercing pain and constipation. (SS, nidāna, 6, 13; śārīra, 4, 52)

AHṛ mentions a few complication in vātaja prameha (not mentioned in CS and SS): udāvarta, dryness (of mouth, palate, and throat), cough and dyspnoea, (AHṛ, nidāna, 10, 24).

Prognosis:

1. The ten kaphaja prameha are curable, because both kapha and medas, etc., are alleviated by the same line of treatment. The six pittaja prameha are yāpya (i.e. they can be palliated, although the treatment has to be continued for the rest of their lives) because the treatment for the vitiated pitta usually aggravates the medas (fatty tissues). The four vātaja pramehas are considered to be incurable because of its deep-seated nature (the involvement of the marrow, of the ojas, etc.,) and the contradiction in treatment, (SS, nidāna, 4, 11, 27, 38).

Pramehas, especially madhu-meha, which are congenital and hereditary are to be considered as being incurable if (all) the prodromal signs and symptoms are severe (intense). However, kaphaja, and pittaja pramehas which through neglect change into vātaja pramehas are not incurable. Similarly, pittaja prameha are curable if the fatty tissues are not excessively vitiated, (CS, chikitsā, 6, 56, 57).

2. A patient suffering from madhu-meha who develops carbuncles and abscesses with all its complications is incurable. All pramehas, if neglected, develop into madhu-meha which is incurable, (SS, nidāna, 6, 24, 27).

Note: According to CS, prameha is a disease that is most given to relapses, (CS, sūtra, 25, 40).

Treatment:

1. Patients suffering from prameha are of two types, the strong and obese, and weak and emaciated.

The emaciated patient is to be given nourishing therapy (bṛmhaṇa) while strong patients can be administered elimination therapy (śodhana). The patient is first to be administered oily preparations to cause purgation and emesis, after which he would requires nourishing treatment. Nourishing treatment has to be administered only after due consideration of the power of digestion, while (improper) eliminative or reducing therapy (apatarpaṇa) engenders abdominal tumours, emaciation, retention of urine, and pain in the penis and urinary blader.

The patient who is too weak to undergo eliminative therapy (śodhana) is advised to partake of the following diet: food easy to digest, preparations of barley, meat-juices of birds of the vishkira and pratuda types and animals of desert areas which are liked by the patient, dry vāṭya, mantha, apūpa with śakthu (barley-meal), gruels (yūsha) of mudga, etc., old rice, āmalaki, bitter vegetables, food prepared with oil of danti, ingudi, atasi and sarshapa; shashṭika rice (which grows in 60 days), and tṛna-dhānya.

Barley which has been soaked overnight in a decoction of triphala is to be administered with honey and sīdhu (a kind of alcoholic drink). Preparations of wheat and bamboo seeds are useful. A decoction of dāru-haridra, devadāru, triphala and mustā or paste of haridra with honey and juice of āmalaki are very useful in prameha.

Eliminative procedures (śodhana), including weight loss and fasting are of unquestioned benefit in kaphaja prameha, while purgation, nourishing treatment (santarpaṇa) and palliation (samśamana) are useful in pittaja prameha.

Decoctions of the following drugs are beneficial in kaphaja prameha when administered with (old) honey: harītaki, kaṭphala, mustā and lodhra; pāṭha, viḍanga, arjuna and dhanvana; haridhra, dāru-haridrā, tagara and viḍanga; kadamba, śāla, arjuna and dīpyaka; dāru-haridrā, viḍanga, khadira, and dhava; dāru-haridra, agnimantha, triphala and pāṭha; pāṭha, mūrva, and gokshura; yavāni, uśīra, harītaki and guḍūchi; chavya, harītaki, chitraka and sapta-parṇa.

The decoctions of these drugs are to be administered with honey in pittaja prameha: uśīra, lodhra, anjana and chandana; uśīra, mustā, harītaki, padmaka and vṛkshaka;

nimba, aruṇa, āmrātaka, harida and utpala; śirīsha, sarja, arjuna and nāga-keśara; priyangu, padma, utpala, and palāśa; asvattha, pāṭha, asana and vetasa or dāru-haridra, utpala and musta.

These drugs can be used in all types of prameha, in the form of mantha with barley or mixed with food. Oils or ghee medicated with these drugs can be used even in vātaja prameha.

The paste of kampillaka, sapta-parṇa, flowers of śāla; and vibhītaka, rohitaka, kuṭaja and flowers of kapittha are to be powdered and administered with honey in kaphaja pittaja prameha.

The paste of the above drugs with the juice of āmalaki can be partaken of at lunch time followed after its digestion by old rice, and meat-juices of desert animals.

Patients suffering from kaphaja prameha with involvement of vāta can be administered oil medicated with drugs indicated in kaphaja prameha, while those suffering from pittaja prameha with the involvement of vāta are to be administered ghee medicated with drugs useful in pittaja prameha.

The decoction of haridra, dāru-haridra, triphala, viśāla and musta can be administered with honey in all cases of prameha.

Persons who are accustomed to regular and varied exercise, vigorous massages, regular baths and application of uśīra, tvak, ela, agaru and chandana will not suffer from prameha, (CS, chikitsā, 6, 15-50).

2. There are two types of prameha, those that are hereditary and those that result from improper food and habits, The patients suffering from the former type will usually be emaciated and active, with a dry skin, poor appetite and excessive thirst.

Those of the latter type are often obese, with an oily skin, voracious appetite and are fond of sleep, sloth and comfort.

Patients of prameha who are emaciated should be given nourishing food and drinks while measures to induces weight loss (such as fasting, eliminative therapy, exercise and intake of bitter substances) are indicated in those who are obese.

The patient (who is obese and strong) should first be anointed with oils (of nikumbha, sarshapa, atasi, etc.,) or with ghee (in cases of pittaja prameha) medicated with priyangu, etc. The patient of kaphaja prameha should then be administered emetics, while purgation is induced in the patient suffering from pittaja prameha. On the eighth day after purgation, the patient is administered āsthāpana enemata with a decoction of drugs of surāsadi group with nāgara, bhadra-dāru, musta, rock salt and honey. If the patient complains of burning pains, an āsthāpana enemata of drugs of the nyagrodhādi group with a little amount of ghee will be found useful.

After the system has been cleansed, the patient can be administered: (a) juice of āmalaki (4 palās, NiS), with haridra (1 karsha, ibid) and honey (1 karsha, ibid) or (b) a decoction of triphala, viśāla, devadāru and musta (with sixteen parts of water, reduced to one-fourth, NiS), (c) paste of one aksha (2 tola) weight of śāla, kampillaha, and mushkaka with honey and juice of āmalaki; and (d) paste of flowers of kuṭaja, kapittha, rohitaka, vibhītaka and sapta-parṇa (with honey and juice of āmalaki, NiS).

The patient is advised to strictly avoid the intake of: souvīraka, tushodaka, śukta, maireya, surā and āsava (which are alcoholic preparations); water, milk, oil, ghee, sugarcane and its products, curds, sweet dishes, sour food, pānaka, gruel (yāvagu) and meat of aquatic and domesticated animals.

These food articles are beneficial in prameha: rice, shashṭika rice, barley, wheat, kodrava, and uddālaka which are all old, dishes prepared from chaṇaka, āḍhaki, kulattha and mudga, leafy vegetables of bitter and astringent taste cooked with oil of nikumbha, ingudi, sarshapa and atasi, and lean meat of desert animals (jāngala) which have anti-diuretic properties, cooked without ghee or sour substances.

Āsavas, arishaṭa, ayaskṛti and lehyas prepared with priyangu, ananta (utpala-sāriva), yūthika, bhārngi, madayantika, manjishṭha, ambashṭha (pāṭha or māchika), bark of dāḍima, śāla-parṇi (or mushali), padma, punnāga, nāga-kesara, dhātaki, bakula, śalmali, śrīveshṭaka (resin of sarala) and mocha-rasa (exudation of śālmali), or with śrngāṭaka, gilodya, bisa-mṛnāla, kaseruka, madhuka, āmra, jambu, asana (bījaka), tiniśa, arjuna, kaṭvanga, lodhra, bhallātaka, palāśa, charma-vṛksha, giri-karnika, śīta-śiva, jala-vetasa, dāḍima, aja-karṇa, indra-vṛksha, rājādāna, gopaghonṭa and vikankata are to be administered. Gruels (yāvagu) or decoctions of the above drugs can also be administered.

Rich patients accustomed to unhealthy food habits and who are averse to taking medicines can be given the aforesaid āsavas thickened with powdered pāṭha, harītaki and chitraka, with liberal amount of honey and food mixed with honey, maricha and kapittha.

Patients suffering from advanced prameha are advised regular physical exercise, wrestling, active sports, riding on horses or elephants, long walks, archery, casting of javelins, etc.

Poor and friendless patients should abandon the use of shoes or slippers and umbrellas, and should live on alms, walking about a hundred yojanas (about 800 miles) or more, without staying for more than one night at a village.

There are some specific treatments for the various kinds of prameha:

(a) Udaka-meha-decoction of pārijāta (pāribhadra, NiS).

(b) Ikshu-meha - decoction of vaijayanti (aranika, NiS).

(c) Surā-meha - decoction of nimba.

(d) Sikatā-meha - decoction of chitraka.

(e) Śanair-meha - decoction of khadira.

(f) Lavaṇa-meha - decoction of pāṭha, agaru and haridra.

(g) Pishṭa-meha - decoction of haridra and dāru-haridra.

(h) Sāndra-meha - decoction of sapta-parṇa.

(i) Śukra-meha - decoction of dūrva, śaivala, plava (gopala-damanaka, or jala-kumbhika, NiS), karanja and kaseruka, or decoction of kakubha and chandana.

(j) Phena-meha - decoction of triphala, āragvadha and mṛdvika, with honey.

(k) Nīla-meha - decoction of triphala, āragvadha, and mṛdvika, with honey.

(l) Nīla-meha - decoction of drugs of sālasārādi group or asvattha.

(m) Haridra-meha - decoction of rāja-vṛksha (kirāmalaka, NiS).

(n) Amla-meha - decoction of drugs of nyagrodhādi group.

(o) Kshāra-meha - decoction of triphala.

(p) Manjishṭha-meha - decoction of manjishṭha and chandana.

(q) Rakta-meha - decoction of guḍūchi, tinduka-asthi kāśmari and kharjūra, with honey.

Even incurable cases can be palliated by the following drugs:

(a) Sarpir-meha - the paste of kushṭa, kuṭaja, pāṭha, hingu and kaṭu-rohini is taken with the decoction of guḍūchi and chitraka.

(b) Vasā-meha - decocotion of agnimantha or simśipa.

(c) Madhu-meha - decoction of khadara and kramuka (pūga-phala, NiS). Śilajatu is extremely efficacious in this disease, (SS, chikitsā, 13).

(d) Hasti-meha - decoction of tinḍuka, kapittha, sirīsha, palāśa, pāṭha, mūrva and dussparsa (durālabha, NiS) with honey.

Note:

1. A person who has the prodromal signs and symptoms of prameha and who passes slightly larger amounts of urine than usual, is considered as being affected with the disease.

2. A person with polyuria, who has only some of the prodromal signs and symptoms is also considered as suffering from the full-fledged disease.

3. A patient of prameha is considered to be cured when the urine is non-slimy, non-turbid, dry and possessed of a bitter and pungent taste (i.e. when it does not attract ants or insects, NiS). (SS, chikitsā, 11; 12, 20; nidāna, 6, 22-23)

3. The decoction of dāru-haridra, devedāru, triphala and musta; or the juice of guḍūchi or juice of āmalaki is administered with honey in prameha.

The well prepared śaktu of yava (barley) which is soaked overnight in a decoction of triphala and dried is administered with honey and sīdhu (an alcoholic preparation). Keeping awake during nights is beneficial in kaphaja prameha. (AHṛ, chikitsā, 12, 6, 15, 33)

4. Equal quantities of rasa-sindūra (rasa-bhasma) and vanga bhasma are administered with honey in vātaja prameha. The diet has to consist of yūsha (gruel) of mudga and āmalaka, and buttermilk. The paste or oil-cake of tila is administered with buttermilk and a very slight amount of hingu. It is better to partake of oil with food, rather than ghee.

The powder of mārkaṇḍi can be partaken of at night with jaggery.

Equal parts of tāmra bhasma and śuddha parada are made into a paste, which is immersed in a decoction or juice of gokshura for 14 days. Later, the paste is kept within a lemon, and boiled for one day (24 hours) with kānjika (in a dolā yantra). A small quantity of this paste is kept within a lemon and a patient suffering from prameha has to place the lemon in his mouth at night and keep on sucking it.

The regular use of vanga bhasṃa with honey is useful in rakta-meha, with the powder of haridra, in śukra-meha, and with tamala, powder of arjuna (bark) and sugar, in madhu-meha. The root juice of śālmali with honey is useful in prameha (as an anupāna). The decoction of the root of śleshmātaka can be administered with ghee at bed-time (night) in rakta-meha. The juice of kūshmāṇda with viḍanga and sugar-candy is useful in rakta-meha, (RRS, 17, 28-39).

5. The powder of triphala or śilājatu or loha (bhasma) or harītaki are to be administered with honey. The decoction of dāru-haridra, yashṭimadhu, triphala and chitraka is also useful in prameha. Śilājatu is useful in prameha, especially in madhu-meha, (CSS, pages. 477, 482).

Classical Prescritptions: Abhraka-bhasma; Āragvadhādi- kvātha-chūrṇa/ Ayaskrti; Chandanādi-chūrṇa; Chandraprabhā-vaṭi; Chatur-mukha-rasa; Devadārvārishṭa; Dhānvantara-ghṛta; Gokshurādi-guggulu; Grahaṇi-mihira-taila; Guḍuchyādi-modaka; Kumāryāsava; Lakshmi-vilāsa-rasa; Loha-bhasma; Madhūkāsava; Mahā-yogaraja-guggulu; Maṇḍura-vaṭaka; Nāga-bhasma; Nāga-vallabha-rasa; Nyagrodhādi-chūrṇa; Prameha-mihira taila; Rajata-bhasma; Sārivādyāsava; Sūraṇa-vaṭaka; Svarṇa-mākshika-bhasma; Svarṇa-vanga; Traikaṇṭaka-ghṛta; Triphala-chūrna; Trivanga-bhasma; Vajra-bhasma; Vanga-bhasma; Vastyāmayāntaka-ghṛta; Yaśada-bhasma; Yogendra-rasa.

Prameha-piḍaka: Dhānvantara-ghṛta; Kaiśora-guggulu; Madhu-snuhī-rasāyana; Navāyasa-chūrṇa; Nyogrodhādi-chūrṇa.

Pratyashṭhila

Western Nosology: Enlarged prostate.

Causative Factors:

Extrinsic: Factors which aggravate vāta.

Intrinsic: Vāta

Symptomatology: A growth similar in shape to that found in ashṭhīla, but which is found in a lateral position (i.e. across the abdomen) and which is painful and obstructs the passage of flatus, urine and faeces is known as prayashṭhīla.

Treatment: The treatment that has been described under gulma and abhyantara-vidradhi should be employed here.

Related Diseases: Ashṭhīla

Ref.: SS, nidāna, 1, 99; chikitsā, 5, 27.

Pratitūnī

Western Nosology: Pain in the anus.

Causative Factors:

Extrinsic: Factors which aggravate vāta.

Intrinsic: Vāta

Symptomatology: Spasmodic splitting pain in the rectal and genital regions which ascend to the intestines (pakvāśaya).

Related Diseases: Tūni

Treatment: The patient is administered hot water with rock salt and unctuous substances (oil, ghee, etc.,) or with powders of drugs of the pippalyādi group, or ghee with hingu and yava-kshāra. The patient can also be subjected to enemata.

Ref.: SS, nidāna, 1, 87; chiktsā, 5, 25.

Pratyādhamāna

Western Nosology: Flatulent gastritis.

Causative Factors:

Extrinsic: See Ādhmāna

Instrinsic: Kapha and vāta

Symptomatology: Flatulent distension of the epigastric region (region of āmāśaya), but without pain in the sides and chest.

Prognosis: Easily curable.

Treatment: The patient is to be administered emesis, and appetizing (dīpana) drugs. He is also advised to fast or subsist on food that is easy to digest.

Related Diseases: Ādhmāna

Ref.: SS, nidāna, 1, 89; chikitsā, 5, 26.

Rāja-yakshma

Synonyms: Sanskrit-Sosha, Kshaya (SS), Roga-rāṭ (AS).

Western Nosology: Consumption, Tuberculosis.

Causative Factors:

Extrinsic:

1. The four main causative factors are excessive exertion, suppression of natural urges, emaciation and improper food.

Under excessive exertion is included activities such as excessive talking, wrestling with a stronger person, carrying heavy loads, swimming for long distances, excessive studying, fasting for many days, injuries etc.

Emaciation may be caused by prolonged grief or anxiety, jealousy, anger, fear, etc., eating too less or eating only dry foods, fasting, excessive sexual intercourse, etc.

By improper food is meant the (regular) intake of food that is incompatible to the person, too less or too much in quantity, which is not prepared properly, which the patient is not accustomed to, etc., and non-observance of the rules for selecting and partaking of food, (CS).

2. The causes are emaciation of body tissues, suppression of the natural urges, trauma in any form and improper food intake, (SS).

Intrinsic: All three doshas, especially kapha, (SS). All three doshas, (CS).

Constituents Affected:

Pathogenesis:

1. If the patient suppresses the urges, due to fear, timidity, shyness, urgent work, etc., the vāta is disturbed and along with the kapha and pitta exerts a harmful influence all over the body, leading to rāja-yakshma.

If the person experiences emaciation of the body tissues, there occurs a diminution in the rasa-dhātu which is present in the heart and aggravation of vāta. This eventually leads to rāja-yakshma. If on the other hand, the person indulges in excessive sexual intercourse, the vāta is disturbed, and exerts an inimical effect on the blood, and on the other two doshas, causing this disease.

By regularly partaking of improper food, the doshas get vitiated, and disturb the body elements (dhātus). These obstruct the body channels, engendering rāja-yakshma. The vitiated doshas may also cause the transformation of food into waste products such as stools, etc., instead of building up the body tissues. This may again cause this disease, (CS).

2. The doshas, particularly kapha get provoked, and obstructing the body channels pave the way to rāja-yaksham, (SS).

Prodormal Symptoms:

1. Catarrh, constant sneezing, hawking of mucus, sweet taste in the mouth, loss of appetite, fatigue at meal times, nausea after eating, regurgitation of food, swelling of the feet and face, paleness of eyes, unusual desire for sex, debility, craving for meat and alcohol, rapid growth of nails and hair, a feeling as if the body is loathsome, increase of fastidiousness to the extent of unjustified criticism in matters regarding food, gazing intently at the hands for long stretches of time, a feeling of disgust, and dreams of dry lakes and ponds, deserted towns and villages, wasted and burnt gardens, of riding on dogs, camels, donkeys, etc., of climbing on heaps of ash, bones, coal, etc., of being touched by snakes, parrots, etc., (CS).

2. Difficulty in breathing, weakness, hawking of mucus, dryness of the palate, vomiting, feeble digestion, catarrh, anaemia (pāṇḍu), sleepiness, paleness of eyes, craving for meat, and dreams of parched rivers, dried up trees, of being borne aloft on a crow, parrot, eagle, etc., and of gales of wind or fire destroying trees, etc., (SS).

3. The patient also feels as if his head is (tightly) wrapped in a piece of cloth, (AS).

Symptomatology:

1. There are three prominent symptoms, viz. pain in shoulders and sides of the chest, burning of hands and feet and fever.

There may also be eleven prominent symptoms, namely, heaviness of the head, cough, dyspnoea, hoarseness, hawking of mucus, vomiting of blood, pain in the sides of the chest, pain in the shoulders, fever, diarrhoea and anorexia.

In the disease caused by over exertion, the patient suffers from yawning, body pain, fever, anorexia, hoarseness, catarrh, dyspnoea, headache, heaviness of the head, and cough which leads to spitting of blood and weakness.

In the disease engendered by suppression of the natural urges, the symptoms are body pain, diarrhoea, dry stools, pain in the sides of the chest, pain in the shoulders, vomiting, headache, cough, dyspnoea, fever, hoarseness, catarrh, anorexia and emaciation.

In rāja-yakshma brought on by emaciation or depletion, the symptoms are weakness of joints, dryness (of skin, etc.,), weakness, wasting of muscles, pain in the sides of the chest, pain in the shoulders, irritation in the throat, congestion in the head, body pain, indigestion, fever, dyspnoea, hoarseness, catarrh and cough which causes urah-kshata (chest injury) leading to spitting of blood and weakness and emaciation.

In rāja-yakshma caused by improper food, the aggravated vāta causes body pain, sharp pain (in any part of the body), irritation in the throat, pain in the sides of the chest, pain in shoulders, hoarseness and catarrh. The vitiated pitta brings about fever, diarrhoea and a feeling of internal heat. The deranged kapha causes catarrh, heaviness of the head, anorexia, salivation, vomiting and cough. Constant cough causes chest injury, leading to spitting of blood and weakness, (CS).

2. If the doshas are moderately provoked, there are six prominent symptoms: Aversion to food, fever, dyspnoea, cough, spitting of blood, and hoarseness.

If the doshas are severely provoked, eleven symptoms are manifested: Hoarseness, sharp pain and pain as of dislocation in the shoulders and sides of the chest (these are caused by vāta); fever, burning pain, diarrhoea and spitting of blood (these are caused by deranged pitta); feeling of congestion in the head, loss of appetite, cough and a sensation of a lump in the throat (these are caused by vitiated kapha), (SS).

3. According to Bhoja, the three most prominent symptoms are cough, fever and haemorrhage, (Madhu-kośa on MN).

4. The main symptoms of rāja-yakshma are feeble digestion, fever, chilliness (lack of vital heat), vomiting of pus and blood, and mental and physical prostration, (RRṢ).

Prognosis: A person who has strength and vitality and in whom there is no depletion of muscular tissue and blood, is curable even if he suffers from all the symptoms of rāja-yakshma, provided there are no arishṭa-lakshaṇas (signs of imminent death). On the other hand, a person who has feeble vitality, and suffers from depletion of strength, muscular tissue and blood is incurable even if he presents only a few symptoms and even if there are no arishṭa-lakshaṇas, (CS, SS).

Note: CS explains in some detail about the various symptoms that are characteristic in rāja-yakshma:

1. Pratiśyāya (catarrh): It is severe, causes emaciation of the body, and is accompanied by headache, heaviness of the body, loss of sensation of smell, fever, cough, hawking of mucus, hoarseness, anorexia, fatigue even without exertion and weakness of sense-faculties.

2. Kāsa (cough): The patient expectorates sputum that is slimy, thick, foul-smelling, yellowish, or pale yellow, etc.

3. Jvara (fever): The fever is accompanied by symptoms like burning of hands, feet, shoulder and sides of the chest.

4. Svara-bheda (hoarseness): There may also be cough and pīnasa (catarrh). If vāta is aggravated, the voice is dry, low, and unsteady; if pitta is deranged, the patient does not speak much, and suffers from burning of palate and throat; if kapha is deranged, the voice is halting and rattling; if blood is vitiated, the patient finds it difficult to speak; if there is also cough, the patient finds it difficult to speak. If there is pīnasa, there are symptoms of aggravated kapha and vāta.

5. Pārśva-sula (pain in the sides of the chest): There is spasmodic feeling of contraction (pressing) and relaxation.

6. Headache: There is a feeling of heaviness and heat in the head.

7. Atisāra (diarrhoea): The stools are slimy.

8. Aruchi (anorexia): The taste may be astringent, bitter or sweet if vāta, pitta and kapha are aggravated, respectively, (CS).

Related Diseases: Dhātu-kshya

Ref.: CS, nidāna, 6; chikitsā, 8, 13-62; SS,

uttara, 41, 3-30; MN, 8; RRS, 14, 1.

Treatment:

I. If the doshas are excessively provoked, the patient is given oleation and fomentation and subjected to mild emesis and purgation. When a person is debilitated, the only thing that sustains him is slightly costive bowels. Diarrhoea in a weak patient of rāja-yakshma proves fatal.

If the patient suffers from depletion of muscular tissues, he should be administered nourishing meat-juices or soups prepared from carnivorous animals, and animals such as barhi, gṛdhra (eagle), ulūka (owl), chāsha, kāka (crow), tittira, varmi, gaṇḍūpada, lopaka, sthūla-nakula, biḍāla (cat), sṛgāla (jackal), sava, śaśa (rabbit), simha (lion), ṛksha, vyāghra, tarakshu, etc. The recipe known as vesavāra prepared from elephant, khangi, turanga, etc., is also useful. Parts covered with flesh are useful in building up muscular tissue.

Meat which is sharp, hot and light is especially useful. The meat of cow, camel, ass, buffalo, swan is also very beneficial. A patient with symptoms of vāta should partake of meat of prasaha, bhūśaya (burrowing), and vārija animals, while patients suffering from symptoms of kapha and pitta should eat meat of pratuda, vishkira, dhanvaja and mṛga-dvija animals. The meat should be prepared in the form of a soup, and should be soft, tasty, aromatic and pleasant. Honey or alcoholic drinks like sīdhu, vāruṇi, prasanna, āsava, arishṭa, etc., should be used as anupāna. However, in patients who are not used to meat, the meat should be given in a concealed form, so that the persons are not aware that they are eating meat. If they come to know that they are being given meat, they may vomit it out or would refuse it.

However, even patients who are being given meat juices, alcoholic drinks, etc., and who bathe in the open will not be cured if they are constantly agitated and if they continue to suppress the natural urges.

Alcoholic drinks which are sharp (tīkshṇa), hot, non-slimy and subtle will open up the obstructed body channels and thus help in building up the body tissues.

The patient should also be administered ghee medicated with meat juices of carnivorous animals and honey; or with drugs and meat juices; or with drugs of the panchakola group, yava-kshāra and milk; or with rāsna, bala, gokshura, sthira, punarnavā, jīvanti, pippali-garbha and milk, These drugs can also be administered with honey or yavāgu (gruel) prepared with these drugs. Red rice is also useful.

The patient should be allowed to partake of food which is pleasing to him. Food should be easy to digest, fresh, tasty and aromatic. He should be exposed to good music, reading from scriptures, and such other pleasant distractions.

The patient should also be massaged with oil and advised a tub bath with water and milk or oils. He should also be gently massaged with a paste of śatapushpa, aśvagandha, apāmārga, balā, sarshapa, vidāri, rice powder, atasi, māsha, tila, barely powder, honey, etc.

The following measures are beneficial in headache, and pain in the shoulders and sides of the chest: External application of paste of śatapushpa, yashṭi-madhu, kushṭha, tagara, chandana and ghee; external application (pradeha) of paste of balā, rasna, tila, yashṭi-madhu, nilotpala and honey or of guggulu, devadāru, chandana, kesara and ghee, or of padma, uśīra, chandana and ghee or dūrva, yashṭi-madhu, manjishṭha, kesara and ghee; sprinkling of milk or a decoction of yashṭi-madhu or of a decoction of chandana, etc., sankara type of fomentation with māsha, kulattha, yava and milk preparation; a nāḍi type of fomentation with decoction of balā, guḍūchi, and madhūka, or balā ghṛta or paste of kharjūra, pippali, drāksha, harītaki, sṛngi, durālabha, honey and ghee or paste of triphala, pippali, musta, sṛngāṭa, guḍa (jaggery), sugar, honey, and ghee or of nāgara, chitraka, lājā, pippali, āmalaka, jaggery, honey and ghee etc. are useful. Massages with oil medicated with chandana etc., or with śata-dhouta ghṛta is also useful. Blood letting can also be carried out.

The following measures are useful in catarrh: The patient is subjected to fomentation, massage, fumigation (dhūma), external application, sprinkling (of decoctions, etc.,) and tub baths. Nourishing food prepared from substances that are salty, sour, pungent and hot, unctuous preparations, meat of lāva, tittiri and draksha, meat juices of goat, etc., with pippali, yava, kulattha, nāgara, dāḍima and āmalaka are useful. Soup of mūlaka (radish) and kulattha (horse-gram) is useful. The patient can also partake of barley, wheat, red rice, etc., and a decoction of panchamūla drugs or of dhānya and nāgara or of tāmalaki.

In hoarseness, the patient can be given errhines (nasya) of ghee medicated with balā, vidāri, madhuka, etc., rock-salt, and ghee or milk medicated with prapouṇḍarīka, yashṭi-madhu, pippali, brhaṭi and bala. Ghee medicated with kharjūra, mṛdvīka, sugar candy, honey nand pipali or with a decoction of daśamūla drugs, pippali and honey can be administered internally.

In cough and dyspnoea, ghee medicated with kharjūra, mṛdvīka, sugar-candy, pippali and honey or with a decocotion of daśamūla drugs, milk, pippali and honey, paste of sitopala (sugar candy), tūga-kshīra, pippali, bahula (maricha), dālchini, honey and ghee; and other measures employed in headache and pain in shoulder and chest are useful.

Vāsā-ghṛta and śatāvari ghṛta are very useful in burning of the hands and feet, fever and spitting or vomiting of blood.

Ghee medicated with jīvanti, yashṭi-madhu, drāksha, fruits of kuṭaja, śaṭi, pushkara-mūla, kaṇtakāri, gokshūra, bala, nilotpala, tāmalaki, trāyamāna, durālabha and pippali is very beneficial in all eleven symptoms of rāja-yakshma.

Ghee medicated with milk and balā, sthira, pṛśni-parṇi, bṛhati, kaṇṭakāri, nāgara, drāksha, kharjūra, pippali and honey is useful in fever, cough and hoarseness. Gruel prepared from goat's milk, meat juices of desert animals, chaṇaka, mudga and makushṭha is also usefıl in these complaints.

In fever, the drugs mentioned in jvara are to be administered with ghee.

In strong persons suffering from hawking of mucus, an emetic prepared with milk, yashṭi-madhu and madanaphala is administered. Gruel mixed with ghee and emetic drugs can also be employed. After emesis, the patient is advised food that is appetizing and easy to digest such as barley, godhūma, madhvika, sīdhu, āsava, arishṭa, meat juices of desert animals, etc.

In patients suffering from diarrhoea with slimy stools, tastelessness and loss of appetite, drugs, and food articles which are binding and appetizing should be employed. Rice water with nāgara and indra-yava (seeds of kuṭaja), or gruel prepared from buttermilk, chāngeri, and dāḍima, or buttermilk with pāṭha, bilva and yavāni or wine with durālabha, fresh ginger and pāṭha or thin gruel with bilva, āmra, jambu and kapittha is useful. The diet can consist of red rice, a decoction of bṛhat pancha-mūla drugs, buttermilk, wine, juice of dāḍima, etc.

In tastelessness or a bad taste in the mouth, the patient is advised to brush his teeth twice a day, with bitter and pungent tooth-brushes prepared from karanja, karavīra, etc. The decoction prepared from these drugs can be used for gargling. The patient should eat food which he is fond of. The drugs which are useful in cleansing the mouth are dālchini, ela, musta, āmalaka, dārvi bark, yavāni, pippali, tintiḍīka, etc. Pills made from these drugs can be kept in the mouth to be chewed, (CS).

II. The patient is to be first administered ghee of goat's or sheep's milk medicated with drugs of vidārigandhādi group. He is then given a mild emetic and laxative. He can also be given āsthāpana enema and errhines. The patient should then partake of barley, wheat, red rice and meat juices of desert animals. If his appetite and digestion are good, the patient is advised to eat nourishing food. Nourishing food is particularly useful if excess sexual intercourse has been the cause for rāja-yakshma.

Meat of animals like kākā, ulūka (owl), nakula (mongoose), biḍāla (wild cat), gaṇḍūpada, vyāla, bileśaya (burrowing animals), ākhku, gṛdhra, etc. are to be fried with mustard oil and given along with rock salt. The meat of desert animals and soup of mudga, and āḍhaki, meat of khara (ass), ushṭra (camel), snake (elephant), aśva (horse), etc., are also to be partaken of. Alcoholic drinks such as arishṭa, mṛdvīka, and madira are drunk (as anupāna). Various preparations of barley that have been previously soaked overnight in water in which the ash of arka and guḍūchi is soaked are useful. The ghee of goat or sheep milk is to be taken during meals. The paste of trikaṭu, chavya, viḍanga, honey and ghee is also beneficial.

Ghee medicated with pippali and meat juices of carnivorous animals is to be administered with honey.

The following recipes are also useful: Paste of drāksha, sugar candy, pippali, til oil and honey; the paste of aśvagandha, tila, māsha, honey and goat's ghee; paste of sugar candy, aśvagandha, pippali, honey and ghee; milk boiled with the powder of aśvagandha; ghee extracted from milk which is boiled with aśvagandha is given with sugar candy and followed by milk; ghee medicated with all the parts of vāsā (including flowers) is administered with honey; all parts of the goat are very useful; garlic can be used as mentioned in the texts; the paste of nāgabala with milk; pippali and śilājatu can also be employed as mentioned in the texts.

The patient can be rubbed with the paste of aśvagandha, barley and punarnava.

The patient should avoid sexual intercourse, grief, anger and criticising other, (SS).

III. The decoction of drugs of the daśamūla group, dhānyaka, pippali and nāgara is useful in fever, dyspnoea, catarth and pain in the sides of the chest. The decoction of aśvagandha, amṛta, bhārngi, daśamūla drugs, vachā, vāsa, ativisha and pushkara are useful in rāja-yakshma, along with a diet of milk. The meat of kapi (monkey), hariṇa or cchāga is dried, finely powdered and administered with goat's milk. The decoction of daśamūla drugs, vachā, rāsna, pushkara, nāgara, and devadāru is useful in headache, pain in the sides of the chest, kāsa and other symptoms of rāja-yakshma. The powder of bark of kakubha (arjuna), nāgabala and kapi-kacchu seeds is boiled in milk, and administered with honey, ghee and sugar in rāja-yakshma. The decoction of daśamūla drugs, pippali, dhānya, nāgara and chatur-jātaka is also very useful. The juice of root, leaves, and tender leaves of madayantika, if taken for a month, will eradicate rāja-yakshma. The powder mixed with the juice of kūshmanda fruit will stop haemorrhage and spitting of blood. The powder of purified iron can be administered with triphala, trikaṭu, śatāvari and balā. The paste of chavya viḍanga and trikaṭu, ghee and honey is also very beneficial. The paste of pippali, drāksha, sugar, honey and til oil, and fresh butter with sugar-candy and honey are also useful, (CSS).

IV. The patient can be administered pārada bhasma with ghee medicated with goat's milk and pippali or pārada bhasma with triphala, purified sulphur, trikaṭu and jaggery. The patient can also be administered loha bhasma with powder of trikaṭu, triphala, chitraka, viḍanga, musta, sugarcandy, and purified śilājatu. These must however be triturated together, mixed with honey and stored in a vessel of kānta (iron), (RRS).

Classical Prescriptions: Agastya-harītaki-rasāyana; Balā-taila; Balā-dhātryādi-taila; Balā-aśvagandhā-lākshādi-taila; Chāgalādya-ghṛta; Chandanādi-taila; Chandana-balālakshādi-taila; Chaturmukha-rasa; Chyavana-prāśa; Daśamūlārishṭa; Drākshārishṭa; Eladi-ghṛta; Guḍūchyādi-modaka; Haratāla-bhasma: Indu-kānta-rasa; Kanta-vallabha-rasa; Kapardika-bhasma; Karpurādi-chūrṇa; Kūshmāṇḍa-rasāyana; Laghu-māliṇi-vasanta-rasa; Mahā-lakshmi-vilāsa-rasa; Mukta-bhasma; Muktā-panchāmṛta-rasa; Mṛgānka-rasa; Nāga-vallabha-rasa; Narasimha-chūṛna; Navaratna-rāja; Pippalādyāsava; Rajata-bhasma; Śatāvari-guḍa; Sitopalādi-chūrṇa; Śiva-guṭika; Svarṇa-parpaṭi; Tāmra-bhasma; Vajra-bhasma; Vaikrānta-bhasma; Vanga-bhasma; Vāsavaleha; Vāsakāsava; Vāsa-chandanādi-taila; Vasanta-kusumākara-rasa; Vidāryādi-kvātha-churṇa; Vidāryadi-ghṛta; Kusumākara-rasa; Vidāryādi-kvātha-churṇa; Vidāryādī-ghṛta; Yaśada-bhasma. Vata-kaphaja kshaya : Rāja-mṛgānka-rasa.

Ref.: CS, chikitsā, 8, 65-189; SS, uttara, 41, 32-58; CSS, pages. 223-225; RRS, 28, 37; 30, 26.

Rakta-pitta

Synonyms: Sanskrit: Lohita – pitta (CS)

Western Nosology: Haemorrhage

Causative Factors:

Extrinsic:

1. Excessive intake of yavaka, uddālaka (the wild variety of kodrava), koradūsha (kodrava) and foods that are very hot and active with pulses like nishpāva, māsha, and kulattha, yava-kshāra, curds, whey, udasvit (a mixture of equal amounts of butter milk and water), katvāra (sour buttermilk) and sour kānji; excessive intake of meat of vārāha (pig), buffalo, sheep, cow and fish with piṇyāka (oil cake), piṇḍālu (a variety of alaku) and dry vegetables or after taking mūlaka, sarshapa, laśuna, karanja, śigru, madhu śigru, bhūstṛna, sumukha, phann jaka (and other varieties of basil), or followed by surā, souvīra, tushodaka (and other types of alcoholic drinks), badarāmla, etc., intake of flour prepations or pastries (pishṭānna) after meals; frequent intake of unboiled milk in large quantities immediately after being exposed to the sun; intake of the rohiṇi kind of fish along with milk, intake of meat of small kapota with mustard oil or yava-kshāra (or alkalies); intake of milk with kulattha, piṇyāka (oil cake), ripe fruit of jambu or lakucha while being exposed to the sun, etc.

Excessive exposure to the sun, and intake of food that is vidāhi (viz. which causes pyrosis), hot, very active or sharp, sour pungent and salty, (CS).

2. Emotions such as anger, grief and fear, excessive exertion, imcompatible food, excessive exposure to the heat of the sun or fire, and regular intake of food articles which are pungent, sour, salty, alkaline (kshāra), hot, sharp and vidāhi, (SS).

Intrinsic: Pitta, (CS, SS).

Constituents Affected: Blood (CS, SS); The liver, spleen and channels that carry blood, (CS).

Pathogenesis:

1. Due to the causative factors, there is aggravation of pitta and through it, of the blood. The pitta then localises in the channels which carry blood, which originate from the liver and spleen. This further vitiates the blood, (CS).

2. The aggravated pitta vitiates the blood, thereby giving rise to this disease. (SS).

Prodroma Symptoms:

1. Loss of appetite, burning pain (in the alimentary tract) after eating, sour and acid, eructations, frequent vomiting, foul appearance of the vomit, hoarseness, debility, burning pain (all over the body), a feeling as if hot smoke was coming out from the mouth, a smell of metal, blood, fish, and raw meat in the mouth, a reddish, green or yellow discolouration of the skin, faeces, urine, sweat, saliva, and waste products of the ears, eyes, nose, etc., appearance of eruptions, body pain,

and frequent dreams of dazzling objects and objects that are red, blue, yellow or gray in colour, (CS).

2. Debility, craving for cold (substances), vomiting, a feeling as if smoke was issuing from the throat and metallic smell of the breath, (SS).

3. Heaviness of the head, cough, dyspnoea, vertigo and fatigue even without exertion, (AS).

Types:

1. Rakta-pitta can be caused by the aggravation of the three doshas, either singly or combined, (CS).

2. Rakta-pitta is of three types depending on the directions of the bleeding, *viz.* it can be upward, or downward or both upward and downward, (CS, SS).

Symptomatology:

1. If rakta-pitta is caused by the deranged vāta, the blood will be grey or brownish in colour, frothy, thin and dry (not sticky). If it has been caused by the aggravated kapha, the blood will be thick, whitish or pale red, oily and slimy. If caused by the provoked pitta, the blood will be pale-red or saffron coloured or blackish, or of the colour of cow's urine, or burning coal or collyrium (anjana) or polished black stone. If the disease has been caused by two doshas, the patient will suffer from symptoms of both the doshas, (CS).

2. The bleeding can occur in an upward direction *viz.* from the eyes, nose, mouth and ears, or in a downward direction *viz.* from the rectum or urethra. If the kapha is deranged (along with the pitta), the bleeding will occur in an upward direction, whereas the derangement of vāta (along with the pitta) will bring about bleeding from the rectum or urethra. If all the three doshas are provoked, there will be bleeding even from the skin, (CS).

3. If the vitiated blood accumulates in the āmāśaya (stomach) there will be bleeding from the upper outlets, while there is bleeding form the rectum or urethra if the deranged blood accumulates in the pakvāśaya (intestines), (SS).

Complications:

1. Debility, loss of appetite, indigestion (or feeble digestion), dyspnoea, cough, fever, diarrhoea, swellings, emaciation, anaemia and hoarseness, (CS).

2. Debility, dyspnoea, cough, fever, vomiting, a state resembling intoxication, lethargy, burning pain, unconsciousness, burning pain (in the alimentary tract) after eating, loss of courage, intolerable pain or distress in the precordial region, thirst, throat-pain, burning pain in the head, spitting of foul sputum, indigestion and loss of sexual desire (libido), (SS).

Prognosis:

1. Cases where bleeding takes an upward direction are curable, because such cases are treated by purgation (which is the main remedial measure employed in vitiation of pitta), whereas cases where bleeding occurs in the urethra and rectum can only be palliated. Patients in whom bleeding occurs both through the upper and lower outlets are incurable, (CS, SS).

2. Cases of rakta-pitta in which the blood is black or blue or many coloured like a rainbow, where the blood sticks to the cloth (even after washing), is very foul smelling and in excessive quantity, where there are all the complications, and where there is loss of strength and depletion of muscular tissue, are considered to be incurable.

Cases where the patient perceives the sky and all the objects as being red, where the blood is black and has a cadaverous odour, where the patient is continuously coughing and emaciating are incurable, (CS).

3. Cases where the blood resembles the washings of meat (*viz.* water in which meat has been washed), decoctions of drugs, filthy water, fat, pus, liver or the ripe fruit of the jambu or is black, blue or many hued like a rainbow, where

it has a cadaverous odour, and where all the complications are present, are incurable, (SS).

4. The disease caused by one dosha is curable, and that caused by two doshas can be palliated. The disease caused by all three doshas is incurable, (CS).

Ref.: CS, nidāna, 2; chikitsā, 4; SS, uttaran, 46; AS, nidāna, 3.

Treatment:

1. This is a dangerous disease which spreads like a forest fire. Treatment should therefore be started immediately, after duly considering the dosage, locality (area affected) and time (season).

In a case of rakta-pitta in a person who has not undergone depletion of strength and muscular tissue, and thus who can undergo santarpaṇa (nourishing) therapy, the blood should not be stopped immediately (with astringents, etc.,). Such sudden suppression of the bleeding often gives rise to galagraha, pūtinasya (a form of nāsa roga), unconsciousness, anorexia, fever, abdominal tumours, enlargement of the spleen, flatulence, kilāsa, dysuria, skin diseases, haemorrhoids, herpes, tinnitus, anal fistula and weakness of mind and sense faculties.

A case of rakta-pitta should first be treated either with langhana (fasting and other emaciating measures) or with tarpaṇa (refreshing or nourishing) therapy, depending on the outlet of bleeding, the dosha affected (usually aggravation of kapha is treated with fasting, etc.,) and the causes.

A case of upward bleeding is treated first with refreshing (nourishing) therapy, while a patient of downward bleeding is administered gruels, etc. For tarpaṇa, the cold infusion of kharjūra, mṛdvīka, yashṭi-madhu, sugar and parūshaka or powder of lājā with honey and ghee is very useful, especially in upward bleeding. In persons with feeble digestion, and those accustomed to sour foods, dāḍima and āmalaka can be added to the above mentioned preparations.

In case of thirst, the patient can drink either cold water or the cold decoction of hrīvera, chandana, uśīra, musta and parpaṭaka.

The diet in rakta-pitta should consist of rice grown in sixty-days (or red rice), nīvara, koradūsha, praśāntika, śyāmāka, priyangu, soup or gruel of mudga, masūra, chaṇaka, āḍhaki, and makushṭaka, the tender leaves of paṭola, nimba, vetra, plaksha and vetasa, leaves of kirātatikta, gaṇḍira and kathillaka, and flowers of kovidāra (a variety of kānchanara), śalmali and kāśmari. These can be prepared in the form of gruel or can be fried with ghee. The meat of pārāvata, kapota, lāva, raktāksha, vartaka, rabbit, kapinjala, eṇa, hariṇa, and kāla-pucchaka, can be taken either as meat-juices or with sugar or after being fried with ghee. These should not be sour. Cases where kapha is provoked are to be given gruels and leafy vegetables, while patients in whom vāta is deranged are to be given meat juices.

Gruels (yavāgu) prepared with the following drugs are beneficial: padma, utpala, kinjalka, pṛśniparṇi, meat juices and ginger; kirātatika, uśīra and mustā; dhātaki, dhanvayāsa, bilva, and meat juices; masūra and pṛśniparṇi; soup of green gram with sthira; the juice of hareṇuka with juice of balā and ghee; or of meat juices of pāravata, etc. These gruels have to be taken cold, after adding honey and sugar.

In cases of constipation, the meat of śaśa (rabbit) can be taken along with vāstuka. In patients suffering from aggravation of vāta, the diet can consist of meat of tittiri with the decoction of undumbara, meat of mayūra with the decoction of plaksha, meat of kukkuṭa with the decoction of nyagrodha (banyan), and meat of vartāka and krakaśa with a decoction of bilva and utpala. In cases of severe thirst, a decoction of bitter drugs or cooling fruit juices or cold infusions of drugs of vidārigandha group is useful. However water should not be drunk in excess.

Strong persons, in whom there has been no

depletion of strength and muscular tissue, and where the doshas have aggravated due to over-nutrition (over-eating, etc.,) and where the doshas have been severely provoked, have to be subjected to purgation (in cases of bleeding from upward outlets), and emesis (in cases where the bleeding is from downward outlets), after duly considering the time and strength (of the patient and disease). For inducing purgation, the patient can be administered trivṛt with harītaki or fruits of āragvadha or roots of trāyamāṇa and gavākshi or āmalaki (fruits), in each case with plenty of honey and sugar. For inducing emesis, the patient can be administered fruit-pulp of madana with honey and sugar, or madana with sugar, sugarcane juice and water or fruits of kuṭaja with mustā, madana, yashṭi-madhu and honey. After the purificatory procedures, patients suffering from bleeding from upward outlets are given refreshing and nourishing food (tarpaṇa), while those suffering from bleeding from downward outlets are given gruels, etc., if vāta is not excessively provoked (if vāta is excessively provoked, the latter patients are also given meat-juices, etc.).

Palliative treatment is however indicated in emaciated and debilitated persons, in persons who have suffered from grief, or who are weakened by lifting heavy loads, travelling, from exposure to sun or fire (for long stretches of time) or by many diseases, pregnant women, elderly people, children, persons who are accustomed to dry and limited food and who are suffering from rāja-yakshma in addition to rakta-pitta. Such persons should not be given emesis or purgation.

The formulations that are used in palliative therapy are: decoction of vāsā, mṛdvīka and harītaki with honey and sugar; decoction of vāsā priyangu, anjana, lodhra and vinaya with honey; decoction of padma, filaments or blossoms of lotus, dūrva, vāstuka, utpala, nāgapushpa and lodhra, the juice of the dung of cow or horse with honey and ghee; the paste of flowers of priyangu, khadira, kovidāra, śālmali and honey; the powder of sṛngaṭāka, lājā, musta, kharjūra, padma, kesara and honey; blood of any desert animal with honey; the paste of uśīra, kulīyaka, lodhra, padma, priyangu, kaṭphala, śankha or gairika with equal amounts of chandan, sugar and rice water; the juice or paste or decoction or infusions of chandana with equal amount of any of the following drugs: kirātatikta, kramuka, musta, prapouṇḍarīka, kamala, nilotpala, roots of hrīvera, leaves of paṭola, durālabha, parpaṭaka, mṛṇāla (lotus stem), arjuna, udumbara, vetasa, dālchini, vaṭa, priyangu, yavāsa, taṇḍulīya, mocharasa or lājālu (namaskāri); the cold infusion of balā, uśīra, chandana, musta, mudga, lājā yava and pippali; the decoction of āmalaka or water in which vaiḍūrya, mukta, precious stones, śankha or gairika (red ochre) has been soaked; sugar cane juice with a decoction of yashṭi-madhu; the filtered upper layer of cold infusion of burnt brick, uśīra, padma, utpala and chandan; with honey and sugar; etc.

The above-mentioned formulations will help in alleviating kapha and improving digestion. If, however, the bleeding does not subside, it indicates that vāta is still provoked. So the patient should be administered goat's milk, or cow's milk boiled with one fifth of water or a decoction of the vidārigandhādi group of drugs along with honey and sugar. The decoction of drāksha, or nāgara, or balā or gokshura or milk boiled with sugar is also useful.

The decoction of śatāvari and gokshura or milk boiled with leaves of śālaparni, pṛśni parṇi, māshaparṇi and mudgaparṇi is very useful in painful bleeding from the urinary tract.

Milk boiled with mocharasa or with tender buds or fresh sprouts of the banyan tree or with hrīvera, nilotpala and nāgara is very useful in bleeding from the rectum.

Ghee medicated with the juice and paste of leaf-stem of palāśa and honey or with paste of kuṭaja or paste of lajjālu, utpala and lodhra or paste of udumbara and leaves of patola is very efficacious in rakta-pitta.

The remedial measures such as massage, sprinkling of decoction, tub baths, enemata, etc., described under pittaja jvara are useful in the diseases also. The medicated ghee prescribed in kshata-kshīṇa is also is useful.

In cases where patients hawk coagulated or thick blood from the throat, the kshāra (ash) of lotus stems or palāśa or priyangu or madhūka or asana is administered with honey and ghee.

In epistaxis, the drugs which have been mentioned above are powdered and used as errhines (avapīḍa). Sugar water medicated with nilotpala, gairika, śankha and chandan, or juice of mango-stone, lājjālu, dhātaki, lodhra and mocha-rasa is used as errhines (nasya) in cases of epistaxis with headache, foul odour from the nose, loss of smell and chronic catarrh. The juice of drāksha and sugarcane, or milk boiled with juice of dūrva, or a decoction of flowers of dāḍima or milk boiled with yashṭi-madhu can also be used as nasal drops.

The patient should also be exposed to a pleasant and cool environment, with plenty of fragrant flowers, leaves of plantain, lotus, etc., ponds, lakes and shady trees, etc., (CS).

2. Bleeding in a strong person should not be stopped (by astringents) at the beginning, as it may give rise to anaemia, sprue (grahaṇi), skin diseases, enlargement of spleen, abdominal tumours and fever. In such (strong) patients, emesis and purgation are induced in bleeding from downward and upward channels respectively. However, debilitated persons are treated with palliative (śamana) therapy.

In strong persons with excessively vitiated doshas, fasting is first to be advised. Later, he is given gruels with a little rice, gruels (yūsha) prepared from meat juices, ghee or oil and aromatic substances, refreshing and nourishing food (such as decoction of mṛdvīka, yashṭi-madhu, etc., with ghee and honey, or preparations of lāja, etc., water boiled with digestive drugs (such as hrīvera, chandan, uśīra, parpaṭa, musta, etc.,) with ghee. After this, the patient is administered laxatives with drāksha, yashṭi-madhu, sugar candy and kāśmari, or emetics with yashṭi-madhu and honey.

The diet has to consist of the following: cold milk, milk boiled with dṛugs having cold potency (like candana), meat juices of desert animals, gruel (yūsha) of satīna, rice which is harvested in sixty days, red rice, paṭola, śeluka, sunishaṇṇaka, yūthika, sprouts of vaṭa nirguṇdi, vegetables with ghee and fruits such as āmalaki and dāḍima, meat juices of pārāvata, and kūrma, gruels with ghee drugs of the utpala group with ghee, milk, honey and sugar, and cold substances.

The following formulations are efficacious: the paste of flowers of madhūka, śigru, kovidāra, or priyangu with honey; the paste of tender leaves of dūrva and vaṭa with honey; fruits like kharjūra with honey; drugs useful in raktātisāra; a piece of sugar-cane without the skin should be crushed, and immersed in cold water in an open earthern vessel for a night, filtered and given with powder of utpala and honey; cold infusions of jambu, āmra and arjuna with honey; the juice of udumbara with honey; paste of the root of trapusha with honey and rice water; paste of yashṭi-madhu, with honey and rice water; paste of chandan, yashṭi-madhu, lodhra, with honey; paste of karanja seeds with sugar and honey; the paste of the pulp of ingudi fruit with yashṭi-madhu and honey; the paste of rock salt and seeds of karanja with curd-cream (dadhi-mastu) which should be administered lukewarm for three days; ghee medicated with milk boiled with the juice of kshīri trees (like vaṭa), with sugar; cold infusion of drāksha, uśīra, padma and sugar, milk with an equal amount of water; paste of seeds of vastuka with honey; paste of taṇḍulīyaka and honey; paste of lājā, rasānjana, sugar and honey; paste of tuga kshīra or vamsalochana with sugar and honey; paste of drāksha, kaṭuka-rohiṇi, yashṭi-madhu, and sugar with cold milk; paste of harītaki, ahimsra and haridra with ghee; the decoction of vāsā with honey and paste of utpala, red earth, priyangu, lodhra, rasānjana, padma-kesara and sugar, in very acute bleeding; the alkaline water prepared form the ash of indīvara with honey; the paste of seeds of karanja and honey; the decoction of jambu, arjuna and āmra; and the paste of roots and flowers of mātulunga with rice water.

In epistaxis, milk or water with sugar should be applied over the nostrils. The patient can also take the juice of drākshā, ghee extracted from milk or sugarcane juice with sugar.

Āsthāpana type of enema can be administered with milk boiled with drugs of the vidarīgandhādi group, drāksha, sugar, honey and ghee. Ghee (medicated with yashṭi-madhu, etc.,) should be used for anuvāsana enema.

In severe bleeding from the rectum, nirūha (āsthāpana) enema should be given with drugs such as priyangu, lodhra, souvīrānjan, gairika, utpala, chandana, sugar, aśvagandha, musta, yashṭi-madhu, lotus stem and sougandhika (a variety of lotus) and milk, honey and ghee. The patient is then sprinkled with cold water, and after he partakes of rice with milk, is administered an anuvāsana enema with ghee medicated with yashṭi-madhu.

In severe bleeding from the urethra, the same drugs can be used for urethral injections.

The above (palliative) measures are useful in menorrhagia and bleeding after any surgical procedures, (SS).

3. The following formulae are useful in rakta-pitta: the paste of leaves of paṭola, loha bhasma and rasa-sindūra; the paste of rasa-sindūra with leaf-juice of vāsā, honey and sugar, which should be taken every morning, even in very severe cases; the paste of leaves of paṭola, purified hingula and honey; the parts of paste of fresh butter, sugar, lājā, and drāksha; the paste of ghee which should be applied on the head (in case of epistaxis); the decoction of drākshā and vāsa with sugar; the juice of vāsa with honey and sugar; the paste of lājā with sugar and juice of vāsa and the paste of āmalaki powder and sugar, (RRS).

Classical Prescriptions: Abhraka-bhasma; Ahiphenāsava; Amṛtaprāśa-ghṛta; Bola-parpaṭi; Chandanādi-taila; Chandana-balā-lākshādi-taila; Chandrakalā-rasa; Dhātryādi-ghṛta; Elādi-guṭika; Guḍūchyādi-modaka; Kankāyana-guṭika; Kumāryāsava; Kuṭajāvaleha; Mahā-tiktaka-ghṛta; Muktā-pishṭi; Nārikela-khanḍa; Nyagrodhādi-kvātha-chūrṇa; Satāvari-guḍa; Trāyantyādi-kvātha-chūrṇa; Tṛṇa-kānta-maṇi-pishṭi; Uśīrasava; Vāsakāsava; Vāsāvaleha; Vāsā-chandanādi-taila; Vāsā-guḍūchyādi-kvātha-chūrṇa.

Rakta-nishṭhīvana: Elādi-guṭika

Ref.: CS, Chikitsā, 4; SS, uttara, 45, 11-45; RRS, 13, 1-22.

Raktātisāra

Western Nosology: Dysenteric diarrhoea

Causative Factors:

Extrinsic: This disease results when a patient suffering from pittaja-atisāra is improperly treated or partakes of food which aggravates pitta instead of being treated (for pittaja-atisāra).

Intrinsic: Pitta

Constituents Affected: Blood

Symptomatology: The patient passes bloody stools, and also suffers from thirst, abdominal pain, pyrosis and severe inflammation around the anus.

Treatment:

1. The patient can be given gruel (peya) prepared from hrīvera, utpala, pṛśniparṇi, musta and goat's milk which is diluted with half the amount of water, (CS, sūtra, 2, 21).

2. Cold goat's milk which is mixed with honey and sugar candy should be used both internally and for washing the anus.

The diet should consist of red rice with milk;

or meat juice of pārāvata, etc., which are fried or cooked with ghee and taken with sugar or cold meat juices of śaśa (hare), pakshi mṛga, or desert animals, which should not be sour, along with ghee and sugar; or of gruel of slightly sour fruits of kāśmari with sugar.

The decoction of nilotpala, mocharasa, dhātaki, padma-keśara (or padma, nāga kesara) and goat's milk can be drunk after the meal which should consist of rice and milk. Debilitated persons can drink this decoction first and follow it up with the meal of rice and milk. Fresh butter can be eaten with sugar and honey before meals. The paste of ghee extracted from milk, meat juices of kapinjala and milk can be administered, with the diet consisting of milk and rice. This is very efficacious and will show a good result in just three days.

The paste of śatāvari and milk can be also be administered with a diet of only milk (and rice). Ghee medicated with śatāvari is also useful. The decoction of fruits of kuṭaja can be administered with ghee and the upper layer of yavāgu (gruel).

The following recipes are useful in arresting the bleeding from the rectum: the paste of priyangu and honey should be taken with rice water, a diet consisting of meat juices of desert animals; the paste of black tila seeds and five parts of sugar should be administered with goat's milk; the paste of chandana, sugar and honey should be given with rice water.

The anus can be washed with a cold infusion of paṭola and yashṭi-madhu or with goat's or cow's milk mixed with sugar and honey, (CS).

3. The following formulations are useful: The paste of bark of śallaki or badara or jambu or priyāla or āmra or arjuna with milk and honey; the leaf juices of tender sprouts of jambu, āmra and āmalaki should be administered with goat's milk and honey; and the paste of bilva, goat's milk, sugar-candy and mocha rasa is administered with powder of kalinga, (CD).

4. The paste of śṛngi (karkaṭa-śṛngi), pāṭha, musta, honey and water, is very useful in raktātisāra in children, (RRS).

Related Diseases: Atisāra

Ref.: CS, chikitsā, 19, 69-70; 71-88; CD, 3, 67-69; RRS, 22, 137.

Romāntika

Western Nosology: Measles

Causative Factors:

Extrinsic: Factors which aggravate kapha and pitta

Intrinsic: Kapha and pitta, (CS, MN).

Symptomatology:

1. Small eruptions (vesicles) all over the body with itching and burning pain. The patient also suffers from thirst, fever, salivation and loss of appetite, (CS).

2. Eruptions (all over the body) which are red (copper coloured) and of the size of hair follicles (roma-kūpa), along with other symptoms like cough and loss of appetite. The formation of the eruptions is preceded by fever, (MN).

Treatment: The patient is to be treated on the same lines as indicated in visarpa, kushṭha, (CS), and masūrika.

Related Diseases: Masūrika

Ref.: CS, chikitsā, 12, 92-93; MN, 54, 13.

Sadyo-vraṇa

Western Nosology: Wounds

Causative Factors:

Extrinsic:

1. Injury caused by various kinds of weapons on different parts of the body; injuries caused by the bites of men, beasts, birds, ferocious

animals, and snakes, injuries caused by a fall, or by pressure or a blow or by burns, application of caustics (alkali), or by poison, strong toxic drugs, and various other kinds of trauma, (SS).

2. Trauma, pressure, or ligature, fall, injuries by fangs, teeth or nails, contact with poisons or fire or weapons, etc., (CS).

Intrinsic: Vāta (SS)

Types:

1. There are six types of external injuries: (a) cchinna (cuṭs); (b) bhinna (punctured or stab wounds); (c) viddham (pierced wounds), (d) kshata (contusions), (e) picchita (crushed wounds), and (f) ghṛshta (lacerated wounds), (SS).

2. There are eight types of sadyo-vraṇa, *viz.* ghṛsṭha, avakṛtta, vicchinna, pravilambita, pātita, viddha, bhinna and vidalita, (AHṛ).

Symptomatology:

I. Cchinna-vṛana: The wound is either oblique or straight, elongated, and the part of the body may be completely severed.

Bhinna-vraṇa: The perforation of any cavity of the body by the sharp end of a lance, spear, sword or horn, attended by a slight discharge (of urine if the bladder is perforated, of blood if the abdomen, liver or spleen is perforated, etc., NiS).

The thoraco-abdominal cavita (koshṭha) consists mainly of the stomach, small intestines (or pancreas), large intestines, urinary bladder, heart, caecum liver, spleen, and lungs.

If any of these organs are punctured, they are filled with blood and there is fever, burning pain, haemorrhages from the urethra, rectum, mouth or nose, dyspnoea, syncope, thirst, flatulent distension of abdomen, aversion to food, constipation, retention of urine, obstruction of flatus, excessive sweating, redness of eyes, the smell of loha (iron) in the mouth, foul odour of the body, chest pain and pain in the sides of the chest.

If the stomach is perforated, it is filled with blood. The person also suffers from vomiting of blood, severe pain and intense flatulent distension of the abdomen.

If the large intestines are injured, there is pain, a sense of heaviness, chilliness and discharge of blood through rectum and urethra. Even if the intestines are not perforated, they are filled with blood, just like an earthern pot with its mouth covered may be filled with water through the pores, (SS).

Vīddha-vraṇa: Any injury inflicted in any part of the body other than the āśayas (cavities) by sharp pointed instruments is known as viddha-vraṇa. The instrument may or may not be extricated, (SS).

Kshatha-vraṇa: A wound that is not exactly a cut nor puncture, but partakes of the nature of both, and which is irregular (or uneven) is known as kshata, (SS).

Picchita-vraṇa: In this type of wound, a part of the body when hit by a blunt weapon or when crushed along with the bone between the folds of a door is extended and covered with blood and bone-marrow, (SS).

Ghṛshṭa-vraṇa: Any part of the body, through friction or any other cause is deprived or denuded of the skin. There is also burning pain and discharge in the affected area, (SS).

II. The symptoms of the eight varieties are as follows:

Ghṛshṭam: Wounds with serous exudate and little blood, which burn and ooze out when excised.

Avakṛttam: Wounds that are deep.

Vicchinnam: Wounds that are even deeper.

Pravilambi: Wounds in which a part of the body is partly severed and is connected only by the bones, or wounds where the bones have been exposed.

Pātitam: Wounds where a part of the body has been completely severed.

Vīddha: Injuries inflicted by sharp-pointed instruments in any part of the body other than the thoraco-abominal cavity (koshṭha).

Bhinnam: Perforated injuries of the koshtha.

Vīdalitam: Wounds which are full of blood and marrow, which are inflicted by blunt weapons, and where a part of the body has been crushed with the bone, (AHṛ).

Prognosis: A bhinna-vraṇa involving the eyes is considered to be very difficult to treat except in cases where the eye-ball is dangling, and is not completely severed from the body.

Cases of perforation of koshṭha (thoraco-abdominal cavity) are incurable if blood accumulates within the body without finding an outlet, if the patient is very pale, has cold extremities and face, cold breath, and blood-shot eyes, (SS).

Complications: visarpa, pakshāghāta, sirāstambha, vertigo, unmāda (insanity) pain, fever, thirst, hanugraha (lock-jaw), cough, vomiting, diarrhoea, hiccoughs, dyspnoea and tremors, (CS).

Note:

1. If any one of the vital organs (marmas), joints, blood vessels or nerves, hard fibrous structures and bones are injured, the persons suffer from vertigo, delirium (incoherent speech), prostration, semi-consciousness, incapacitation, increase in body heat, debility, syncope, gasping for breath, severe pain, symptoms caused by aggravation of vāta, flow of blood that resembles water in which meat has been washed, and weakness of all sense organs.

If the sirās (blood vessels or nerves) are injured, there is copious bleeding of red blood, headache, blindness (andhya), adhimantha (eye-disease), timira (eye-diseases), depletion of body tissues, ākshepaka, burning pain, pakshāghāta, ekānga-vikara (hemiplegia), hiccoughs, dyspnoea, cough, anaemia and even death.

If the hard fibrous structures such as tendons and ligaments are injured, the patient suffers from deformity and weakness of the affected limb, loss of function of the limb and severe pain, while the wound takes a long time to heal.

If the joints are injured, there is intense sweating, severe pain, debility, breaking pain and swelling in the joints and loss of function of the affected joints.

If the bones are injured, there is severe pain, both in the day and night, without relief in any postion, thirst, prostration and painful swelling, (SS, śutra, 14, 30; 25, 34-39).

Ref.: SS, chikitsā, 2, 3-22; 1, 3; CS, chikitsā, 25, 7; AHr, uttara, 26, 2-5.

Treatment:

1. In cases of cchinna, bhinna, viddha and kshata types injuries, there is bleeding which aggravates vāta. Therefore the patient has to be administered potions of unctuous substances (like ghee), while the injured part has to be sprinkled with warm ghee or oil. Poultices of vesavāra (paste of boiled meat) and kṛśara (gruel prepared from tila, rice and māsha) mixed with unctuous substances can be applied externally. The part can also be fomented and plastered with unctuous substances. The patient can also be administered enema, with ghee or oil medicated with drugs that alleviate vāta.

In cases of picchita and ghṛshṭa wounds, there is not much bleeding, but there is burning pain and pāka (suppuration). In order to alleviate these symptoms and to reduce the body heat in that region, the area can be washed and plastered with cold substances.

Specific treatment in cchinna-vraṇa: An open wound situated at the sides of the head should be sutured and bandaged firmly (gāḍha-bandha). An ear that has been severed should be brought to its original position and sutured, while oil medicated with drugs that alleviate vāta should be poured into the ear. A cut in the laryngeal prominence (adam's apple) should be sutured and bandaged, even if it was allowing air to pass through it. The wound has then to be washed and sprinked with goat's ghee. The patient should eat his food, defecate, and urinate while lying on his back, until the wound has healed.

Wide-mouthed and lateral wounds on the extremities have to be sutured after the joints have properly set. They have to be bandaged with the vellitaka-bandha, and sprinkled with oil. The gophana-bandage can also be used.

A person with a wound on his back should lie on his back, while he should lie on his face and abdomen if he has been injured in the chest.

In cases where a limb has been completely severed from the body, the part should be cauterised with hot oil, and bandaged with a kośa-bandha. The part should then be plastered and washed with drugs that facilitate healing.

Oil boiled with milk and chandana, padmaka, lodhra, nilotpala, priyangu, haridra and yashṭi-madhu is very useful in promoting healing of wounds.

Oil medicated with chandana, karkaṭa-śṛngi, māshaparṇi, mudgaparṇi, guḍūchi, hareṇu, mrṇala (lotus stalk), triphala, padmaka, nilotpala, milk, ghee, animal fat and marrow is also useful in promoting the healing of wounds, when used externally.

Specific treatment in bhinna-vraṇa: In cases of injury to the eyes, where the eyeball is dangling, it should be replaced in the original position without disturbing the blood-vessels and nerves. It should be covered by a lotus leaf, and gently pressed with the palm. The eyes should then be filled with ghee mentioned below, the ghee can also be used as nasya:

Goat's ghee should be medicated with milk, yashṭi-madhu, nilotpala, jīvaka and ṛshabhaka, and boiled with ghee.

In cases of a perforated wound in the abdomen from which lumps of fat are discharged, the lumps have to be dusted with the alkali (ashes) of sarja, arjuna, etc., and black clay. A ligature should be tied around the lump, and this should then be excised with an instrument heated red hot. The wound is then plastered with honey. The patient should partake of ghee after the digestion of the food (previously taken). Milk medicated with sugar, yashṭi-madhu, and castor oil or with a decoction of gokshura, lāksha and caster oil can be drunk instead of ghee. This alleviates pain and burning. The lumps of fat may, if unexcised, cause flatulence, pain and even death.

In cases of perforated wounds, where the stomach is filled with blood, emesis is to be employed. If the large intestines are filled with blood, purgation is to be prescribed, along with āsthāpana enema with hot, purifying drugs (such as cow's urine), without unctuous substances. The diet should consist of boiled rice or gruel with barley, kola, kulattha and rock-salt, without unctuous substances. If there is copious haemorrhage, the patient may drink blood.

If parts of the intestines have bulged out from the wound without being injured, they can be gently re-introduced and placed in their original position, Even if the intestines are perforated, large black ants should be made to bite the perforated parts, after which their heads should be cut off. The intestines can then be re-introduced. They have to be washed with milk, lubricated with ghee, and gently re-introduced with the palms, with trimmed nails. If the intestines can be only partly introduced, the patient can be made to retch by tickling the interior of the throat, or he can be sprayed with cold water or lifted into the air and shaken, so that the intestines slip into the original position.

If the wound is too narrow to admit the reintroduction of the intestines, it should be widened by making a few incisions. The opening of the wound should then be sutured, bandaged with a silk cloth dipped in ghee, and plastered with oil medicated with barks of aśvakarṇa, dhava, śālmali, mesha-śṛngi, śallaki, arjuna, vidāri and kshīri (trees which exude resin) trees and root of bala. The patient should be internally administered warm ghee with castor oil for easy defecation and passage of flatus.

If the testicles protrude from the scrotum, the eyes and legs should be sprinkled with cold water, and the testicles re-introduced in the proper position. The scrotum is then sutured in the manner of tuna-sevani, and bandaged with a gophaṇa-bandha and a restraining apparatus to prevent the scotum from jerking. The wounds should not be lubricated with unctuous substances. Oil medicated with tagara, manahśila, agaru, ela, jāti flower, chandana, padmaka, devadāru, guḍūchi and tuttha should be applied.

Oil medicated with samanga, haridrā, padma, triphala, trikaṭu, trimada, tuttha, viḍanga, kaṭuka, harītaki, guḍūchi and karanja or with tāliśa, padmaka, jaṭāmāmsi, hereṇu, agaru, chandana, haridra, dāru-harida, seeds of padma, uśīra and yashṭi-madhu is useful in promoting the healing of wounds.

Picchita wounds should be treated as in a case of bhagna.

Specific treatment in ghṛshṭa-wound: The pain has to be relieved by means of applications of yashṭi-madhu, etc., and the wound has to be dusted with powders (of śāla, sarja, arjuna, etc.,).

In cases of dislocation, the patient should be kept immersed in a tub full of oil, and should be made to partake of meat-juices.

Medicated ghee that has been mentioned in the treatment of pittaja-vidradhi can be used in wounds.

Wounds should be immediately washed with warm ghee, or oil or balā-taila.

Drugs that are astringent, sweet, cold and unctuous should be used for a week, (SS).

2. External wounds should be treated by application of medicated pastes and by anti-toxic measures. If these measures fail to cure the sadyo-vraṇa, the patient is to be treated as indicated in śārīra-vraṇa, depending on which dosha is mainly aggravated, (CS, SS).

3. Immediately after the injury, when there is severe pain, the affected part should be sprinkled with warm ghee medicated with madhu-yashṭi or by balā-taila. In order to decrease or arrest the rise in body heat at that area, it can be plastered or washed with substances that are astringent, cold, sweet and unctuous.

For promoting the healing of wounds, the part can be anointed with a paste of honey and ghee; or any cold drugs that alleviate pitta. In cases where there is inflammation and swelling (saṃrambha), the patient should be subjected to emesis, purgation, fasting and bloodletting, and should be asked to partake of proper food.

The above measures are especially useful in ghṛhta and vidalita wounds where there is less bleeding and rapid inflammation (pāka).

In all other types of injuries, there is excessive bleeding, which leads to aggravation of vāta, which in turn causes severe pain. In such cases, drugs and substances that alleviate vāta should be used for sneha-pāna (internal administration of unctuous substances), affusions, fomentation, plasters, poultices and sneha-basti.

These measures have to be continued for seven days. If the injury has not healed, measures useful in śārīra-vraṇa are to be employed, (AHṛ).

4. The wound can be washed with the leaf-juice of apāmārga, which acts as a styptic. The paste of musta with ghee (preferably śata-dhouta ghee) is also very useful. In cases of injuries by instruments, the wound has to be plastered with karpūra and cow's ghee (preferably śata-dhouta ghee). The juices of śarapunkha, kākajangha or lājjalu are also useful in promoting healing of wounds.

A person suffering from injuries in the koshṭha (thoraco-abdominal cavity) should be administered a decoction of vamśalochana, eraṇḍa, gokshūra, dālchini, pāshaṇa-bheda, rock-salt, and hingu, which will help in the discharge of blood that is accumulated within, (CD).

Related Diseases: Śarīra-vraṇa

Ref.: SS, chikitsā, 1, 4; 2; CS, chikitsā, 25, 8; AHṛ, uttara, 26, 6-13, CD, 44, 50-64.

Sanniruddha-guda

Synonyms: Sanskrit: Baddha-guda (CD, 55, 39).

Western Nosology: Anorectal stricture

Causative Factors:

Extrinsic: Suppression of natural urges and all factors which aggravate vāta.

Intrinsic: Vāta

Symptomatology: The aggravated vāta localises in the rectal region and constricts the rectal passage, due to which the stools are passed with difficulty.

Prognosis: This is difficult to cure.

Treatment: The patient can be treated as in a case of niruddha-prakāśa. The appliance sanniruddha-guda-yantra can be used for gradually enlarging the constricted passage.

Ref.: SS, nidāna, 13, 55-56; chikitsa, 20, 47; sūtra, 7, 13.

Sanyāsa

Western Nosology: Coma

Casuative Factors:

Extrinsic: Improper food habits and daily regimen, and errors of judgement in a person whose mind is over come by rajas (passion) and moha (ignorance), (CS).

Intrinsic: All three doshas, (CS, SS).

Pathogenesis: The disturbed doshas, either individually or combined affect the channels which convey blood, rasa (nutrient fluid) and cognition and thereby cause total loss of consciousness, (CS).

Symptomatology: Absolute unconsciousness where the person becomes like a log of wood which leads to death unless treated early, (CS, SS).

Prognosis: Difficult to cure, (SS, CS). The presence of flatulent distension, salivation and dyspnoea render the case incurable, (SS).

Treatment:

1. The treatment should be begun at the very earliest. The following measures are to be employed: application of medicated collyrium, the avapīḍa and pradhamana kinds of errhines, fumigation (dhūma), pricking the body with needles, application of heat, causing pain in the nail bed, plucking the hairs from the head and body, biting the patient, rubbing the body with the fruits of ātmagupta, etc.

Very strong alcoholic drinks mixed with pungent drugs should be frequently fed to the patient. The juice of mātulunga with nāgara, or wine or sour kānji with souvarchala salt or with hingu and trikaṭu should also be administered until the patient regains consciousness.

After the patient regains consciousness, he should be made to partake of food that is easily digested. He should then be exposed to music, pleasing words, to words and action that stimulate his memory, pleasant scenes, etc. He should be then given purgation, emesis, fumigation, collyrium, medicated gargles bloodletting and massage. He should be made to exercise, (CS).

2. Treatment should be started immediately. The following measures are to be employed: strong collyriums, massage, fumigation, pricking needles into the nail bed, instrumental and vocal music, pleasant words, roughly shaking the patient, rubbing the fruits of ātmagupta on the body, etc.

After the patient regains consciousness, he should partake of food that is easy to digest. He should be administered strong purgatives and emetics.

He should be administered śilājatu with triphala, chitraka, nāgara and sugar continuously for a month. Old ghee is particularly useful, (SS).

Related Diseases: Mada, Mūrccha

Ref.: CS, sūtra, 24, 25-27, 42-53; SS, uttara, 46, 20-24; AS, nidāna, 6, 36.

Sirā-graha

Causative Factors:

Extrinsic: All factors that aggravate vāta

Intrinsic: Vāta

Constituents Affected: Blood

Pathogenesis and Symptomatology: The aggravated vāta affects the blood (and its channels) and causes dryness, blackish discolouration and pain in the blood vessels situated on the neck.

Prognosis: This is considered to be incurable.

Ref.: AS, nidāna, 15.

Śiro-roga

Western Nosology: Headache

Causative Factors:

Extrinsic: Suppression of the natural urges, loss of sleep during the night, sleeping during the day-time, intoxication, speaking loudly (or in a shrill tone), exposure to frost and wind, excessive sexual intercourse, exposure to strong, unpleasant smells, dust, smoke, dew and the sun, drinking excess of cold water, excessive intake of food that is hard to digest and sour, and of rhizomes, head injury, production of āma (undigested food), excassive weeping, forcibly suppressing tears, mental stress, cloudy weather, and seasonal variations (or failure to adapt to the weather, or follow the correct regimen). These are the common causes for diseases of the head.

The particular causative factors responsible for diseases of the head caused by vāta are: speaking too much and too loudly, loss of sleep, indulgence in pungent alcoholic drinks, exposure to cold winds, suppression of the natural urges, excessive sexual intercourse, fasting, head-injury, excessive emesis or purgation, lifting or carrying heavy loads, excessive weeping, grief, fear and anxiety and excessive walking (or exertion).

The causes responsible for head diseases caused by pitta are: anger, intake of food that is pungent, sour, salty and alkaline (kshāra), alcoholic drinks, and exposure to sun and fire.

The causes of diseases of the head caused by kapha are: a sedentary and luxurious life style, excess of sleeping, intake of food that is unctuous and hard to digest and over-eating.

The intake of tila, milk, and jaggery, and stale and unwholesome food, and eating before the digestion of the previous meal will further aggravate the vitiation of doshas in a person who is already sick, and brings about krimija type of head disease.

Intrinsic: All three doshas.

Types:

1. There are five diseases of the head i.e., those caused by the vitiation of each of the three doshas, by the derangement of all the doshas and that caused by krimi, (CS, sūtra, 19, 4).

2. There are eleven diseases of the head. They are the diseases caused by vāta, pitta and kapha, by all three doshas combined, by vitiated blood, caused as a result of kshaya (rāja-yakshma or emaciation), or due to worms (krimi), and the four types known as sūryāvarta, ananta-vāta, ardhāvabhedaka and śankhaka, (SS).

Pathogenesis and Symptomatology: The aggravated doshas vitiate the blood which courses through the head and engenders diseases of the head, (CS).

Vātaja-Śiro-roga:

1. Pricking pain in the temples, tearing pain in the nape of the neck, severe pain and burning in the forehead and between the eye brows, pain in the ears, tinnitus aurium, a sensation as if the eyes are being torn out, and the head is whirling around, a dislocated feeling in all the joints, throbbing or pulsation of the blood vessels and stiffness of the neck. There is amelioration from unctuous and hot substances, (CS).

2. There is pain which occurs without any tangible cause, which is worse at night, and with relief from heat and pressure (bandaging), (SS).

Pittaja-Śiro-roga:

1. Burning and aching pain in the head, burning of the eyes, thirst, vertigo, sweating and craving for cold, (CS).

2. The head feels as if it is stuffed with burning coal, there is burning of the eyes and nose, and relief at night and from cold, (SS).

Kaphaja-śiro-roga:

1. Dull pain and numbness in the head, a sensation as if the head is wrapped in a wet cloth, heaviness of the head, lethargy, drowsiness and loss of taste, (CS).

2. Heaviness of the head, swelling around the eyes and face, dull aching pain in the head, and a sensation as if the head is full of cold water, and as if the head and throat are stuffed with mucus, (SS).

Tridoshaja-śiro-roga:

1. In head-diseases caused by all the doshas, there is pain, tremors and vertigo (caused by vāta), burning pain, thirst and a feeling of intoxication (due to vitiated pitta) and heaviness of the head and lethargy (due to deranged kapha), (CS).

2. There will be symptoms that are characteristic of derangement of all three doshas, (SS).

Krimija-śiro-roga:

1. This diseases which is caused by krimi is associated with serious symptoms. There will be stabbing and cutting pain, itching, swelling, foul odour, and at times, the organisms even show themselves, (SS).

2. There is pricking and bursting pain, a feeling as if the contents of the head are being eaten up, discharge of water and blood from the nose, and such other serious symptoms, (CS).

Raktaja-śiro-roga: This type of headache is caused by the depletion of kapha and the fatty tissues all over the body, or due to trauma, and usually precedes rāja-yakshma. There will be severe pain which increases even after fomentation, vomiting, fumigation, errhine therapy and blood letting, (SS).

Sūryāvarta: There will be deep seated pain around the eyes and eyebrows which is mild in the morning (at sun-rise), increases as the day progresses and subsides after sun-set. It sometimes reduces with heat and at other times with cold. It is caused by the derangement of all three doshas, (SS).

Ananta-vāta: There is severe pain in the region of the neck, and occipital region, which extends forwards to the region of the eyebrows and temples, throbbing in the cheeks, lock-jaw and eye diseases. It is caused by vitiation of all three doshas, (SS).

Ardhā vabhedaka:

1. There is intensive pricking and tearing in one half of the head, and vertigo. The pain recurs periodically, or once in a fortnight or once in ten days. This is also caused by the vitiation of all three doshas, (SS).

2. There is severe semi-lateral headache, with severe pain in the neck, eyebrows, temples, ears, eyes and forehead. The disease, if untreated, may damage the faculties of vision and hearing. There may also be burning pain. The disease may be caused by vāta alone or combined with kapha, (MN).

Sankhata:

1. The deranged vāta along with the vitiated kapha, pitta and blood causes severe pain in the head and especially in the temples, (SS).

2. There is severe pain, burning sensation, redness and swelling in the temples. The swelling spreads all over the head and throat, (MN).

Prognosis:

1. The diseases known as kshayaja-śiro-roga, krimija-śiro-roga, sūryāvarta and śankhaka are all very difficult to cure, (SS).

2. The disease known as śankhata usually proves to be fatal in three days. If however the patient survives for three days, he can be cured, (MN).

Ref.: CS. sūtra, 17, 8-29; chikistā, 26, 118; SS, uttara, 25, 2-18; MN, 60, 1-15.

Treatment:

1. The patient suffering from vātaja-śiro-roga is subjected to oleation, fomentation and errhine therapy, and is administered drugs and advised food that alleviates vāta. Poultices composed of drugs that alleviate vāta can also be used.

The flesh of fish and other animals and drugs belonging to the jīvanīya group are fried in oil, and used when luke-warm, as poultices (upanāha). Milk medicated with rāsna, sthirā (śālaparni), etc., is used as nasal drops. Oil medicated with rāsna, kākoli, kshīra-kākoli and sugar, or with bala, madhūka, yashṭi-madhu, vidāri, chandana and utpala or with jīvaka, ṛshabhaka, drāksha and śarkara, is boiled along with milk and meat juices of desert animals. This oil can be used for errhine therapy. The medicinal ghee known as mayūra-ghṛta is very useful (for internal use). Another medicinal ghee known as mahā-mayūra-ghṛta is also used for errhine therapy, massage and internal use. Ghee medicated with the meat of ākhu, kukkuṭa, hamsa (swan) and śaśa (rabbit) is also useful in vātaja-śiro-roga.

The measures useful in pittaja-śiro-roga are application and sprinkling of cold drugs, errhine therapy, drugs that belong to the jīvanīya group, and internal and external use of milk, or ghee, and other drugs that alleviate pitta. External application of milk or ghee medicated with chandana, uśīra, yashṭi-madhu, balā, kaṇṭakāri, utpala, etc. Ghee medicated with dālchini, tamala-patra, sugar and rice-water can be used for avapīḍa-nasya. Ghee medicated with yashṭi-madhu, chandana, sāriva and milk or with sugar, drāksha and madhūka can also be used for errhine therapy, (nāvana).

The patient suffering from kaphaja-śiro-roga is subjected to fomentation, fumigation, nasal drops, pradhamana kind of errhines, and external and internal use of drugs that alleviate kapha. Old ghee can be used internally, and enema of tīkshṇa (active) drugs can also be given.

The patient suffering from burning pain caused by the vitiation of kapha and vāta can be subjected to bloodletting. Fumigation with drugs such as eraṇḍa, nalada, wool, guggulu, agaru, and chandana, or kushṭha, tagara, etc., is also useful.

Errhine therapy using active drugs is very useful in krimija-śiro-roga. The decoction or powder of tvak, danti, kaṇṭakāri, karanja, viḍanga, navamālika, fruits of apāmarga, seeds of nakta-māla and śirīsha, kshavaka, aśmantaka, bilva, haridra, hingu and yūthika can be used as nasal drops and for pradhamana type of errhines respectively. The avapīḍa kind of errhine with the fruits of śigru and karanja and trikaṭu, and gargling with the decoction of śukta, tiktaka, honey, etc., are also useful, (CS).

2. In vātaja-śiro-roga, the patient is treated along the same lines as in vāta-roga. The patient can partake of mudga kulattha and māsha, without being mixed with other substances, as well as pungent and hot drugs mixed with ghee, followed by milk. These should be eaten only at night. Til oil with milk or the paste of tila seeds with milk can also be eaten. The head should be washed or sprinkled with warm milk medicated with drugs that alleviate vāta. A warm plaster composed of the same drugs boiled with milk can be applied externally. A plaster of a paste of boiled flesh or fish or with kṛśara (gruel prepared from māsha, tila and rice) and rock-salt, or with the paste of chandana, utpala, kushṭha and pippali. After the patient has been oleated, oil medicated with kulira (crabs) is used for nasya therapy.

Milk diluted with half its quantity of water is to be boiled with drugs of varuṇādi group, and taken down from the fire after the evaporation of the water content. Ghee extracted from this milk is again medicated with drugs of the kākolyādi group. This ghee is very efficacious when used as a nasya in vātaja-śiro-roga. The ghee extracted from milk (which has been boiled with drugs of the varūṇādi group) can be used internally with sugar. Balā taila and traivṛta ghee can be used internally, for massage, as nasya, for sprinkling and for administering enema. The diet has to consist of milk, medicated with drugs that alleviate vāta and unctuous meat-juices.

The measures useful in pittaja and raktaja-śiro-roga are sprinkling of cold drugs, such as milk, sugar cane juice, dhānyāmla, honey, sugar water, etc., and application of drugs saturated with ghee. The paste of nala, vetasa, raktotpala, chandana, nilotpala, padma, vamśa, śaivala, yashṭi-madhu, mustā, etc., with ghee can be applied externally. Drugs belonging to the kākolyadi group can be used as plasters, and ghee medicated with these drugs can be used as nasya. Ghee extracted from milk, fat of desert animals is used as nāsya. The patient can also be administered āsthāpana enema and sneha-basti. Milk medicated with drugs of the utpalādi group can be used for asthāpana basti. The diet has to consist of meat-juices of desert animals, ghee, ghee extracted from milk and medicated with drugs of kākolyādi group, sugar, etc.

The measures useful in kaphaja-śiro-roga are: strong gaṇḍūsha, emesis, śiro-virechana, etc. The patient should be given potions of pure ghee, and should be frequently subjected to fomentation. Oily substances, extract of heart wood of madhūka can be used for śiro-virechana. The barks of ingudi or mesha-sṛngi can be used for the same purpose.

The above mentioned barks can also be used for smoking of fumigation. The powder of kaṭphala can be used as snuff. Drugs that alleviate kapha should be used for gargling. The paste of sarala, kushṭha, śārngeshṭa, deva dāru, rohisha, salt and alkaline water (kshārodaka), can be applied externally. The diet can consist of yavā, rice harvested in sixty days, trikaṭu, yava-kshāra, paṭola, kulattha and mudga (soup), etc.

The internal use of old ghee is very useful in tridosha-śiro-roga.

The patient suffering from kshayaja-śiro-roga should be given nourishing drugs and food. Ghee medicated with drugs that alleviate vāta, and that which belongs to kākolyādi group can be used both for internal use and as nasya. Any medicated ghee that is useful in kshaya-kāsa is useful in this disease also.

In a case of krimija-śiro-roga, the patient is administered nasya of animal blood. The worms would be attracted and intoxiciated by blood and would come down where they can be (manually) extracted. The seeds of small variety of śigru, kāmsya and nīla can be used for śiro-virechana. Drugs that are vermicidal (like viḍanga) can be mixed with cow's urine and used for avapiḍa nasya. The diet that is indicated in krimi-roga is to be partaken of.

The sūryāvarta kind of headache should be treated with errhines, etc. The diet has to consist of boiled rice, milk, ghee and meat-juices of desert animals.

The measures useful in ardhāvabhedaka type of headache are: avapīḍa nasya of sirīsha and seeds (fruits) of mūlaka, or of bamboo root and camphor or of vachā and pippali, or of yashṭi-madhu and honey or of manahśila or of chandana and honey, is to be followed by nasya of ghee medicated with drugs of kākolyādi group. The paste of sāriva, utpala, kushṭha, yashṭi-madhu, kānji, oil and ghee can be applied externally. This can be used even in kaphaja-śiro-roga.

The above measures are useful in sūryāvarta type of headache also.

The patient suffering from ananta-vāta is to be treated along the same lines as sūryāvarta. Bloodletting by vensection is beneficial. The diet has to consist of drugs and food that alleviate vāta and pitta, madhu-mastaka, sanyāva, ghṛta-pūra, etc.

In śankhaka type of head disease, ghee extracted from milk is used both internally and for nasya. The diet should comprise of unctuous food and unctuous meat-juices of desert animals. The paste of śatāvari, black tila seeds, yashṭi-madhu, nilotpala, dūrva and punarnava or of mahāsugandha (utpala-sāriva) or of palindi and kānji can be applied over the affected area. Cooling washes and applications, and avapīda-nasya used in sūryāvarta are also useful.

In all cases of śiro-roga, excepting krimija and kshaya types, strong śiro-virechana drugs mixed with honey and oil should be administered. This should be followed by nasya of mustard oil.

If the above therapeutic measures fail, the patient should be subjected to bloodletting after oleation and fomentation, (SS).

3. In vātaja-śiro-roga, the paste of kushṭha, root of eranḍa and kānji or paste of flowers of muchukunda can be applied externally. Milk medicated with drugs of panchamūla group can be used for nasya.

The procedure known as śiro-basti which is very useful in vātaja-śiro-roga is now described: A strip of leather which is eight finger-breadth wide is bound on top of the head, and the joints can be sealed with the paste of māsha. The basin-like hollow on top of the head (which is enclosed on all sides by the leather) is filled with warm oil. The oil can be allowed to remain there for 1, 1 1/2 or 3 hours. According to some authorities, the oil should be allowed to remain for 500 mātras in kaphaja-śiro-roga, 800 mātras in pittaja-śiro-roga and 1000 mātras in vātaja-śiro-roga.

In pittaja-śiro-roga, the patient can be administered a purgative composed of triphala, mṛdvīka, sugar cane root, or a decoction of these drugs with milk and ghee etc. Application of a paste of śata-dhouta-ghṛta relieves the burning pain. The paste of the lotus stalk, lotus root, śāluka, chandana, utpala and kesara or of āmalaki and nilotpala can be applied along with some unctuous substances.

The measures useful in kaphaja-śiro-roga include fasting, fomentation (svedana),drugs that are dry, hot and digestive, strong avapīḍa-nasya, fumigation, gargling with hot and active drugs etc. The paste of pippali, musta, nāgara, yashṭi-madhu, śatapushpa, utpala, kushṭha and water is very useful (when used externally). The paste of devadāru, tagara, kushṭha, jaṭāmamsi, nāgara, and kānji is also useful (when applied externally).

The nasya of a decoction of trikaṭu, pushkara, haridra, rasna, devadāru, and aśvagandha, or of powders of nāgara mixed with milk is also efficacious (in tridoshaja-śiro-roga).

In krimija-śiro-roga, the patient is administered nasya of trikaṭu, karanja, seeds of śigru and goat's urine, or of oil medicated with seeds of apāmārga, trikaṭu, haridra, kshavaka, hingu, viḍanga and cow's urine.

The nasya of sugar and kunkuma, which are both fried in ghee is very useful in all varieties of head-diseases.

The nasya of expressed juices of tender leaves of āragvadha, mixed with fresh butter and seeds of apāmarga is useful in sūryāvarta. The decoction of daśamūla drugs mixed with ghee and rock-salt is also used as nasya in ardhāvabhedaka and sūryāvarta. The decoction of daśamūla drugs mixed with ghee and rock-salt is also used as nasya in ardhāvabhedaka and sūryāvarta. Avapīḍa nasya with (juice of) vachā and pippali or of sirīsha and mūlaka is useful in sūryāvarta. Poultices composed of meat of desert animals can be applied in sūryāvarta and ardhāvabhedaka. The paste of sāriva, utpala, kushṭha, yashṭi-madhu, kānji, honey and ghee is useful in sūryāvarta and ardhāvabhedaka (for external use).

The measures useful in anantavāta are: draughts of milk with sugar, or coconut water with sugar, nasya of cold ghee or cold water; venesection; the measures useful in sūryavarta; food articles that alleviate vāta and pitta, etc.

In śankhaka, the patient is given nasya of ghee extracted from milk, (CD).

4. The nasya (errhines) of a decoction of juice of fruit and root of giri-karṇika, or a paste of jaggery, seeds of karanja and hot water is used in ardhāvabhedaka. The paste of maricha and juice of bhṛngarāja is useful in relieving head-diseases (when applied externally).

Equal parts of rasa-sindūra, abhraka bhasma, tīkshna-loha-bhasma, kānta-bhasma and tāmra are triturated together with the juice of snuhi for 24 hours. This has to be administered for a week, in sūryāvarta and other head-diseases. The paste of maricha and juice of śigru leaves is used as nasya in ardhāvabhedaka. The paste of juice of kumkuma and honey is useful in head-diseases, (RRS).

Classical Prescriptions: Asaṇa-bilvādi-taila; Balā-dhātryādi-taila; Bhṛngarāja-taila; Mṛdvīkārishṭa; Rāsnādi-chūrṇa; Shaḍ-bindu-taila; Triphalādi-taila, Tunga-drumādi-taila.

Sirogata-vāta: Nārāyana-taila.

Siro-ruja: Balā-dhāthryadi-taila; Godanti-bhasma; Kāyyonnyādi-taila; Manjishthādi-taila.

Vātaja-siro-roga: Kaccūradi-chūrṇa.

Siro-dāha: Balā-dhātryadi-taila

Ref.: CS, chikitsā, 26, 158-186; SS, uttara, 26; CD, 57; RRS, 24, 72-78.

Sīrshāmbu-roga

Causative Factors:

Extrinsic: Excessive indulgence in alcoholic drinks, intake of incompatible food, impure water, exposure to intense cold, and head-injury.

Intrinsic: Vāta

Pathogenesis: The deranged vāta causes gradual accumulation of water in the brain.

Prodromal Symptoms: Excessive sleepiness, weakness, defaecation of very hard stools, foul odour of breath and a coated tongue.

Symptomatology: Severe headache, defaecation of black stools, scanty urine, acuteness of hearing and vision, rapid pulse, dryness and burning of the skin, vomiting, deformity of the inner cavity of the eye, discolouration of face, grinding of teeth during sleep, itching of the lips, reddish discolouration of eyes, flapping of the wings of the nose, paralysis (pakshāghāta) and incoherent speech.

Prognosis: Difficult to cure.

Treatment: The patient should be administered medicines which are purgative, diuretic and cleanse the blood.

The head should be carefully shaved, and covered with a cloth previously soaked in hot water. The juice of coconut should be given to drink frequently. Small doses of rasa-sindūra should be administered.

The decoction of revatchini, kachora, śyāma, trivṛt, harītaki, āmalaki, sāriva, dhānyaka, yashti-madhu, kaṭuki, mustā, haridra, dāru-haridra, dālchini, ela and teja-patra should be administered with yavakshāra.

Equal quantities of rasa-sindūra, yava-kshāra, revatchini, ela, dālchini, teja-patra, bhārngi, harītaki and indravāruṇi should be given with milk.

Ghee medicated with kumkuma, sāriva, drāksha, jīvanti, harītaki, viḍa (salt), teja-patra and root of paṭola is also very useful in this disease and all other diseases of the head.

If these therapeutic measures fail to produce any improvement, the patient should be referred to a good surgeon who will remove the excess accumulation of water.

The patient should partake of food that is easy to digest and nourishing.

The prescriptions named rasa-taila and vahnībhāskara-rasa are also useful.

Ref.: BR, pages. 189-190.

Śīta-pitta

Western Nosology: Urticaria

Causative Factors:

Extrnsic: Exposure to cold winds.

Intrinsic: All three doshas, particularly pitta, (MN).

All three doshas but predominantly vāta, (CSS).

Prodromal Symptoms: Thirst, tastelessness, nausea, debility, heaviness of body, reddish discolouration of eyes.

Symptomatology: Swelling confined to the outer regions of the skin, similar to that produced by the sting of a wasp, with itching, pricking pain, vomiting, fever and a sensation of heat.

Related Diseases: Udarda, Koṭha

Note: Udarda which is very similar to śīta-pitta is caused by the provocation of kapha. The swelling is reddish in colour, has a depression at its center, and is usually circular in shape. Itching is also present.

Ref.: MN, 50, 1-5; CSS, page, 621.

Treatment:

1. The patient can be subjected to emesis by administering the decoction of paṭola, vāsa and nimba, and purgation by administering the decoction of triphala, pippali and purified guggulu.

The following formulations are useful: the decoction of triphala with honey; decoctions which are useful in visarpa; the paste of āmalaki, jaggery, trikaṭu and sugar, the decoction of yavāni with yava-kshāra and trikaṭu; the paste of dīpyaka with jaggery, which should be taken for a week; the paste of fresh ginger with old jaggery; the fruits of kāśmari which has to be boiled in milk and given; and mahā-tiktaka ghṛta.

The paste of siddhārta, haridra, tila seeds, prapunnāṭa and kaṭu-taila can be used for external application, (CSS).

2. The patient is made to vomit by administering the decoction of leaves of paṭola and bark of nimba. The body is to be massaged with kaṭutaila, and washed with hot water. The paste of dūrva and haridra, can be applied over the affected area.

The root of agnimantha is made into a paste with ghee and administered (internally) for seven days. This is very efficacious.

In śīta-pitta, the patient is to be massaged with the paste of til oil, rock-salt and yava-kshāra. The paste of dried ripe fruits of kāśmari can also be used. The diet has to predominantly consist of milk. The soup of dried mūlaka and juice of kulattha, and meat juices of lāva and tittiri is also to be eaten regularly, (CD).

Ref.: CSS, page, 621-622; CD, 51, 1-12.

Classical Prescription: Haridrā-khaṇḍa

Śīta-vāta

Causative Factors:

Extrinsic: All factors that aggravate vāta.

Intrinsic: Vāta

Symptomatology: Coldness of limbs, formication, throbbing or tremors, headache, pain in the eyes and lethargy.

Ref.: RRS, 21,2.

Treatment: The patient should be treated as in vāta-roga.

Ślīpada

Synonyms: Vernacular: Hasti-pāda (Madhu-kośa, MN). Pāda-valmīka (Kaiyadeva, 8, 261).

Western Nosology: Elephantiasis

Causative Factors:

Extrinsic:

1. This disease is common in damp and cold places and in areas where there are lakes, ponds and rivers, (SS; Ahṛ, sūtra, 5, 10).

2. The rivers originating from the Pāriyātra (Western Vindhya ranges), Vindhyā and Sahyādri ranges are unhealthy, and give rise to this disease, (CS, sūtra, 27, 212).

Intrinsic: All three doshas particularly kapha (SS); kapha (CS).

Constituents Affected: The sixth layer of the skin, rohiṇi (stratum reticular) (SS, śārīra, 4, 4); blood and flesh (CS); and muscular and fatty tissue (paushkalāvata, Chkp. On CS).

Pathogenesis and Symptomatology:

1. The deranged doshas move downwards, and localize in the groin, thigh, knee and leg, and gradually gives rise to swelling around the feet.

The symptoms differ according to the predominant dosha involved. In slīpada caused by deranged vāta, the swelling is rough, blackish in colour, hard and uneven, and begins to crack or burst. There will be pricking pain in the affected area.

In ślīpada engendered by aggravated pitta, the swelling is yellowish in colour and slightly soft. There will be fever and burning pain (in the affected area).

In ślīpada brought about by the vitiated kapha, the swelling will be white, unctuous (or oily), slightly painful, and will appear like a big knotty growth with small thorn-like projections and will feel heavy.

A few authorities claim that a similar swelling can occur even around the hands, ear, eyes, nose and lips, (SS).

2. Swelling localised in the regions of leg (jangha), calf and fore-foot (prapāda), (CS).

3. A similar swelling can occur around the neck, groins, leg, lips, ears, and hands. (Paushkalāvata, Chkp. On CS).

Prognosis:

1. Patients who have suffered from the disease for more than one year, in whom the swelling is very large, resembling a big ant-hill with many pores and proliferations are incurable, (SS).

2. Those cases of ślīpada which are caused by aggravated kapha, with exudation, in a person who has a kapha constitution, and who is accustomed to food and regimen that aggravate kapha, and those cases characterized by all symptoms are incurable, (MN).

Ref.: SS, nidāna, 12, 10-15; CS, chikitsā, 12, 98; AS, uttara. 34; MN 39, 7.

Treatment:

1. In ślīpada caused by aggravated vāta, the affected area is massaged or rubbed with oil or ghee and fomented. Later, the veins situated at a distance of four finger breadths above the ankle should be opened.

After the patient has been restored to his original state of health, he should be given (āsthāpana type of) enema. He should be administered (internally), for a month, castor oil mixed with cow's urine. The diet should mainly consist of rice with milk that has been medicated with nāgara (ginger). Traivṛta ghṛta can also be used. Cauterization with fire can also be employed.

In a case of ślīpada engendered by deranged pitta, the vein situated below the ankle should be opened. The other measures useful in this disease are those described under pitta-roga, visarpa and pittaja arbuda.

In a case of ślīpada caused by vitiated kapha, the surgeon should open the vein of the first toe. The patient can be administered (internally) decoctions of drugs that alleviate kapha, with honey, or the paste of harītaki and cow's urine. The paste of kaṭuka, guḍūchi, nāgara, viḍanga, deva-dāru and chitraka or of chitraka and deva-dāru should be applied over the affected area. Til oil medicated with viḍanga, maricha, arka, nāgara, chitraka, deva-dāru, elavāluka and the five salts should be given internally. The diet should mainly consist of cooked barley.

The other formulations useful in ślīpada are: mustard oil; the expressed juice of pūti-karanja; the expressed juice of putranjīva; the above-mentioned juices along with kevuka and biḍa salt; alkaline water (kshāra-kalpa) prepared from the ashes of kākādani, kākajangha, bṛhati, kanṭakāri, flowers of kadamba, mandāri, kaṭukālābu and śukanāsa with cow's urine; and the expressed juices of kakodumbarika and śukanāsa and the decoction of madana fruit with cow's urine; etc.

The ashes of dravanti, trivṛt, danti, nīli, vṛddha-dāru, saptala and śankhini should be dissolved in cow's urine and boiled with the decoction of triphala. This will also be efficacious in ślīpada (when taken internally).

Oils medicated with the above drugs (i.e. kākādani, etc., can be used for massage and as nasal drops, (SS).

2. The remedial measures useful in the disease are drugs and a regimen that alleviate kapha, bloodletting, and external application of paste of sarshapa (mustard), (CS).

3. The patient should be given emesis, and anuvāsana type of enema. The expressed juice of fresh ginger is useful when administered internally, (Ahṛ).

4. The general remedial measures are: fasting, application of medicinal plasters, fomentation, purgation, measures to alleviate kapha and bloodletting.

The following plasters (lepa) can be used for external application: the pastes of dhattūra, eranḍa, nirgunḍi, punarnava, śigru and sarshapa; the paste of root bark of white arka with kānji (sour gruel); the paste of chitraka or devadāru or sarshapa and śigru, with cow's urine; and the paste of majishṭha, yashṭi-madhu, rāsna, himsra, punarnava and kānji, in pittaja ślīpada.

The following prescriptions are to be administered internally: equal quantities of the powder of haridra and jaggery, with the anupāna of cow's urine; or the fruit-pulp of harītaki which should be fried in castor oil and administered for only a week with cow's urine; or a dish prepared from māsha and godhāvati root, which relieves the fever in slīpada; or the juice of guḍūchi and til oil which should be taken regularly (for a few months), etc., (CD).

5. Tāmra bhasma and purified pārada should be repeatedly separately triturated with the juice of nāgavalli, pāṭha, punarnava and tanḍulīyaka, seperately for three days each. The two masses are then triturated together with cow's urine, and subjected to heat in a chakra-yantra for twenty-four hours. This medicine is to be administered with honey for a month. The anupāna should consist of the paste of khadira-sāra, sallaki-sāra, asana with honey and cow's urine.

The paste of guḍūchi, kaṭuka, nāgara,

viḍanga and devadāru with cow's urine can be used externally.

Ref.: SS, chikitsā, 19, 52-69; CS, chikitsā, 12, 98; AHṛ, sūtra, 18, 2; 19, 9; 6, 165; CD, 42, 1-16; RRS, 25, 58-61.

Classical Prescriptions: Bṛhat-manjishṭhadi-kvātha-chūrṇa; Kānchanāra-guggulu; Rāsnadi-kvātha-chūrṇa; Śūla-vajriṇi-vaṭika; Sūraṇa-vaṭaka.

Snāyuka

Synonyms: Sanskrit: Tantu-roga (CSS, 62, 5-6; BP, chikitsā, 57, 8).

Western Nosology: Guinea-worm infestation.

Causative Factors:

Intrinsic: All three doshas.

Pathogenesis and Symptomatology: The vitiated doshas bring about a swelling in the limbs, which spreads like visarpa, and later bursts. The hard fibrous structures (snāyu) wither away, and thread-like, round, white-coloured worms emerge and gradually eat away into the surrounding areas. When these worms disappear, the swelling also subsides, but the worms emerge in a different area. If the worms are mistakenly cut into pieces, in the regions of the arms or legs, there will be contraction (sankocha) and lameness in the affected areas.

If vāta is predominantly affected, the swelling will be painful, dry and blackish in colour. If pitta is mainly involved it will be blue or yellow in colour, and attended by burning pain. If kapha is mainly vitiated, the swelling will be large and will feel heavy; if blood is excessively vitiated, the swelling will be reddish in colour.

Ref.: BP; MN, pariśishṭa.

Treatment:

1. The diseases is to be treated along the same lines as in visarpa, (MN, BR).

2. The affected area is to be smeared with medicated oils and ghee, fomented and plastered with the appropriate drugs (depending on the doshas involved), (BP).

3. The flowers of kumbhika are extremely efficacious (when given internally). The oil named asparśāri-vātari-taila is used externally, (RRS).

Ref.: BP; MN, ibid; RRS, 25, 55, 77.

Śotha

Synonyms: Sanskrit: Syayathu, Śopha

Western Nosology: Inflammation: swelling.

Classification:

1. Śotha may be either nija (endogenous) or āgantu (exogenous). The former kind (endogenous) may be caused by the vitiation of vāta, or pitta or kapha. The endogenous swellings are again of three types, the swelling that is generalised (affecting the whole body), or localised (affecting a particular part of the body) or affecting one half of the body (e.g., swelling of upper extremities or lower extremities), (CS).

2. Śotha is mainly of two kinds: that which is localised (avavaya-samuttha), (see vraṇa-śotha), and that which is generalised (sarvasara). The former kind of swellings (localised) are again of six types, those causes by the vitiation of vata, pitta, or kapha, or all three doshas or blood or by trauma. The latter (endogenous) swellings are of five types: swelling engendered by vitiated vāta, or pitta or kapha or all three doshas combined or caused by toxicosis (visha), (SS).

Causative Factors:

Extrinsic:

1. The exogenous swellings may be caused by excision, incision, injuries, fractures, excessive pressure, abrasions, assaults, etc., or through contact with the flowers and fruits of

bhallātaka, ātmagupta, bristles of insects, leaves of poisonous plants and creepers, or wine, sweat or mere contact with poisonous animals, bites or scratches of poisonous animals, burns, contact with snow, etc., (CS).

The endogenous swelling (nija-śotha) may be caused by improper administration of snehana (oleation), svedana (sudation), emesis, purgation, āsthāpana and anuvāsana types of enemata, śiro-virechana, etc., as a complication or concomitant of vomiting, alasaka, visūchika, dyspnoea, cough, diarrhoea, tuberculosis (śosha), pāṇḍu (anaemia), udara (ascites), fever, pradara (excessive bleeding from vagina), anal fistula, haemorrhoids, skin diseases, urticaria, etc., or due to suppression of vomiting, sneezing, eructations, ejaculation, flatus, urine and stools, due to weakness caused by fasting, or religious observances (karma), or walking for long distance, excessive intake of food that is hard to digest, sour, salty, of flour preparations, fruits, leafy vegetables, curds, alcoholic drinks, germinated grains, and meat of aquatic or fresh-water animals, eating mud, excessive use of salt, pressure by the foetus, due to abortion, improper regimen during puerperium, etc.

Endogenous swellings may also be caused by intake of toxic substances (gara-visha) incompatible food (viruddhāhāra), by inactivity and intake of caustics (kshāras), sour, hot, sharp and heavy food, and in persons who have become weak and emaciated due to eliminatory (śodhana) procedures, diseases or fasting, (CS).

2. Exertion by persons who have become emaciated (due to fasting, exertion, purificatory procedures, etc.,) excessive intake of flour preparations, greens, leafy vegetables and salt, excessive use of sour substances by emaciated persons, eating of mud, kaṭa-śarkara or meat of aquatic or fresh-water animals, sexual intercourse by a person suffering from ajīrna, intake of incompatible food, joltings from riding on animals, etc., (SS).

Pathogenesis:

1. The provoked vāta localises in the peripheral blood vessels (or nerves), vitiates the blood, kapha and pitta, is obstructed by them, diffuses and causes śotha.

When the doshas are localised in the upper part of the body, they cause śotha of the upper limbs. If they are localised in the regions of vāta, they engender swelling of the lower limbs. If the doshas are situated in the torso (middle of the body), swelling occurs in that region. If the doshas are localised in one limb, śotha of that limb occurs, (CS).

Prodromal Symptoms: Increased body temperature or heat, burning pain (davathu) and dilatation of blood-vessels (sirāṇām āyāmah), (CS).

General Symptoms: Swelling, a sense of heaviness (in the affected area), variability or changeableness, heat, thinning of blood vessels (sirā-tanutvam), discolouration of skin and horripilation, (CS).

Symptomatology:

I. Sarva-sara śotha (generalised swellings):

Vāta-śotha:

1. The swelling is either bluish, brown or skin coloured, appears and disappears rapidly, is variable, mobile, rough, dry and cracked, pits on pressure but immediately regains its normal shape when the pressure is removed, and there are symptoms like pulsation, numbness, amelioration of swelling during the night, formication (sensation as if ants are crawling on the affected area), tingling sensation and cutting, pressing and pricking pain. The swelling (and other symptoms) are relieved by pressure and oily and hot applications, (CS).

2. The swelling is brownish or blackish in colour, variable, soft and is attended by pricking, and other kinds of pain, (SS).

Pitta-śotha:

1. The swelling is blackish, yellow, blue or coppery in colour, is hot to touch, soft, tender, covered by tawny or coppery coloured hairs, appears and disappears rapidly, and commences from the middle portion of the body. There is burning pain, sloughing, offensive odour, sweating, yellow discolouration of the eyes, face and skin, thirst, fever, diarrhoea, vertigo, and a tendency to suppuration and aggravation from heat, (CS).

2. The swelling is yellowish or bloody, soft, rapid in growth, and is attended by various kinds of burning pains, (SS).

Kapha-śotha:

1. The swelling takes a long time both to appear and disappear, is pale-yellow or white in colour, is heavy, smooth, oily, firm, compact, covered with white hairs, not sensitive to pressure or heat, cold to touch, pits on pressure, itches, does not bleed even when incised, but oozes out a sticky fluid after a long time, and is aggravated at night. The patient also suffers from pāṇḍu (anaemia), loss of appetite, salivation, sleepiness, vomiting and weak digestion, (CS).

2. The swelling is pale-yellow or white in colour, oily, hard, cold, slow in spreading, and is attended by itching, (SS).

Sannipātaja-śotha:

The swelling caused by the aggravation of all the doshas has many of the symptoms and signs of all the three types described above, (SS).

Visha-nimitta-śotha:

This kind of swelling may occur as a result of internal and external use of toxic agents (garavisha), by making use of unclean or polluted water, by bathing in polluted water, by bathing in a polluted tank, etc., by dusting the body with powders that have come into contact with poisonous animals, or by contact with weeds and plants that have been poisoned by contact with urine, faeces or semen of poisonous animal, etc.

The swelling is soft, spreads or increases rapidly, is pendulous, may or may not spread to other parts of the body, and is attended by inflammation, suppuration and burning pain, (SS).

II. Avayava-samuttha-śotha (localised swellings):

1. The aggravated pitta localises in the parotid region after fever, and causes a swelling in that is very difficult to cure.

The other localised swellings are adhimāmsa, arbuda, pliha, tila-kālaka, vyanga, nīlika, śankhaka (see siro-roga), gulma, vṛddhi, udara, ānāha, visarpa, gala-gaṇḍa, upa-jihvaka (see mukha-roga), gala-śuṇḍika (see ibid), etc., (CS).

2. Localised swellings caused by vāta are blackish or brown in colour, rough, variable, and are attended by pricking and other kinds of pain causes by vāta.

Localised swellings caused by pitta are yellowish or bloody, soft, rapid in growth, and are attended by burning pain.

Localised swellings caused by kapha are pale yellow in colour, hard, oily, cold to the touch, slow in development and are attended by itching.

Localised swellings caused by all three doshas have all the signs and symptoms of the three types described above.

Localised swellings caused by vitiated blood are black in colour, and have all the symptoms seen in pitta-śotha.

Localized swelling caused by injury, are reddish in colour, and have symptoms that are seen in pittaja and raktaja-śotha, (see vraṇa-śotha), (SS).

Complications: Vomiting, difficulty in breathing, distaste for food, thirst, fever, diarrhoea and weakness, (CS).

Prognosis:

1. The swelling that commences in the perineal region and is accompanied by all the complications is very difficult to cure. The swelling that commences in the feet and spreads upwards all over the body in males, and which commences in the face in females, is also difficult to cure.

The swelling that occurs in a person debilitated and emaciated by disease, which affects the vital organs, which is covered over by prominent streaks (or ridges), from which discharge takes place, and which spreads all over the body, in a debilitated person is considered to be incurable.

The swelling that is caused by any one dosha, which is of recent onset, which occurs in a person who is strong and well-built (not emaciated) is easily curable, (CS).

2. The swelling that is generalised (occurs all over the body), and that which affects the middle part (trunk) of the body is curable with difficulty. The swelling that begins at the lower extremeities and spreads upwards is fatal (in males, according to NiS). A case of śotha that is accompanied by dyspnoea, thirst, weakness, fever, vomiting, aversion to food, hiccoughs, diarrhoea and cough is also fatal, (SS).

Related Disease: Vraṇa-śotha

Ref.: CS, sūtra, 18, 3-33; chikitsā, 12, 4-16; SS, sūtra, 17, 3-4; uttara, 23, 3-9.

Treatment:

1. The swelling engendered by āma (the undigested food) should be treated by fasting, and administration of digestive drugs. The swellings caused by excessively aggravated doshas should be treated by purificatory procedures (śodhana). Patents suffering from śotha of the head, lower limbs and upper extremities should be subjected to śiro-virechana (errhines), purgation ad emesis respectively. Śotha that is caused by excessive dryness or oilyness should be treated with measures that increase unctuousness or dryness respectively. Patients suffering from constipation along with vāta-śotha should be administered a nirūha type of enema, while those suffering from vāta and pitta śotha should be administered ghee medicated with bitter drugs. Cases of śotha with synocope, restlessness, burning pain and thirst, and which necessitate śodhana should be administered milk with cow's urine. Śotha engendered by kapha should be treated with alkalies (kshāras), and drugs that are pungent and hot mixed with butter-milk, wine or cow's urine.

A person suffering from śotha should avoid coitus, dry leafy vegetables, newly harvested rice, products of jaggery, flour preparations, curds, preparations of tila, alcoholic drinks, sour substances, dhāṇa (fried barley or rice), vallūra (dried flesh), intake of meat of aquatic, wet-land and domesticated animals, of food that is hard to digest, unwholesome and irritant (vidāhi), mixtures of wholesome and unwholesome food articles, and sleeping during the day.

Patients suffering from kapha-śotha may be administered the powder of trikaṭu, trivṛt, kaṭuka-rohiṇi, purified loha powder along with decoction of triphala, or powder of harītaki with cow's urine.

The powder of harītaki, ginger, devadāru and punarnava with cold water, or with cow's urine is useful in śotha caused by all the doshas. After the medicine has been digested, the patient may take a bath and partake of food mixed with milk.

A person suffering from vāta-śotha can be administered milk medicated with punarnava, ginger, and musta or milk medicated with mayūraka, pippali, pippali roots and ginger. Persons suffering from śotha caused by vāta and pitta should be administered milk medicated with danti, trivṛt, trikaṭu, and chitraka, or milk medicated with a decoction of deva-dāru and ginger or with śyāma, eraṇḍa, and maricha or with dālchini, deva-dārū, punarnava and ginger or with guḍūchi, ginger and danti. Alternatively, the patient may live on meat of camel or camel's milk for seven days, or on cow's milk with an equal amount of cow's urine or on buffalo's milk, or on cow's urine with milk of any other animals, while avoiding all other food and drinks. If the patient passes stools that are diarrhoeic and heavy, he can drink buttermilk medicated with honey, sourvarchala salt and trikaṭu. If the stools are undigested or loose or hard, the patient can be administered harītaki with jaggery or jaggery with ginger. In constipation and obstruction of flatus, castor-oil can be given with milk or meat-juices, before meals. Alocholic drinks like wine and arishṭa of good quality can be administered in cases of śotha with obstriction of channel, feeble digestion and loss of appetite.

A person suffering from śotha should be administered equal quantities of ārdraka (fresh ginger) or nāgara (dry ginger) and jaggery, in doses of two tolas. The dosage can be gradually increased over a month, until the patient takes twenty tolas. Every day, after the digestion of this medicine, the person can eat gruel, milk and meat-juices and boiled rice.

The juice of fresh ginger and (dry) ginger can be taken in a similar manner. After the digestion of each dose, food should be taken with milk.

The juice (or decoction) of triphala with śilājatu is very useful in tridoshaja śotha.

The decoction of paṭola roots, devadāru, danti, trāyanti, pippali, haritaki, visāla (indravāruṇi?), madhu-yashṭi, kaṭuka-rohini, chandana, nichuka and dāru-haridra should be administered with a kuḍava of ghee in cases of śotha. Ghee prepared with eight parts of water, chitraka and yava-kshāra is also very useful.

Cow's milk is stored in a vessel which is plastered internally with the paste of chitraka, and is converted into curds. The ghee extracted from this is very useful in śotha.

A gruel (yavāgu) prepared with jīvanti, ajāji, śaṭhi, pushkara-mūla, ajamoda, chitraka, pulp of bilva, yava-kshāra, and vṛkshāmala, fried with ghee and oil is very useful. Gruel medicated with the pancha-kola drugs is also beneficial. The patient can also partake of soup of kulattha with pippali, soup of mudga with yava-kshāra and trikaṭu, meat-juices of desert and vishkira, animals, meat of the tortoise, godha, śikhi, and śallaka, souvarchala salt, gṛnjanaka, paṭola, vetra, nimba, vāyasi, mūlaka, nimba and such other vegetables, and old barley and rice.

A person suffering from vāta-śotha can make use of oleation, affusions, applications and fomentations as external measures of treatment. The medicated oil known as śailayādi-taila can be used for external application. The patient can be fomentated using water that has been boiled with leaves of vāsa, arka, karanja, śigru, kāśmari and arjaka, and should bathe in water that has been heated by exposure to the sun. He should then anoint himself with aromatic drugs.

In pitta śotha, oil medicated with chandana, padmaka, bālaka, manjishṭa, lotus stalks, vetasa and barks of milky trees can be used for application. After applying this oil, the person can the bathe in water that has been heated by the sun rays, and has been medicated with chandana, uśīra and padmaka. The person can also bathe in milk, or a deoction of barks of milky trees, and can then apply the paste of chandana.

In kapha-śotha, oil medicated with pippali, sand (quartz), old oil-cake, bark of śigru and umā (linseed) can be used for application. The decoction of kulattha, nāgara and cow's urine can be used for affusion, while the paste of chaṇḍā and agaru can be applied.

A paste of the pulp of vibhītaka is useful in relieving burning and pain in all kinds of śotha. The paste of yashṭi-madhu, musta, leaves of kapittha and chandana can be applied in śotha with eruptions.

The formulations such as gaṇḍīra-arishṭa, ashṭa-śata-arishṭa, kshāra-gutika, punarnava-arishta, phala-trika-arishṭa, chitrakādi-ghṛta, kamsa-harītaki, pancha-gavya-ghṛta, mahā-tiktaka ghṛta, tiktaka-ghṛta etc., have also been recommended, (CS).

2. A person suffering from śotha should be asked to strictly avoid coitus, food that is sour, hard to digest and salty, curds, jaggery, milk, ghee, animal fat (vasā), and flour prepartions (pishṭa), sleep during day, alcoholic drinks, eating mud, and meat of animals other than desert animals.

A patient of vāta-śotha should be administered castor-oil or traivṛta for a fortnight or for a month. Those suffering from pitta-śotha should be administered ghee medicated with a decoction of drugs of the nyagrodhādi group. Ghee medicated with drugs of the āragvadhādi group should be administered in kapha-śotha. Ghee prepared from one āḍhaka of milky exudation of snuhi, twelve āḍhakas of kānji and (one-fourth the quantity of ghee) paste of danti and dravanti is to be administered in tridoshaja-śotha. The remedial measures useful in visha can be employed in śotha that has been engendered by visha.

The following prescriptions are generally useful in all the five varieties of śotha: the four types of medicated ghee ending with tilvaka-ghṛta which have been described in the treatment of udara; the daily use of the preparation known as navāyasa with honey; the powders of viḍanga, ativisha, kuṭaja-fruit, devadāru, ginger and maricha with hot water; the powders of trikaṭu, yava-kshāra and purified loha with a decoction of triphala; cow's urine with an equal quantity of milk; the paste of equal amount of harītaki and jaggery; the powder of devadāru and nāgara with warm water; guggulu with cow's urine or with a decoction of punarnava; sṛngavera (ginger) with an equal quantity of jaggery; the daily use of a month of a decoction of punarnava or paste of punarnava roots followed by milk medicated with ginger; ghee medicated with the decoction of punarnava and trikaṭu, with a diet consisting of mudga, boiled and fried; milk medicated with pippali, pippali roots, chavya, chitraka, apāmārga and punarnava; milk medicated with māshaparṇi, murangi (śobhānjana) roots and ginger, milk medicated with punarnava, ginger, devadāru and māshaparni; milk medicated with trikaṭu, eraṇḍa, and śyama roots; the paste of alābu and vibhītaka fruits with rice water, a diet of soup of mudga medicated with yava-kshāra, pippali, maricha and ginger, with only a little amount of unctuous substances, and without salt; with dishes prepared from barley or wheat; affusions (parisheka) with a decoction of vṛkshaka (kuṭaja), arka, karanja, nimba and punarnava; plasters (pradeha) composed of sarshapa, suvarchala salt, rock salt and kākajangha, etc.

A strong patient can be repeatedly subjected to emesis, purgation and āsthāpana enema, snehana (oleation), svedana (sudation), and bloodletting. Poultices can also be applied, (SS).

3. The formulations that are generally useful in generalised śotha are: the paste of sthala-padma and milk; the paste of nāgara and punarnava (with cow's urine); the decoction of vāsa (bark), guḍūchi and bhaṇṭāki (bṛhati?) with honey; the decoction of punarnava with the paste of bhūnimba and nāgara; the ash of kokilāksha with water or cow's urine; the milk medicated with devadāru, punarnava and nāgara; milk medicated with chitraka, trivṛt and devadāru; ghee boiled with the decoction of panchakola drugs and kulattha and paste of punarnava; ghee boiled with the decoction of dasamūla drugs and paste of nāgara; ghee medicated with a decoction and paste of mānakanda; milk boiled with sthala-padma and trikaṭu; the powder of jaggery, pippali and śuṇṭhi; the paste of guggulu with cow's urine; milk boiled with pippali; a paste of equal parts of harītaki and jaggery; a paste of jaggery and nāgara; the expressed juice of bilva-leaves with powder of maricha; guggulu with a decoction of daśamūla, or cow's urine or a decoction of punarnava, devadaru, and nāgara; the

expressed juice of ārdraka with old jaggery, a diet consisting of goat's milk; the decoction of punarnava, nimba, paṭola, nāgara, kaṭuki, guḍūchi, devadāru and harītaki; the powder of ajāji, pāṭha, musta, panchakola drugs; kaṇṭakāri, haridra, bhū-nimba and nāgara with warm water; and a decoction of harītaki, devadāru, yashṭi-madhu, kaṭuki, danti, pippali, paṭola, chandana, daru-haridra, trāyamāṇa and indra-vāruṇi.

Equal parts of jaggery and fresh ginger or jaggery and dry ginger or jaggery and harītaki or jaggery and pippali are taken in doses of one tola the first day, and gradually increased (by one tola) until a dose of twelve tolas are taken. It has then to be gradually decreased. This can be done for a fortnight or a month. It is especially useful in diseases caused by kapha and vāta.

The decoction of daśamūla drugs or of śuṇṭhi, punarnava, pancha-mūla drugs and eraṇḍa is very useful in vāta-śotha. The decoction of trivṛt, guḍūchi and triphala or powder of triphala mixed with cow's urine is very useful in pitta-śotha. The decoction of pṛshniparṇi, musta, udīcya and nāgara is also useful in pitta-śotha, (CD).

4. The external application of a paste of punarnava, vachā and dhānya is very useful in swelling in pregnant women.

The patient can be administered pārada bhasma with the decoction of nāgara, bhūnimba and cow's urine, and paste of nimba, āmalaka and kankushṭa, (RRS).

Ref.: CS, chikitsā, 12, 16-71; SS, chikitsā, 23, 10-13; CD, 39, 1-40; RRS, 83; 30, 46.

Classical Prescriptions:

Śotha: Ajamodādi-chūrṇa; Ardha-bilva-kvātha-churna; Avittolādi-bhasma; Chandana-balā-lākshādi-taila; Dantyārishṭa; Daśānga-lepa; Daśamūla-harītaki; Dhānvantara-ghṛta; Dugda-vaṭi; Gandharva-hasta-taila; Guḍa-pippali, Huta-bhugādi-chūrṇa; Kadalī-kshāra; Loha-bhasma; Lohāsava; Lokanātha-rasa; Mahā-panchagavya-ghṛta; Maṇḍūra-bhasma; Maṇḍūra-vaṭaka; Punarnavādi-maṇḍūra; Puṭapakva-vishama-jvarāntaka-lauha; Rasa-parpaṭi; Sapta-viṁśatika-guggulu; Śothaghna-lepa; Śukumśra-ghṛta; Śūla-vajriṇi-vaṭaka; Sūraṇa-vaṭaka; Sushka-mūlaka-taila; Svarṇa-bhūpati-rasa; Svarṇa-mākshika-bhasma; Tāmra-bhasma; Triphala-guggulu; Uśirāsava; Vajra-bhasma; Vajraka-kshāra; Vāri-soshaṇa-rasa; Vāsakāsava; Viḍanga-lauha; Viḍangādi-lauha.

Sarvānga-śotha: Punarnavādi-kvātha-chūrṇa; Punarnavāshṭaka-kvātha-chūrṇa.

Sparsā-vāta

Synonyms: Sanskrit: Supta-vāta

Causative Factors:

Extrinsic: Factors which aggravate vāta.

Intrinsic: Vāta

Symptomatology: Pricking pain all over the body, occasional burning pains, and appearance of circular anaesthetic patches on the skin.

Treatment: One karsha each of purified pārada, loha bhasma and purified hingula, one pala each of black abhraka bhasma, and powders of maricha and pippali, and two palas each of tāmra bhasma and purified gandhaka are to be taken and triturated in the usual manner, seven times each with juices of nimbūka, dhattūra, arka, vāsa, kupīlu and karavīra. The triturated bolus is then subjected to heat in a bāluka yantra for two days. This medicine if taken with one karsha of pippali powder and one nishka of purified vatsanābha powder is very useful in this disease.

Eight parts of rajata bhasma and purifed bhanga are triturated with one part of rasa-sindūra. This can then be administered with jaggery, in the morning. If this medicine is taken continuously for two months, it will relieve this disease.

The patient can also be administered a decoction of āragvadha, while its paste can be applied externally.

As an alternative measure, the powder of seeds of chakramarda can be taken with cow's urine. The paste of chakra-marda seeds, and milky exudation of arka and snuhi can be applied on the affected areas.

Eight parts of purified pārada and twelve parts of purified mercury are triturated with two parts of purified seeds of kupīlu, three parts of trikaṭu, three parts of triphala powder, one part each of purified bhallātaka powder, root powder of chitraka, mustā, kushṭha, root powder of pippali, nāgakesara, aśvagandha, reṇuka, purified vatsanābha, and twenty-four parts of jaggery. This medicine is very useful in sparśa-vāta.

Equal quantities of purified manahśila, haratāla and gandhaka are taken and triturated seven times with the decoction of hiyāvali (?). This can then be administered every day.

The milky exudation of arka is to be rubbed on the anaesathetic patches until blisters form. A medicated ghee can then be applied over the affected area. By this method, the anaesthetic patches will be removed.

According to some authorities, the patient has to be subjected to bloodletting (in the affected area) after which purified mercury can be used both internally and externally.

One part of purified mercury and eight parts of purified sulphur are triturated, mixed with a decoction of chitraka and subjected to heat in an iron vessel. After evaportion of the water content, the mass is triturated with the powder of purified vatsanābha. While taking this medicine, the patient has to be on a diet of milk, rice and ghee.

Equal quantities of purified sulphur and mercury are triturated for three days with a decoction of the seeds of palāśa. One sixteenth part of powder of purified kupīlu is mixed with this mass. This medicine has to be taken in a dosage of one nishka, daily for three months.

An oil prepared from the paste of equal quantities of dālchini, tejpatra, ela, purified tuttha, aśvagandha, karavīra, nāgakesara, bhoja patra and kākamachi, and eight parts of the juice of arka leaves, can be used for external application.

Ref.: RRS, 21, 12-40.

Classical Prescriptions: Sparśa-vāta: Visha-tinḍuka-taila

Stana-kīlaka

Causative Factors:

Extrinsic: The intake by a lactating mother (or wet-nurse) of dirt, insects, bits of grass, paddy-husks, hairs, bone, and wool along with her food (regularly).

Intrinsic: All three doshas, but mainly vāta.

Pathogenesis and Symptomatology: The intake of these indigestible particles will aggravate vāta, which in turn affects the channels that carry the rasa-dhātu (nutrient fluids), and hence the breasts are especially affected (it is the nutrient fluid, rasa-dhātu, that is responsible for the production of breast-milk).

The symptoms are: indigestion, restlessness, fatigue, a sensation of vague, undefined disease, loss of taste, pain in the joints, body pain, headache, ineffectual sneezing, hawking of mucus, fever, with thirst, diarrhoea, suppression or retention of urine, stiffness of the body, exudation from the breasts, prominence of the blood-vessels of the breasts; the breasts become swollen, tender and painful, and feel hot.

If pitta is mainly affected, there will be speedy ripening and suppuration. If kapha is mainly provoked, the disease drags on for a long time. If vāta is involved, the disease will soon run its course.

Related Diseases: Stana-śopha, Stana-vidradhi

Treatment: The patient is internally administered ghee (either alone or medicated with suitable drugs). This causes softening of the breast-tissues. The breasts should be gently squeezed, and the milk extracted. Cold applications and sprinkling (of cold substances) is also useful. The patient is also administered mild purgatives, and is advised nourishing and light food.

The disease can also be treated on the same lines stana-vidradhi.

Ref.: KS, sūtra, 21, 19.

Soma roga

Synonyms: Sanskrit: Bahu-mūtra roga, (BR).

Causative Factors:

Extrinsic: Excessive sexual intercourse, grief, fatigue, administration of purgative drugs, garadosha (poisoning), (CSS, MN).

Constituents Affected: The watery elements of the body, (CSS, MN).

Pathogenesis and Symptomatology: The watery elements of the body will be disturbed and eliminated through the urinary tract. The urine will be clear, cold, odourless and whitish. Urination will be profuse, painless and the urge cannot be controlled. The patient becomes debilitated, suffers from dryness of the mouth and throat, a feeling of hollowness in the head, syncope, yawning, delirium or irrelevant speech, dryness of skin, and is not satisfied by sweet dishes, gruels or any food, (CSS, MN).

The patient also suffers from intense thirst, (BR).

Treatment:

1. Ripe fruits of kadalī (banana) are administered along with juice of āmalaki, honey and sugarcandy.

The fine power of māsha, madhuka (liquorice), vidāri, and sugarcandy is administered with honey and milk, early in the morning.

Ripe fruits of banana, vidāri and śatāvari are administered with milk early in the morning.

If the patient suffers from painful urination, the powder of the leaves of ela is administered with taruṇī (a kind of alcoholic drink), (CSS).

2. The juice of āmalaki with honey, or the juice of vāsā with yava-kshāra, or stems of tāla, tender fruit of kharjūra, and ripe kadalī fruit with milk; all these recipes are very useful.

The powders of triphala, bamboo leaves, mustaka, and pāṭha can be administered with honey and ghee.

Any one of the following drugs can also be used: vaṭa (banyan tree), udumbara, asvattha, priyāla, lāksha, vetasa, āmra, the two varieties of jambu, badara, madhūka, tinduka, arjuna, tilvaka, kaṭuka, kadamba, kimśuka and sirīsha.

Purified haratāla, mercury and sulphur, loha bhasma, abhraka bhasma and vanga bhasma, all these are triturated and about one ratti can be administered with honey. The powder of dried fig fruit (udumbara-phala) can be taken with honey as anupāna, (BR).

Treatment: Meat, barley, wheat, milk from which cheese has been extracted, various leafy vegetables, fruits such as kadali, walking without slippers, exercise and tranquility of mind are all beneficial, (BR).

Sugarcane and its products, excessive intake of water, unripe fruits, laziness, sleep during day-time, and emotions such as fear, anger and grief are to be avoided, (BR).

Note:

1. This disease is peculiar to women, (CSS, MN, BR).

2. The advanced stage of this disease is known as mūtrātisāra, (CSS, BR).

Ref.: CSS, pages. 781-782; MN, 72; BR, pages. 482-485.

Classical Prescriptions: Guḍuchyādi-mọdaka; Vasanta-kusumākara-rasa.

Stana-vidradhi

Synonyms: Sanskrit: Stana-roga, Stana-śopha

Causative Factors:

Extrinsic:

1. The same factors which cause nāḍi-vraṇa, (SS).

2. Intake of state, very hot, dry food and food which is heating (i.e. causes pyrosis), improper postures during sleeping, etc., and a lack of proper hygiene, (AHṛ).

3. Trauma, (SS, AHṛ).

Intrinsic: The disease may be caused by the aggravated vāta, pitta, or kapha, or all three doshas combined, (SS, AHṛ).

Constituents Affected: Blood and flesh (muscular tissues), (SS).

Pathogenesis and Symptomatology:

1. This diseases does not occur in unmarried women. It is however seen most in pregnant women, and in women soon after parturition. The symptoms are the same as those described under external vidradhi.

The aggravated doshas affect the breasts, regardless of whether there is lactation or not, and cause this disease, (SS).

2. The common symptom is hard swelling of the breasts. If vāta is mainly provoked there will be severe pain, blackish or brown discolouration and irregularity in shape. The swelling will ripen and suppurate slowly. There will be pricking and cutting pain, vertigo, flatulence, pulsation (in the affected area) and crepitation or sound (on pressing the swelling).

If pitta is mainly involved, the swelling will ripen and suppurate rapidly. There will be burning pain in the affected area, thirst, syncope and fever.

If kapha is mainly involved, the swelling will be pale-white in colour, and will feel heavy. There will also be salivation or hawking of mucous, itching, chilliness, yawning and loss of appetite. The swelling will ripen and suppurate slowly.

If the swelling results due to an injury, the symptoms will be similar to those seen in the pittaja type.

If all three doshas are involved, the symptoms of all three types will be present, (AHṛ).

Related Diseases: Stana-kīlaka, Bāhya-vidradhi

Ref.: SS, nidāna, 10, 15-17, 26-27; AHṛ, nidāna, 11, 1-20.

Treatment:

1. The patient should first be administered ghee. Later, in the evening, she must be given a mild emetic composed of a decoction of nimba with honey and pippali. The next day, the patient should be advised to partake of red rice with soup of mudga. The emetics can be continued for three to six days.

As an alternative, the patient can be administered ghee medicated with triphala, or a decoction of bhārngi, ativisha, vachā, devadāru, pāṭha, kaṭu-rohini and drugs of the mustakādi group of drugs, or a decoction of drugs of the āragvadhādi group with honey.

The measures that are useful in external vidradhi are also to be employed. However, poultices should not be used, since any light bandage around the breasts may be followed by sloughing of the affected area. If suppuration has already commenced, an operation should be made in the affected area, avoiding the milk-ducts and the nipple with the areola. In all cases, milk should be expressed from the breasts (by gently pressing the breasts), (SS, AHṛ).

2. The application of a paste of the root of viśāla (indravāruni) or paste of haridra and flowers of dhattūra is useful in alleviating the pain and swelling, (CD).

3. A paste of the root of ekavīra and goat's urine is to be applied externally. It will promote rapid suppuration. The paste of powders of yashti-madhu, nimba, haridra, nirgundi and dhātaki is applied, in order to facilitate healing. The external application of oil medicated with a decoction of the bark of kuruvaka is also useful, (RRS).

Ref.: SS, chikitsā, 17, 42-47; AHr, chikitsā, 13, 28; CD, 63, 53; RRS, 25, 12-14, 53.

Sthaulya

Synonyms: Medo-roga

Western Nosology: Obesity

Causative Factors:

Intrinsic: Kapha and rasa-dhātu (CS, SS)

Extrinsic:

1. Overeating, excessive intake of food which is heavy (hard to digest), sweet, cold and unctuous; lack of exertion, total sexual abstinence, sleep during the day, constant cheerfulness, absence of mental activity and heredity (bīja-svabhāva), (CS).

2. Excessive intake of food articles that aggravate kapha, overeating, lack of exertion and sleep during daytime, (SS).

Constituents Affected: Medas (fatty tissues), (CS, SS).

Pathogenesis and Symptomatology:

1. Due to the causative factors, only medas develops in the body and not the other dhātus. The medas also obstructs the channels in the body, due to which the vāta is impeded in its movements and is restricted to the koshṭha (abdominal visceral organs). In the koshṭha, the vāta stimulates the functioning of the agni (digestive power), and as a result, there is voracious appetite. The increased intake of food causes accumulation of fat and flesh in the regions of the buttocks, abdomen and breasts.

The obese person is comparatively short lived due to the fact that the other dhatus do not develop to the same extent as the medas. Due to excessive accumulation of fat and heaviness, the person is slow in movements. The obstructions of the sukra-mārga (the channels of the reproductive organs) by the fat makes the persons incapable of successful coitus. The person is also debilitated and suffers from excessive appetite and thirst. The obese person also sweats a lot, due to the inherent nature of medas and as a result, emits bad body odour, (CS).

2. As a result of the causative factors, the āmaanna-rasa, the body fluids that contain āma (the macro molecules from improperly digested food of improper assimilated products of digestion) circulates throughout the body and due to its sweet taste and viscosity (ati-snehāt), promotes the development of medas (adipose tissue) and thus obesity. Obesity brings about in its wake distressing symptoms like difficulty in breathing (panting on exertion), thirst, sleepiness, increased appetite, sweating, foul body odour, heaviness of limbs and indistinct speech. Due to the disproportionate growth of medas, the person is weak and incapable of carrying out his duties. The obstructions of the channels (receptor-channels) by the kapha and medas, causes difficulty in conceiving, and the other dhātus do not develop normally, leading to a short life. The obese person quickly falls prey to diseases like prameha-piḍaka (diabetic carbuncles), fever, bhagandara (anal fistula), vidradhi (abscesess), vāta diseases etc. The main cause for all these troubles is the obstruction of the srotas (receptor channels) by medas, (SS).

Prognosis: It is far easier to cure a cause of kārsya (emaciation, thinness) than it is to cure sthauya. Thinness is also less harmful that obesity. The line of treatment for obesity should consist of measures to diminish medas vāta and the agni (digestive power). If langhana (emaciating) measures are adopted, the medas would be reduced, vāta and agni will increase and if brmhana (nourishing) measures are adopted, the medas will increase, even if agni and vāta reduced. This is the reason for the difficulty in curing obesity, (CS, SS, AHr).

Treatment:

1. The obese person should partake of food that is hard to digest, but is non-nourishing (emaciating), and which reduces vāta, kapha and medas. The person should also be administered enema with drugs that are dry (rūksha), hot and sharp (tīkshna), and should also be rubbed (udvartana) with dry drugs. The person should also be administered drugs such as gudūchi, bhadra-musta and triphala; takrārishta; honey; vidanga, nāgara, yava-kshāra, kāla-loha-raja (black loha chūrna or mandūra) with honey, yava-chūrna and āmalaki; the brhat pancha-mūla drugs with honey; śilājatu and the juice of agni-mantha.

The diet should consist of praśātika, priyangu, śyāmāka, yavaka, yava, jūrnahva, kodrava, mudga, kulattha, chakra-mudga, seeds of ādhaki, patola and āmalaki, etc., and madhūdaka (honey water). Arishtas are also useful in obesity.

The obese person should be asked to indulge in coitus, should exercise, keep awake during nights and should have some mental activity.

The purificatory precedures (śodhana) also help in reducing weight, (CS).

2. All efforts should be made to prevent this disease by avoiding the causative factors.

An obese person should be administered substance like śilājatu, guggulu, cow's urine, triphala, loha-raja, rasānjana, honey, yava, mudga, kora-dūshaka, śyāmāka, uddālaka, etc., and drugs that are rūksha (dry), and cchedanīya. The person should also have regular exercise and should be administered lekhana-basti, (SS).

3. The preparation known as vyoshādi-yoga is very useful in this disease, (AHr).

4. The following recipes are useful in sthaulya:

(a) Water mixed with honey should be taken first thing in the morning.

(b) Hot anna-manda (thin rice gruel).

(c) The powders of chavya, jīraka, trikatu, hingu, souvarchala and chitraka should be taken with musta and śaktu.

(d) Śilājatu is taken along with the juice of agnimantha.

(e) The paste of badari leaves taken with sour gruel.

(f) Medicines such as vidangādya-taila; amrtādya-guggulu; nāvaka-guggulu; loha-rasāyana and triphalādya-taila, (CD).

5. The following preparations are beneficial in obesity :

(a) Daily intake of ginger juice with honey.

(b) The medicine, agni-kumāra-rasa.

(c) Purified guggulu is first triturated with castor oil, and powders of triphala, trikatu and vidanga. This is then administered with pārada-bhasma.

(d) Pārada-bhasma can also be given with purified guggulu and honey-water (madhūdaka), (RRS).

Ref.: CS, sūtra, 21; 16, 13-16; SS, sūtra, 15, 32; 24, 9; AHr, 14, 25-28; CD, 36; RRS, 18, 177-178; 30,58-59.

Classical Prescriptions: Arogya-vardhini-gutika; Kārpurādyarka; Loha-bhasma; Mahā-lakshmi-vilāsa-rasa; Tāmra-bhasma; Vanga-bhasma; Vajra-bhasma; Vyoshādi-guggulu.

Śūla

Western Nosology: Abdominal pain

Causative Factors:

Extrinsic:

1. Suppression of the natural urges (especially suppressing stools, urine and flatus), overeating, indigestion, eating before the digestion of the previous meal, intake of incompatible food, fatigue, drinking too much liquid when one is hungry, intake of germinated grains, flour products (pishtānna), dry foods, dry meat, etc., (SS).

2. The causes for vātaja-śūla are: excessive exertion, travelling and sexual intercourse, keeping awake during nights, drinking too much cold water, intake (in excess) of kalāya, mudga, ādhaki, dūsha, vallūraka and dry vegetables; very dry food, eating before the digestion of the previous meal, intake of food that is bitter and astringent and of germinated grains, intake of incompatible food, suppression of natural urges, grief, fasting, injury, excessive laughing or talking.

The causes for pittaja-śūla are: anger, exposure to sun and fire, fatigue, excessive indulgence in sex, and excessive intake of kshāras (alkalies), sharp (active) and hot food articles that cause a burning sensation (in the alimentary tract), oil, nishpāva, pinyāka, soup of kulattha, souvīra (a kind of fermented drink), alcoholic drinks, and food-articles that are sour and punget.

The causes for kaphaja-śūla are: excessive intake of meat of aquatic animals, kilāta, milk products, meat-juices, dishes made from flour, krśara (gruel prepared from rice, tila and māsha), and other factors that aggravate kapha, (MN).

Classification: There are eight types, viz. pain caused by vāta, pitta, or kapha, or all three or combined, or by āma, (MN).

Pathogenesis and Symptomatology:

1. The aggravated vāta accumulates in the koshtha, and causes severe pain which interferes with breathing.

If vāta is mainly involved, the pain is severe while the stomach is empty. The limbs are benumbed, and the patient finds it difficult to breathe, and to eliminate stools, urine and flatus.

If pitta is mainly involved, there is severe pain, syncope, burning pain, thirst, craving for cold substances and amelioration by cold.

If kapha is mainly involved, the patient suffers from nausea if the abdomen is pressed, and feels as if the abdomen is full, and limbs heavy, (SS).

2. In vātaja-śūla, there is sharp pain in the precordial region, sides of the chest, back, sacrum and region of the urinary bladder. The pain aggravates after digestion of food, during the evening, and during rains and cold weather. The pain is spasmodic. There is also constipation and obstruction of flatus, pricking pain, and amelioration of pain from rubbing the abdomen, fomentation, massage (with oil) and intake of unctuous and hot substances.

In pittaja-śūla, the pain is concentrated around the umbilical region. There is also burning pain thirst, syncope, sweating and vertigo. The pain is aggravated in the afternoon, midnight, during digestion of food and in śarad season (Winter), and ame-liorated by cold applications, cold weather and intake of cold and sweet substances.

In kaphaja-śūla, the pain is worse just after eating, in the early morning, in spring and śiśira season (the season that precedes spring). The patient also suffers from nausea, cough, debility, loss of taste, salivation, heaviness of head, and a feeling as if the stomach and abdomen are full.

In śūla caused by āma (undigested food), the patient suffers from flatulence, nausea, vomiting, heaviness, salivation and other symptoms of aggravated kapha, (MN).

In śūla caused by kapha and vāta, the pain is localised in the precordial region, sides of the chest, back and around the urinary bladder.

In śūla caused by kapha and pitta, the pain is concentrated in the region between the chest and umbilicus and in the abdomen.

The śūla caused by vāta and pitta is attended by fever and a burning sensation.

Prognosis:

1. The disease caused by all three doshas is incurable, (SS).

2. The disease that is brought about by the aggravation of only one dosha is easily curable, while the disease caused by the vitiation of two doshas is curable with difficulty. The disease caused by all three doshas is incurable, (MN).

Related Diseases: Gulma, Parināma-śūla, Anna-drava śūla and Pārśva-śūla.

Ref.: SS, uttara, 42, 77-87; MN, 26, 1-14.

Treatment:

1. A patient suffering from vātaja-śūla should be first subjected to hot fomentation. The patient should partake of pāyasa (rice boiled with milk), krśara-pinda (balls prepared from gruel of tila, rice and māsha), unctuous food and unctuous meat-juices. The leaves and stalk of trivrt, the sprouts of chirabilva fried with oil, meat-juices of desert animals cooked with oil, meat of burowing animals, and other food articles which are hot and unctuous are to be eaten. Alcoholic drinks like surā, souvīra, chukra, etc., curds, buttermilk diluted with half its quantity of water, curd-whey (mastu), and rock-salt or souvarchala salt can also be eaten.

The following formulations are useful in vāta śūla: gruel of kulattha medicated with dādima, etc., and other sour fruits; gruel prepared with meat-juices of lāva with rock-salt and maricha; the paste of vidanga, śigru, kampilla, harītaki, trivrt, tulasi, sallaki, amla-vetasa and souvarchala salt, with wine; the powders of prthvīka (hingu-patrika), ajāji (a variety of jīraka), chavika, yavāni, trikatu, chitraka, pippali fruits, root of pippali and rock-salt, with milk or with juice of mātulunga or with gruel of badara along with hingu and sugar.

The patient suffering from pittaja-śūla is first administered a mild purgative, and is given cold water to drink. The patient is advised to eat only cold substances, and avoid everything hot. Vessels of copper, silver or precious stones should be filled with water and placed over the painful area. The patient is also administered jaggery, red rice, barley, milk, ghee, meat of desert animals and mild purgatives; gruels prepared from meat of desert and carnivorous animals are useful. Fruits such as parūshaka, mrdvīka, kharjūra and aquatic fruits are to be taken with sugar.

The person suffering from kapha-śūla, and in whom the pain aggravates soon after eating should be made to vomit by administering a decoction of madana and pippali. Dry fomentation is also useful.

The following formulae are also useful in kaphaja-sūla: a decoction or paste of nāgara and pippali; decoction to pāṭha, vachā, trikaṭu, kaṭu-rohini and chitraka; gruel prepared from mudga etc., and katheruka (arjaka); and the fine powder of pippali, svarjika-kshārā, yava, and chitraka with hot water, (SS).

2. The general remedial measures in this disease are: emesis, fasting, fomentation, drugs that are digestive, powders of kshāras (alkalies), use of anal suppositories and pills. The fomentation can be carried out by using kṛśara, pāyasa, flour and unctuous meat preparations.

The recipes useful in vāta-śūla are: the decoction of bala, punarnava, eraṇḍa, bṛhati, kaṇṭakāri, goksura, rock-salt and hingu; the powders of hingu, prati-visha, trikaṭu, vachā, souvarchala salt, and harītaki with hot water, on an empty stomach; the powders of tumburu, harītaki, hingu, pushkara, and the three salts with barley water, the powders of yavāni, hingu, rock-salt, yava-khsāra, souvarchala salt and harītaki with the upper clear layer of wine; the decoction of nāgara and root of eraṇḍa with hingu and souvarchala salt; the decoction of eraṇḍa, and yava with hingu and souvarchala salt; pills prepared from hingu, amlavetasa, trikaṭu, yavāni, the three salts and juice of bījapūra; the paste of the root of bījapūra and ghee; the paste of root of bilva, tila, eraṇḍa and kānji with hot water; which is applied locally; and the paste of tila seeds which is also applied externally.

The following formulations are useful in pitta-śūla: the cold gruel of yava with honey; the expressed juice of āmalaki, vidāri, trāyamāṇa or go-stana (grapes) with sugar, the expressed juice of śatāvari with honey; the decoction of bṛhati, kaṇṭakāri, gokshura, eraṇḍa, kuśa, kāśa and ikshu; the cold decoction of śatāvari; yashṭi-madhu, vāṭya, kuśa and gokshura with honey, jaggery and sugar; the decoction of triphala, nimba, yashṭi-madhu, kaṭuki and āragvadha with honey; castor oil with the decoction of yashṭi-madhu; the decoction of triphala and āragvadha with sugar and honey; and the paste of the powder of āmalaki with honey.

The formulations useful in kaphaja-śūla are: gruel medicated with pancha-kola drugs; the powders of pancha-kola drugs, the three salts and hingu with hot water; the decoction of roots of bilva and eraṇḍa, chitraka, nāgara and hingu with rock salt; the powders of musta, vachā, kaṭuka-rohini, harītaki and mūrva with cow's urine; the decoction of daśamūla drugs with yava-kshāra; the powder of vachā, musta, chitraka, harītaki and kaṭuki with cow's urine; the juice of mātulunga or decoction of śigru with yava-kshāra and honey, etc.

The treatment in āma-śūla should be the same as in kaphaja-śūla.

The formulations useful in all kinds of śūla are: the decoction of chitraka, root of pippali, eraṇḍa, nāgara, and dhānya with hingu, viḍanga and dāḍima; the powders of ajamoda, rock salt, harītaki and nāgara; the bhasma of mṛgaśṛnga with ghee; the paste of juices of vidāri and dāḍima with trikaṭu, rock salt and honey; the paste of purified manḍūra and triphala with honey and ghee; the paste of śankha bhasma, rock salt, hingu, trikaṭu and hot water; the paste of loha bhasma, triphala, honey and ghee; harītaki which is boiled in cow's urine and dried is taken with loha bhasma and jaggery.

In sūla caused by vāta and kapha, the paste of laśuna and wine is very useful. The decoction of paṭola, triphala and nimba, with honey is useful in śūla caused by kapha and pitta.

The person suffering from śūla should strictly avoid exercise, sexual intercourse, wine, salt, pungent food, pulses, suppression of natural urges, grief and anger, (CD).

3. The kshāra (ash) of amlika taken with water is very useful in śūla. The paste of fried borax, rasa-sindūra and yavakshāra with honey, is administered with a diet consisting of the gruel of meat of jambu and ghee.

The paste of rocksalt and ghee; the paste of roots of devadāru and vaṭa with hot water; souvarchala salt with hot water; the paste of root of indravāruṇi, trikaṭu and hot water, etc., are all efficacious in śūla, (RRS).

Ref.: SS, uttara, 42, 88-116; CD, 26, 1-86; RRS, 18, 101, 162-165.

Classical Prescriptions: Ajamodādi-chūrṇa; Bhāskara-lavaṇa-chūrṇa; Chandraprabha-vaṭi; Chitraka-chūrṇa; Dhātri-lauha; Gṛha-dhūmādi-lepa; Hingvādi-chūrṇa; Hingu-vachādi-chūrṇa; Hingvāshṭaka-chūrṇa, Indu-kānta-ghṛta; Kaṇṭakaryāvaleha; Loha-bhasma; Miśraka-sneha; Mūsta-karanjādi-kvātha-chūrṇa; Nārīkela-khaṇḍa; Narīkela-lavaṇa; Navaratna-rāja-mṛgānka-rasa; Panchasama-chūrṇa; Pradarāri-launa; Pradarāntaka-lauha; Prabhanjana-vimardana-taila; Pūga-khanda; Rasa-parpaṭi; Saptāmṛta-lauha; Samudrādya-chūrṇa; Śatapushpārka; Siddha-prānesvara-rasa; Sūla-haraṇa-yoga; Sūla-vajriṇi-vaṭaka; Sushka-mūlaka-taila; Vajraka-kshāra;

Viḍanga-lauha; Yava-kshāra.

Amaja-śūla: Chitrākadi-chūrṇa; Gagana-sundararasa.

Vāta-śūla: Rāsnairaṇḍādi-kvātha-chūrṇa; Vāta-vidhvamsana-rasa.

Svara-bheda

Western Nosology: Hoarseness

Causative Factors:

Extrinsic:

1. Speaking at a very high pitch (or loudly), reciting or singing for long stretches of time, intake of poisons, exposure to cold, etc., (SS).

2. MN which has incorporated the verses from SS refers to trauma as one of the causes.

Intrinsic: All three doshas.

Pathogenesis: The three doshas get aggravated, and after localising in the laryngeal, oral and nasal passages (svara-vaha-srotas) engender hoarseness.

Types:

1. Hoarseness can be of six types, three types due to the vitiation of the three doshas separately, one type due to the aggravation of all three doshas, one kind that results from kshaya (tuberculosis) and one kind that is caused by medas, (SS).

2. Hoarseness can occur due to the aggravation of vāta, pitta or kapha, or due to vitiated blood, or as a result of (chronic) cough, or accompanied by pīnasa, (CS).

Symptomatology:

Vātaja svara-bheda:

1. There is blackish discolouration of the eyes, face, urine and stools, and the voice is broken and indistinct, (SS).

2. The voice will be dry, weak, and tremulous, (CS).

Pittaja svara-bheda:

1. There will be yellowish discolouration of the eyes, face, urine and stools, and burning pain in the larynx while speaking, (SS).

2. The patient suffers from burning in the palate and throat (including larynx), and has an aversion to speaking, (CS).

Khaphaja-svara-bheda:

1. The throat is constantly obstructed by phlegm, and the voice is low and faltering (slow). These symptoms are better during the daytime, (SS).

2. The voice is interrupted, muffled (vibhaddha) and husky, (CS).

Tridoshaja svara-bheda: The patient suffers from symptoms present in the three types mentioned above. The voice is very indistinct, (SS).

Kshayaja svara-bheda: The patient feels as if smoke is coming out from the mouth and throat. The voice gradually becomes lower and lower until it finally disappears, (SS).

Medoja svarabheda: There is an increase in fatty tissues within the throat, and as a result, the patient speaks very indistinctly. There is also a sticky feeling in the throat, lips and palate, (SS).

Raktaja svara-bheda: Due to the obstruction of the throat by the vitiated blood, the voice is very feeble, and the patient can only speak with difficulty, (CS).

The patient suffering from excessive cough also suffers from hoarseness. The hoarseness that is concomitant with pīnasa (catarrh) is often caused by the aggravation of vāta and kapha, (CS).

Note: CS has described these types of svara-bheda in the chapter dealing with rāja-yakshma (tuberculosis), because svara-bheda is one of the most prominent symptoms in that disease.

Prognosis: The tridoshaja and kshayaja svara-bheda are considered to be incurable. The disease is also incurable if it occurs in debilitated, aged or emaciated persons, if it is very chronic, if it is congenital or if it occurs in obese persons, (SS).

Ref.: SS, uttara, 53, 3-7; CS, chikitsā, 8, 53-55; MN, 13.

Treatment:

1. The patient has to be subjected to oleation that should be followed by emesis, purgation and enemas. Later, nasya (errhine) therapy, avapīḍa nasya, medicinal gargles and gaṇḍūsha, fumigation or smoking of medicinal cigars and lehyas (linctus) are to be employed. The measures that are useful in śvāsa and kāsa can also be used.

In vātaja svara-bheda, the patient can be administered ghee medicated with the expressed juices of kāsa-marda, vārtāka, and bhṛngarāja, after meals. Ghee medicated with ārtagala (kakuba), or goat's milk medicated with yavakshāra, ajamoda or with chitraka and āmalaka or with devadāru and chitraka can be administered with honey. The anupāna (post-prandial drink) can be warm water or rice with jaggery and ghee.

A person suffering from pittaja svara-bheda should be given ghee followed by a draught of milk as anupāna. The diet can consist of pāyasa (rice and milk preparation) along with ghee and yashṭi-madhu. The paste of drugs of the kākolyādi group (without guḍūchi), honey and ghee or powder of śatāvari or bala with honey and ghee is also very useful.

In kaphaja svara-bheda, the patient can be administered pungent drugs like trikaṭu with cow's urine or a paste of such drugs with til oil and honey. Pungent food can also be partaken of.

A case of medoja-svara-bheda should be treated as described for kaphaja svara-bheda.

In a case of hoarseness resulting from talking at a very high pitch (or loudly), milk boiled with the decoction of sweet drugs (belonging to kākolyādi group) can be administered with sugar and honey, (SS).

2. The patient can be advised gargles (kavala) with til oil with salt in vātaja svara-bheda; ghee with honey in pittaja svara-bheda and honey with yava-kshāra and pungent drugs in kaphaja-svara-bheda.

The following preparations are useful generally in svara-bheda: the powder of equal quantities of chavya, amla-vetasa, trikaṭu, amlika, tālīsa, jīraka, vamśalochana, chitraka, dālchini, teja-patra and ela with jaggery; powders of equal quantities of ajamoda, haridra, āmalaki, yava-kshāra, and chitraka with honey and ghee; the paste of fruits of vibhītaki, rock-salt, pippali powder and butter-milk; the powder of āmalaki with cow's milk; the paste of leaves of badara which have earlier been fried in ghee, with rock salt; ghee medicated with juice of kaṇṭakāri and paste of rāsna, vātya (bala), gokshura and tirkaṭu; ghee medicated with juices of bhṛngarāja, guḍūchi, vāsā, daśamūla drugs, and kāsa-marda, and paste of pippali, and with honey.

The paste of khadira with til oil or of harītaki with pippali or harītaki with nāgara (ginger) can be kept in the mouth and sucked.

A person suffering from kaphaja svara-bheda can be administered the paste of pippali, root of pippali, maricha and ginger with cow's urine, (CD).

3. The expressed juice of āmalaka can be administered with milk in hoarseness, (RRS).

Ref.: SS, uttara, 53, 8-53; CD, 13; RRS, 25, 45.

Classical Prescriptions: Bhṛngāmalākadi-taila; Chyavana-prāśa.

Śvāsa

Western Nosology: Dyspnoea

Causative Factors:

Extrinsic:

1. Exposure to dust, smoke, and strong wind; residing in a cold climate, using cold water, excessive exertion, coitus, walking for long distances, excessive intake of dry foods, irregular or incompatible food, til oil, nishpāva, māsha, piṇyāka (til paste), flour preparations, lotus rhizomes (śālūka), food that is heavy, vishṭambhi (hard to digest), and irritant (vidāhi), meat of aquatic and wet-land animals, curds, raw milk and foods that are abhinshyandi (which cause coating on blood vessels) and which aggravate kapha, excessive purificatory procedures (ati-śodhana) and apatarpaṇa (fasting, etc.,).

Śvāsa can also result from (improperly treated) āma, ānāha, debility, injury to vital organs, atisāra, jvara, cchardi (vomiting), pratiśyāya (catarrh), kshata-kshaya, rakta-pitta, udāvarta, visūchika, alasaka, paṇḍu and toxicosis, and from trauma and various kinds of constriction or obstruction (vibandha) affecting the chest and throat, (CS).

2. All the factors that are responsible for causing hikka, (SS).

Intrinsic: Prāṇa-vāta (SS, nidāna, 1, 13), Prāṇa-vāta and kapha, (SS, CS).

Pathogenesis:

1. The vāta that is localised in the respiratory tract is aggravated, and disturbs or affects the kapha that is localised in the chest, and thus śvāsa is produced.

The vāta in association with kapha obstructs the respiratory passages, is itself obstructed, and spreads in all directions, engendering śvāsa.

The disease mainly originates in the region of pitta (mainly the organs involved in digestion), and dries up the rasa and other dhātus (body tissues), (CS).

2. The aggravated prāṇa-vāta in association with the deranged kapha is responsible for causing this disease, (SS).

Types: There are five kinds of śvāsa, namely mahā-śvāsa, ūrdhva-śvāsa, cchinna-śvāsa, tamaka-śvāsa, and kshudra-śvāsa. There is another variety of tamaka-śvāsa, which is known as pratamaka-śvāsa, (CS, SS).

Prodromal Symptoms:

1. Flatulence (ānāha), pain in the sides of the chest, discomfort in the cardiac region and disorders of respiration (prāṇasya-vilomatvam), (CS).

2. Discomfort (or pain) in the cardiac region, disinterest in food (aversion to food), restlessness, flatulence (ānāha), bad taste in the mouth and pain in the sides of the chest, (SS).

Symptomatology:

Mahā-śvāsa:

1. In this disease, expiration is very difficult, and the patient who will be struggling to breathe will breathe incessantly with a sound like that produced by an intoxicated bull. The patient will be devoid of knowledge and understanding, his eyes will be restless, his face distorted, his stools and urine suppressed, his voice low and weak, and thus his general condition will be wretched. The sound of his laboured breathing can be heard even from a distance, (CS).

2. The patient will be unconscious, his eyes swollen and there will be a loud rattling sound (in his throat). There will be pain in the sides of the chest and dryness of the throat. The patient will be lying with his body stretched backwards, (SS).

Ūrdhava-śvāsa:

1. The patient's mouth and respiratory passages will be filled with mucus (kapha), and the inspiration will be prolonged, while he will be unable to breathe out. The eyes will be turned upwards and will be restless, turning

and tossing. The patient will be in a semi-conscious condition but will be suffering, There will also be dryness of the mouth, restlessness and anxiety, (CS).

2. The vital organs will be affected, and the patient will be lying inert, with his eyes constantly fixed upwards. He will also be unable to speak, (SS).

Cchinna-śvāsa:

1. In this condition, the respiration will be interrupted while there is breaking pain in the vital organs (marmas, such as heart), and great distress. At times, it will seem as if the patient is unable to breathe. The patient will also suffer from flatulence (ānāha), sweating, spells of fainting, burning in the urinary bladder, restless and red (injected) eyes, emaciation, dryness of mouth, discolouration and delirium.

2. The respiration will be painful and interrupted, and accompanied by distension of the abdomen and burning in the region of the urinary bladder, (SS).

Tamaka-śvāsa:

1. The aggravated vāta reverses its usual course, localises in the respiratory passages, vitiates the kapha (that is present there), and causes nasal catarrh (pīnasa). This is followed by difficulty in breathing with a wheezing sound (ghurghurakam). The dyspnoea may become very severe, even threatening the life of the patient, and on such occasions, the patient faints. There will also be cough, and the patient may even faint occasionally during the paroxysms of cough. If the patient is able to expectorate, there will be transient relief, while inability to expectorate increases the suffering. The throat will be affected, and the patient can only talk with difficulty. The patient will also suffer from sleeplessness, as lying down increases the dyspnoea. The sitting position and hot drinks and food bring relief. The eyes will be wide open, the forehead will be covered with sweat, and there will be dryness of the mouth, and short periods of relief. The disease is aggravated by cloudy, cold and rainy weather, cold winds, and foods that aggravate kapha, (CS).

2. The person suffers from dyspnoea in bed weather and this is usually accompanied by thirst, sweating, weakness, nausea (vamathu) and rattling in the throat. There is also cough with expectoration, aversion to food and aggravation after loud talking and lying down, and relief after expectoration, (SS).

Pra-tamaka-śvāsa: In this condition, the dyspnoea is accompanied by fever and syncope, (CS, SS).

San-tamaka śvāsa: This (a kind of tamaka-śvāsa) is caused by udāvarta, inhalation of dust, ajīrṇa, old age or due to suppression of natural urges. The symptoms increase at night, and are relieved by cold substances. The patient feels as if he is submerged in a sea of darkness, (CS).

Kshudra-śvāsa:

1. There is slight difficulty in breathing which is caused by the intake of dry foods or is due to exertion. This is due to the vāta that is aggravated in the koshṭha (thoraco-abdominal cavity). There is no weakness, or any other general distress, nor does it interfere with the normal intake of food and drink or cause distress in the sense-organs or any pain, (CS).

2. There is slight difficulty in breathing that is caused by undue exertion, and is relieved after taking rest, (SS).

Prognosis:

1. Mahā-śvāsa, ūrdhava-śvāsa and cchinna-śvāsa are considered to be incurable. Tamaka-śvāsa can be palliated if it is chronic, and cured if it is acute or of recent origin. Kshudra-śvāsa is easily curable.

However, all the five types of śvāsa are curable in persons having a strong constitution provided all the symptoms enumerated above are not present, (CS).

2. Kshudra-śvāsa is easily curable, while tamaka-śvāsa can be cured with difficulty, except in debilitated persons. The three other kinds are incurable, (SS).

Related Diseases: Hikka

Ref.: CS, chikitsā, 17, 6-20, 45-67; SS, uttara, 51, 4, 14.

Treatment:

1. Persons suffering from this disease should be treated without losing time, since the disease if neglected or improperly treated, will aggravate and may prove fatal.

The person has first of all to be massaged with oil medicated with rock-salt, and then fomented by means of nāḍi, prastara and sankara types of sudation (svedana) with unctuous substances. By these measures, the kapha (mucus) that has hardened will be liquified, the respiratory passages are soothened (softened) while the vāta will be restored to its normal condition. Immediately after sudation, the patient should partake of unctuous food, meat juices of fish or pig or the upper layer of curds. This results in increase of mucous. The patient is then administered an emetic consisting of rock-salt, pippali, honey and drugs that do not aggravate vāta. After emesis, there will be relief from suffering, the respiratory passages will be clear, and the movement of vāta will be unimpaired. If there is still a residue of morbidity, the patient should smoke a medicated cigar composed of haridra, teja-patra, root of castor, lāksha, manah-śila, haritāla, devadāru, and jaṭāmamsi, and ghee. The fumes of barley mixed with ghee can also be inhaled. The fumes of bee's wax, sarja-rasa (resin of sarja) and ghee, or of horns, hairs or sinews of cow or of śyonāka, eraṇḍa, the dried stems of kuśa, padmaka, guggulu, agaru, śallaki and ghee, may also be used.

Śvāsa that is a concomitant of svara-kshīṇa (laryngeal affections), diarrhoea, rakta-pitta and dāha (burning pain) should be treated by drugs, food etc., that are sweet, unctuous and cold. However, sudation (svedana) is contra-indicated in debilitated, emaciated and dried up individuals, in pregnant women, in persons of pitta constitution and in persons who are prone to suffering from burning pain, haemorrhages and excessive sweating. If sudation has to be done, they should be made to sweat only for a short time by sprinkling warm unctuous substances, or by application of utkārika poultices mixed with sugar. Fomentation has to be done on the chest and throat. An utkārika composed of tila seed, atasi seeds, māsha, godhūma (wheat) powder, sour drugs or milk, and unctuous substances can be applied as poultices.

If the patient is suffering from acute fever and āma-dosha (indigestion), he should be subjected to dry sudation (rūksha-sveda) and fasting, or can be administered emesis with salt water, after careful examination.

If the purificatory procedures aggravate vāta, the patient should be made to partake of meat juices, and should be massaged with substances that are luke warm. If the person suffers from udāvarta and adhmāna (flatulent distention of the abdomen), he should be prescribed a diet comprising of mātulunga, amla-vetasa, hingu, pīlu, viḍa-salt and boiled rice.

Among persons suffering from śvāsa, some possess a strong constitution and excess of kapha, while others are debilitated and suffer from aggravation of vāta. The former patients can be administered emesis, and purgation, followed by a suitable diet, fumigation (dhūma) and linctuses (lehya). The latter kind of patients, as well as those who are aged or very young should be given nourishing foods, meat-juices, soups and unctuous preparations that alleviate vāta.

Purificatory procedures should not be employed on persons who do not have liquified mucous, who have not been fomented and who are debilitated.

Persons suffering from śvāsa, especially if they are debilitated, can partake of the following:

meat-juices of peacock, partridge, cock and desert animals boiled with a decoction of dasāmūla drugs or soup of kulattha (horse-gram); soup prepared from the decoction of kaṇṭakāri, pulp of bilva, karkaṭa, durālabha, gokshura, guḍūchi, kulattha and chitraka; nāgara (ginger), rock-salt and pippali that has been fried in ghee; soup prepared from the decoction of rāsna, bala, drugs of laghupanchmūla group, mudga, and chitraka; soup prepared from tender leaves of mātulunga nimba and kulaka, mudga, trikaṭu and yava-kshāra; soup prepared from yava-kshāra; rock salt, śigru, and maricha; soup prepared from leaves of kāsamarda and śigru; soup prepared from dry radish; soup prepared from vārṭaka (brinjal) mixed with curds, trikaṭu and ghee; rice that is harvested in sixty days, preparations of wheat or barley; gruel (yavāgu) prepared from hingu, souvarchala salt, ajāji, viḍa salt, pushkara-mūla, chitraka, and karkaṭa-śrngi; and gruel or a decoction of daśamūla drugs; śaṭi, rāsna, pippali root, pushkara, śṛngi, tāmalaki, guḍūchi, mātulunga and amalavetasa are mixed with hingu, viḍa-salt and ghee and are to be used along with food and drink.

If the patient is very thirsty, he can drink the decoction of daśamūla drugs or devadāru or madira wine. The supernatent layer of wine (surā) should be mixed with the fine powders of pāṭhā, madhurasa, rāsna, sarala and devadāru, and a little quantity of rocksalt. This can be drunk by a person suffering from śvāsa. The juice of mātulunga or aranāla (kānji) mixed with hingu, souvarchala salt, kola, samanga (lajjālu), pippali and balā or hot water medicated with the paste of bhārngi and nāgara, or of maricha and yavakshāra or with davadāru, chitraka, sāriva and mūrva may be drunk.

In cases of śvāsa which are marked by symptoms of aggravated pitta, utkārika prepared from madhūlika, vamśalochana, nāgara and pippali, and cooked in ghee can be administered. If there is aggravation of vāta, the meat of svavidha (porcupine) and rabbit and the blood of śallaka may be cooked with ghee and pippali, and administred. In cases where there is aggravation of vāta and pitta, the patient can be administered the juice of suvarchala, milk and ghee medicated with trikaṭu, followed by a dish of boiled rice. In cases where there is aggravation of kapha and pitta, the expressed juices of sirīsha flowers or of saptaparṇa may be mixed with pippali and honey and administered. A patient with profuse expectoration (bahu-kapha) should partake of the kshāra (alkali) of aśvagandha mixed with honey.

Persons suffering from śvāsa with concomitant symptoms of cough and hoarseness should be given emesis with drugs that alleviate vāta and kapha, while those suffering from tamaka-śvāsa should be subjected to purgation (by drugs that alleviate vāta and kapha).

The powder of equal quantities of śati, choraka, jīvanti, dālchini, musta, pushkara, surasā (tulasi), tāmalaki, ela, pippali, agaru, ginger and bālaka (hrivera) and eight parts of sugar is useful in most cases of tamaka-śvāsa.

Treatment with drugs that are nourishing (and palliative) is not followed with many adverse effects, while karśaṇa (deletion) therapy can cause many adverse effects, (CS).

2. Patient possessing a strong constitution should be subjected to mild emesis and purgation. Old ghee medicated with harītaki, viḍa salt and hingu is considered to be very useful in most cases of śvāsa, kāsa, hikka and hṛdroga.

The following formulations are useful in śvāsa: old ghee medicated with souvarchala salt, harītaki and bilva; old ghee medicated with a paste of drugs of the pippalyādi group and a decoction of drugs of vidārigandhādi group and the five salts; ghee boiled with four parts of water, two parts of milk and himsra, viḍanga, pūtika (chira-bilva), triphala, trikaṭu and chitraka; the decoction of all parts of vāsā boiled with milk, and taken with honey, when cold; ghee boiled with four parts of water, and a paste of karkaṭaka-śṛngi, madhūika, bhārṇgi, ginger, rasānjana, sugar, musta, haridra, and yashṭi-madhu; ghee boiled with two parts of water and paste of suvahā (godhāpadi), kālika, bhārgni, śukākshya(?), jala-vetasa fruit, kākādani, ginger, punarnava, bṛhati and kanṭakāri; ghee medicated with souvarchala salt, yava-kshāra, kaṭuka, trikaṭu, chitraka, vachā, harītaki, and viḍanga; ghee boiled with twice the quantity of the decoction of sāriva; til oil boiled with ten parts of expressed juice of bhṛngarāja; expressed juice of sour fruits (such as dāḍima, bījapūra, etc.) with meat-juices of vishkira birds, unctuous substances and rock-salt; soup of kulattha with heads of eṇa deer, the paste of timira seeds, karkaṭaka-śṛngi, honey and ghee; the paste of durālabha, pippali, kaṭuka, haritaki, honey and ghee; paste of bharngi bark, ginger, sugar, bark of śallaka, honey and ghee; the paste of saptaparṇa flowers, pippali, mastu (curd-cream) and honey; with a diet of roasted barley; the paste of powdered barley previously soaked in the juice of tender twigs of arka, and honey; the tarpaṇa (saktu) of barley; potion of flowers of kadali, kunda and sirīsha, pippali, karkaṭa-śṛngi, durālabha, honey and ghee; the paste of haridra, maricha, drāksha, jaggery, rāsna, pippali, śāli and tila oil; and utkārika prepared from seeds of ankoṭha; and a bolus prepared from a paste of kanṭakāri that should be equal to the size of āmalaka fruit, half that quantity of hingu and honey.

The patient can partake of old ghee, pippali, soup of kulattha, meat juices of desert animals, surā wine, souvīraka, hingu, honey, juice of mātulunga, drāksha, āmalaka and bilva.

The patient can also be subjected to only fomentation (snigdha-sveda) with til oil and salt, which will liquify the hardened kapha and also alleviate vāta. This should be followed by a diet of boiled rice and meat juices.

The patient can smoke a medicated cigar prepared from manahsila, devādaru, haridra, teja-patra, guggulu, lāksha, and root of red castor plant, in cases where there is aggravation or obstruction of vāta and kapha. The fumes obtained by burning ghee, barley, bee wax, and resin of śāla are also useful, (SS).

3. Drugs such as śaṭi, pushkara-mūla, amla-vetasa, ela, hingu, agaru, surasa (tulasi), tāmalaki, jīvanti and chandana are very efficacious in śvāsa, (CS, sūtra, 4, 8-16).

4. The paste of the root of indra-vāruṇi, devadāru, trikaṭu and sugar is useful in ūrdhava-śvāsa.

One part of purified pārada is triturated with two parts of purified sulphur, and the juice of kumāri for three hours. Then three parts of purified copper leaves are taken to cover and enclose the bolus. This is then heated in a handika-yantra. The mixture is then powdered and can be administered in case of śvāsa in doses of two gunja.

The paste of purified sulphur, maricha powder and ghee or the paste of purified manahśila, hingu, viḍanga, maricha, kushṭha, rock-salts, honey and ghee is also very useful.

The decoction of kaṭuki, harītaki, bhārngi, vachā, and ginger is administered with jaggery in śvāsa in pregnant women, (RRS).

Related Diseases: Kāsa (SS), Hikka (CS)

Ref.: CS, chikitsā, 17, 70-124; SS, uttara, 51, 15-56; RRS, 13, 48-52; 22, 86.

Classical Prescriptions: Abhraka-bhasma; Agastya-harītaki-rasāyana; Amṛta-prāśa-ghṛta; Apāmārga-kshāra; Aśva-kanchuki-rasa; Balā-taila; Bāla-chaturbhadrika-chūrṇa; Bhārngi-guḍa; Chandanādi-chūrṇa; Chandana-balā-lākshadi-taila; Chandrāmṛta-rasa; Chitraka-harītaki; Chyavana-prāśa; Daśa-mūlārishṭa; Daśamula-harītaki; Daśamūla-kaṭutrayādi-kvātha-chūrṇa; Daśamula-kvātha-chūrṇa; Dhānvantara-guṭika; Elādi-chūrṇa; Eladi-gūṭika; Godanti-bhasma; Gorochanādi-vaṭi; Grahaṇi-mihira-taila; Jātiphalādya-chūrṇa; Kanakāsava; Kānta-vallabha-rasa; Kanta-karyāvaleha; Kaphaketu-rasa; Karpūrādi-chūrṇa; Kasturyādi-guṭika; Khadirādi-vaṭi; Kumara-kalyāṇa-rasa; Kumāryāsava; Kūshmaṇḍa-rasāyana; Laghu-chinchādi-leha;

Lavangādi-vaṭi; Loha-bhasma; Pippalyādi-lauha; Prāṇada-guṭika; Rasa-māṇikya; Sapta-vamśatika-guggulu; Soubhāgya-vaṭi; Shaṭpala-ghṛta; Śiva-gutika; Śṛnga-bhasma; Sūraṇa-vaṭaka; Svārṇa-bhasma; Svarṇa-vanga; Śvāsa-kuṭhāra-rasa; Tālisadi-chūrṇa; Tāmra-bhasma; Vaikrānta-bhasma; Vanga-bhasma; Vāsa-kshāra; Vāsavaleha; Vāsa-chandanādi-taila; Vātagni-kumāra-rasa; Yakṛdari-lauha.

Pittaja-śvasa: Sitopalādi-chūrṇa

Tamaka-śvāsa: Balā-jīrakadi-kvātha-chūrṇa; Nāyopayam-kvātha-chūrṇa; Malla-sindura; Śiva-guṭika.

Ūrdhva-svasa: Vidāryādi-kvātha-chūrṇa.

Tālu-kaṇṭaka

Synonyms: Tālu-pāta

Causative Factors:

Intrinsic: Aggravated kapha.

Symptomatology:

1. There is a depression in the region of the tālu (anterior fontanel). The infant has an aversion to breast milk, drinks with difficulty and suffers from loose, watery stools, thirst, pain in the throat, mouth and orbital region, vomiting and rattling in the throat, (MN).

2. There is a depression in the tālu (anterior fontanel) along with thirst, inflammation (vipāka) of the affected area (tālu), aversion to breast milk, constipation, vertigo, dryness of the mouth, itching, weakness of the neck, vomiting, eye diseases, etc.

Treatment:

1. The infant should be administered the paste of harītaki, vachā, kushṭha and honey with breast milk, (CD).

2. The affected area (the tālu) should be gently rubbed with the paste of yava-kshāra and honey or of śuṇṭhi, pippali, rock salt and cowdung water. The paste of harītaki, vacha, kushṭha and honey should be given internally with breast milk, (RRS).

Ref.: MN, 68, 12-13; RRS, 22, 143-146; CD, 64-47.

Tila-kālaka

Western Nosology: Non-elevated mole

Causative Factors:

Intrinsic: Vāta and pitta, (SS), Pitta, (CS).

Constituents Affected: Blood (CS, SS)

Pathogenesis and Symptomatology: The blood is dried by the aggravated vāta and pitta, due to which blackish, painless, non-elevated marks the size of tila seeds are formed on the skin, (SS).

This diseases is caused by the drying up of the aggravated pitta and the vitiated blood, (CS).

Related Diseases: Mashaka, Nyaccha, Nīlika

Ref.: SS, nidāna, 13, 43; CS, sūtra, 18, 25.

Treatment: The affected areas has to be gradually cauterized by fire or by employing alkalies, (SS, sūtra, 12, 10; chikitsā, 20, 32).

Tūni

Western Nosology: Pain in bladder and anus.

Causative Factors:

Extrinsic: Factors which aggravate vāta.

Intrinsic: Vāta

Symptomatology: Splitting pain that radiates downwards from the rectum and urinary bladder towards the perineum (gudopastha).

Related Diseases: Prati-tūni

Ref.: SS, nidāna, 1, 86.

Treatment: The patient is to be administered hot water with rock-salt and some unctuous substances (like ghee or oil). The powder of drugs of pippalyādi group or ghee medicated with hingu and yava-kshāra can be administered. The patient can also be administered enema, (SS, chikitsā, 5, 25).

Udara

Causative Factors:

Extrinsic:

1. The general causes are excessive intake of food that is hot, salty, alkaline, irritant, dry and sour, administration of poisons, improperly done purificatory procedures (śodhana), intake of incompatible and unclean food, emaciation due to disease such as enlargement of the spleen, haemorrhoids, grahaṇi, suppression of the natural urges, neglecting severe disease, obstruction of the rectum by hard stools or hair in the ingested food, ulceration and perforation of the intestines, diseases affecting the channels of the body, excessive āma, dehydration, overeating, etc. A person suffering from poor digestion is especially susceptible to this disease.

Causes for vātaja udara are: excessive exertion, suppression of natural urges, mal nourishment, intake only of dry food and other factors that cause emaciation.

Causes for pittaja udara are: exposure to sun, excessive intake of food that is pungent, irritant, salty, hot and sharp, over-eating and eating before the digestion of the previously eaten meal.

Causes for kaphaja udara are: lack of physical exertion, sleep during the day-time, excessive intake of curds, milk, meat of aquatic and wet-land animals, and food that is sweet, unctuous and slimy.

Causes for tridoshaja udara: intake of heavy, incompatible and unwholesome food by a person with poor digestion, or administration of slow poisons or menstrual blood, faeces, urine, bones, etc., by a woman.

Causes for plīhodara: excessive exertion or jolting immediately after meals, excessive riding on animals, lifting heavy weights, excessive coitus, walking for long distances, and emaciation due to diseases.

Causes for baddha-gudodara: obstruction of the gastro-intestinal tract by particles of hair eaten along with food, paralysis of the intestines and the disease udāvarta.

Causes for chidrodara: Injury to the intestines by sand, gravel, straw, pieces of wood, thorns, etc., ingested along with food, over-eating or yawning vigorously.

Causes for jalodara: drinking excessive amounts of water soon after partaking unctuous substances (sneha-pāna) or by a debilitated and emaciated person with a very poor digestion, (CS).

Excessive intake of unwholesome food by a person with poor digestive powers, intake of dry, putrid (unclean) food and improper administration of oleation, sudation, emesis, purgation and enema.

Causes for tridoshaja udara: intake of contaminated water, dūshi-visha, gara-visha and menstrual blood, nails, hairs and urine along with food and drink.

Causes for plīhodara: excessive intake of irritant and abhishyandi food.

Causes for parisrāvi udara: injury to the intestines by sharp objects ingested along with food.

Causes for dakodara: drinking large amounts of cold water immediately after oleation (internal use of unctuous substances), anuvāsan or nirūha basti, or emesis or purgation, (SS).

Classification:

1. There are eight types of udara - that caused by the aggravation of vāta, pitta, kapha, all

three doshas, plīhodara (caused by disorders of the spleen), baddhodara (due to intestinal obstructions), chidrodara (due to intestinal perforations) and jalodara (ascitis), (CS, sūtra, 19, 4).

2. SS also descibes eight kind of udara — three kinds of udara are caused by the vitiation of the three doshas, while the fourth kind is caused by the vitiation of all the three doshas. The four other kinds are plīhodara (caused by disorders of the spleen), baddha-guda-udara (due to intestinal obstruction), āgantuka or parisrāvi udara (caused by injury to intestines) and dakodara (ascites).

Pathogenesis:

1. Due to intake of improper food by a person with poor digestion, the food will not be digested, and this undigested food will vitiate the prāṇa and apāna vāṭa, and the digestive fire, and will obstruct the upper and lower parts of the gastro-intestinal tract. It will then penetrate the area in between the skin and flesh and cause distension of the abdomen. The aggravated doshas obstruct the sweat glands and their ducts and channels that carry fluid, vitiate the prāṇa and apāna vāta and the digestive fire, and engender these diseases, (CS).

2. The anna-sāra (lymph-chyle) will penetrate into the gastro-intestinal tract being stimulated thus by the aggravated vāta, and localizing interior to the skin, causing distention all over the abdomen, (SS).

Prodromal Symptoms:

1. Loss of strength, complexion and appetite, erasure of wrinkles (on the skin), appearance of ridges or grooves on the abdomen, swelling of the lower limbs (feet), acidity immediately after the digestion of food and pain in the region of the urinary bladder, (SS).

General Symptomatology:

1. Flatulent distension and meteorism of the abdomen, swelling of the hands and feet, poor digestion, emaciation and smoothness of cheeks (slakshṇa-gaṇḍatva), (CS).

2. Flatulent distension of the abdomen, difficulty in moving about, weakness, poor digestion, swelling of extremities, constipation, retention (or suppression) of urine, thirst and burning pain, (SS).

Pathogenesis and Symptomatology:

Vātaja udara:

1. The aggravated vāta localising in the abdomen, chest, urinary bladder and rectal region enfeebles the digestive fire, adversely affects the kapha, draws it out of its usual position, is obstructed by it, and gets blocked in between the skin and the flesh.

The patient suffers from swelling of the abdomen, hands, feet and scrotum, bursting pain in the abdomen, unpredictable increase and decrease (of the symptoms), sharp pain in the abdomen and sides of the chest, udāvarta, body pain, pain in the joints, dry cough, emaciation, debility, anorexia, poor digestion, obstruction of stools, urine and flatus, brownish-black discolouration of nails, eyes, face, skin, urine and stools, flatulent colic and rumbling sound in the abdomen. The abdomen is covered by a network of thin, dark veins, and on percussion produces a tympanitic sound, (CS).

2. The abdomen is distended at the sides, posterior part and umbilical region and is covered with dark veins. There is piercing and splitting pain, flatulent colic and tympanitic sound on percussion, (SS).

Pittaja-udara:

1. The aggravated pitta obstructs the normal functioning of vāta and kapha, is itself displaced from its position, impairs the digestive fire and gives rise to udara.

The patient suffers from burning pain, fever, thirst, syncope, diarrhoea, vertigo, pungent taste in the mouth, yellowish or green discolouration of nails, eyes, face, skin, faeces and urine, while the abdomen is covered by a network of blue, yellow, coppery or green veins. There is also sweating, burning pain, local heat, softness (of the affected area), and rapid suppuration, (CS).

2. The patient suffers from yellow discoloration of the eyes, faeces, urine, nails and face. The abdominal region is hot and covered by a network of yellowish veins. There is also fever, thirst and burning pain. The symptoms increase rapidly, (SS).

Kaphaja-udara:

1. The aggravated kapha obstructs the (abdominal) channels. The passage of vāta is thus obstructed, and the patient falls prey to udara.

The patient suffers from heaviness of the body, anorexia, indigestion, body pain, numbness, swelling of the hands, feet, scrotum and thighs, nausea (utkleśa), sleepiness, cough, dyspnoea, and whitish discolouration of nails, eyes, face, skin, urine and faeces; the abdomen is heavy, hard, firm, feels as if covered by a wet cloth, and is covered over by a nework of whitish veins, (CS).

2. The patient suffers from debility, and whitish discolouration of nails and face. The abdomen is greatly swollen, cold, unctuous, heavy, firm and covered by white blood-vessels. The symptoms increase gradually, (SS).

Tridoshaja-udara:

1. The three doshas are aggravated and gradually localise in the abdomen.

The patient suffers from symptoms of all the three types descibed above, (CS).

2. The aggravated three doshas will vitiate the blood and cause a severe swelling of the abdomen, with symptoms of all the three types described above. There is a burning sensation (in the abdomen), thirst and dryness (of mucous membranes). The patient becomes pale, and emaciated. The symptoms increase in cold and damp weather, (SS).

Plīhodara:

1. Due to the causative factors, either the spleen (that is situated in the left hypo-chondrium) is displaced and swollen, or there is an increased amount of blood formed from the nutrient fluids, and this causes swelling of the spleen.

The spleen becomes hard, like a stone, and gradually increases in size until it resembles a tortoise. If this is neglected, the spleen further increases in size, and occupies the flanks and abdomen, and displaces the agni-adhiṣṭāna (gastro-intestinal place of digestion).

The patient suffers from debility, anorexia, indigestion, constipation, retention of urine, fainting spells, thirst, body pain, vomiting, syncope, cough, dyspnoea, mild fever, ānāha, loss of appetite, emaciation, bad taste in the mouth, pain in the joints and flatulent colic. The abdomen is brownish or discoloured, and covered by bluish, green, yellow, veins. The liver may also be affected in a similar manner, but the symptoms will be the same as in plīhodara, (CS).

2. The kapha and blood are excessively aggravated and cause enlargement of the spleen. There is mild fever, excessive emaciation, debility and swelling in the left hypo-chondrium. The patient is also very pale, suffers from symptoms of kapha and pitta, and poor digestion.

If the liver is similarly affected, the disease is known as yakrt-dālyudara, (SS).

Baddha-guda-udara (or baddhodara); Tricho bezoar; Intestinal obstruction:

1. The apāna-vāta is aggravated (by the obstruction of the gastro-intestinal tract, impairs the digestive fire, and further obstructs the passage of faeces, kapha and pitta, thus causing udara.

The patient suffers from thirst, burning pain, fever, dryness of the mouth and palate, weakness of thighs, cough, dyspnoea, weakness, anorexia, indigestion, constipation, retention of urine, flatulent distension of the abdomen, vomiting, sneezing, headache, and pain in the cardiac region, umbilical region and rectum. The abdomen is tympanitic, firm and covered by a network of bluish and brown veins. There is also a protuberance above the umbilicus, shaped like a cow's tail, (CS).

2. There is constipation, with difficult evacuation of scanty stools, and swelling of the abdomen in between the cardiac region and umbilicus. There is also faecal vomiting, (SS).

Cchidrodara: (Perforation)

1. The rasa (the intestinal contents) flows out of the perforations, causes suppuration, and fills up the intestines and rectum, causing udara.

There is swelling mainly below the umbilicus, and accumulation of fluid there. The stools are slimy, offensive, undigested, reddish, blue or yellowish in colour. The patient also suffers from hiccoughs, dyspnoea, cough, thirst, or cloudiness of mind, anorexia, indigestion and debility, (CS).

2. A watery fluid flows out copiously from the perforations and accumulates in the abdomen. There is thus swelling of the abdomen below the umbilicus, with burning and severe pricking pain and oozing of fluid from the anus, (SS).

Jalodara: Ascites

1. The aggravated vāta and the kapha along with the watery fluid, obstructs the gastro-intestinal tract, and causes ascites.

The patient suffers from loss of appetite, thirst, discharge of (watery) fluid from the anus, abdominal pain, dyspnoea, cough and debility. The abdomen is full of watery fluid, and is covered by a network of many hued blood-vessels, the swollen abdomen resembling a bladder full of fluid.

If this disease is not treated before the collection of water, the doshas become further liquified, while the sweat is also obstructed and increases the fluid that is accumulating. The abdomen thus becomes rounded, heavy, firm, soft to touch, without any wrinkles and producing no sound on percussion. The network of veins also disappears, (CS).

2. The fluid transuding through the wall of the channels (that carry fluid) accumulates in the abdomen, which becomes greatly swollen, especially around the umbilicus, rounded and glossy on the surface. It particularly resembles a water-drum, as it fluctuates under pressure, oscillates and produces sound on percussion, (SS).

Complications:

Vomiting, diarrhoea, tamaka (dyspnoea, tamaka-śvāsa), thirst, cough, hiccoughs, debility, pain in the sides of the chest, anorexia, hoarseness, retention or suppression of urine, etc, (CS).

Prognosis:

1. All cases where there is marked collection of fluid, and cchidrodara are incurable. Baddagudodara is incurable after a fortnight. Vātaja-pittaja-tridoshaja, types of udara, plīhodara and jalodara are progressively more difficult to cure.

The patient who suffers from swelling around the eyes, crookedness or deformity of genital organs, moist and softened skin, loss of strength, feeble digestion, emaciation, bloodlessness, swelling of all the vital organs, dyspnoea, hiccoughs, restlessness, thirst, syncope, vomiting and diarrhoea is very difficult to cure.

Those cases of udara which are recent, where there is no collection of fluid and which occur in strong persons are curable.

Cases of udara where there is no collection of fluids are characterized by absence of swelling, brownish colour of the skin (over the abdomen), presence of tympanitic sounds (on percussion), presence of a network of veins, the peristaltic wave going to the rectum returns to the umbilicus and subsides, presence of colicky pain in the cardiac region, umbilical region, groins, waist and rectum, forceful elimination of flatus, good digestion, loss of taste, scanty urine and well formed stools. Such cases are to be taken up for treatment, (CS).

2. All the types of udara if neglected culminate in jalodara, which is very difficult to cure, (SS).

Ref.: CS,chikitsā, 13, 20-58; SS, nidāna, 7.

Treatment:

1. In vātaja-udara, a patient who is strong enough should be subjected to oleation (snehana), and then sudation. He should then be given purgation by means of unctuous preparations. After purgation, his abdomen should be tightly bandaged, so that it will not become distended again. Purgation should be done daily in order to avoid the obstruction of the gastro-intestinal tract. After samsarjana (post purificatory measures), he should be given milk in order to increase his strength. This should be gradually reduced before the patient develops an aversion to milk. Gruels (yūsha) or meat-juices mixed with sour and salty substances should be administered in order to improve his digestion. If there is udāvarta, the patient should be oleated, fomented and subjected to āsthāpana enema. Anuvāsana enema is also useful in patients suffering from tremors (pulsations), convulsions (ākshepa), pain in the joints, bones, sides of the chest, back and sacrum, constipation, dryness (dehydration), but whose digestion is good. The nirūha-enema should consist of strong purgative drugs and daśamūla drugs, while the anuvāsana enema should consist of castor oil or til oil medicated with sour substances and drugs that alleviate vāta. Persons who are aged, very young, delicate, who are not suitable for being administered purgatives, who are weak, or in whom there is very slight or very severe aggravation of vāta should be treated with pallatives (śamana), medicated ghee, gruels, boiled rice, meat-juices, medicated milk, enemata, and massages.

In pittaja-udara, strong persons can be administered purgatives even at the beginning, while debilitated persons should be first administered anuvāsana enema and later cleansed by means of kshīra-basti (milk-enema). After the patient recovers his strength and power of digestion, he should again be given purgatives composed of unctuous substances, such as castor oil mixed with milk and a paste of trivṛt or a decoction of āragvadha with satala and trāyamaṇa. If vāta or kapha are also aggravated, the above-mentioned purgatives can be administered with ghee medicated with bitter drugs or with cow's urine. The patient should be repeatedly subjected to the process of milk-enema, and purgation.

In kaphaja-udara, the patient has to be subjected to snehana, svedana and purificatory measures, after which the samsarjana treatment can be done by means of boiled rice medicated with drugs that are pungent, alkaline and that alleviate kapha. The patient can also be administered cow's urine, arishṭas, preparation of ayaskṛti, and potions of oil medicated with alkalis.

The tridoshaja-udara should be treated with all the above mentioned measures, except where there are complications, in which case, the disease is to be considered as incurable.

In a case of plīhodara, the physician should be aware that the symptoms of udāvarta, pain and ānāha, burning pain, fainting spells, thirst and fever, and heaviness, anorexia and hardness are caused by the aggravation of vāta, pitta and kapha respectively. The patient is to be subjected to snehana, svedana, purgation, nirūha, anuvāsana and venesection on the left hand. The formulation known as shaṭpala-ghṛta, or a course of pippali or of jaggery and harītaki or kshāras or arishṭas can be employed. The patient can be administered the powders of pippali, nāgara, danti, chitraka, and viḍanga with hot water; the powders of viḍanga, chitraka, nāgara, rock-salt, and vachā which are to be fried in ghee and administered with milk; small pieces of rohitaka creeper which may be soaked for seven days in a decoction of harītaki or cow's urine while the diet should consist of meat-juices of desert animals; ghee (weighing one prastha) is boiled with the decoction of twenty-five palas of rohitaka bark and two prasthas of kola, and paste of one pala each of panchakola drugs and rohitaka bark. This ghee can be administered in suitable dosages. In cases of plīhodara where pitta is aggravated, ghee medicated with drugs of jīvanīya drugs, milk-enemas, blood-letting and (internal use of) milk are useful. All patients suffering from plīhodara should partake of gruels prepared from meat-juices and appetizing drugs, and light, easily digested food. Yakṛt-dālyudara should be treated similarly.

In baddha-guda-udara, the patient should be given sudation therapy and then administered nirūha enema consisting of cow's urine, strong drugs, oil and salt, followed by anuvāsana enema, a laxative diet and strong purgatives. The remedial measures that alleviate vāta and are useful in udāvarta are also useful.

In cchidrodara, the patient is treated along the same lines as in kaphaja-udara, the sole exception being that sudation is contra-indicated. The fluid should be drained out as it collects. The patient who is afflicted with cough, thirst and fever, who is emaciated, has a very poor digestion, who is not able to eat, and who also has enfeebled sense organs, pain and dyspnoea is incurable.

In jalodara, the patient should be administered drugs that remove the water-content, kshāras and drugs that are strong, mixed with cow's urine. The diet should consist of food that is appetizing, and which alleviates kapha. The intake of fluids and water should be gradually curtailed.

In all types of udara, the diet should consist of substances that are appetizing and easy to digest, and red rice, barley, mudga, meat of desert animals and birds, milk, cow's urine, honey, sīdhu, āsava, arishṭa, alcoholic drinks, gruels, boiled rice, and soup prepared from substances that are slightly sour, pungent, and unctuous, and meat-juices, etc., prepared from pancha-mūla drugs.

The patient should strictly avoid meat of aquatic and wet-land animals, leafy vegetables, flour preparations, tila, food that is hot, salty, sour, hard to digest and irritant, water, and exertion, sleep during daytime and travelling.

Buttermilk that is sweet, not very thick, from which butter has been removed and which has been medicated with trikaṭu, rock-salt and kshāras can be used regularly as a drink, A person suffering from vātaja-udara should drink buttermilk that has been medicated with rock-salt and pippali, while those suffering from pittaja-udara should take it medicated with yashṭi-madhu and sugar. In kaphaja-udara, it should be mixed with rock-salt, yavāni, ajāji, and trikaṭu or with honey, and it should be lukewarm. In plīhodara, it should be medicated with honey, til oil, vachā, nāgara, śata pushpa, rock-salt and kushṭha, while in jalodara, it is given with trikaṭu. In baddhodara, buttermilk is mixed with hapusha, yavāni, ajāji and rock-salt, and in cchidrodara, with honey and pippali. Buttermilk acts like ambrosia in people with diarrhoea, poor digestion, anorexia, heaviness of body, and in diseases caused by vāta and kapha.

Camel's milk, likewise is very beneficial in patients afflicted with swelling, ānāha, pain, thirst, and syncope, and the milk of cow, goat and buffalo is beneficial in emaciated persons.

A paste of devadāru, palāśa, arka, hasti-pippali, śigru, aśvagandha and cow's urine can be applied over the abdomen. The decoction of vṛschikāli, vachā, kushṭha, panchamūla drugs, punarnava, bhūtika (ajamoda), nāgara, and dhānya or of palāśa, kattṛna and rāsna or the eight types of urine can be used as affusion (for sprinkling).

Various kinds of ghee preparations such as snuhi-kshīra ghṛta, pancha kola ghṛta, nāgara ghṛta, chitraka ghṛta and yavādya ghṛta are useful in persons who are dried up, and in whom vāta is greatly provoked. After these ghṛtas have enhanced the strength, and relieved the aggravated vāta, the loosened morbidity can be eliminated by purgatives. The powder of one part each of paṭola-root, haridra, viḍanga, triphala, dālchini, two parts of kampillaka, three of nilini, and four of trivṛt can be administered along with cow's urine. After the cessation of purging, the patient can partake of meat juices of desert animals, thin gruel, and milk boiled with trikaṭu for six days. The procedure can be repeated. The above mentioned powder is very useful in udara.

The powder of indra-vāruṇi (gavākshi), śankhini, danti, tilvaka bark and vachā can be taken with water, cow's urine, grape juice or juice of kola, karkaṇḍu or sīdhu wine. The powders known as nārāyaṇa-chūrna and hapushādya-chūrṇa are also very useful. The powders of nīlini, nichula, trikaṭu, sarjika-kshāra, yāva-kshāra, the salts and chitraka can be administered with ghee.

After the administration of the medicated ghee, the patient can partake of gruel or sweetened milk or delicious meat-juices. After this has been digested, he can be purged, and can drink water boiled with ginger, and on the next day, can take thin gruel (peya), and on the day after, soup of kulattha.

A person afflicted with udara who has been subjected to these purificatory procedures, and who partakes of meat of jāngala (desert animals) can be administered milk with the paste of chitraka and devadāru, or milk with hasti-pippali and nāgara, for a month, or milk with viḍanga, chitraka, danti, chavya and trikaṭu, or the decoction of triphala, rohitaka and danti, mixed with yava-kshara and trikaṭu. The patient can also be administered cow's urine or harītaki followed by milk, or the milk and urine of buffalo, avoiding solid food, for a week, or camel's milk for a month, or goat's milk with trikaṭu for three months. He can also take the course of one-thousand harītaki fruits, or a course of śilājatu keeping himself on a diet of milk, or a course of guggulu. Milk with an equal amount of ginger juice or oil medicated with ginger juice is also useful.

Oil extracted from the nuts of danti and dravanti is useful in tridoshaja udara, abdominal pain, ānāha and constipation. It has however to be taken along with mastu, gruel or meat-juices. In vātaja udara, oil extracted from the seeds of mūlaka, sarala and madhu-śigru can be used for massage and internal use.

Gruel (yavāgu) prepared from shashṭika-rice that has been soaked in cow's urine, and milk can be eaten followed by sugarcane juice in all cases of udara. The tender leaves of śankhini, snuhi, trivṛt, danti and chira-bilva can be administered before meals in persons who are constipated and pass hard stools. After the problem of constipation has been relieved, the patient can drink milk with cow's urine. Oil medicated with bilva-kshāra can be administered in cases where there is pain in the sides of the chest and chest pain. Strong patients can be given castor oil, if the vāta has been obstructed (by kapha or pitta).

If all the above measures fail, a patient can be asked to eat a fruit that has been bitten by a venomous snake. After there has been improvement, the patient has to be sprinkled with cold water, and asked to partake of milk or gruel. For a month after this he can partake of barley and vegetables like maṇḍūka-parṇi, trivṛt, and vāstuka or bāla-śaka and its juice (or decoction), boiled without salt, sour drugs or unctuous preparations. He can regularly drink camel's milk.

In baddha-udara and chidra-udara, an incision whose width is four finger breadths, can be made on the left side, below the umbilicus, the intestines inspected and the obstructing matter (like hair, etc.,) removed. In cases of perforation, big ants should be made to bite the injured area, and after the perforations have been closed, their bodies should be cut off.

In ascites, the fluid should be drained out by inserting a canula (nāḍi), on the left side of the abdomen, below the navel. The abdomen is then bandaged firmly with a cloth. The patient should then fast, and drink gruels devoid of salt and unctuous substances. He should then subsist on a milk diet for six months. For three months, he can partake of milk with gruel, and for three more months, he can partake of śyāmāka, koradūsha, and milk without salt. Milk is very useful in patients suffering from ascites, (CS).

2. The person suffering from udara should strictly avoid food that is hard to digest, abhishandi, dry, unctuous, all kinds of meat, or irritant food, and bathing. However, shashtika rice, barley, wheat and nīvara are beneficial.

In vātaja-udara, the patient is to be given snehana by means of ghee medicated with drugs of the vidāri-gandhādi group, and purged by ghee boiled with tilvaka. Āsthāpana and anuvāsana enemas can be given using oil of danti, and a decoction of drugs of the vidāri gandhādi group. A sālvana upanāha (poultice) can be applied on the abdomen. The patient can also be fomented regularly. The diet should consist of meat juices of desert animals, and milk boiled with drugs of the vidāri gandhādi group.

In pittaja udara, the patient is oleated with ghee boiled with sweet drugs, purged with ghee boiled with syāma, triphala and trivṛt, and administered asthāpana and anuvāsana enema using a decoction of drugs of the nyagrodhādi group with sugar, honey and ghee. The abdomen can be plastered with a poultice consisting of pāyasa. The diet should consist of milk boiled with drugs of the vidāri-gandhādi group.

In kaphaja-udara, the patient is oleated using ghee medicated with a decoction of drugs of the pippalyādi group, purged using ghee boiled with gum of snuhi, given āsthāpana and anuvāsana enema with a decoction of drugs of the mushkakādi group mixed with trikaṭu, yava-kshāra, oil and cow's urine. A poultice consisting of śāna, atasi, dhātaki, sarshapa, kiṇva, mūlaka and bījaka can be applied over the abdomen. The patient is fomented regularly. The diet should consist of yūsha (gruel) of kulattha or pāyasa with trikaṭu.

In dūshyodara, the patient is purged for a month or a fortnight with ghee medicated with juices of śankhini and saptala or ghee medicated with mahā-vṛksha, milk, wine, and cow's urine. The paste of aśvamāra, gunja and kākādani root should be taken internally with wine. Sugarcane stalks or fruits of creepers (such as karkaṭi) should be made to be bitten by kṛshṇa-sarpa, and this should be eaten by the patient. Poisonous roots or barks can also be administered. However, this disease is very hard to cure.

All udaras are caused by the aggravation of vāta, and accumulation of water products. Hence purgative (anulomana) drugs are very useful.

The patient can be administered the medicines known as harītaki ghṛta, chavyādi ghṛta, mahā-vṛksha ghṛta and anaha varti. A suppository known also as ānāha-varti can be used.

The following recipes and formulations are useful in udara: castor oil is to be taken either singly or with cow's urine or milk for a month or two, while avoiding drinking water; the urine of a buffalo can be taken with buffalo's milk for a week, avoiding all other food; camel's milk can be taken for a fortnight, avoiding all other food and water; a course of pippali (as descibed in the treatment of vāta roga) taken for a month; oil extracted from danti can be used (internally) with rock-salt and ajamoda; the above mentioned oil can be boiled with the juice of fresh ginger in cases of abdominal pain; milk medicated with fresh ginger juice; milk with the paste of chavya and fresh ginger or of sarala, devadāru and chitraka; the parts of murangi (śobhanjana), śālaparṇi, śyāma, punarnava and milk; oil extracted from seeds of jyotishka with milk, mixed with svarjika-kshāra and hingu; the paste of harītaki and jaggery; one thousand pippali fruits soaked in milky juice of snūhi can be gradually consumed; an utkārika prepared from harītaki and pippali which are soaked in the milky juice of snuhi; the decoction of purgative drugs with devādaru and fresh ginger, etc.

In plīhodara, the patient is oleated, fomented and asked to partake of curds (with boiled rice). The veins that are found in the left elbow internally are to be opened. The enlarged spleen should be rubbed firmly with the palms. The patient can then be administered the kshāra of śukti found in the sea (marine oyster shell) with milk, or hingu and souvarchala salt with milk; or filtered pālaśa kshāra or yava-kshāra; the alkaline water of palāśa (-kshāra) with a liberal amount of yava-kshāra; the kshāras of pārijāta, ikshuka and apāmārga, fried in oil and mixed with gruel of śobhanjana, rock-salt, pippali and chitraka; the kshāra of pūti-karanja which is filtered through kānji, taken with viḍa-lavaṇa and pippali. The medicated ghee known as shatpala-ghṛta is also very useful.

These measures are useful in yakṛt-dālyudara also. However, in this disease, venesection can be done in the veins of the right hand. After slightly bending the wrist of the left hand downwards, the vein that connects the thumb (of the left hand) should be cauterised with a heated sara, in plīhodara.

In cases of baddhaguda and parisrāvi-udara, the patient has to be oleated and fomented. His abdomen should then be massaged with oil. An incision is made on the left side of the abdomen below the umbilicus, about four finger breadths to the left of the median line. The intestines are then gently drawn out, and any foreign matter such as hair or stones, etc., is removed. The intestines are then lubricated with honey and ghee, and gently replaced within the abdominal cavity. The incision should be sewn up. In parisrāvi-udara, the two ends of the injured (perforated) intestines should be pressed together and large black ants applied, so that they bite the correct spot. The incised part should be plastered with black earth mixed with yashṭi-madhu, and bandaged. The patient should then retire to a chamber that is not exposed to draughts of air, and should sit in a tub full of oil or ghee. He should partake of only milk.

In dakodara, the patient is massaged with oil prepared from drugs that alleviate vāta, and fomented by means of hot water. The surgeon should then make an incision by an instrument known as vrīhi-mukha, on the left side of the abdomen, below the umbilicus, about four finger-breadths away from the median line. The incision should be about the breadth of a thumb, in depth. A tube open at both ends is then introduced, so that the accumulated fluid is drained out. The puncture is then lubricated with rock-salt and oil and duly bandaged. If all the fluid is drained out in a day, the patient may suffer from thirst, fever, body pain, diarrhoea, dyspnoea, cough or burning of the soles, or there may be a fresh collection of fluid. Therefore small amounts of fluid can be drained out at intervals of three, four, five, six, eight, ten, twelve or sixteen days. The abdomen is then bandaged with a piece of flannel, silk-cloth or leather, in order to prevent flatulent distension. For six months (after tapping), the patient should partake of milk or meat-juices of desert animals. For another three months, the patient can partake of milk diluted with an equal amount of water along with sour fruits or meat-juices of desert animals. For the next three months, the diet should consist of food that is easy to digest and wholesome, (SS).

3. In every case of udara, the patient is first administered purgatives, such as castor oil with cow's urine or cow's milk.

A paste of equal quantities of jaggery and ginger is useful in all udaras. The paste of khadira and devadāru can be taken along with cow's urine. A fine powder of pippali can be triturated or soaked in milky juice of snuhi and administered with buffalo's urine. The paste of pārada bhasma can be trituruated with sudhā-kshāra, and given with harītaki and fresh butter, (RRS).

Ref.: CS, chikitsā, 13, 59-194; SS, chikitsā, 14; RRS, 19, 3-40; 30, 43.

Classical prescriptions: Arka-lavaṇa; Bhallātaka-rasāyana; Dadhika-ghṛta; Daśamūla-harītaki; Daśamūla-panchakoladi-kvātha-chūrṇa; Daśamūla-śhaṭpala-ghṛta; Dugdha-vaṭi; Gandharva-hasta-taila; Icchābhedi-rasa; Kalyāṇaka-guḍa; Lakshmī-vilāsa-rasa; Loha-bhasma; Mahā-panchagavya-ghṛta; Maṇibhadra yoga; Nārāyaṇa-chūrṇa; Nimbādi-chūrṇa; Punaravāsava; Punarnavādi-kāvātha-chūrṇa; Punarnavāshṭaka-kvātha-chūrṇa, Rohitākarishṭa; Saptasāra-kvātha-churṇa; Śankha-drāvaka; Shaṭpala ghrta; Śiva-guṭika; Sukumāra-ghṛta; Śūla-vajriṇi-vaṭaka, Tāmra-bhasma; Vajra-bhasma; Vajra-kshāra; Yava-kshāra;

Jalodara: Rasa-pushpa; Tamra-bhasma; Vāriśoshana-rasa; Daśamūla-panchakolādi-kvātha-chūrṇa.

Plīhodara: Arka-lavaṇa; Kadali-kshāra; Kānta-vallabha-rasa; Khadirārishṭa; Śūla-vajriṇi-vaṭika; Yaṛt-śūla-vināśini-vaṭika.

Mahodara: Indukānta-ghṛta

Yakṛt-plīhodara: Abhayā-lavaṇa; Lokanātha-rasa.

Vātodarā: Navaratna-rāja-mṛgānka-rasa.

Ulbaka-roga

Synonyms: Sahaja, Ambu-pūrṇa

Western Nosology: Asphyxia neonatorum

Type: This disease occurs in new-born babies (AS).

Causative Factors: Failure to vomit the garbhāmbhasa (amniotic fluid) or the accumulated mucus in the throat, (AS).

Symptomatalogy: The deranged rasa (body fluids) obstructs the channels of the heart (and circulation). The newborn infant, with clenched hands, suffers from heart diseases (hṛdroga). ākshepaka (convulsions), dyspnoea, cough, fever, vomiting etc., (AS).

Treatment: The bottom of a spindle (tarku) is heated red-hot and immersed in kaṭu-taila. A few drops of that oil is given to the infant.

The powders of trikaṭu, harītaki, vachā and haridra are made into a paste with breast milk and administered to the baby, (CD).

Ref.: AS, uttara, 2, page. 32; CD, 64, 2-3.

Upadamśa

Western Nosology: Venereal diseases

Causative Factors:

Extrinsic: Excessive sexual intercourse, total abstinence from sex, frequent sexual intercourse with a woman who has long been chaste or who has not had coitus for a long time or a menstruating woman, or a woman who has rough, long or densely compressed pubic hairs or with a woman who has hairs within the vagina or who has a very small vaginal orifice, or with a woman who is not inclined to sex, sexual intercourse without inclination, intercourse with a woman with unclean genital organs or who washes herself with impure water, or with a woman suffering from yoni-roga (diseases of female genital organs), introducing the penis into any natural orifice of the body other than the vagina, by getting the penis scratched or bitten, or if the penis is in contact with bristles of śūka (a kind of poisonous insect), practising masturbation, sexual intercourse with animals, washing the genitals with filthy water, failure to wash the genitals after coitus, suppressing ejaculation, or any pressure or injury to the genital organs, (SS).

Pathogenesis: These factors cause aggravation of the doshas which localise in the penis, which may or may not be injured, and bring about a swelling in that region, (SS).

Types: The disease is of five types. It can be caused by the aggravation of vāta, pitta or kapha, or all three doshas or by the vitiation of blood, (SS).

Symptomatology:

Vātaja-upadamśa: various types of pain, cracks in the skin (of penis, prepuce, etc.,), roughness of genital organs, numbness and rough swelling of penis.

Pittaja-upadamśa: Fever, swelling which is red like the ripe udumbara fruit, severe burning pain and speedy suppuration.

Kaphaja-upadamśa: Itching, hard and unctuous looking swelling.

Tridoshaja-upadamśa: Presence of the above symptoms, gangrene (avadaraṇa) of the penis, infestation with parasites and death.

Raktaja-upadamśa: All the symptoms of pittaja-upadamśa will manifest in a severe form, fever, burning pain, śosha (dryness or emaciation), blackish vesicles appear in the region, and there is excessive bleeding, (SS).

Prognosis:

1. The tridoshaja-upadamśa is considerd to be incurable, while raktaja-upadamśa can be palliated, (SS).

2. The vātaja, pittaja and kaphaja upadamśa are curable, (AS).

Ref.: SS, nidāna, 12, 7-9; AS, uttara, 38. pages. 284-285.

Treatment:

1. A person suffering from a case of curable upadamśa should be subjected to oleation (snehana) and sudation (svedana) after which blood has to be let out from the vein found in the centre of the penis, either though leeches or venesection. If the doshas are excessively vitiated, emesis and purgation should also be carried out. These measures will soon relieve the pain and swelling. If the patient is too weak to be administered purgation, nirūha-type of enema can be employed.

In a case of pittaja-upadamśa, a paste of gairika, rasāñjana, yashṭi-madhu, sāriva, uśīra, padmaka, chandana, and nilotpala and ghee (or oil), or a paste of padma, nilotpala, mṛṇāla (lotus stem), sarja, arjuna, vetasa, yashṭi-madhu, and ghee can be applied over the affected area. The area can be washed with ghee, milk, sugar (solution), sugarcane juice, solution of honey or a cold decoction of vaṭa, etc.

In kaphaja-upadamśa, the paste of the bark of śāla, aśva-karṇa, aja-karṇa and dhava, sūra (wine), flour, and hot oil or a paste of haridra, ativisha, musta, surasa, deva-dāru, teja-patra, pāṭha and pattūra can be applied externally. The affected area can be washed with a decotion of drugs of the surasādi group or āragvadādi group.

All these measures are to be employed in cases of non-suppurated upadamśa. The physician should try to arrest the suppurative process, because suppuration in the veins, ligaments, skin and flesh would destroy the penis. Therefore as soon as the suppurative process commences, an incision should be made, and the pus drained out. The incised area should be plastered with the paste of tila seeds, honey and ghee. The decoction of karavīra leaves, jāti leaves, āragvadha leaves or vaijayanti (agnimantha) leaves should be used to wash the incised area.

The fine powders of sourāshtri, gairika, tuttha, pushpa-kāsīsa, rock-salt, lodhra, rasāñjana, dāru-haridra, haritāla, manahśila, hareṇu and ela should be mixed with honey and used (for external application).

The incised area should be constantly washed with a decoction of fresh leaves of jambu, āmra, sumana, nimba, śveta (sveta-syanda) and kāmbhoji and barks of sallaki, badara, bilva, palāśa, tinisa and the milky trees, and triphala. Oil medicated with the above drugs and goji (gojihva), viḍanga, yashṭi-madhu and drugs of elādi group is very useful in fecilitating the healing process.

The powder of equal amounts of svarjika-kshāra, tuttha, kāsīsa, śaileya, rasānjana and manahśila is very useful in ulcers. The ashes of gundra, harītala and manahśila are also useful. The paste of bhṛngaraja (juice), triphala, danti, tāmra (bhasma) and iron (loha bhasma) is also very efficacious in upadamśa.

Even incurable cases of raktaja and tridoshaja upadamśa should be treated with the above measures, depending upon the doshas that are mainly involved.

A case of tridoshaja-upadamśa should be treated as indicated for dushṭa-vraṇa. The putrid (gangrenous) portion of the penis should be cut off, and the remining part cauterized with a jambvoshtha instrument, made red hot in a fire. Later, a paste of honey and ghee should be applied. Medicated oils and plasters should be used for promoting healing, ropaṇa, (SS).

2. The person suffering from upadamśa can be internally administered the decoction of paṭola, nimba, triphala and guḍūchi or of khadira and asana with guggulu. Ghee medicated with bhūnimba, triphala, nimba, paṭola, karanja, jāti, khadira and asana or with karanja, nimba, arjuna, śāla, jambu and vaṭa is also efficacious (when used internally).

The ash (soot) obtained by burning triphala powder in a frying pan is to be applied over the ulcer of upadamśa along with honey, in order to hasten the healing. The upadamśa can also be washed with a decoction of triphala or juice of bhṛngarāja. The paste of rasānjana, sirīsha bark, harītaki and honey or of pūga fruit and root of karavīra can be applied externally. The fine powders of babbūla leaves, or of bark of dāḍima can be sprinkled over the affected area. The diet should consist of yavā (barley) and well-water, (CD).

3. In a case of upadamśa, blood should be let out from the vein that runs along the dorsal aspect of the penis. The patient should then be administered bola-baddha rasa with honey. A paste of the root of matsyākshi can be applied externally. If there are swollen glands along the knee and thigh, the paste of yavā and chinchā (amlika) can be applied. The paste of sour gruel (kānji) and sea salt can also be applied externally.

Bola-baddha rasa: Equal parts of pārada bhasma (rasa-sindūra), and purified vatsanābha, and two parts of purified sulphur, and one part each of bola, purified haratāla (or haratāla bhasma), hingu, karkoṭi, svarṇa-mākshika (bhasma), haridra, kaṇṭakari, yava-kshāra, lāngali root powder, rock-salt and sāra (essence, heart wood) of madhuka are together triturated in the prescribed manner with the juice of ārdraka (fresh ginger) for seven days and made into small pills, (RRS).

Classical Prescriptions: Bṛhat-manjishṭhādi-kvātha-chūrṇa; Sārivādyāsava.

Upadamśaja-Vraṇa: Tutthādi-lepa

Ref.: SS, chikitsā, 19, 25-51; CD, 47; RRS, 13, 37-38; 25, 73-74.

See also: Vidradhi, Śiro-roga

Upa-śīrshaka

Western Nosology: Cephal-hematoma.

Causative Factors:

Intrinsic:

1. The aggravated vāta (AHṛ)

2. All the three vitiated doshas (CS).

Type: This is a congenital disease (AHṛ).

Symptomatology: There is a painless swelling that is not discoloured in the cranial bone (Kapāla).

Treatment: The infant should be treated with

drugs and other measures that alleviate vāta. If it starts to suppurate, it should be treated like a vidradhi.

Ref.: CS, chikitsā, 12, 75; AHṛ, uttara, 23, 21; 24, 20.

Urastoya

Western Nosology: Pleurisy.

Causative Factors:

Extrinsic: Debility or anaemia due to diseases like intermittent fever, diarrhoea, dysentery (pravāhika), enlargement of spleen, pāṇḍu (anaemia), arbuda, heart diseases, phiranga, ascites, and diseases of liver and kidneys.

Exposure to cold, injury, fever, sannipāta jvara, tuberculosis, diseases of the lungs, and anaemia and swelling caused by diseases of liver.

Pathogenesis: There is accumulation of fluid in the pleura, similar to that seen in jalodara.

Symptomatology: There is severe pain and swelling (oedema) in the lungs (pleura), which may fluctuate, increasing some times and decreasing at other times. If it progresses, a yellowish fluid accumulates, being preceded by fever.

The other symptoms seen are fever, dyspnoea, swelling in the sides of the chest, restlessness, dry cough, thirst, debility, feeble digestion, paleness (of mucous membranes and skin), anorexia, depression (dainya), displacement of the heart, very feeble or rapid pulse, friction sound heard below the scapula, gradual decrease in the rate of respiration, dull sound heard on percussion, severe pain while coughing, deformity of the sides of the chest and drowsiness.

Treatment:

1. The patient has to be treated with drugs that are diuretic and that alleviate kapha. The patient has to strictly avoid cold water, exposure to cold air and use of drugs and food that are abhishyandi, (that cause coating on blood vessels). If the patient is thirsty, he can partake of small amounts of water which has been boiled and reduced to one-fourth its quantity, or warm milk which has been diluted.

The expressed juice of punarnava with yavakshāra has to be administered twice a day, for some days. The drugs, and regimen which have been described under śotha, mūtra-kṛcchra, kāsa, śvāsa, hṛdroga and rāga-yakshma can be judiciously employed in this disease also.

The patient should avoid exertion, coitus, use of cold water, sleep during daytime, grief and anger, for one year after he has been cured.

The formulation known as sudhānidhi-rasa is very useful. If these medicines do not have any effect, the fluid has to be carefully drained out, by using an instrument known as trikūrchaka, (BR).

Ref.: BR, pages. 439-441.

Classical Prescriptions: Sṛṅga-bhasma; Vāriśoshana-rasa.

Uru-stambha

Synonyms: Sanskrit-Āḍhya-vāta (AHṛ, nidāna, 15, 51).

Western Nosology: Stiffness of the thighs; Paraplegia.

Causative Factors:

Extrinsic: Over exertion, fright, sleeping during the day, loss of (night) sleep, suppression of natural urges, fasting, partaking of food before the digestion of the previously eaten food, overeating, intake of meat of domesticated, aquatic and wet-land animals, flour preparations (pishṭa), stale wine, and food which is unctuous (oily), hot, very easy to digest and cold, (CS).

Intrinsic: Vāta (CS, sūtra, 20, 11); Kapha (CS).

Constituents Affected: Medas (fatty tissues), (CS).

Pathogenesis: The āma (undigested food) along the medas obstructs the functions of the vāta and other doshas, which localise in the lower limbs, especially in the thighs and legs. The aggravated kapha and medas overpower vāta and pitta, and render the thighs immobile on account of its coldness and rigidity, (CS).

Prodromal Symptoms: Fever, sleepiness, self-absorption, anorexia, horripilation, vomiting, weakness of thighs and legs and staimitya (immobility or a sensation as if covered by a wet cloth), (CS).

Symptomatology: Involuntary (or uncontrollable) spasms and weakness (of the affected limbs), a sense of heaviness, contraction (sankocha), burning sensation, numbness, tremors, pulsation, breaking and piercing pains, and a sensation as if the thighs and feet have been broken. The patient feels pain when putting his feet on the ground, cannot perceive the sensation of cold, and feels as if he has no control over the function of standing, pressing or walking, (CS).

Prognosis: Recent cases are curable. Cases in which there is burning sensation, pain and tremors are considered incurable, (CS).

Ref.: CS, chikitsā, 27, 8-19; AHṛ, nidāna, 15, 47-51.

Treatment: The person suffering from this disease should not be subjected to oleation and emesis, because these two procedures will aggravate kapha. Purgation, on the other hand, will not have any effect on the kapha that has been localised on the lower limbs.

Therefore the patient has to be judiciously treated with palliative drugs (samśamana), and measures which expel kapha from its seat (of thighs, etc.,) and help in its dehydration (śoshaṇa).

For the purpose of dehydration (of the kapha), the person should partake of yava, śyāmāka, kodrava, leafy vegetables cooked with water and oil, but without salt, tender leaves of sunishaṇṇaka, nimba, arka, vetra, and āragvadha, vayasi (kāka-machi), vāstuka, kulaka (kāravellaka) and other bitter substances.

The following recipes are also useful: drugs such as kshāra (yava-kshāra), harītaki, madhuka and pippali; the paste of samanga (lajjālu), śālmali, bilva and honey; the paste of śrīveshṭaka, udīchya, devadāru, tagara and honey; the paste of chandana, dhātaki, kushṭha, tālīśa, nalada (jaṭāmāmsi) and honey; the paste of musta, harītaki, lodhra, padmaka, kaṭuka-rohiṇi and honey; the paste of devadāru, haridra, dāru-haridra, vachā, kaṭuka-rohiṇi and honey; the paste of pippali, pippali roots, sarala, devadāru and honey; the paste of chavya, chitraka roots, devadāru, harītaki and honey; the paste of bhallātaka, pippali, pippali roots and honey; the powders of śārngeshṭa (gunja), madana, danti, vatsaka (kuṭaja) seeds, vachā, mūrva, āragvadha, pāṭha, karanja and kulaka (kāravellaka) with honey or water; or with honey and whey (dadhi-maṇḍa); the powders of mūrva, ativisha, kushṭha, chitraka, and kaṭu-rohiṇi with honey, or water or honey and whey; the paste of guggulu which has been previously soaked in cow's wine overnight; the powders of svarṇa-kshiri, ativisha, musta, tejovati, vachā, devadāru, chitraka, kushṭha, pāṭha, kaṭuka-rohiṇi with honey or with water and honey; the paste of phali, vyāghra-nakha, nāga-keśara and honey; the powders of triphala, pippali, musta, chavya and kaṭu-rohini with honey; oil medicated with pīluparṇi, payasya, rāsna, gokshura, vachā, sarala, agaru and pāṭha with honey; mustard oil medicated with kushṭha, śrī-veshṭaka, udīchya, sarala, devadāru, nāga-kesara, ajagandha, and aśvagandha, with honey; oil boiled with two palas of rock-salt, five palas of ginger, two palas of granthi (pippali-roots) and chitraka each, twenty bhallataka stones and two ādhakas of kānji; and one prastha of oil medicated with a pala each of pippali roots and nāgara, eight palas of katvara (buttermilk) and equal amount of curds.

If there is excessive depletion of tissues, after these medicines, the patient can be nourished with old rice and meat of desert animals. If the person suffers from aggravation of vāta, pain and sleeplessness, he can be subjected to oleation and sudation by drugs that alleviate vāta.

In order to expel the aggravated kapha, the patient can be massaged with the mud of ant hills, the powdered root, bark or fruit of karanja or with powdered brick. The powders of aśvagandha, root, arka roots, nimba roots or devadāru roots should be mixed with honey, sarshapa (mustard) oil, mud of ant hill, and massaged over the affected area. The paste of danti, dravanti, surasa (tulasi) and sarshapa can be applied externally. The affected area can be washed or sprinkled with a hot decoction of leaves, fruits or roots of tarkāri, śigru, tulasi, dry ginger, kuṭaja and nimba. The paste of sarshapa seeds which have previously been soaked in cow's urine can be applied externally. The paste of kuṭaja, surasa, kushṭha, aromatic substances, tumburu, śigru, himsra, arka roots, mud of ant-hills, kuṭheruka, curds and rock-salt can be applied externally. The decoction of śyonāka, khadira, bilva, kaṇṭakāri, bṛhati, sarala, asana, sobhānjana, tarkāri, gokshura, surasa, arjaka, agnimantha and karanja can be used as affusions (parisheka).

The patient should be advised to walk or indulge in some exercise in order to alleviate kapha. Then he can be advised to walk on uneven ground full of gravel and sand, or to swim in a river against the current, or in a pond with pure water.

All measures which alleviate kapha and do not aggravate vāta should be employed, (CS).

2. The patient can be administered the decoction of chitraka, indrayava, pāṭha, kaṭuka, ativisha, and haridra; or the paste of trikaṭu, chitraka, musta, triphala, viḍanga and guggulu, (AHṛ).

3. The patient can be administered śilājitu, guggulu, pippali or nāgara with cow's urine or a decoction of daśamūla drugs; or the paste of triphala, kaṭuka and honey; or vardhamāna pippali with honey or jaggery, (CD).

Ref.: CS, chikitsā, 27, 20-62; AHṛ, chikitsā, 21, 45-50; CD, 24.

Classical Prescriptions: Maṇḍūra-vaṭaka; Śiva-guṭika; Viḍangārishṭa.

Utphullika

Western Nosology: Nephritis.

Type: This disease occurs in children.

Symptomatology: The child suffers from flatulent distension of the abdomen (ādhmāna), difficulty in respiration and swelling (śvayathu) of limbs. (There is swelling of right abdomen according to KBT).

Treatment: Bloodletting can be done using leeches. The mother or wet nurse is to be given the powders of karkoṭa, nāgara, kankola, megha and ativisha with milk. This will eliminate the defects in the breast-milk. The decoction of bilva root, nīrada (musta), vṛkshi, triphala and two varieties of simhika (brhati and kaṇṭakāri) is given to the child with jaggery. The powders of pippali, granthika, viśva, trāyamaṇa, dārvika, pathyebha, pippali, bhārngi, lavanga, borax, kumārī, bāla-haritaki and rock salt are administered with goats urine, (YR, KBT).

Ref.: YR, bāla-roga, KBT, 6.

Valmīka

Western Nosology: Dermatitis verrucosa

Causative Factors:

Intrinsic: All three doshas.

Symptomatology: Knotty growths which in their appearance resemble ant hills, are found in the palms, soles, joints, around the neck, and in the regions above the clavicles; they develop gradually and have many outlets. There is also pricking pain, discharge, burning pain and itching.

Prognosis: Knotty growths appearing on the palms and soles, attended with swelling, and with many openings are considered to be incurable.

Treatment: These growths have to be excised, and cauterized by fire or kshāra (alkali). They are then subjected to cleansing (śodhana) and healing (ropaṇa) measures, as in the case of arbuda.

In cases where the growths are found in regions that are not vital (amarma), and where they are not too large, the patient has to be subjected to eliminative procedures (such as emesis, purgations, etc.,) which are to be followed by bloodletting. The paste of roots of kulattha, danti and śyāma (a variety of trivṛt), and guḍūchi, rock salt, palala (paste of tila seeds) and śaktu (fried and powdered barley) can be applied externally over the affected area. Poultices prepared from the same drugs mixed with only unctuous substances should be applied when warm. When the growths are ripe (after they have suppurated), the sinus or the course of the pus channels should be ascertained and the ulcer opened and cauterized. After the putrid flesh (dushṭa-māmsa) has been removed, an alkali (kshāra) should be applied. After the ulcer has been cleansed, it has to be plastered with healing drugs. Neem oil medicated with sumana (jāti leaves), granthi, bhallātaka, manahśila, the black variety of sāriva, sukshma-ela, chandana and agaru can be used for this purpose.

Ref.: SS, nidāna, 13, 9-10; chikitsā, 20, 48-56.

Classical Prescription: Vajra - bhasma

Vāta-rakta

Synonyms: Sanskrit: Vatāsra, khuḍa, Āḍhya-vāta, Āḍhya-roga, Vāta-balāsa

Western Nosology: Gout; Arthritis

Causative Factors:

Extrinsic:

1. This disease commonly occurs in delicate, obese, and pleasure-loving persons and those who are accustomed to improper food and life style.

Excessive exertion, overeating, excessive intake of food that is hot, and hard to digest, etc., are also responsible for causing this disease, (SS, chikitsa, 5).

2. This disease also occours due to excessive intake of salty food, (CS, sūtra, 26, 43, 3).

3. Riding on animals such as elephants, horses, etc., for long distances, exposure to heat (of sun and fire), excessive intake of food that is sharp, hot, sour and caustic (kshāra) and vegetables, (SS, nidāna,1, 42).

4. Excessive (and regular) intake of food articles that are salty, sour, pungent, caustic, greasy, and hot, of kulattha, māsha, nishpāva, leafy vegetables, oil cakes, sugarcane, meat of aquatic and wet-land animals, mūlaka, food that is stale and dry, of curds, aranāla, souvīra, śukta (vinegar), buttermilk, alcoholic drinks, of food that is incompatible, eating before the digestion of the previous meal, overeating, anger, sleep during daytime, keeping awake at nights, injury, fasting, intake of food that is dry, astringent, pungent, and bitter, riding on animals, swimming and excessive travelling.

This disease usually occurs in persons who are delicate, who lead a very sedentary life, and who are used to sumptous food, with plenty of sweet dishes, (CS).

Intrinsic: Vāta, (SS).

Constituents Affected: Blood (CS, sutra, 24, 12).

Pathogenesis:

1. The aggravated vāta is obstructed by the deranged blood, and thus it further vitiates the blood. Due to the fluidity and flowing of blood and the subtle and all pervasive nature of vāta, they spread all over the body, through the circulatory channels, and localise in the joints, (CS).

2. The aggravated vāta is obstructed by the deranged blood, further vitiates the blood, and gives rise to this disease, (SS).

Prodromal Symptoms:

1. The hands and feet are first affected. There is pricking and burning pain, stiffness, itching, swelling, roughness of skin, pulsation of blood vessels, tremors of the snāyus (hard fibrous structures), weakness of limbs, and sudden appearance of brownish-grey circular patches on the palm, soles, fingers, toes, ankles, wrists, etc., (SS).

2. Absence of or excessive sweating, blackish discolouration, numbness, extreme tenderness, weakness, of joints, lethargy, weakness, appearance of eruptions, pricking pain, pulsation, breaking pain, heaviness and numbness of knee, legs, thigh, waist, shoulders, hands, feet and joints, itching, frequent spasmodic pain in the joints, discolouration, and appearance of circular patches, (CS).

Classification:

1. Vāta-rakta may be either superficial or deep-seated. When it is superficial, the skin and muscles are affected. However, the deeper parts are affected in the latter kind of vāta-rakta, (CS).

2. According to SS, there is one vāta-rakta. The superficial parts of the body are affected in the early stages. The deeper parts are affected in the chronic stage.

Symptomatology:

1. In the superficial type of vāta-rakta, there is itching, burning sensation, pain, pricking pain, pulsation, contraction, extension and greyish, red or coppery discolouration.

In vāta-rakta that is deep-seated, there is swelling, rigidity (or stiffness), hardness, intense pain within the joints, greyish or coppery discolouration, burning, pricking pain, pulsation and suppurative tendency.

The disease manifests in the joints, especially of the hands, feet, fingers and toes, from where it spreads (all over the body).

There is burning and cutting pain in the joints, bones and bone-marow and deformity within the joints. There is also lameness and khanja.

If vāta is excessively aggravated, there is distension of the veins, sharp and pricking pain, pulsation, blackish discolouration and dryness of the swelling, fluctuation in the swelling, contraction of blood vessels, fingers, toes and joints, intense pain, stiffness of the body, contraction (deformity) and aversion to cold.

If there is extreme derangement of blood, there is swelling with agonising pain, pricking pain, copper-coloured discolouration, tingling sensation, itching, softening and no relief either from unctuous or dry substances.

If pitta is vitiated, there is a burning sensation, pain, syncope, perspiration, thirst, vertigo, feeling of intoxication, reddish discolouration, suppuration, atrophy and destruction.

If kapha is excessively aggravated, there is heaviness, greasiness, numbness, dull pain and a sensation as if enveloped by a moist cloth, (CS).

2. The prodromal signs and symptoms appear in an intensified form. If proper treatment is not given, there is deformity, (SS).

Complications:

1. Loss of vitality, wasting of muscles, thirst, fever, syncope, dyspnoea, cough, stiffness, anorexia, indigestion, contraction, metastasis (visaraṇa), (SS).

2. Insomnia, anorexia, dyspnoea, koṭha (putrefaction) of muscles, stiffness of the head (and neck), syncope, a feeling of intoxication, pain, thirst, fever, clouded sensorium (moha), tremors, hiccoughs, lameness, visarpa, suppuration, pricking pain, debility, deformity of fingers and toes, appearance of vesicles and arbuda, and injury to vital organs, (CS).

Prognosis:

Cases where there is aggravation of only one dosha, which are recent and where there are no complications are curable. That disease that is characterised by aggravation of two doshas, and where there are few complications, can be palliated. The disease that is caused by the aggravation of all three doshas and where all the complicating symptoms are present is incurable, (CS).

Ref.: CS, chikitsā, 29, 5-34; SS, nidāna, 1, 42-43; chikitsā, 5, 3-6.

Treatment:

1. Due to the fact that the blood channels are obstructed by the aggravated vāta, and that this in turn further vitiates the pain, blood-letting by means of venesection or leeches, etc., is indicated. Leeches are to be employed where there is pricking pain and burning pain. The gourd or horn can be used in cases where there is numbness, itching and tingling. Venesection or cupping can be done where the symptoms are shifting (from one joint to another). However, bloodletting is contra-indicated in atrophy (or emaciation), in cases where vāta is excessively provoked and where there is dryness. Bloodletting in such cases causes deep-seated swelling, stiffness, tremors, disorders of blood vessels and hard fibrous structures (snāyu), fatigue, contraction (of limbs, etc.,) lameness, vāta-roga and even death. Bloodletting is indicated only in persons who are rich in the unctuous principle.

In general, a person suffering from vāta-rakta should be oleated, and then administered unctuous purgatives or dry and mild purgatives, followed by frequent enemata. Non-irritant affusions, massages, external applications, food and unctuous substances are also useful.

The superficial type of vāta-rakta should be treated by means of external applications, massages (by medicated oils), affusion and use of poultices. The deep seated disease is treated by purgation, āsthāpana enema, and potions of unctuous preparations.

Cases of vāta-rakta where there is aggravation of vāta are treated by the internal use, massage and enema of ghee, oil, vasā (fat) and majja (marrow), and poultices that are tepid. Cases where there is aggravation of pitta and vitiation of blood are to be treated by administering purgatives, potions of ghee and milk, affusions, enemata and cool and refreshing applications.

Cases where there is aggravation of kapha are to be treated by mild emesis, limited use of affusions and unctuous preparations, fasting and luke-warm external applications.

Cold applications in cases of vāta-rakta caused by aggravation of vāta and kapha lead to an increase in burning pain, swelling, pain, itching and stiffness, while hot applications in vāta-rakta caused by vitiation of blood and pitta bring about burning pain, softening and bursting.

The patient may be administered ghee medicated with milk, yashṭi-madhu, srāvaṇi, kshīra-kākoli, jīvaka and ṛshabhaka, or ghee medicated with drāksha, yashṭi-madhu, and sugar, or parūshakadi ghṛta, jīvanīya ghṛta, sthirādi ghṛta and chatush-sneha. The patient can also partake of milk boiled with the expressed juice of guḍūchi.

The patient can also be administered til oil mixed with milk and sugar, or milk mixed with ghee, or sugar and honey, or milk boiled with a decoction of śālaparṇi and sugar-candy or milk medicated with nāgara and pippali or medicated with balā, śatāvari, rāsna, daśamūla drugs, pīlu, śyāma, eraṇḍa and śālaparṇi (in cases where vāta is aggravated).

In cases where the vāta has been obstructed by

pitta and blood, the patient can partake of udder-warm milk with cow's urine or udder-warm milk with powder of trivṛt.

In severe cases, the patient can be purged by using milk mixed with castor-oil, which should be followed by a diet of rice and milk. The decoction of harītaki with ghee or grape juice mixed with trivrt powder can be administered, followed by the anupāna of milk. The purgative drink composed of a decoction of kāśmari, trivṛt, drāksha, triphala and parūshaka mixed with honey and rock-salt can also be administered.

Patients in whom kapha is aggravated are to be administered a decoction of triphala with honey or a decoction of āmalaki, haridra and musta.

The patient can also be given enema of milk and ghee for eliminating the faecal matter. The nirūha and āsthāpana enema are useful in case of pain in the hypochondriac region, groins, sides of the chest, thighs, joint, bones and abdomen, and in udāvarta.

Oil medicated with one āḍhaka of aranāla (kānji) and one-fourth the quantity of sarja-rasa is useful in relieving fever, burning sensation and pain. The medicated oils known as madhu-parṇyādi taila, sukumāraka taila, amṛtādya taila, mahāpadma taila, khuḍḍaka-padma taila, madhuka taila and balā-taila (prepared one thousand or one-hundred times), and piṇḍa taila are useful in administering enema, nasya (errhines), massage and affusions, and for relieving burning and pain.

For alleviating the pain in vāta-rakta, the decoction of milk and daśamūla drugs is useful. Warm ghee can also be used for affusion. Ghee, oil, etc., medicated with sweet drugs can also be used for affusing the affected area, in relieving stiffness, convulsion and pain. Oil medicated with the milk of cow, sheep and goat or with drugs of jīvanīya group or pancha-mūla group can also be used. Grape-juice, sugarcane juice, curds, whey, sour kānji, rice-water, honey-water and sugar water can be used for the purpose of affusion.

In cases of burning, the cold infusion of kamala, nilotpala, chandana, etc., are useful. In cases where there is redness, pain and burning pain, bloodletting is resorted to. The paste of aśvattha bark, yashṭi-madhu, jaṭāmāmsi, śatāvari, udumbara and dūrva, or aquatic drugs or barley powder mixed with yashṭi-madhu, ghee and milk or ghee medicated with drugs of jīvanīya group can be applied externally. The paste of tila, priyāla, yashṭi-madhu, lotus bulb, vetasa root, and goat's milk is useful in relieving redness and burning. The paste of prapouṇḍarīka, manjishṭha, dāru-haridra, yashṭi-madhu, chandana, sugarcandy, masūra, uśīra, padmaka, and śaktu is useful in relieving swelling, spreading affections, pain and burning pain, and where there is vitiation of blood and pitta.

Poultices of pāyasa of mudga, oil or ghee, drugs that alleviate vāta, or of a paste of tila and sarshapa, or of vesavāra composed of flesh of aquatic, wet-land and prasaha animals, is useful in vāta-rakta with aggravation of vāta.

Ghee boiled with cow's urine, alkali (kshāra) and surā wine is used in massaging in cases where there is swelling, heaviness, itching and aggravation of kapha. Ghee medicated with padmaka, dālchini, yashṭi madhu, sarīva and madhu-śukta can be used for affusion and massage in similar cases.

The paste of soot, vachā, kushṭha, śatapushpa, haridra and dāru-haridra, is useful in vāta-rakta characterised by aggravation of vāta and kapha. The paste of tagara, dālchini, śatapushpa, etc., kushṭha, musta, hareṇuka, devadāru, and shell rubbed with sour drugs is also useful. The paste of seeds of madhu-śigru and kānji can also be applied.

An iron vessel should be plastered within with a paste of equal parts of triphala, trikatu, tejapatra, ela, dālchini, vamśalochana, chitraka, vachā, viḍanga, pippali roots, kāsīsa, vāsā bark, ṛddhi, tāmalaki and chavya, in the morning. At noon, the patient should eat out of that vessel. But the patient should avoid curds, śukta (vinegar), kshāras and substances that are incompatible.

Even severe cases of vāta-rakta can be alleviated by partaking of a decoction of aśvattha, with honey. The use of guggulu, śilājatu, honey, old barley, wheat, sīdhu, arishṭa, āsavas, etc., is also very useful.

The patient can partake of a diet composed of old barley, wheat and nīvara, oil, rice that is harvested in sixty days, meat of vishkira and pratuda animals, the soup of āḍhaki, chaṇaka, mudga, masūra, makushṭhaka, etc., with ghee, vegetables such as sunishannaka, vetra, kākamāchi, śatāvari, vāstuka, upodika, etc., souvarchala salt, etc., and milk of cow, buffalo and goat.

The patient should avoid sleep during the day, exposure to heat (of the sun and fire), exercise, coitus, and food that is pungent, hot, hard to digest, salty, sour and abhishyandi, (CS).

2. The first remedial measure that is to be employed is bloodletting in smallquantities, and over many days. However, bloodletting is contra-indicated in persons in whom vāta is aggravated, who are emaciated and driedup. The patient can then be subjected to emesis (purgatives, enemata, etc.,) and post-purificatory procedures.

Patients in whom there is aggravation of vāta have to be administered potions of old ghee; goat's milk boiled with half its quantity of oil and yashṭi-madhu; goat's milk boiled with pṛśniparṇi, sugar, honey and sweet drugs, goat's milk boiled with ginger (śuṇṭhi), śṛngāṭaka and kaseruka, or with śyāma, rāsna, sushavi, pṛśniparṇi, pīlu, śatāvari, gokshura and daśamūla drugs; oil medicated with the paste of yashṭi-madhu, meshaśṛngi, gokshura, sarala, bhadradāru, vachā and surabhi (rāsna) and milk boiled with one-eighth part of a decoction of daśamūla drugs; oil medicated with the paste of drugs of the kākolyādi group and a decoction of śatāvari, apāmārga, ajamoda, yashṭi-madhu, kshīra-vidāri, balā, atibala and drugs of tṛna panchamūla group; or hundred times prepared (śatapāka) balā-taila. The affected part can be affused with milk boiled with the roots of drugs that alleviate vāta (daśamūla drugs) or with sour liquids such as surā, souvīra, etc. The paste of yava, yashṭi-madhu, eraṇḍa, tila and punarnava can be applied externally. The powders of barley, wheat, tila and mudga should be seperately mixed with the paste of kākoli, kshīra-kākoli, jīvaka, ṛshabhaka, balā, atibalā, lotus bulb, lotus stalk, pṛśniparṇi, mesha-śṛngi, priyāla, sugar, kaseruka, surabhi and vachā and boiled with milk, ghee, oil, animal fat or marrow. This can be applied as poultices. A vesavāra prepared from fish and powders of barley, wheat, tila, mudga and māsha can also be applied (as poultices). A poultice composed of bilva pulp, tagara, devadāru, sarala, rāsna, hareṇu, kushṭha, śata-pushpa, ela, surā wine and curd whey can also be applied. The paste of madhu-śigru roots mixed with juice of mātulunga, rock-salt, and ghee or of tila seeds alone can also be applied.

A patient of vāta-rakta in whom there is severe aggravation of pitta should be administered the decoction of draksha, ārvetaka (kiramālaka), kaṭphala, payasya, yashṭi-madhu, chandana and kāśmari mixed with sugar and honey; or the decoction of śatāvari, yashṭi-madhu, paṭola, triphala, and kaṭurohiṇi; or the decoction of guḍūchi; or the decoction of chandana, etc., is useful in pittaja-jvara, with honey and sugar; or ghee medicated with drugs of the sweet and bitter (paṭoladi) group; etc. The decoction of lotus bulbs, lotus stalks, white chandana, and padmaka, and half the quantity of milk or the decoction of milk, sugarcane juice, yashṭi-madhu, sugar and rice water or decoction of drākshā and sugarcane with kānji, wine and whey can be used for affusing the part. Ghee medicated with drugs of jīvanīya drugs or śatadhouta ghṛta or ghee medicated with drugs of kākolyādi group can be used externally. The tepid paste of rice harvested in sixty days, fresh vetasa, tālīsa, sṛngāṭaka, padma seeds, haridra, gairika, saivala, padma, lotus leaves, etc., and kānji and ghee can be applied.

In cases where there is excessive vitiation of blood, the same treatment is useful. Bloodletting and very cold external application can be employed.

Patients in whom the kapha is excessively vitiated can be administered the decoction of āmalaka and haridra sweetened with honey; or the decoction of triphala; or the paste of yashṭi-madhu, śrngavera, harītaki, kaṭuka-rohini and honey; the paste of harītaki and jaggery mixed with cow's urine or any other suitable liquid; etc. The affected area can be affused with the decoction of drugs that alleviate kapha along with oil, cow's urine, kshārodaka, surā, śukta, etc. The hot decoction of drugs of the āragvadhādi group can also be used. Ghee medicated with yashṭi-madhu, sāriva, padma, whey, cow's urine, surā and śukta can be applied externally. The paste of tila, sarshapa, atasi, barley, śleshmātaka, kapittha, madhu-śigru and cow's urine, kshārodaka, etc., can be applied. The pastes of white sarshapa, tila and aśvagandha, priyāla, seluka and kapittha, or of madhu-śigru and punarnava, or of trikaṭu, kaṭurohiṇi, pṛthakparṇi, bṛhati and kshārodaka, or of śālaparṇi, pṛśniparṇi, bṛhati, kaṇṭakāri and milk can be applied.

All cases of vāta-rakta can be treated by administering the mixture of jaggery and harītaki, or pippali with milk or water. The number of pippali fruits can be increased by five or ten every day for ten days, and thereafter it should be successively decreased (in a similar manner). The diet while taking this course should consist of milk and rice. Ghee cooked in milk and boiled with drugs of jīvanīyādi can be used externally. The paste of māshaparṇi, sahadeva, chandana, mūrva, musta, priyāla, śatāvari, kaseruka, padma, yashṭi-madhu, śatapushpa, vidāri, kushṭha and milk can be applied with ghee. The paste of saireyaka, vāsā, balā, atibalā, jīvanti, sushavi, and goat's milk, or of kāśmari, yashṭi-madhu, and cow's milk can be applied. Piṇḍa taila prepared from manjishṭha, bee wax, sarja rasa, sāriva, and milk can be applied. Old ghee boiled with the juice of āmalaki can be used internally. Old ghee boiled with drugs of jīvanīya group or kākolyādi group or with sushavi paste and decoction, or with a decoction of kāravellaka or bala taila can be used for affusion, tub baths, enemata and for internal use.

The diet has to consist of rice harvested in sixty days, barley, wheat, old rice and meat juice of desert animals boiled with milk or soup of mudga without sour substances. Blood-letting is also useful. Severe cases can be treated with emesis, purgation, āsthāpana and anuvāsana enemata.

The patient should avoid coitus, exertion, anger, food that is hot, sour, salty, hard to digest and abhishyandi and sleep during day, (SS).

3. The patient can be administered the following prescriptions: the decoction of guḍūchi, nāgara and dhānyaka; the decoction of guḍūchi with guggulu; the decoction of vāsa, guḍūchi, āragvadha and castor oil; the paste of muṇḍi, honey and ghee followed by a decoction of guḍūchi; the paste of three or five harītaki fruits (crushed) and jaggery, followed by a decoction of guḍūchi; castor oil with guḍūchi; the expressed juice, paste powder or decoction of guḍūchi, taken regularly; the decoction of paṭola, kaṭuka, śatāvari, triphala and guḍūchi; the decoction of āmalaki, haridra, and musta or of kokilāksha, pippali and guḍūchi in cases marked by aggravation of kapha; the mixture of ghee and jaggery; ghee medicated with a paste and decoction of guḍūchi; ghee medicated with milk and śatāvari, etc.

The paste of wheat flour, ghee and goat's milk or goat's milk and castor-seeds can be applied externally; oil medicated with milk and expressed juice of guḍūchi is also very useful. Oil medicated with grape juice or with yashṭi-madhu and kāśmari juice is also useful, (CD).

4. The patient can be administered trinetra

rasa, śūla-gaja-kesari-rasa and udaya-bhāskara-rasa. Pārada bhasma may be triturated with jaggery, harītaki and a decoction of guḍūchi and then administreated. The cold decoction of kokilāksha roots, guḍūchi, ginger and haridra is useful. The patient can first be administered triyoni-rasa followed by the powders of harītaki, āmalaki, guḍūchi, kaṭuka, and five parts of nimba with water. The patient should avoid sūraṇa, masha, vṛntāka and rājika, etc., (RRS).

Ref.: CS, chikitsā, 29, 35-160; SS, chikitsā, 5, 7-17; CD, 23; RRS, 21, 43-46; 170-171; 30, 57.

Classical Prescriptions: Amṛta-ghṛta; Balā-guḍūchyādi-taila; Bṛhat-guḍūchyādi-taila; Bṛhat-manjishṭhādi-kvātha-chūrṇa; Haratāla-bhasma; Kaiśora-guggulu; Kushṭha-rākshasa-taila; Madhu-snuhi-rasayana; Madhu-yashṭyādi-taila; Mahā-yogarāja-guggulu; Mṛgānka-rasa; Navaratna-rāja; Nimbādi-chūrṇa; Piṇḍa-taila; Rāsnairaṇḍādi-kvātha-chūrṇa; Sārivadyāsāva; Simhanāda-guggulu; Śiva-guṭika; Somarāji-taila; Gṛhadhūmādi-lepa; Vāṭari-guggulu; Vātaraktāntaka-rasa; Visha-tinḍuka-taila.

Vāta-roga

Diseases engendered by deranged vāta.

Causative Factors:

1. Excessive intake of food articles that are dry, cold and very easy to digest, eating less than the required quantity, excessive sexual intercourse, keeping awake at nights, loss of blood, wrong treatment, excessive use of purificatory procedures (such as emesis and purgations), fasting, swimming, walking for long distances, excessive exertion, depletion of body tissues, fear, grief, anger and anxiety, emaciation as a result of disease, sleep during daytime, suppression of natural urges, trauma (of any sort), sleeping or sitting in unnatural postures, and accumulations of āma (the undigested food), (CS).

2. Excessive exertion such as wrestling with a stronger person, running and swimming, excessive sexual intercourse, studying for long stretches of time, injuries, keeping awake at nights, lifting heavy weights, travelling for long distances on animals, excessive intake of food that is pungent, astringent, bitter, dry, light and cold and dried vegetables, vallūra (dried meat), varaka, uddālaka, koradūsha, śyāmaka, nīvara, mudga, masūra, aḍhaki, hareṇu, and nishpāva, fasting, overeating, eating at irregular timings, suppression of urges (of stool, urine, ejaculation of semen, vomiting, sneezing, etc.,) etc.

Vāta is normally aggravated in the cold season, in cloudy and windy weather, during the rains, at dawn, afternoon and after the digestion of food, (SS, sutra, 21, 19-20).

Pathogenesis: The vacant spaces (vacuities) in the body are filled up by the aggravated vāta, and innumerable disease are caused:

I. CS has enumerated eighty diseases caused by vāta alone. They are:

1. Nakha bheda (splitting of nails)
2. Vipādika (cracks in the soles)
3. Pāda-śūla (pain in the foot)
4. Pāda-bhramsa (foot drop)
5. Pada-suptata (numbness of foot)
6. Vāta-khuḍḍata (club foot)
7. Gulpha - graha (stiffness of ankle-joint)
8. Piṇḍikodveshṭana (cramps in the calf)
9. Gṛdhrasi (sciatica)
10. Jānu-bheda (genu varum)
11. Jānu-vislesha (genu valgum)
12. Ūrustambha (paraplegia)
13. Ūrusāda (weakness of thighs)
14. Pāngulya (lameness of both legs)
15. Guda-bhramsa (anal prolapse)
16. Gudārti (tenesmus)
17. Vṛshaṇākshepa (pain in scrotum)
18. Śepha-stambha (loss of erection)
19. Vankshaṇāha (tension of groin)
20. Śroni-bheda (pain in the pelvis)
21. Vid-bheda (hard lumpy stools)
22. Udāvarta (mis peristalsis)

23. Khanjatva (lameness of the leg)
24. Kubjatva (kyphosis)
25. Vāmanatva (dwarfism)
26. Trika-graha (arthritis of sacro-iliac joint)
27. Pṛṣṭha-graha (lumbago)
28. Pārśvāvamarda - (pleuritic pain)
29. Udaraveshṭa -(abdominal cramp)
30. Hṛnmoha & hṛdrava (palpitation)
31. Vaksha-uddharsha (chest pain)
32. Vaksha-uparodha (stiffness of thoracic cavity)
33. Hanu-bheda (pain in jaw)
34. Osṭha-bheda (cracks in lip)
35. Akshi-bheda- (pain in the eyes)
36. Danta-bheda -(toothache)
37. Danta-śaithilya -(looseness of teeth)
38. Mūkatva -(aphasia)
39. Vāk-sanga (stammering)
40. Kāshayāsyata (astringent taste in the mouth)
41. Mukha-śosha (dryness of the mouth)
42. Arasajnata (loss of sense of taste)
43. Ghrāṇa-nāśa (loss of sense of smell)
44. Karṇa-śūla (otalgia)
45. Aśabda-śravaṇa (auditory hallucinations)
46. Uchai-śruti
47. Bādhirya (deafness)
48. Vartma sankocha (contraction of eye-lids)
49. Vartma-stambha (ptosis)
50. Timira
51. Akshi-śūla
52. Akshi-vyudāsa (ptosis)
53. Bhrū-vyudāsa
54. Śankha-bheda (pain in temples)
55. Lalāta-bheda (frontal headache)
56. Śiro-ruk (headache)
57. Keśa-bhumir-sphuṭana (dandruff)
58. Ardita (facial paralysis)
59. Ekāngaroga
60. Sarvānga-roga (paralysis)
61. Paksha-vadha (hemiplegīa)
62. Ākshepaka (convulsions)
63. Daṇḍaka (tonic spasms)
64. Tama (fainting)
65. Bhṛama (vertigo)
66. Vepatha (tremors)
67. Jṛmbha (yawning)
68. Hikka (hiccoughs)
69. Vishāda (depression)
70. Ati-pralāpa (irrelevant speech)
71. Roukshya (dryness)
72. Pārushya (roughness)
73. Śyāvaruṇa-bhāsata (greyish-brown discolouration)
74. Asvapna (insomnia)
75. Anavastitha-chittatva (unstable mind)
76. Vaksha-toda (chest pain)
77. Bāhu-śosha (atrophy of arm)
78. Grīvāstambha (stiff-neck)
79. Manyā-stambha (torticollis)
80. Kaṇṭhodhvamśa (hoarseness)

Almost all diseases of vāta are characterised by looseness, prolapse, diffusion or seperation, contraction, rupture or division, weakness, horripilation, thirst, tremors, varta, movement, pricking pain, agitation, roughness, dryness, non-sliminess, porosity, brownish discolouration, astringent taste in the mouth, dryness of the mouth, numbness contraction, stiffness, deformity, etc., (CS, sūtra, 20, 11-12).

The aggravated vāta also causes contraction, stiffness of joints, aching pain in bones and joints, horripilation, irrelevent speech or loquacity, stiffness of fingers, back and head, deformity, emaciation, insomnia, abortion, amenorrhoea, sterility, tremors, numbness, tics (hundana) affecting the head, nose, eyes and neck, debility, convulsions, pricking pain, etc.

The aggravated vāta localising in the gastro-intestinal tract and thoraco-abdominal cavity causes constipation, retention or suppression of urine, bradhna, heart-disease, abdominal tumours, haemorrhoids, and pain in the sides of the chest.

If the vāta that pervades the entire body is affected, it causes tremors, breaking pain, all varieties of pain and a sensation as if all the joints are dislocated.

If the vāta that localises in the rectum is affected, it causes constipation, retention or suppression of urine, obstruction of flatus, pain, flatulent distension of the abdomen, formation of calculi, pain and atrophy of leg, thighs, sacral region, back and sides.

If the vāta that is situated in the stomach is deranged, it causes dyspnoea, dryness of the mouth and throat, cough, visūchika, thirst, eructations, and pain in the cardiac region, umbilical region, sides of the chest, and abdomen.

The vāta that is located in large intestines, if provoked, will cause a rumbling sound in the abdomen, abdominal pain, flatulence, dysuria, constipation, and pain in the sacrum.

The vāta that is localised in the sense organs will destroy the sense-faculties if provoked.

If the vāta present in the skin is deranged, it causes dryness, fissures and numbness of skin. The skin is black, shrivelled, and stretched and red. There is also pain in the joints.

If the deranged vāta affects the blood, it causes intense pain, fever, discolouration of skin, etc., emaciation, anorexia, stiffness of the body after meals and appearance of boils all over the body.

If the aggravated vāta affects the flesh and fatty tissues, there is heaviness of the body, intense pricking pain, aching pain as if beaten by a blunt instrument, and extreme weakness.

If the aggravated vāta affects the bones and marrow, there is breaking pain in the bones and joints, loss of flesh, weakness, insomnia and constant pain.

If the aggravated vāta affects the śukra (reproductive element), it causes premature ejaculation, retention of semen, abortion, and foetal deformities.

If the aggravated vāta affects the hard fibrous structures, it causes antarāyāma, bāhyāyama, khalli, kubjatva, etc.

If the deranged vāta affects the blood vessels and nerves, there is mild pain, swelling, atrophy, pulsation, numbness (or loss of pulsation), and dilatation and contraction (of the vessels).

If the aggravated vāta affects the joints, it causes swelling of the joints which feel as if they are full of air, and painful extension and flexion.

When the vāta is obstructed by the aggravated pitta, there is burning pain, thirst, abdominal pain, vertigo, desire for cold, and heart-burn on eating foods that are pungent, sour and salty.

If the vāta is obstructed by the kapha, it causes chilliness, heaviness of the body, colic, desire for fasting (for eating less), exertion, and dry and hot foods and relief from eating pungent food.

If the vāta is obstructed by the vitiated blood, there is swelling in between the skin and flesh, with burning pain and redness, and circular eruptions or rashes. If the vāta is obstructed by the deranged medas, it causes a swelling that is greasy, soft, cold, and which shifts (from place to place), and anorexia. If the vāta is obstructed by the bones, there is pricking and splitting pain, weakness and relief with pressure and warmth. When the vāta is occluded by the marrow, there is deformity (vināma), yawning, pain and colic with relief on being pressed with the palms. If the vāta is occluded by the reproductive tissues or in the seminal passages, there is either no discharge of semen or premature ejaculation or sterility. If the vāta is obstructed by food, there is abdominal pain on eating, which subsides after digestion of food. If the vāta is occluded by urine, there is retention of urine, and distension of the urinary bladder. If the vāta is obstructed by the faeces, there is severe constipation with griping pain. The unctuous food that is partaken of is at once digested, but the stools are dry. There is also pain in groins, hips and back, cardiac troubles and movement of vāta in the opposite direction.

The five types of vāta may also obstruct each other. If the vyāna is obstructed by prāṇa, there is impairment of all sense-faculties, loss of memory and weakness. If the prāṇa is obstructed by vyāna, there is excessive sweating, horripilation, skin diseases and numbness. If the samāna is occluded by prāṇa, there is slurring or stammering speech, and dumbness. If the apāna is obstructed by samāna, there will be grahaṇi, heart troubles, pain in the stomach and palpitation. If the udāna is enveloped by prāṇa, there is heaviness of the head, catarrh, dyspnoea, heart disease and dryness of the mouth. If the prāṇa is enveloped by udāna, there is loss of enthusiam, strength, immunity and complexion, and even death. If the apāna is enveloped by udāna, there is vomiting, dyspnoea, etc. If the udāna is occluded by apāna, there is stupefaction, feeble digestion, and diarrhoea. If the apāna is occluded by vyāna, there is vomiting, flatulent distension of the abdomen, udāvarta, abdominal tumours and griping pain. If the vyāna is enveloped by apāna, there is excessive discharge of flatus, urine and semen. If the vyāna is obstructed by samāna, there is syncope, lethargy, irrelevant loquacious speech, debility, feeble digestion and weakness. If the vyāna is obstructed by udāna, there is stiffness, feeble digestion, lack of perspiration, laziness and ptosis, (CS).

II. The aggravated vāta which localises in the stomach causes vomiting, moha (stupefaction) syncope, thirst, palpitation, and pain in the sides (of the chest). If it localises in the large intestines, it causes rumbling in the abdomen, pain in the umbilical region, ānāha, dysuria, constipation and pain in the scrotum. The sense faculties are destroyed if they are affected by aggravated vāta. If the aggravated vāta affects the skin, it causes discolouration, pulsation, dryness, numbness, tingling, pricking pain and cracking (of the skin). If the aggravated vāta affects the blood, there are ulcers, and knotty and painful tumours if the flesh is affected. If the meda (fatty tissues) are affected, it causes knotty growths that are mildly painful and do not ulcerate. The aggravated vāta if localised in the blood vessels and nerves causes varicosities, painful stiffness or neuralgia. If the hard fibrous structures are affected, there is stiffness, tremors, pain and convulsions. The vāta sometimes affects the joints causing painful swelling (of joints). If the deranged vāta localises in the bones, it causes asthi-śosha (necrosis), and breaking pain. If the marrow is involved there is severe pain which is not relieved in any position. If the reproductive element is affected, there is scanty, excessive or defective emission of semen.

The aggravated vāta first affects the lower and upper extremities, and head and then extends to all the dhātus. Later the whole body will be affected, causing stiffness, convulsions, numbness, swelling and pain, (SS).

Prognosis: Vāta-rogas which are of recent origin which occur in persons who are endowed with a strong constitution, and where there are no complications are curable, (CS).

Complications: If the various kinds of occlusions are not treated, the patient will suffer from heart disease, abscesses, enlargements of the spleen, abdominal tumors and diarrhoea, (CS).

Ref.: CS, chikitsā, 28, 15-37; 60-71; 201-214; 236; SS, nidāna, 1, 21-31.

Treatment:

I. The patient who suffers from aggravation of vāta without any kind of obstruction should be oleated with substances like oil, ghee, fat or marrow (which are given orally). After the patient has recovered from the strain, he should again be oleated with milk, gruel (yūsha) or meat-juices of domesticated, aquatic or wet land animals, mixed with sour and salty substances. The patient should later be administered anuvāsana enema, nāvana (errhines) and demulcent food. The patient is then fomented by means of nāḍī, sankara and prastara kinds of sudation therapy. By these processes, even a deformed and stiff limb can be brought back to normal. The patient should be repeatedly subjected to oleation and sudation therapy.

If these measures are not sufficient to remove the diseased condition, the patient can be purified by means of mild drugs mixed with unctuous substances. He can be administered ghee medicated with tilvaka or sātala or castor oil with milk. These are especially useful if vāta is aggravated by the excessive use of unctuous, sour, salty and hot food.

A person who is too weak to be purged can be given nirūha-enema after which he can partake of food mixed with substances that are appetizing and digestive. When the patient's digestion has been stimulated, he can again be subjected to oleation and sudation.

The person has to partake of substances that are sweet, sour, salty and unctuous. He can be subjected to errhine therapy and fumigation.

In cases where the aggravated vāta has localised in the gastro-intestinal tract and thoraco-abdominal cavity, the patient can be administered alkalies (yava-kshāra) mixed with drugs that are appetizing, digestive or sour.

In cases where the vāta has localised in the rectum and large intestines, the patient can be treated as in udāvarta. When the vāta has been provoked all over the body, the patient can be massaged and administered anuvāsana enema. If the skin has been affected, fomentation, massage with oil or ghee, tub baths and tasty food are useful. If the blood has been affected by the deranged vāta, cold applications, purgation and blood-letting are employed; when the flesh and fatty tissues are affected, the patient can be subjected to purgation, nirūha enma and palliative drugs. When the bones and marrow are affected, the patient can be oleated both internally and externally. If the śukra (reproductive element) is affected, the patient can partake of aphrodisiac food and drink. If the passage of semen is obstructed, the patient can be purged. If the foetus is too small (and does not grow) or if the child emaciates, milk medicated with sugar, kāśmari, and yashṭi-madhu can be administered (either to the pregnant woman or to the child). Milk boiled with śālaparṇi is useful in cases where the heart has been adversely affected by the aggravated vāta. If the aggravated vāta localises in the region of the umbilicus, fish boiled with unripe bilva fruits is taken. If there are cramps in any part of the body, poultices can be applied. If any part of the body is stiffened or contracted, it can be massaged with oil medicated with rock-salt and māsha. If the aggravated vāta affects the arms or head, errhines, and potions of unctuous preparations after meals are useful. If the regions below the umbilicus are affected, the patient can be administered enemata and avapīḍa errhine.

In every case of vāta-disease, the following are useful: ghee, oil, marrrow and fat (used either internally or externally), affusions, massages, enemata, unctuous fomentations, residing in a place free from draughts, warm clothing, nourishing food and food or meat-juices or milk mixed with substances that are sweet, sour and salty.

Meat-juices of goat's head or of wet land and aquatic animals boiled with the decoction of balā or drugs of pancha-mūla or daśamūla drugs, and mixed with unctuous substances, sour curd and trikaṭu are useful. The same flesh can be crushed, steamed, freed from bones and made into poultices with ghee, oil and sour drugs. For tub-baths, medicated oil, ghee or a decoction of leaves can be used. Affusions are applied only after the patient has been massaged.

The decoction of meat of aquatic and wet-land animals, drugs of daśamūla group, śatāvari, kulattha, badara, māsha, tila, rāsna, yava, balā, vasā, (animal fat), curds, kānji and sour drugs can be used for administering nāḍi-sveda. The paste of these drugs can be used as poultices; ghee or oil medicated with these drugs can be used for massaging the body. The paste of musta, kiṇva (yeast), tila seeds, kushṭha, devadāru, rock-salt, curds, milk, oil, ghee, fat and marrrow can also be used as a poultice. The painful part of the body can be plastered with the utkārika, vesavāra, milk, māsha, tila, boiled rice, eraṇḍa seeds, wheat, yava, kola and drugs of the śālaparṇi group, and bandaged with castor leaves. The next morning, the bandage can be removed. The part should then be affused with milk and water, and poulticed. It must be bandaged by a strip of hide containing hair only during the daytime. The cold paste of oil seeds and sour drugs can be applied.

Ghee of one prastha quantity should be boiled with the decoction of one droṇi of water, four palas of daśamūla drugs, and one prastha of yava, kola and kulattha, milk and paste of drugs of jīvanīya group, khārjura, kāśmari, drāksha, badara and phalgu. The ghee can be used internally, for massage and enemata. Ghee medicated with chitraka, nāgara, rāsna, pushkara, pippali and śaṭhi is also useful.

Oil medicated with the roots and leaves of nirguṇḍi can be used internally, for massage and as ear drops. Oil medicated with kulattha and stone of kārpāsa is also very useful. Curds should be stored in a vessel for three days with an equal amount of milk and expressed juice of mūlaka. Oil boiled with this and with the paste of yashṭi-madhu, sugar, rāsna, rock-salt, fresh ginger and dried ginger is very useful in vāta-diseases. Very old piṇyāka (oil cakes) are to be boiled with a decoction of pancha-mūla drugs. One prastha of oil boiled with the decoction and eight parts of milk is also very useful. Oil boiled with the decoction of yava, kola, kulattha, gaja-pippali, dried radish, bilva and sour solution (i.e. kānji or curds) and paste of trikaṭu and sour fruits is also useful, especially in the cold season. One āḍhaka of oil should be boiled with one tulā of a decoction of sahachara, ten palas of paste of mūlaka and four times the quantity of milk. This oil should be administered with eighteen palas of sugar in severe vāta-rogas. One prastha of oil is to be boiled with one prastha of a decoction of gokshura, equal quantity of milk, eight palas of ginger (dry) and eight palas of jaggery. This oil is given internally. After its digestion, the patient can partake of milk with gruel (peya). The medicated oils known as balā-taila, amṛtādi-taila, rāsna-taila, mūlakādya-taila, mūlaka-taila and vṛsha-mūlaka-taila can also be used. Oil medicated with a decoction of yava, kola, kulattha, fish, śigru, bilva, radish, curds and milk or medicated with laśuna (garlic) and the other drugs is very useful. This oil can be administered to a woman just after menstruation in cases of sterility.

There is no medicine that is as efficacious in vāta-diseases as oil. The efficacy of oil is enhanced when it is boiled with drugs that alleviate vāta. The more it is boiled, the more efficacious it becomes.

In cases where the vāta has been obstructed by pitta, hot and cold lines of treatment should be employed alternately. Ghee medicated with drugs of the jīvanīya group, meat of desert animals, barley, rice, yāpana and milk enema, purgatives, and milk medicated with balā and pancha-mūla drugs are all useful. Milk, ghee or oil boiled with yashṭi-madhu and bala can be used for affusion. The decoction of pancha-mūla drugs or just cold water can also be used for that purpose.

In cases where the vāta has been obstructed by kapha, strong fomentation, emesis, nirūha enema, purgation, a diet of yava, flesh of desert animals and birds, ghee, oil, and sarshapa-oil are all useful. If vāta is obstructed by both kapha and pitta, pitta should first be subdued.

If both vāta and kapha are aggravated, the patient can be given nirūha-enema with cow's urine. If both vāta and pitta are aggravated, nirūha-enema of milk can be given. This can be followed by anuvāsana enema prepared from sweet drugs. If vāta is obstructed by blood, the treatment indicated in vāta-rakta can be employed. If vāta is obstructed by āma, the patient is treated on the same lines as in prameha and medas (obesity). If the vāta is obstructed by flesh, sudation, massages with oil, etc., meat-juices, milk and unctuous medications are useful. If vāta is occluded by food, emesis and drugs that are light, appetizing and digestive are employed. If it is obstructed by urine, diuretics, sudation and urethral douches are employed. If obstructed by faecal matter, castor oil and unctuous therapy as recommended in udāvarta is useful.

Cases of occlusion of vyāna by prāṇa are treated by measures useful in diseases of the head, eyes, ears, nose and mouth. Cases of obstruction of prāṇa by vyāna are treated by unctuous purgation. In cases where samāna is enveloped by prạna, all four kinds of unctuous therapy and yāpana-enema are useful. Cases where apāna is enveloped by samāna are treated by ghee medicated with appetizing drugs. The obstruction of udāna by prạṇa is remedied by reassurance and treatment of diseases of parts above the clavicles. Cases where prạṇa is enveloped by udāna are healed by affusion with cold water and reassurance. If apāna is obstructed by udāna, enemata and laxative drugs are used. In cases of udāna enveloped by apāna, emesis and food that is appetizing and constipative (astringent) is recommended. If vyāna is obstructed by apāna, unctuous laxatives (anulomana) are administered. If vyāna is enveloped by apāna, measures that are astringent are useful. Cases of obstruction of vyāna by samāna are remedied by food that is easy to digest, and exercise. Cases of vyāna being obstructed by udāna are treated by light and wholesome food.

A course of rasāyana drugs, or śilājatu or guggulu with milk is useful in such conditions. Or a patient can partake of chyavana-prāśa or abhayāmalaki while living on a diet of milk.

In cases of occlusion of vāta by pitta, measures are employed which alleviate pitta and do not aggravate vāta. Similar measures are used if vāta is obstructed by kapha, (CS).

2. Cases where the large intestines have been affected by the aggravated vāta are treated by administering enema of active and sharp drugs mixed with salt. If the bladder has been affected, diuretics are employed. If the aggravated vāta has adversely affected the skin, flesh, blood and blood-vessels (and nerves), potions of unctuous substances, massage with medicated oils, poultices, massages, external applications and blood-letting are useful. If the hard fibrous structures, joints and bones have been affected, internal use of unctuous substances, poultices, cauterization, bandaging (the affected part), massage (without oil) are recommended. If the aggravated vāta is localised in the bones, a perforation is made through the skin, flesh and the affected bone, and a tube open at both ends is inserted through it. The aggravated vāta should be sucked out. If the aggravated vāta affects the whole body, the treatment should consist of avagāha, kuṭi, karshu and prastara types of fomentation, massage with oil, enemata and venesection. If only a part of the body has been affected, blood-letting by śṛnga (horn) is useful.

In a case of supta-vāta (numbness of the body), frequent blood-letting, and application of a paste of salt, oil and soot (āgāra-dhuma) are beneficial.

Milk boiled with the decoction of drugs of pancha-mūla group, sour fruits (such as dāḍima), meat-juices mixed with unctuous substances and gruel prepared from dhānyas (grains such as kulattha) and unctuous substances are all useful in diseases of vāta.

A poultice known as sālvaṇa-upanāha which is prepared from drugs of the kākolyādi group, drugs that alleviate vāta, sour drugs, meat of wet-land and aquatic animals, unctuous substances and salt, is to be applied warm. It is very efficacious in all vāta-diseases. It is to be applied on any part of the body that is contracted, painful or numb and the part is firmly bandaged with a piece of linen or woolen cloth. The affected part may also be rubbed with this poultice and inserted into a sheath made out of cat or mongoose skin or of camel or deer hide.

If the shoulder, chest, neck or sacral region is affected by the vitiated vāta, emesis and errhines are efficacious. If the aggravated vāta localises in the head, it can be subdued by bloodletting and śiro-basti for a period of 100 mātras (time taken to utter one-hundred short vowel sounds). Unctuous enema is very efficacious in all diseases of vāta.

The general remedial measures in all diseases of vāta are: oleation, sudation, massage with unctuous substances, enemata, purgation with unctuous substances (such as castor oil), śiro-basti, rubbing of oil on the head, unctuous fumigation, gaṇḍūsha with warm unctuous substances, oily errhines, a diet consisting of meat-juices, sour fruits, milk, unctuous substances, and salt, affusion with warm liquids, gentle (dry) massage, the use of kunkuma, agaru, kusṭha, teja-patra, ela and tagara, wearing of woolen, silken, cotton or any thick garments, residing in places free from draughts, or in an inner chamber, sleeping on soft beds, bathing in the heat of a fire, abstinence from coitus, etc.

The medicated ghees known as tilvaka-ghṛta, aśoka-ghṛta and ramyaka-ghṛta are used as unctuous purgatives in vāta-diseases. The medicated oils known as aṇu-taila, sahasra-pāka-taila, and śata-pāka-taila are also very useful. The salt preparations known as patra-lavaṇa, kāṇḍa-lavana and kalyāṇaka-lavaṇa are also very efficacious. A course of guggulu is also very useful. It can be taken with a decoction of triphala, dāru-haridra and paṭola or with a decoction of kuśa roots or with cow's urine or with warm water. After this medicines has been digested, the patient can partake of boiled rice with soup, milk or extract of meat, (SS).

3. The general remedial measures in vāta-rogas are: oleation, sudation, mild purificatory procedures, food articles that are sweet, sour, salty and hot, massage with and without unctuous substances, bandaging the affected part, suddenly inducing fear (trāsana), affusions, alcoholic drinks prepared from jaggery and flour, enema consisting of oily and hot substances, a comfortable life style, use of unctuous substances medicated with drugs that are appetizing and digestive, and anuvāsana enema of fat or meat-juices, (AHṛ).

4. The mixture of chitraka, indrayava, pāṭha, kaṭuka, ativisha and harītaki is very useful in all vāta-rogas, especially where the stomach has been affected. Castor oil can be administered with the decoction of daśamūla drugs or a decoction of dry ginger in waist pain. Milk boiled with drugs of pancha-mūla drugs or balā is useful. The drugs that are efficacious in vāta-diseases are aśvagandha, balā, daśamūla drugs, ginger and rāsna. The formulations that are useful are āditya-pāka-guggulu, trayodaśānga-guggulu, aśvagandhādya-ghṛta, daśamūlādya-ghṛta, chāgalādya-ghṛta, elādi-taila, mahā-bala-taila, vishṇu-taila, nārāyaṇa-taila, mahā-nārāyaṇa-taila, aśvagandha-taila, mūlakādya-taila, rasona-taila, ketakādya-taila, saindhavādya-taila, māsha-taila, triśati-prasāraṇi-taila, mahā-māsha-taila, chatuh-sneha, kubja-prasāraṇi-taila, etc., (CD).

5. Pārada-bhasma can be administered with the oil of laśuna. The gruel prepared from drāksha and yashṭi-madhu is useful in diseases of vāta occuring in pregnant women. The remedy known as vātāri-rasa is very useful in diseases of vāta, (RRS).

Ref.: CS, chikitsā, 28, 75-245; SS, chikitsā, 4; 5, 42-43; AHṛ, sūtra. 13; CD, 22; RRS, 21, 3-7; 22, 98; 30, 55.

Classical Prescriptions: Aśta-varga-kvātha-chūrṇa; Asvagandhādyarishṭa; Balā-taila; Balā-dhātryādi-taila; Balāśvagandhā-lākshādi-taila; Chintāmaṇi-chaturmukha-rasa; Daśa mūlarishṭa; Daśamūla-kaṭu-trayādi-kvātha-chūrṇa; Devadarvārishṭa; Dhānvantara-taila; Gandharva-hastādi-kvātha-chūrṇa; Haratāla-bhasma; Indu-kānta-rasa; Karpāsasthyādi-taila; Kottam-chukkādi-taila; Kshīra-balā-taila; Kumaryāsava; Laghu-vishagarbha-taila; Lakshmī-nārayaṇa-rasa; Laśunādi-ghṛta; Mahā-vishagarba-taila; Maha-yogarāja-guggulu; Mṛgānka-rasa; Nāga-vallabha-rasa; Nārāyana-taila; Nāvaratna-raja; Prabhanjana-vimardana-taila; Prāṇada-guṭika; Prameha-mihira-taila; Sahacharadi-taila; Siddha-prāṇeśvara-rasa; Svarṇa-bhasma;

Vidārika

Causative Factors:

Intrinsic: Kapha and vāta

Symptomatology: There is a painless, hard and long (or big) cylindrical swelling in the groin or axillae, which is accompanied by fever.

Treatment: The disease is treated according to the doshas involved. Bloodletting can be done. Piṇḍa (lump) kind of poultices can be applied over the swelling. After the swelling suppurates, it should be treated as in a case of vraṇa.

Ref.: CS, chikitsā, 12, 89-90.

Vidradhi

Western Nosology: Abscess.

Causative Factors:

Extrinsic:

1. The causes for internal vidradhi are: excessive sexual intercourse, excessive exertion, suppression of natural urges, and intake of food that is hard to digest, incompatible, unwholesome, unpalatable, dry, unclean and irritant (vidāhi), (SS).

2. Suppression of natural urges, excessive exertion, such as lifting heavy weights, excessive coitus, sleeping or lying down in unnatural postures, intake of large quantities of strong alcoholic drinks, or food that is incompatible, impure, unwholesome, unpalatable, very cold, irritant, hot, too dry and stale, and eating before the digestion of the previous meal. These are the causes for internal vidradhi, (CS).

Constituents Affected:

1. Skin, hard fibrous structures and flesh (muscles) in external vidradhi, and blood and flesh in internal vidradhi, (CS).

2. Skin, blood, flesh, bones and fatty tissues. (SS); superficial and deep fascia, (SS, śārīra, 4, 4).

Classification: Vidradhi may be either internal or external, (SS, CS). External vidradhi are of six types, namely, those that are caused by the vitiation of the three doshas, either individually or together, that which is caused by deranged blood, and that kind which is the result of trauma, (SS).

Pathogenesis:

1. When the aggravated doshas localise in the flesh and blood, within the body, they bring about internal vidradhi, (CS).

2. Due to the action of the deranged doshas, a swelling is formed, and this gradually increases in size, becomes deep seated, and results in (external) vidradhi. The doshas vitiated by the respective causes bring about a hard tumour like vidradhi in the interior of the body, which in shape resembles an anthill, (SS).

Symptomatology:

1. The external vidradhi which has a shape resembling a tendon is very painful. The discharge from the vātaja-vidradhi is thin, ununctuous, brownish-black in colour and frothy. The discharge from pittaja-vidradhi resembles the decoction of tila, māsha or kulattha. The discharge from kaphaja-vidradhi is whitish, thick, slimy and copious. The discharge from the tridoshaja-vidradhi partakes of the nature of all the three kinds described above.

The internal vidradhi is often very deep seated and causes severe pain in the heart, groins and kloma, liver, spleen, abdomen, kidneys, umbilicus, and urinary bladder. In vātaja-vidradhi, there is pulsating, splitting, and cutting pain, vertigo, ānāha and sound (on percussion). In pittaja-vidradhi, there is fever, thirst, burning pain, cloudiness of sensorium and syncope. In kaphaja-vidradhi, the patient suffers from yawning, nausea, anorexia, stiffness, and chilliness. The tridoshaja vidradhi is marked by excruciating pain. When the internal vidradhi ripens, there is pain as if one is being incised by a sharp instrument, burning pain as if there is a lighted torch within, and biting pain, as if one has been bitten by a scorpion.

If the (internal) vidradhi occurs in the heart, there is palpitation, dyspnoea (tamaka), fainting spells, and cough. If it is found in the kloma (laxynx, trachea and bronchi), there is thirst, dryness of the mouth and galagraha. If the vidradhi occurs in the liver, there is dyspnoea (śvāsa), and if in the spleen, impeded respiration (expiration). If the vidradhi occurs in the abdomen, the patient suffers from pain in both sides of the abdomen and deep within the shoulder. If the kidneys are the seat of the vidradhi, there is stiffness in the back and waist. If the umbilical region is involved, there are hiccoughs, and weakness in the thighs if the groin is involved. If the vidradhi occurs in the urinary bladder, there is dysuria, putrid urine and constipation with putrid stools.

After the internal vidradhi suppurates and breaks open, there will be discharge through the mouth (if the vidradhi occures in the upper region of the body), through the rectum (if the lower regions were affected) and through both the lower and upper orifices if the vidradhi was in the umbilical region, (CS).

2. The external vidradhi is usually deep seated, painful, and may be elongated or rounded. The vātaja-vidradhi is usually brownish-black in colour, rough, very painful, and very variable as far as the swelling and suppuration is concerned. The pittaja-vidradhi is blackish or of the colour of ripe udumbra (fruit), rapid in growth and suppuration, and is accompanied by fever and burning. The kaphaja-vidradhi is whitish or pale-yellow in colour, slightly painful, numb, slow to grow and mature, attended by itching, and shaped like a saucer. The tridoshaja-vidradhi is of varying colour, has varying discharges, is attended by different kinds of pain, is raised at the top, large and irregular in shape. In vidradhi caused by trauma, the aggravated vāta, pitta and the deranged blood causes a vidradhi that is similar to pittaja-vidradhi, and is accompanied by fever, thirst, and burning pain. The raktaja-vidradhi is blackish, is surrounded by black vesicles, is similar to pittaja-vidradhi, and is accompanied by fever, pain and severe burning sensation.

The internal vidradhi may occur in the rectum, the orifice of the urinary bladder, the umbilical region, abdomen, groin, kidneys, liver, spleen, heart and kloma (larynx, trachea and bronchi). The symptoms are similar to those observed in external vidradhi. If the vidradhi is situated in the rectum, there is obstruction of flatus; if in the urinary bladder, dysuria and scanty urination, if in the umbilical region, hiccoughs; and a rumbling sound in the abdomen and flatulence, if it occurs in the abdomen. If the vidradhi occurs in the groin, then there is intense pain in the back and waist. If the kidneys are the seat of vidradhi, there is constriction in the sides (of the abdomen), and dyspnoea if the vidradhi occurs in the spleen. If the heart is the seat, then there is severe chest pain and drawing pain all over the body. If the vidradhi is situated in the liver, there is dyspnoea and intense thirst. The latter symptom is present if the vidradhi occurs in the kloma.

A women suffers from raktaja-vidradhi if there has been an abortion; or due to improper regimen after parturition. This is accompanied by burning pain and fever. A vidradhi can also be caused in a woman who has delivered normally, if there are any blood clots within the body, (SS).

Complications: Flatulent distension of abdomen, suppression of urine, vomiting, hiccoughs, thirst, pain and dyspnoea, (SS, sūtra, 33, 22).

Prognosis:

1. The tridoshaja kind of external-vidradhi is considered to be incurable.

The cases of internal-vidradhi that occur in the vital areas of the body are very difficult to cure. The cases in which there is discharge (of pus, etc.,) from the lower orifices are curable, while those cases where there is discharge from the upper orifices are incurable. The vidradhi which occur in the heart, umbilicus and urinary bladder are incurable. Usually, even the vidradhi found in other parts of the body are incurable if there is an incision made from the outside, (SS).

2. The internal-vidradhi that mature in the heart, umbilicus and urinary bladder, as well as those which are caused by the aggravation of all three doshas are incurable. The other kinds are all curable provided they are treated by an experienced physician from the very beginning, (CS).

Ref.: SS, nidāna, 9; CS, sūtra, 17, 90-103.

Treatment:

1. The treatment should start with oleation and purgation. Vidradhi should be treated along the same lines as gulma, (CS).

2. The (external) vidradhi which have not yet matured are to be treated as described in sopha (i.e. from apatarpaṇa up to purgation).

A vātaja-vidradhi should be plastered with a warm paste of roots of drugs that alleviate vāta, and ghee, oil, and fat. A poultice composed of the meat of aquatic and wet-land animals, drugs of the kākolyādi group, salts, unctuous and sour substances should be applied. The area should be fomented by using pāyasa, kṛśara, milk and vesavāra. Bloodletting can also be employed. When the vidradhi matures (inspite of these measures), it should be incised, and later washed with the decoction of pancha-mūla drugs. Oil medicated with salt, yashṭi-madhu and drugs of the bhadradārvādi group can be used externally. The wound can be purified by using traivraṭa ghee and purgative drugs. Healing can be promoted by using trivrṭa ghee with drugs of the pṛthakparṇi group.

A pittaja-vidradhi should be plastered with a paste of lāja, sugar, yashṭi-madhu, and sāriva or a paste of uśīra, chandana, payasya and milk. The decoction or cold infusion of yava-kshāra, sugarcane juice and milk or ghee medicated with drugs of the jīvanīya drugs and sugar can be used for affusion (sprinkling). The paste of harītaki, trivṛt and honey can be administered internally. Leeches can be used for bloodletting. If the vidradhi matures, it should be lanced, and the wound washed with a decoction of trees with milky exudation or of aquatic bulbs (such as kumuda). The plaster of tila, yashṭi-madhu, honey and ghee can be applied and bandaged with a thin cloth. Ghee medicated with propouṇḍarīka, manjishṭha, yashṭi-madhu, uśīra, padmaka, haridra and milk is used for promoting the healing of the wound. Ghee medicated with kshīra-vidāri, pṛthak-parṇi, lajjālu, lodhra, chandana and tender leaves of drugs of nyagrodhādi group can also be used (for promoting the healing).

A kaphaja-vidradhi should be fomented by means of heated brick, stone, cow dung cakes, husks, ash or cow's urine. The use of decoctions, emesis, plasters, poultices, and bloodletting by alābu is also advised. The vidradhi when mature is lanced, and later washed with a decoction of drugs of the āragvadhādi group. The wound is filled (or plastered) with the paste of haridra, trivṛt, śaktu, tila, and honey and bandaged. The oil medicated with kulattha, danti, trivṛt, śyāma, arka, tilvaka, cow's urine and rock-salt is useful in purifying and promoting the healing of the wound.

A raktaja vidradhi or vidradhi caused by any trauma should be treated as in a case of pittaja vidradhi.

A medicated ghee known as karanjādya-ghrta is very useful in all cases of vidradhi.

In a case of internal-vidradhi that has not matured, the patient is administered the decoction of drugs of the varuṇādi group or ūshakādi group. Ghee medicated with drugs of the two groups mentioned above and purgative drugs should be administered daily, in the mornings. This will usually cure recent cases of internal vidradhi. The patient can be subjected to āsthāpana and anuvāsana enema with the drugs of the same two groups. The drugs of these two groups and the bark of madhu-śigru can be used internally and externally. The madhu-śigru can also be administered with water (in pittaja-vidradhi), dhānyāmla (in vāitaja-vidradhi) and cow's urine (in kaphaja-vidradhi) or with alcoholic drinks. The patient can also be administered śilājatu, guggulu, nāgara or devadāru with other drugs depending on which dosha is aggravated. Oleation therapy, poultices and laxative drugs are to be employed.

An internal-vidradhi that has suppurated and bulged out should be incised and treated as in the case of vraṇa. If there is discharge (of the contents of the vidradhi) through the upper or lower orifices, drugs of the varuṇādi group or madhu-śigru can be administered with maireya, kanji, wine or āsava. The diet should consist of rice boiled and cooked in a decoction of śigru roots and mustard, yava (barley), gruel of kola and kulattha, etc. The medicated ghee known as tilvaka-ghṛta should be taken every morning. Ghee medicated with a decoction of drugs of trivṛtādi group can be used similarly. The physician should try his best to prevent the suppuration of an internal vidradhi, (SS).

3. The docoction of śigru, vachā, asvattha, hingu and rock salt is very useful (when used internally) in vidradhi. The decoction of bark of varuṇa, hingu, kāsīsa, rock-salt and śilājatu is also very useful (in internal vidradhi). The formulations known as sarvāmaya-hara rasa and sarveshvara-parpaṭi are also very useful, (RRS).

4. The patient can be administered purified guggulu or castor oil with a decoction of punarnava, devadāru, nāgara and daśamūla drugs (in vātaja-vidradhi); the decoction of triphala with a paste of trivṛt (in pittaja-vidradhi); guggulu with cow's urine or with the decoction of triphala, śigru, varuṇa and daśamūla drugs (in kaphaja-vidradhi); the decoction of śobhānjana with hingu and rock-salt which can be taken every morning; the expressed juice of śigru root with honey (in internal-vidradhi); the decoction of white punarnava roots and varuṇa roots (in non-suppurated vidradhi); and powder of pāṭhā roots with honey and rice water (in internal vidradhi), (CD).

Ref.: CS, sūtra, 17, 103; SS, chikitsā, 16; RRS, 18, 2-27; CD,43.

Classical Prescriptions: Dhānvantara-ghṛta; Gandharva-hasta-chūṛna; Misraka-sneha; Trāyāntyādi-kvāta-chūṛna; Viḍangārishṭa.

Vāta-vidradhi: Prabhanjana-vimardana-taila

Vilambika

Causative Factors: This disease occurs if the three kinds of ajīrna (āmājīrna, vidagdhājīrṇa and vishṭabdhā jīrṇa) are neglected or improperly treated.

Intrinsic: Kapha and vāta

Symptomatology: The undigested or improperly digested food is not eliminated either through the upper or lower outlets of the body (i.e. neither vomited out, nor is eliminated through the rectum but is retained within the body)

Prognosis: This condition is very difficult to treat.

Treatment: Curable cases of this disease are to be treated on the same lines as in visuchika.

Ref.: SS, uttara, 56, 9, 12.

Visarpa

Synonyms: Parisarpa (that which spreads in all directions), (CS).

Western Nosology: Herpes zoster

Causative Factors:

Extrinsic: The excessive intake of stale alcoholic drinks, of greens and vegetables that are irritating, of heat-producing rāga and shāḍavas, of food that is salty, sour, pungent and hot, of (sour) curds, whey, śukta (vinegar), surā (wine) and souvīra, of laśuna (garlic), flesh of domesticated and wet-land animals, of pastries prepared from tila, māsha, kulattha and oils, of food that is unclean, uncooked (or improperly cooked), incompatible and unpalatable (or unwholesome), eating before the digestion of the previous meal, excessive loss of blood (atyādāna), sleep during the day, overeating, injuries, excessive exposure to sun, fire and wind, toxicosis, etc., (CS).

Intrinsic: All the three doshas, (CS).

Constituents Affected:

1. The fifth layer of skin known as vedini (Stratum pappilare), (SS, śārīra, 4, 4).

2. The blood, skin, flesh and lasika (serous exudate), (CS).

3. Skin, flesh and blood, (SS).

Classification:

1. There are seven kinds of visarpa. There are four types caused by the aggravation of vāta, pitta, kapha and all three doshas combined. The other three types are āgneya-visarpa (caused by vāta and pitta), granthi-visarpa (caused by kapha and vāta) and kardama-visarpa (caused by kapha and pitta), (CS).

2. There are five types of visarpa, four that are caused by the aggravation of the three doshas, seperately and combined, and visarpa that is caused by injuries, (SS).

3. Visarpa can be either external or internal, (CS).

Pathogenesis:

1. The aggravated doshas affect the skin, blood and flesh, and cause a swelling that is extensive, not very much elevated and which spreads all over the body, (SS).

Prodromal Symptoms: Appearance of reddish circular patches, thirst, fever, arati, (restlessness), burning pain and amelioration by cold and sweet substances, (KS).

Symptomatology:

1. Vātaja-visarpa:

1. The swelling is soft, blackish in colour, rough, and is accompanied by body pain, vātaja-jvara, and breaking and pricking pain (all over the body), (SS).

2. The patient suffers from vertigo, burning pain, thirst, pricking and cramping pain, body pain, tremors, fever, tamaka (dyspnoea), cough, weakness and pain in the joints, anorexia, indigestion, obscuration of vision, watering of the eyes, formication, constipation, retention of urine and obstruction of flatus.

The swelling is brownish or grey, and is attended by pricking and splitting pain, contractions, pulsation and horripilation. If it is not properly treated, the affected area is covered by thin, blackish or brown vesicles which rapidly suppurate, the discharge being scanty, thin, brownish and non-slimy, (CS).

2. Pittaja-visarpa:

1. There is fever, and a rapidly suppurating swelling that is inflamed, burns, and is covered by vesicles. It is reddish in colour, (SS).

2. The patient suffers from fever, thirst, syncope, clouded sensorium (moha), vomiting, anorexia, body pain, sleeplessness, restlessness, vertigo, obscuration of vision, headache, delirium, sweating, a sensation of intense heat (within the body), craving for cold and cold water, greenish or yellow discolouration of the skin, urine, faeces and eyes, etc.

The affected area is swollen, is copper-coloured, green, yellow, blue, black or blood-red in colour, and is covered over by vesicles which are also of the same colours (described above). There is intense burning pain, (CS).

3. Kaphaja-visarpa:

1. The swelling is cold, does not suppurate rapidly, is unctuous, whitish in colour, is only mildly painful but is attended by intense itching, (SS).

2. The patient suffers from fever with chills,

heaviness of the body, lethargy, drowsiness, anorexia, sweetish taste in the mouth, coating of the tongue, hawking (of mucous), vomiting, poor digestion, a sensation as if covered over by a moist cloth, debility and paleness of eyes, nails, urine and faeces.

The affected area is swollen, greasy, yellowish-white in colour, not reddish, slow to suppurate and is attended by numbness, heaviness, stiffness and slight pain. It is covered over by white or pale-yellow vesicles (sphoṭa) which have a thick outer layer. The discharge (from the vesicles) is white, slimy, thick, ropy and unctuous. The area is then covered by a network (of slough) which has a thick covering which firmly adheres to the body, (CS).

4. Tridoshaja-visarpa:

1. The disease is deep-seated and has the signs and symptoms of the three types described above, (SS).

2. This disease affects the entire body, manifests all the signs and symptoms, spreads very rapidly and is fulminating, (CS).

5. Agni-visarpa:

The patient feels as if his entire body is covered by red hot coals. There is also vomiting, diarrhoea, syncope, burning pain, fever, dyspnoea, anorexia, splitting pain in the joins, thirst, indigestion, body pain, etc.

The affected area becomes blackish, resembling the colour of extinguished embers of a fire, or is excessively red, and is covered over by blisters (similar to those in burn injuries). The disease spreads rapidly and affects the vital areas. This causes clouded sensorium, hiccoughs, dyspnoea and sleeplessness. Due to prolonged lack of sleep, the person becomes apathetic and is unable to find comfort in any position. The patient is unable to sit or recline, and will take to bed. Due to extreme suffering and debility, he will be semi-conscious, and can be roused only with difficulty, (CS).

6. Kardama-visarpa:

The general symptoms are fever with chills, heaviness of the head, burning pain, debility, a sensation as if the body is covered by a moist skin, drowsiness, lethargy, clouded sensorium, anorexia, delirium, poor digestion, splitting pain in the bones, syncope, thirst, coating of the vessels, weakness of sense faculties, lack of interest in life, sub sultus tendinum (anga-vikshepa), body pain, restlessness (arati) and anxiety. Generally this disease affects the āmāśaya (stomach) and is localised.

The affected area is swollen, greasy, appears to be studded with red, yellow or white eruptions, or is dark-blue or black in colour, dirty, hot, heavy and afflicted by a dull pain. The suppuration is deep seated. There is no discharge, but the affected area is moist, soft and slushy, with putrified flesh and skin, which pits on pressure, and peels off, exposing the blood vessels (nerves) and hard fibrous structures. There is also a putrid smell. The patient is often bereft of consciousness, (CS).

7. Granthi-visarpa:

The aggravated vāta obstructed by the kapha engenders a garland of knotty tumours in the regions of kapha (such as the chest, mouth, etc.), which are slow to suppurate. In plethoric persons, it affects the blood and causes a garland of knotty growths involving the blood-vessels (and nerves), hard fibrous structures, flesh and skin, which are severely painful, reddish in colour, and may be big or small, rounded or elongated.

The patient also suffers from fever, diarrhoea, cough, hiccoughs, dyspnoea, emaciation, discolouration (of skin, etc.), anorexia, indigestion, salivation, vomiting, syncope, body pain, drowsiness and arati, (CS).

8. Kshataja-visarpa:

The doshas especially pitta are excessively vitiated in a person with an open wound, this affects the blood, and causes a swelling that is grey or reddish in colour, with high fever, burning pain, and suppuration. The swelling is covered over by blackish vesicles that resemble kulattha pulse, (SS).

Prognosis:

1. The vātaja, pittaja and kaphaja types of visarpa are curable. Agni-visarpa and kardama-visarpa can be cured by the systematic application of remedial measures, if the vital organs are not involved, and if the blood vessels (and nerves), hard fibrous structures and flesh are not softened. The granthi-visarpa is curable if there are no complications (such as fever, diarrhoea, cough, hiccough, etc.,). The tridoshaja-visarpa is incurable, (CS).

2. The vātaja, pittaja and kaphaja types of visarpa are curable. They are however difficult to cure, if the vital organs are affected. Vātaja-visarpa is considered to be incurable if blisters appear on the cheeks. In pittaja-visarpa, if the dosha is excessively aggravated and there is destruction of blood vessels (and nerves) and flesh, and the affected area (or the swelling) is like blackish slime (kardama), it is incurable. The tridoshaja and kshataja-visarpa are incurable, (SS).

Difference Between Internal and External Visarpa:

Internal visarpa is characterized by injury to vital organs, stupefaction, dilation of the body-channels (or passages), thirst, irregular elimination (of urine, stools, etc.), and loss of digestive power, (CS).

Ref.: CS, chikitsā, 21, 11-42; SS, nidāna, 10, 3-8; KS, sūtra, 25, 25.

Treatment:

1. In cases of visarpa that appear in the locations where kapha is present, and where there is āma, fasting, emesis, bitter drugs and external use of drugs that are dry and cold are to be employed. In visarpa that is found in the habitats of pitta, the same measures, in addition to blood-letting and purgation are to be employed. In visarpa that affects the regions where vāta is situated, rūkshaṇa therapy is to be used first. Oleation is not advised in the early stages of even visarpa caused by pitta and vitiated blood.

Ghee medicated with bitter drugs is advised in vātaja and pittaja visarpa where the doshas are not excessively vitiated. If pitta is excessively aggravated, purgation is useful. Ghee that is not purgative should not be used as it obstructs (the passages), and causes destruction of skin, flesh and blood. Therefore, in most cases of visarpa, purgation should be the first measure, and can be followed by bloodletting.

Persons suffering from kaphaja and pittaja visarpa should be administered enemata composed of madana, yashṭi-madhu, nimba and kuṭaja fruits. An emetic compound of paṭola, nimba, pippali, madana and indrayava is also useful in visarpa.

A patient of visarpa can be administered the decoction of musta, nimba, paṭola, chandana and nilotpala, or of sāriva, āmalaka, uśīra and musta or of kirāta-tikta, lodhra, chandana, durālabha, nāgara, stamens of lotus, nilotpala, vibhītaka, yashṭūi-madhu and nāga-kesara, or of prapouṇḍarika, yashṭi-madhu, nilotpala, lotus stamens, nāga-keśara, guḍūchi, and lodhra, or a cold infusion of drāksha, parpaṭaka, nāgara, guḍūchi, and dhanvayāsa which quickly relieves the thirst also, or the decoction of paṭola, nimba, dāru-haridra, kaṭuka-rohiṇi, madhu-yashṭi and trāyamāṇa, or the above decoction mixed with triphala, masūra soup and ghee. The decoction of paṭola leaves, mudga, and juice of āmalaka with ghee can also be administered.

The patient can be administered the mahā-tikta-ghṛta (which is very useful in pittaja-kushṭha) as a purgative. The trāyamāṇa-ghṛta which is useful in gulma can also be used. The powder of trivṛt can be administered with ghee, milk, or hot water or grape-juice. Milk boiled with trāyamāṇa is also useful as a purgative. Ghee medicated with a decoction of triphala and powder of trivṛt is useful both as a purgative and for relieving fever. The juice of āmalaka can also be given with ghee. It can be given with trivṛt also if the patient is costive.

In cases where the blood has been vitiated in the peripheral areas of the body, bloodletting can be done in the very beginning. It can be done by using a horn (vishāṇa), by leeches or alābu if there is aggravation of vāta, pitta and kapha respectively.

External applications can be used only after the above mentioned purificatory measures, or in mild cases, at the beginning. The paste of udumbara bark, yashṭi-madhu, nilotpala, lotus stamens, nāga-keśara, priyangu and ghee, or of tender aerial roots of vaṭa, pith of banana plant, lotus nodes and śata-dhouta ghee, or of kālīya, yashṭi-madhu, hema (nāga-kesara), vanya, chandana, padmaka, ela, lotus stalk, priyangu and ghee or of śādvala, lotus stalks, śankha, chandana, utpala, vetasa-roots and rice, or of sāriva, lotus stamens, uśīra, nilotpala, manjishṭha, chandana, lodhra and harītaki or of jātāmāmsi, hareṇu, lodhra, yashṭi-madhu, padmaka, dūrva, sarja-rasa and ghee, or of barley flour, śaktu and ghee, or of fried barley flour, yashṭi-madhu, śatavāri and ghee, or of balā, niltopala, śālūka, śatāvari, agaru, chandana, lotus stalks and biśa (lotus tubers), or of barley flour, yashṭi-madhu and ghee, or of hareṇu, masūra, mudga, white śāleya, and ghee or of mud at lotus roots, mukta (pearl), śankha, pravāla, gairika and śukti, each mixed with ghee, or of prapounṭarīka, yashṭi-madhu, bala, śālūka, utpala, banyan leaves, dugdhika and ghee, or of biśa (lotus tubers), lotus stalks, ghee, and kaseruka, or of śatāvari, vidāri and ghee, or of śaivala, nala roots, gojihva, vṛsha-karṇika, indrāṇi with ghee or of sirīsha bark, balā and ghee, or of tender leaves of vaṭa, udumbara, plaksha, vetasa and asvattha, along with the barks and ghee, are all extremely useful in visarpa that is caused by aggravated vāta and pitta.

The following pastes are useful for external application in kaphaja-visarpa: The paste of triphala, padmaka, uśīra, samanga (namaskāri), karavīra, nala roots and sāriva; the paste of khadira, saptaparṇa, musta, āragvadha, dhava, kuranṭaka and devadāru; the pastes of āragvadha leaves, sleshmātaka bark, indrāṇi-śāka, kākāhva, sirīsha flowers, śaivala, nala roots, śatavāri, priyangu, triphala, yashṭi-madhu, prapouṇḍarīka, hrīvera, dāru-haridra, etc., either together or individually or in combination; but mixed with ghee. In vātaja and pittaja visarpa, pure śatadhouta-ghṛta can be applied.

In visarpa characterized by aggravated vāta, pitta and blood, the affected area can be sprinkled (or affused) with cold milk, or cold ghee, or a decoction of yashṭi-madhu, or a cold decoction of pancha-valkala, etc.

A fine powder of the drugs (used for application) can be used for dusting over the affected area. Ghee medicated with juice of dūrva is useful in promoting the healing of wounds. The powders of dāru-haridra bark, yashṭi-madhu, lodhra and nāga-kesara, or of paṭola, nimba, triphala, yashṭi-madhu and nilotpala can be used for dusting, or as a lotion. The paste should not be applied very thick, but should be as thick as one-third of the thickness of the thumb, should not be too unctuous, or too dry, not too watery nor too viscid. A number of thin coatings should be applied at frequent intervals. But in kaphaja-visarpa, a thick paste is to be applied and removed when dry.

A person suffering from granthi-visarpa which is marked by aggravation of pitta and blood should be treated by fasting, drying procedures (rūkshaṇa), affusions, external applications (of pancha-valkala), venesection, bloodletting by leeches, emesis, purgation, medicated ghees, bitter drugs, etc. If there is severe pain, a hot poultice composed of utkārika or unctuous vesavāra is applied. The area can be affected with hot oil medicated with daśamūla drugs, or with cow's urine or a hot decoction of medicinal leaves. A tepid paste of aśvagandha can also be applied. The hot pastes of dry radish, or bark of karanja (naktamāla), or bark of vibhītaka can be applied. The paste of balā, nāgabalā, harītaki, bhūrja patra, vibhītaka, bamboo leaves and agnimantha or of danti, chitraka root-bark, sudhā, exudation of arka, jaggery, bhallātaka fruit-stone and kāsīsa can be applied.

In a case of granthi-visarpa which breaks open (suppurates), the patient can partake of soup of radish, kulattha, yava-kshāra and dāḍima, preparations of wheat or barley with sīdhu, honey and sugar, vāruṇi-maṇḍa with honey and juice of mātulunga, triphala powder or decoction with honey and pippali, śaktu with musta and bhallātaka and honey; śilājatu with devadāru and guḍūchi, etc. Fumigations, errhines etc., described in the treatment of gulma are also useful.

In spite of all these measures, if the swelling is hard, and does not subside, it has to be cauterised by caustics or heated instruments of gold or they can be made to suppurate, and should be removed after incising them. Later, the treatment useful in vraṇa should be employed. Oil medicated with the paste of kampillaka, viḍanga, dāru-haridra, and karanja-fruits is useful in ulcers seen in granthi-visarpa.

The diet is described below. Persons who have fasted should partake of mantha that is not unctuous along with honey and sugar, mantha that is mixed with dāḍima and āmalaka, is sweet, and only slightly sour, a drink prepared from fruits of parūshaka, mṛdvīka and kharjūra, and refreshing paste of barley and rice with ghee. After these have been digested, the patient can eat old boiled rice with soups prepared from mudga, masūra, chaṇaka, dāḍima, paṭola and āmalaka, but which should not be sour. The meat-juices of desert animals can be taken with parūshaka, drāksha, dāḍima and āmalaka, but without any oily substances. Barley and wheat can be given to a person who does not like rice or for whom it is not suitable.

Persons suffering from visarpa should avoid food and drinks that are irritant and incompatible, sleep during the day, exertion, exposure to sun and wind and anger, (CS).

2. All cases of visarpa have to be generally treated with (internal use of) ghee medicated with appropriate drugs, affusions and external applications.

In a case of vātaja-visarpa, the drugs of bhadra-dārvādi and pippalyādi groups, and drugs such as musta, śatāhva, devadāru, kushṭha, vārāhi, kustumbara and kṛshṇagandha should be used for preparing a decoction, or for affusions and external application. The drugs of bṛhat-pancha-mūla, laghu-pancha-mūla, kantaka-pancha-mūla and vallī-pancha-mūla should be used for preparing ghee, oil, for affusion and for external application.

In pittaja-visarpa, a cold paste of kaseru, śṛngāṭaka, padma, guṇḍra, śaivāla, mud found near lotus and ghee can be applied on the affected area. The cold paste of hṛīvēra, lāmajjaka, chandana, souvirānjana, mukta, gairika, milk and ghee or prapouṇḍarīka, yashṭūi-madhu, payasyā (kshīra-vidāri), manjishṭha, padmaka, chandana, and sugandhika (utpala-sarīva) can be applied. A decoction of drugs of the nyagrodhādi group can be used for affusing the part, while ghee medicated with the same drugs can be administered internally. The affected area can also be affused with cold milk, water mixed with madhūka, sugarcane juice, etc. The ghee known as gouryādi-ghṛta is also very useful.

In a case of kaphaja-visarpa, a paste of ajagandha, aśvagandha, sarala (trivṛt), kālā (kāsamarda), ekaishika (śatavāri, NiS), ajasṛngi and cow's urine can be applied externally. Other drugs such as kālānusāri (tagara), agaru, chocha (dālchini), gunja, rāsna, vachā, sītasiva, indraparṇi (langali), pālindi, munjata, matri-kadamba (alambusha), etc., are useful.

Drugs of varuṇādi group are also very useful in visarpa. The patient can also be subjected to purificatory procedures and bloodletting. If the swellings suppurate, they are to be treated as described in the treatment of vraṇa (śārīra-vraṇa), (SS).

3. Equal amounts of purified mercury, sulphur, kānta-loha-bhasma, tīkshṇa-loha-bhasma, abhraka-bhasma, purified vatsanābha and svarṇa-mākshika-bhasma are triturated with the juice of the stem of vandhya-karkoṭaki, and the mass is then subjected to heat (in a bhūdara-puṭa) for twenty four hours. This is very useful in visarpa.

The two medicated oils known as eraṇḍa-bījādi taila are also useful, (RRS).

Ref.: CS, chikitsā, 21, 43-144; SS, chikitsā, 17, 2-16; RRS, 20, 1-5.

Classical Prescriptions: Dasānga-lepa; Haratāla-bhasma; Kāsīsa-bhasma; Loha-bhasma; Kāsīsadi-ghṛta; Mahā-tiktaka-ghṛta; Nalpamarādi-taila; Tiktaka-ghṛta; Triphala-ghṛta; Trāyantyādi-kvātha-chūrṇa; Vajraka-ghṛta.

Visphoṭaka

Western Nosology: Pemphigus vulgaris

Causative Factors:

Extrinsic: Intake of incompatible food, (CS, sūtra, 26, 102).

Intrinsic: Pitta, (SS).

Constituents Affected: Blood (SS)

Symptomatology:

1. The entire body or parts of it are covered with vesicles that resemble blisters caused by burn injuries, accompanied with fever, (SS).

2. The entire body is covered by vesicles, with redness, fever and thirst, (CS).

Related Diseases: Visarpa

Ref.: CS, chikitsā, 12, 90; SS, nidāna, 13, 18.

Treatment:

1. The disease is treated as described in the treatment of pittaja visarpa. Ghee that has been medicated with sweet drugs is used to promote healing of vesicles that have suppurated, (SS).

2. The remedial measures useful in visarpa and kushṭha are to be employed in this disease also, (KS, CS).

Related Disease: Visarpa

Ref.: SS, chikitsā, 20, 7-8; CS, chikitsā, 12, 93; KS, khila, 14.

Visūchika

Western Nosology: Gastro-enteritis

Causative Factors:

Extrinsic:

1. This disease results if the three kinds of ajirṇa (āmājīrṇa, vidagdhā jīrṇa and vishṭabdhājīrṇa) are neglected or improperly treated and is caused only in people who have no self control (in eating), (SS).

2. This disease is caused by the accumulation of āma-dosha in the body, which in turn is caused by overeating, (CS).

Intrinsic: Vāta, (SS). All three doshas, (CS).

Pathogenesis: If the patient who has eaten his fill of solid food partakes of liquid food in excessive amounts, all the doshas will be aggravated, and will interact with the undigested food, (CS).

Symptomatology:

1. Pricking pain all over the body, vomiting, diarrhoea, syncope, thirst, abdominal pain, vertigo, breaking pain (in the leg, NiS), yawning, burning sensation, discolouration (of skin, etc.), tremors, pain in the cardiac region and headache, (SS).

2. Vomiting and diarrhoea. The aggravated

vāta causes abdominal pain, ānāha, body pain, dryness of mouth, syncope, vertigo, irregular digestion, pain in the sides of the chest, back and waist, and stiffness and contraction of the blood vessels. The vitiated pitta causes fever, internal heat, thirst, diarrhoea, clouded sensorium, vertigo and delirium (irrelevant speech), while the deranged kapha causes vomiting, anorexia, indigestion, fever with chills, lethargy and heaviness of the body, (CS).

Complications: There are five complications namely sleeplessness, restlessness, tremors, suppression of urine, and unconsciousness, (MN).

Prognosis: The patient who has blackish (blue) discolouration of teeth, tips and nails, who is semi-conscious, has (severe) vomiting, very feeble voice, a feeling as if all the joints are dislocated and sunken eyes is to be considered as being incurable, (SS).

Related Diseases: Alasaka, Ajīrṇa

Ref.: CS, vimāna, 2, 7, 11; SS, uttara, 56, 3-6; 11; MN, 6.

Treatment:

1. The patient has to be cauterized near the heels, subjected to dry fomentation, strong emesis, fasting until digestion of the food, drugs and measures that are digestive, and purgation. These measures will immediately relieve the syncope, diarrhoea, etc. The patient can also be administered āsthāpana enema. These measures are all purificatory.

For palliative purposes, the patient can be administered the following prescriptions: the powder of harītaki, vachā, hingu, indrayava, gṛnjana, souvarchala salt and ativisha with warm water; the paste of biḍa salt and jaggery (with hot water, NiS); the paste of sarshapa, jaggery and hot water; the paste of rock-salt, hingu and kānji; the paste of trikaṭu, triphala, trimada and bījapūra with ghee; the paste of trikaṭu, rock-salt and milky exudation of snuhi; kalyāṇaka-ghṛta with rock-salt; the paste of pippali, ajamoda and kshavaka with kānji; the paste of pippali and juice of ghoshaka; the paste of pippali, nāgara and hot water; and the paste of trikaṭu, fruits of kāranja, haridra root, and juice of mātulunga, which is to be applied as collyrium.

When the patient regains his appetite, he can partake of gruels, etc., composed of drugs that are appetizing and digestive, (SS).

2. The patient is first advised to fast, and later (when he regains his appetite), he can partake of gruels, etc., which are usually administered after purgation. If the patient complains of a sense of heaviness in the stomach, and loss of appetite, he should be administered drugs that are appetizing and digestive. Food should never be partaken of when there is indigestion. The digestive fire will be unable to digest the undigested food (āma), food and medicines simultaneously. Drugs and other measures that are either contrary to the cause and symptoms or which have a similar effect should be employed.

After the digestion of the āma, and when the patient regains his appetite, he should be massaged with oil, administered āsthāpana and anuvāsana enema and oleated internally (sneha-pāna) after due consideration of the affected doshas, medicines used, the place, time, strength (of the patient), the constitution, the food to which the patient is accustomed, mental strength (fortitude), etc., (CS).

3. The patient can be massaged with the warm paste of chukra-taila, kushṭha and rock-salt. This will relieve khalvi (cramps) and abdominal pain.

The internal use of a decoction of karanja, nimba, śikharī, guḍūchi, arjaka and kuṭaja is useful, (CD).

4. The patient can be administered pārada-bhasma with pippali and hingu, (RRS).

Ref.: SS, uttara, 56, 12-19; CS, vimāna, 2, 13; CD, 6, 85-90; RRS, 30, 34.

Classical Prescriptions: Ahiphenāsava;

Bilvādi-guṭika; Karpurāsava; Laśuṇādi-vaṭi; Mṛgamadāsava; Mṛta-sanjīvani-sura; Mustakārishṭa; Rasa-pushpa; Sanjīvani - vaṭi; Viḍanga-lauha.

Viśvāchi

Causative Factors:

Extrinsic: Factors that aggravate vāta.

Intrinsic: Vāta.

Symptomatology: The aggravated vāta affects the tendons (or cord like nerves) running along the dorsum of the upper limbs, connecting the palm and finger, rendering the limbs paralysed.

Treatment: The patient is treated along the same lines as are indicated in vāta-roga and gṛdhrasi.

Ref.: SS, nidāna, 1, 75; chikitsā, 5, 23.

Vivṛta

Causative Factors:

Extrinsic: Factors that aggravate pitta

Intrinsic: Pitta

Symptomatology: The body is covered by circular patches of eruptions with open outlets and which resemble in colour the ripe fruits of udumbara. There is also severe burning pain. (SS).

The eruptions are accompanied by fever, (AS).

Treatment: The person suffering from this disease is treated as described in the treatment of pittaja-visarpa. After the eruptions have suppurated, ghee prepared from drugs of the sweet group (kākolyādi group) is used in order to promote healing, (SS).

Ref.: SS, nidāna, 13, 7; AS, uttara, 36; SS, chikitsa, 20, 7-8.

Vraṇa

Synonym: Nija-vraṇa

Western Nosology: Ulcers

Causative Factors:

Extrinsic: Factors which aggravate the three doshas, (CS).

Intrinsic: The three doshas, either individually or conjointly, and vitiated blood.

Location:

1. The vraṇas may locate in, or affect the skin, māmsa (flesh or muscles), sirā (blood-vessels), snāyu (hard fibrous structures), asthi (bones), articulations, koshṭha (thoraco-abdominal cavity or visceral hollow organs) and marmas (vital organs), (SS).

2. The locations for the vraṇas are: skin, blood-vessels, flesh or muscle, meda (fatty tissues), bones, hard fibrous structures, vital organs (marmas) and inner organs (of thoraco abdominal cavity), (CS).

Pathogenesis: The three doshas are provoked by their respective aggravating factors, and locating in the external areas of the body produce ulcers of various types, (CS).

Types:

1. The ulcers are mainly of six types, namely those caused by the vitiation of vāta, pitta, kapha, all three doshas, blood or caused by injury (sadyo-vraṇa), (SS).

2. The ulcers are of three types, those caused by aggravated vāta, pitta or kapha.

The ulcers are also of different kinds depending on whether they are amenable to surgery or not, benign or malignant (dushṭa), affecting vital organs or not, open or closed, hard or soft, with or without discharge, with or without deep burrows (sinuses), depressed or elevated, simple or chronic, or regular and irregular, (CS).

Symptomatology:

1. The vraṇa caused by vitiated vāta is reddish, tawny, blackish or bone-coloured, and is characterised by pain which is shifting and occurs without any apparent cause or modality, throbbing, tension, pricking and drawing pain and a discharge which is rough, brownish or frosty in colour, resembling curd cream, or water in which meat, or paddy-husks or kshāras (caustics) are washed.

The pittaja-vraṇa is blue, yellow, greenish, black, brownish, red or flame-coloured, is rapid in growth, is surrounded by yellow boils, and is characterised by burning pain, as if a piece of red-hot coal or kshāra was placed on the skin, either localised or all over the body; increase of heat (and body temperature); a sensation as if inhaling smoke or fumes (dhumāyana); and a discharge which resembles the gomeda stone; cow's urine, a decoction of conch-shell, madhvika wine or oil.

The kaphaja-vraṇa is whitish, unctuous or greenish in colour, is hard and thick, is covered over by a network of blood-vessels and hard fibrous structures (snāyu), and is characterised by coldness, rigidity, intense itching, heaviness, numbness, a sensation as if the ulcer was plastered over and a discharge resembling butter, kāsīsa (iron sulphate), bone-marrow, coconut water or rice paste.

The vraṇa engendered by vitiated blood is very similar to that caused by pitta and the additional characteristic is that is has the odour of raw meat.

The vraṇa caused by the aggravation of all the doshas has features of all the three types mentioned earlier, and the discharge resembles coconutwater, juice of ervarū (snake cucumber, cucumis utilissimus Roxb), upper layer of gruel, or gruel of mudga or liver.

The vraṇa caused by vitiated blood looks like red coral, is covered by black pustules and boils, has a caustic smell, is painful and sometimes bleeds. There is a sensation as if it emits heat.

The vāta-pitta vraṇa is characterised by pricking pain, burning pain, yellowish or brownish-red colour, feels as if it is emitting heat and has a yellow or tawny discharge.

The vāta-kapha vraṇa is characterised by itching, pricking pain, scanty and periodical (intermittent) discharge which is cold, slimy and scanty and is dry, heavy and hard.

The pitta-kapha vraṇa is heavy, hot, and is characterised by burning pain and yellow, grey discharge.

The vāta-rakta vraṇa is dry, thin, feels numb, is red and bloody in colour and exhibits intense pricking pain and bleeding.

The pitta-rakta vraṇa is soft, resembles the upper layer of ghee, has a fishy odour and has a hot, blackish discharge.

The kapha-rakta vraṇa is firm, bloodred, slimy, unctuous, exhibits itching, heaviness and a bloody grey discharge.

The vāta-pitta-rakta vraṇa is characterised by throbbing, pricking pain, burning, a sensation as if emitting smoke and a yellow, thin, bloody discharge.

The vāta-kapha-rakta vraṇa is characterised by itching, throbbing, horripilation or tingling and a grey, thick, bloody discharge.

The pitta-kapha-rakta vraṇa is inflamed, injected, and exhibits burning, itching and has a grey, thick, blood discharge.

The discharge from the vraṇa located in the skin is yellowish, watery and has a slight smell of raw meat.

The discharge from the vraṇa located in the blood vessels is thin, profuse, purulent, stringy (avalambi), brown and resembles dew (ava-syaya).

The discharge from the vraṇa located in the hard fibrous structures is unctuous, thick and resembles bloody mucus (singhaṇaka).

The discharge from the vraṇa located in the

bones is unctuous, bloody and mixed with bone-marrow.

There is no discharge from the vraṇa located in the articulations when the ulcer is pressed, but when the limb is flexed, expanded, raised or lowered, or when running or straining at passing stools, there is discharge of slimy, stringy, bloody pus.

The discharge from the vraṇa located in the koshṭha (visceral hollow organs) consists of pus mixed with blood, urine, faeces or watery fluid.

The discharge from the vraṇa located on the vital organs depends on the organs affected.

Vraṇas which are too narrow, too wide, too hard or soft, greatly elevated or depressed, too cold to touch or too warm, which are black, red, yellow or white coloured, which exhibit unusual features, which are covered by offensive pus, flesh, blood vessels, hard fibrous structures, etc., which are very painful and attended by burning pain, pāka (inflamation), redness, itching, swelling, are sorrounded by boils and exude offensive (vitiated) blood and are very chronic are known as dushṭa-vraṇas (malignant ulcers), (SS).

2. The details about the vranas are to be elicited by observation, interrogation and palpation. By observation the age, the colouration, the general state of the body and sense organs can be known. The interrogation has to be regarding the aetiology, the kinds of sensation or pain, the modalities (sātmya, the aggravating and ameliorating factors) and appetite. Palpation helps to assess the softness or hardness, heat or coldness, etc.

The vāta vraṇa is hard to touch, indurated, and is characterised by intense pain, pricking pain, throbbing, dusky discolouration and scanty discharge.

The symptoms of pitta vraṇa are thirst, stupefaction (moha), fever, perspiration, burning pain, suppuration, tissue destruction and offensive (putrid) odour and discharge.

The kapha vraṇa is characterised by slimy, thick discharge, greasiness, sense of heaviness, dull pain, moistness, pale (whitish) discolouration, slight softening and chronicity.

The vraṇas which are white (pale), have depressed edges, elevated or thickened edges, are yellowish-red, blue or dusky red, covered with pustules, which exude red, black, offensive pus, which recur frequently and which are kumbhī-mukha (pin-pointed?) are to be known as being dushṭa (malignant).

Complications:

1. The complications (upadrava) of vraṇas are: visarpa, pakshāghāta, sīra-stambha, apatānaka, moha, unmāda, severe pain, fever, thirst, hanu-graha, cough, vomiting, diarrhoea, hiccoughs, dyspnoea and tremors, (CS).

2. The complications which may afflict the patient suffering from vraṇa are: fever, diarrhoea, mūrccha, hiccoughs, vomiting, anorexia, dyspnoea (śvāsa), cough, thirst and indigestion, (SS).

Prognosis:

1. A vraṇa which is confined to the skin is very easily amenable to treatment. The rest of the vraṇas which are located in the blood-vessels, etc., and those which suppurate spontaneously (without any external application) are difficult to cure. A patient who is self-controlled and leads a disciplined life and is treated by a competent physician is easily cured.

A vraṇa in a person who is young, strong, muscular and calm is easily curable, (for more details see SS, sūtra, 23).

A vraṇa which is located in the gluteal region, or around the anus and genital organs, or on the back, forehead, cheek or lips, or around the external ears or on the testes or abdomen, inside the cavity of the mouth, or on the nape of the neck or above the clavicles is easily curable.

A vraṇa which is located in the eyes, in the gums, the nostrils, the outer canthus of the eye, inside the ears, abdomen, umbilical region, on the sutures of the body, hips, ribs, arm pits, chest, breasts, sides or on the joints, and those vraṇas which secrete frothy blood or pus with a gurgling sound or contain any foreign matter within are healed with difficulty.

A vraṇa in a person suffering from kushṭha (chronic skin ailments), toxicosis (poisoning), śosha (tuberculosis), madhumeha (advanced diabetes) and a vraṇa which appears on a pre-existing one are cured with difficulty.

A vraṇa which is located in the large intestine with a discharge similar to the washings of paddy-husks; which is located in the liver or spleen and exudes a discharge resembling ksharodaka (water in which caustics are dissolved) and one which is located in the stomach and trika-sandhi (intra-scapular region or sacral region) with a discharge similar to washings of kalāya (pisum sativum) are incurable.

A vraṇa which does not present signs and symptoms of any of the doshas, which assumes a dark brown colour along the edges, which is evenly elevated along the margins, which is painless, does not secrete, and which is soft and smooth like the base of the tongue is regarded as being a śuddha-vraṇa (healthy or cleansed ulcer).

A vraṇa which is dove-coloured (kapota-varṇa, yellowish, dusky), has no secretion along the margins, is hard, firm and is surrounded by shreds of dead skin and presents signs of healthy granulation is in the process of healing.

A vraṇa which has its edges firmly adhered together, which does not exhibit pain or swelling, which is not knotty or glandular to touch and which has left a cicatrix of the same hue as the surrounding skin is to be considered as being perfectly healed, (SS).

2. A vraṇa which occurs in young and intelligent patients, which is of recent origin, which presents no complications (upadrava), which occurs in favourable seasons and which is located in the skin and flesh (māmsa) and in easily accessible areas, is easily cured.

If the above factors are lacking, the vraṇa is difficult to cure.

The factors which delay healing of vraṇa are: worm infestation, improper bandaging, over-eating, indigestion, intake of improper food, grief, anger, sleep during daytime, exertion, coitus, toxic conditions, injury by nails or excessive pressure by skin and hair, excessive oleation, emaciation caused by over drugging with medicines, deep-seatedness of the vraṇa and softening of the blood vessels and hard fibrous structures, (CS).

Ref.: SS, sūtra, 21, 40; 22; 23; 28, 10; chikitsā, 1; CS, chikitsā, 25.

Treatment:

I. There are sixty surgical and therapeutic methods which can be employed in vraṇa. They are:

1. Apatarpaṇa (fasting or partaking of less food and food that is very easily digested).
2. Ālepa (applications of plasters)
3. Parisheka (irrigation or spraying)
4. Abhyanga (anointing or massaging with oil)
5. Sveda (fomentation or sudation)
6. Vimlāpana (resolution by massaging)
7. Upanāha (application of poultices)
8. Pāchana (hastening suppuration)
9. Visrāvaṇa (evacuating or draining)
10. Sneha (internal use of unctuous substances, medicated, oils, etc.)
11. Vamana (inducing emesis)
12. Virechana (inducing purgation)
13. Cchedana (excision)
14. Bhedana (opening of an abscess)
15. Dāraṇa (causing bursting of abscess by medicinal applications)
16. Lekhana (scraping)
17. Āharaṇa (extraction)
18. Eshana (probing)
19. Vyadhana (puncturing)
20. Vidrāvaṇa (inducing discharge or

liquifying)
21. Sīvana (suturing)
22. Sandhāna (helping adhesion)
23. Pīḍana (pressing)
24. Śoṇitasthāpana (arresting bleeding)
25. Nirvāpaṇa (soothing applications)
26. Utkārika (application of massive poultices)
27. Kashāya (employing medicinal decoctions)
28. Varti (plugging or applying lint)
29. Kalka (employing pastes)
30. Ghṛta (using medicated ghee)
31. Taila (using medicated oils)
32. Rasa-kriya (using drug-extracts)
33. Avachūraṇa (dusting medicinal powders)
34. Vraṇa-dhūpana (local fumigation)
35. Utsādana (inducing granulation)
36. Avasādana (reducing exuberant granulation)
37. Mṛdu-karma (softening the affected area)
38. Dāruṇa-karma (inducing firmness of soft parts)
39. Kshāra-karma (using caustics)
40. Agni-karma (cauterization)
41. Kṛshṇa-karma (increasing pigmentation or darkening the skin)
42. Pāṇḍu-karma (reducing pigmentation)
43. Pratisāraṇa (rubbing with medicinal powders)
44. Roma-sanjanana (inducing regrowth of hair)
45. Lomāpaharaṇa (depilation)
46. Vasti-karma (using enematics)
47. Uttara-basti-karma (urethral and vaginal injections)
48. Bandha (bandaging)
49. Patrādāna (applying certain leaves)
50. Kṛmighna (anthelminthic or vermifugal measures)
51. Bṛmhaṇa (increasing corpulence)
52. Vishagna (using anti-toxic medicines)
53. Śiro-virechana (applying nasal drops)
54. Nasya (using errhines)
55. Kavala-dhārana (retaining certain drugs in the mouth or gargling)
56. Dhūma (smoking medicated cigars)
57. Madhu-sarpi (employing honey and ghee with other drugs)
58. Yantra (mechanical contrivances)
59. Āhara (suitable diet)
60. Rakshā-vidhāna (using amulets, etc. as a psychological measure)

Of these measures, kashāya, varti, kalka, ghṛta, taila, rasa-kriya and avachūraṇa are used to purify (cleanse) the ulcer and aid in granulation. The measures of cchedana, bhedana, lekhana, āharaṇa, eshaṇa, vyadhana, vidrāvaṇa and sīvana are surgical measures.

The first twelve measures beginning from apatarpana and ending in virechana are very useful in the cases of vraṇa. In fact, apatarpaṇa is the principal and generally applicable measure in vraṇa.

The eight surgical measures are described in detail in SS, sūtra 25. The methods of bandaging (bandhana) are elaborated in SS, sūtra 18. The āhāra (suitable diet) and regimen are described in SS, sūtra 19. The rakshā-vidhāna (measures to induce a sense of psychological well-being) are elaborated in SS, sūtra 19 and 5. The methods of śoṇitasthāpana (of arresting bleeding) are described in SS, sūtra 14 and the kshāra-karma (methods of using caustics) in SS, sūtra 11.

The severe pain caused by surgery is relieved by applying tepid ghee boiled with yashṭi-madhu.

The dāraṇa measure (which involves the application of drugs in order to cause the bursting of an abscess) is to be adopted in children, timid, weak or aged patients, in women and in swellings which are located in the vital organs. For details see SS, sūtra 37.

Utsādana: For inducing granulation, alepa (plasters) and ghee medicated with drugs such as apāmārga, aśvagandha, tāla-patri, suvarchala and drugs of the kākolyādi group are applied. Meat of carnivorous animals is also enjoined.

Avasādan: For reducing exuberant granulation, drugs like kāsīsa, rock-salt, kiṇva, vachā, haridra and dāru-haridha are powdered and applied with honey.

Mṛdu-karma: For softening the hardened, indurated areas, plasters, oil, ghee etc., should be used tepid (both internally and externally). Oil, ghee, etc., medicated with drugs that reduce vāta, and sprinkling of such substances are useful. Tight bandaging will also help.

Dāruṇa-karma: Where the skin and ulcers are too soft, they can be hardened by dusting the powders of bark of dhava, priyangu, aśoka and rohiṇi, triphala, flowers of dhātaki, lodhra and sarjarasa.

Kṛshṇa-karma: For increasing pigmentation of white scars, bhallātaka oil (extracted as described in SS, chikitsā 1, 90-93) should be applied, along with the burnt ashes of hoofs of animals.

Pāṇḍu-karma: For imparting normal skin colour to a dark scar, the fruit of rohiṇi (harītaki, kaṭu-tumbi or kataka-phala) is soaked in goat's milk for seven days and then applied along with the same milk. Many other drugs can also be used for this purpose, (SS, chikitsā, 1, 96-100).

Roma-sanjanana: The paste of hasti-danta-maśī and rasānjana can be applied with goat's milk for stimulating the growth of hair where desired. Other measures are also described, (SS, chikitsā, 1, 102-103).

Romāpaharaṇa: For removing hair from an area, the paste of bhallātaka oil with milky exudation of snuhi can be applied. There are many other drugs which can be used for this purpose, (ibid, 104-108).

Patra-dāna: The leaves of eraṇḍa, bhūrja, pūtika, haridra, etc., should be used for bandaging in vāta-vraṇa. In pitta-vraṇa, the leaves of kāśmari, kshīri trees, etc., are used, while in kapha-vraṇa, the leaves of pātha, mūrva, guḍūchi, haridra, etc., are used. Only those leaves which are soft and tender are to be used.

The diet should always consist of food which is easily digestible, (SS).

In vraṇas, the first thing to be done is to carry out the purifying procedures such as emesis, purgation, enemata or nasal drops (errhine-therapy) depending on the area where the vraṇa is located. The śodhana therapy is done only where the doshas are greatly provoked. In cases where the morbidity is slight, langhana alone will be sufficient. If vāta is predominantly affected, decoctions and medicated ghee are to be administered.

The six surgical procedures which can be employed in vraṇa are: pātana (incision), vyadhana (puncturing), cchedana (excision), pracchana (scarification), sīvana (suturing) and lekhana (scraping). (For details see CS, chikitsā, 25, 55-61).

Ulcers with a wide interior and narrow opening should be subjected to pīḍana (compression). For this purpose a dry paste of kalaya, masūra, godhūma and hareṇu can be used.

For reducing the burning and heat, the following drugs can be used as a paste or for sprinkling: śālmali-bark, root of balā, tender leaves of nyagrodha or drugs of nyagrodha group or balā group.

The vraṇas caused by aggravated blood and pitta should be washed with śata-dhauta-ghee or cold milk or a decoction of yashṭi-madhu.

If loose strips of skin and flesh are hanging from the ulcer, they should be anointed with ghee and honey, replaced and bandaged. The ulcer should then be dusted with powders of phalini, lodhra, kaṭphala, samanga and dhātaki.

Ulcers heat rapidly if dusted with powders of pancha-valkala trees and śukti or powders of dhātaki and lodhra.

Vāta-vraṇas which are very painful, dry and stabdha (indurated) should be subjected to sankara-sveda and if they are painful and burn, they should be anointed with the paste of fried atasi, tila and milk. Sprinkling the vraṇa with a decoction of milk boiled with daśamūla drugs or warm oil or milk will also relieve pain.

The burning and pain will also be reduced by applying a warm paste of yava, yashṭi-madhu, tila and ghee. An upanāha (poultice) of tila, and mudga-pāyasa is also useful. (For details about probes, see CS, chikitsā, 25, 80-82).

Drugs which are śodhana (purificatory or cleansing) should be used in vraṇas characterised by offensive odour, discoloration, severe pain and excessive discharge. The decoction of triphala, khadira, nyagrodha group of drugs, bala, kuśa, nimba and kola leaves can be used for this purpose. The paste of tila, rock-salt, haridra, dāru-haridra, trivṛt, yashṭi-madhu, leaves of nimba and ghee can also be applied.

The vraṇa which is not very red (inflamed), nor too pale, not very painful or darkish in colour, and which is neither elevated nor depressed is considered to be healthy, and should be treated with healing medicines (ropaṇa) such as a decoction of nyagrodha, udumbara, aśvattha, kadamba, plaksha, vetasa, arka, karavīra and kuṭaja. The prescriptions like chandanādi-yoga, prapouṇḍarikādya-taila, kampillādya-taila, etc. can be used. Oil medicated with dūrva-juice, kampillaka or dārvi-paste is also efficacious.

The leaves of kadamba, arjuna, nimba, paṭola, pippala or arka can be used for covering the vraṇa. In cases where the ulcers are depressed, drugs of the stanya group, jīvaniya group and bṛmhanīya group should be used.

Vraṇas become hard (firm) when exposed to the fumes of aromatic drugs and sāra (pith), and soft when exposed to fumigation with ghee, bone-marrow and fat. Fumigation is used for relieving pain, discharge, foul odour, worm infestation, softness, etc.

Vraṇas which are painful, hard, indurated and dry should be plastered with the paste of yava and ghee.

The powders of kakubha, udumbara, aśvattha, lodhra, jambu and kaṭphala should be dusted on vraṇas in order to hasten healing.

The cicatrice will quickly regain skin colour if anointed with the paste of iron, iron-sulphate (kāsīsa) and flowers of triphala.

The patient of vraṇa should avoid food that is sour, salty, pungent, spicy and hard to digest, sexual intercourse, and sleep during day-time, (CS).

The vraṇas which are dushṭa (malignant) and which are found in persons suffering from kushṭha and prameha, should be treated by drugs of the surasādi group and āragvadhādi group. These can be used in the form of external washing, ointment, medicated ghee, oil, rasa-kriya (extracts), powders and varti (plugs). Such vraṇas should be washed periodically with a decoction of leaves of paṭoli and nimba. The decoction of bark of nyagrodhādi group of drugs is used for washing vraṇas which have been purified (i.e.which are śuddha).

Vraṇas which have a narrow opening, and which are located in vital organs and joints, should be purified by using a varti (plug) of trivṛt, danti, lāngali, honey and rock-salt.

Vāta-vraṇas which are marked by severe pain and discharge should be fumigated by burning yava, ghee, bhūrja, madana, sūrahva and srīveshṭaka.

The daśamūla drugs and drugs of the vāta-hara group are useful in vāta-vrana, drugs of nyagrodhādi and padmakādi in pitta-vrana and drugs of āragvadhādi in kapha-vraṇa, (AHr.).

Tāmra bhasma which has been well triturated with the juice of madayanti, punarnava and mesha-śṛngi is very efficacious in purifying vraṇas and in speeding up the healing process.

The paste of paṭola and nimba leaves, yashṭi-madhu, haridra, tila, trivṛt and danti also helps in the rapid healing of ulcers. The paste of nimba leaves, tila, honey and ghee; of apāmārga leaves and leaf-juice or of powders of seeds of apāmārga are also useful. The external application of jatyādi-ghṛta is also beneficial, (RRS).

Ref.: SS, chikitsa, 1; CS, chikitsā, 25; AHṛ, uttara 25; RRS, 24, 92-101.

Classical Prescriptions: Chatur-mukha-rasa; Jātyādi-ghṛta; Kānchanāra-guggulu; Kāsīsa-bhasma; Kunkumādi-taila; Mṛdvīkarīshṭa; Nyagrodhādi-kvātha-chūrṇa; Rasa-pushpa; Sindhūrādi-lepa; Vajraka-taila.

Dushṭa-vraṇa: Āragvadhādi - kvātha-chūrṇa, Pancha-tiktaka-ghṛta; Somarāji-taila.

Vraṇa śotha

Western Nosology: Abscess; inflammatory swellings.

Causative Factors:

Intrinsic: The three doshas and vitiated blood (SS).

Constituents Affected: The swelling is confined to the skin and flesh (muscles, māmsa), (SS).

Classification: There are six kinds of vraṇa-śotha, namely vātaja, pittaja, kaphaja, that are caused by vitiated blood, tridoshaja and that which is of traumatic origin, (SS).

Symptomatology: The swelling is wide (extended), elevated, even or uneven in its surface and restricted in area (localised). For symptoms of the six types, see śotha.

The vraṇa-śotha can be divided into three types, depending on its progress, namely āma-vraṇa-śotha, (immature or un-suppurated swelling), pachyamāna-vraṇa-śotha (suppurating-swelling) and pakva-vraṇa-sotha (fully suppurated swelling), (SS).

The vātaja-vraṇa-śotha, sometimes suppurates fast and sometimes slowly, the pitta-vraṇa-śotha always suppurates speedily and the kaphaja-vraṇa-śotha is very slow in suppurating, (MN).

The āma-vraṇa-śotha (immature swelling) is characterised by absence of discolouration, slightness of swelling, slight local heat and pain, hardness and coldness.

The pachyamāna-vraṇa-śotha is characterised by pricking pain, formication, biting pain, tearing and aching pain, burning, local heat, sucking pain, which is not relieved by assuming any posture (i.e.while lying down, sitting or walking about). The swelling is distended (like an inflated leather bag). There is also fever, discolouration of skin, anorexia, and thirst.

The pakva-vraṇa-śotha is marked by relief of pain, decrease in the swelling, whitish discolouration, appearance of wrinkles over the affected area, signs of fluctuation on palpating with fingers, paroxysmal pricking pain, itching, restoration of appetite and amelioration of all distressing symptoms. The swelling pits on pressure and regains its original shape when the pressure is removed.

It is sometimes difficult to ascertain the exact state of a swelling (i.e.whether it is pakva or not) in cases of kaphaja-vraṇa-śotha, where the swelling affects the deeper tissues and in swellings caused by trauma. But the absence of discolouration, coldness of the swelling (i.e. absence of local heat), slightness of pain, hardness and firmness would definitely indicate the state of the śotha.

In swellings, there can be no pain without vāta, no suppuration without pitta and no formation of pus without kapha.

Ref.: SS, sūtra, 17; MN, 41.

Treatment:

1. Incising or opening of an āma-vraṇa-śotha-causes injury to the flesh (muscular tissues), blood vessels, hard fibrous structures, joints and bones, excessive bleeding, severe pain, and many complications, such as kshataja-vidradhi.

Not opening a vraṇa-śotha even when it is fully pakva is also dangerous, as the pus bereft of an external opening will burrow within the tissues and form sinuses which are much more difficult to treat.

Before incising a vraṇa-śotha, the patient should be asked to partake of a good meal in order to keep up his strength. He should also be given strong wine so that he can withstand the pain better.

Every vraṇa-śotha, whether extensive or small, goes on to suppuration if not treated, and may eat into the deeper tissues.

Even if ālepana (application of plasters), blood-letting or śodhana (purificatory procedures) does not relieve (or abort) the suppuration, it ensures that the swelling suppurates quickly, and is marked by a restricted, small base and formation of a head (elevation).

There are seven methods of handling this disease, namely: vimlāpana (kneading the affected part) avasechana (bleeding, blood-letting), upanāha (poulticing), pāṭana (opening or incision), śodhana (purificatory procedures), ropaṇa (medicines to aid healing) and vaikṛtāpaha (re-pigmentation of the cicatrix), (SS).

2. The physician should realise that vraṇa-śotha is the premonitory sign (pūrva-rūpa) of vraṇa. The swelling can be aborted at the very beginning by blood-letting. If there is excessive morbidly, śodhana can be done, and if the morbidity is less, langhana (depletion theory).

The external application of the following drugs relieve the burning, local heat, pain and may also disperse the swelling; paste (pralepa) of barks of nyagrodha, udumbara, aśvattha, plaksha and vetasa with ghee; the paste (pradeha) of vijayā, yashṭi, vīra, viśa-granthi, śatāvari, nilotpala, nāgapushpa and chandana; and the paste (pradeha) of śaktu, ghee, yashṭi and sugar.

If the swelling is not dispersed by these measures, it should be made to suppurate by applying the following poultices: the poutice prepared from ghee or oil and śaktu-pinda (roasted paddy grain) applied warm; or the poultice prepared from atasi-seeds (linseed), tila, śaktu-piṇḍa, kiṇva, sour curds, kushṭha and rock-salt.

Once the swelling is fully mature it can be opened surgically. In delicate and weak patients, drugs such as umā, guggulu, milky exudation of soudha, dung of cock and pigeon, palāśa-kshāra, hema-kshīri and mukūlaka (jayapāla) are used for making the swelling burst on its own, (CS).

3. In vātaja-vraṇa-śotha, the paste (pralepa) of mātulunga, agnimantha, bhadradāru, śuṇṭhi, ahimsrā and rāsna or paste of bark of śākhotaka, kānji (sour gruel) and ghee can be applied with good effect.

In pittaja-vraṇa-śotha, the paste of cold (śīta-vīrya) drugs such as dūrva, nala-root, yashṭi and chandana can be applied.

The paste of ajagandha, aśvagandha, kala, sarala, aja śṛngi and ekisika is useful in dispensing kaphaja-vraṇa-śotha.

The pastes of drugs should not be applied at night, and should not cover the head (opening) of the localised swelling.

In cases where the swelling is hard and only slightly painful, the area should be anointed with any medicated oil (which relieves vāta and kapha), and later fomented (subjected to svedana). The area is then gently kneaded with the finger or a bamboo stick.

In suppurating swelling that occurs in delicate, feeble persons and women, and which are located over vital organs, surgery is contra indicated. Instead a paste prepared by rubbing the horn of a cow with water is rubbed over the swelling which then bursts open, (CD).

Ref.: SS, sūtra, 17; CS, chikitsā, 25, 44-54; CD, 43.

Related Diseases: Vraṇa; Nāḍi-vraṇa; Śotha;

Śadyo-vraṇa.

Vṛddhi

Western Nosology: Swellings of the scrotum.

Causative Factors:

Extrinsic: Constantly suppressing the urge to urinate causes mūtra vrddhi. Lifting heavy weights, wrestling with a strong opponent, falling from a height and such other severe exertion causes antra-vṛddhi, (SS).

Pathogenesis: The aggravated doshas move downwards, localise in the scrotal vessels (or testicular vessels) and cause them to swell. Only one half of the scrotum may be affected, (SS).

Classification: The disease is of seven types. It may be caused by the deranged vāta, pitta, kapha, the vitiated blood, or fat. The other two types are mūtraja-vṛddhi and antra-vṛddhi, (SS).

Prodromal Symptoms: Pain in the urinary bladder, waist, scrotum and penis, swelling of the scrotum and obstruction of flatus, (SS).

Symptomatology:

Vāta-vṛddhi:

1. The scrotum is distended like an inflated air-drum, is rough and marked by varying kinds of pain (such as pricking pain, cutting pain, etc.,), (SS).

2. The pain occurs without any apparent cause, (AS).

Pittaja-vṛddhi: The scrotum assumes the colour of ripe udumbara fruit, and the swelling increases rapidly and as rapidly suppurates. There is also fever, burning pain and local heat, (SS).

Kapha-vṛddhi:

1. The swelling is hard, cold, slightly painful and itches, (SS).

2. The swelling is also greasy (unctuous), (AS).

Rakta-vṛddhi: The swollen scrotum is covered over with black vesicles. In all other respects it resembles pitta-vṛddhi, (SS).

Meda-vṛddhi:

1. The swollen scrotum resembles the fruit of tāla, is soft, unctuous, slightly painful and itches, (SS).

2. In other respects, it resembles kapha-vṛddhi, (AS).

Mūtra-vṛddhi: There is swelling of the scrotum, painful urination and pain in the testicles. The swelling bears a resemblance to a water bag and fluctuates, (SS).

Antra-vṛddhi: The aggravated vāta causes the protrusion of a part of the large intestines into the groins, in the form of a knotty growth. If this is not treated, part of the intestines descends into the scrotum, which becomes elongated, swollen and resembles a bladder inflated with air. It ascends upwards under pressure, with a peculiar sound, and again descends when the pressure is withdrawn, (SS).

Complications: The swollen scrotum is covered with a network of dry, blackish or brown veins, in antra-vṛddhi, (AS).

Prognosis: Antra-vṛddhi is considered to be incurable, (AS, SS).

Ref.: SS, nidāna, 12, 3-6; AS, nidāna, 11, 23-33.

Treatment:

1. In all cases of vṛddhi other than antra-vṛddhi, the patient should avoid riding on animals, exertion, coitus, suppression of natural urges, fasting, walking for long distances and intake of food that is hard to digest.

In vāta-vṛddhi, the patient has to be first oleated with traivṛta-sneha and then subjected to sudation. He should be purged by using the oil expressed from kośāmra, tilvaka and eraṇḍa seeds. As an alternative, castor-oil can be administered with milk for a month. Later, the patient can be given nirūha enema with a decoction and pastes of drugs that alleviate vāta. Food comprising of boiled rice and meat-juices can be partaken, followed by anuvāsana-enema of oil medicated with yashṭi-madhu. Unctuous poultices and applications of drugs that alleviate vāta are also useful. The swelling can be made to suppurate and then incised, and treated as a vraṇa (ulcer).

A case of pitta-vṛddhi which has not suppurated is treated on the same lines as for pitta-granthi. If it suppurates, it should be incised, and cleaned with honey and ghee; oil medicated with healing drugs is applied externally.

In rakta-vṛddhi, blood can be let out by employing leeches or purgation can be administered with honey and sugar. All other measures are similar to what is described in the treatment of pittaja-granthi.

In conditions of kapha-vṛddhi, the pastes of cow's urine and hot drugs (such as drugs of vachādi, pippalyādi and mushkākādi groups or ajagandhādi group) can be applied. The decoction of dāru-haridra can be administered internally with cow's urine. All measures that are useful in kaphaja-granthi should be employed except vimlāpana (application of pressure). If the swelling suppurates, it should be incised and cleansed (purified) with the appropriate drugs. Oil medicated with sumana, arushka, ankhoṭha and sapta-parṇa can be used for this purpose.

The meda-vṛddhi should be fomented and plastered with drugs of the surasādi group, or with drugs used for śiro-virechana (errhine) mixed with warm cow's urine. It should then be fomented and bandaged with a piece of cloth. The patient should then be reassured, and the growth (swelling) should be opened with a vṛddhi-patra (knife) carefully avoiding the testicles and the median line (of the perineum). The accumulated fatty tissue should be removed, a paste of kāsīsa and rock-salt should be applied, and the part bandaged. The wound should then be purified. Oil medicated with manahśila, haratāla, rock-salt and arushkara can be used for promoting healing.

In a case of mūtraja-vṛddhi, the part is fomented and bandaged with a piece of cloth. The swelling should be punctured on the under-surface, on either side of the rapha with a vrīhi-mukha instrument. A tube open at both ends should be introduced, and the liquid drained out. The tube is then removed, and the scrotum bandaged with sthagika-bandha. The incidental ulcer is purified and healed.

A patient suffering from antra-vṛddhi should first avoid the factors responsible for the disease. If the scrotum has not yet been affected, the swelling is to be treated as indicated in vāta-vṛddhi. If the swelling is situated at the groin, then it can be cauterised with the ardha-indu-vakra instrument. The veins at the temples, just above the ears, on the side opposite to the antra-vṛddhi should be opened, avoiding the sevani (raphe). The thumb of the side other than where the vṛddhi is located should be incised at its middle and cauterized.

In vāta-vṛddhi and kapha-vṛddhi, the same process can be carried out, but in additon the snāyu (hard fibrous structures) should be cut off, (SS).

2. The decoction of rāsna, yashṭi-madhu, guḍūchi, eraṇḍa, balā, gokshura can be administered with castor oil in antra-vṛddhi. Castor oil can also be given with milk medicated with balā in cases of antra-vṛddhi attended with flatulent distension of the abdomen, and pain. The patient can also be administered harītaki that has been soaked in cow's urine with rock-salt and oil (castor oil) every morning in vāta-vṛddhi and kapha-vṛddhi. Harītaki that has been soaked in cow's urine can be roasted in castor-oil and administered with rock-salt, followed by a draught of hot water in chronic cases. The decoction of triphala with cow's urine or the paste of sarala, agaru, kushṭha, devadāru, nāgara, cow's urine and kānji is useful in kapha-vṛddhi and vāta-vṛddhi. The pulp of harītaki can be fried in castor oil and administered with pippali and rock-salt in

vṛddhi. The paste of ghee and rock-salt can be placed within a conch-shell and exposed to the sun for a week. This can then be administered in chronic vṛddhi. The root-powder of aindhri is to be rubbed with castor oil and administered with milk.

The paste of root-bark of rūpika (arka) and kānji or of vachā, and sarshapa can be applied externally, (CD).

3. The constant use of powder of dāru-haridra with cow's urine is recommended in antra-vṛddhi. The formulation known as vātāri-rasa can be given with honey, followed by the anupāna of castor oil and cow's milk. This can be used for a month (in cases of vṛddhi). The expressed juices of fresh ginger can be administered every morning with til oil, in antra-vṛddhi. Oil medicated with a decoction of triphala is also useful in antra-vṛddhi. The meat-juices of mayūra and tittiri are useful in antra-vṛddhi. Oil or ghee boiled with the meat-juices of tāmra-chūḍa, curds, kānji, madira and juices of mātulunga is efficacious in antra-vṛddhi. The meat-juices of vārtāka and kukkuṭa can be partaken in such cases, (RRS).

Ref.: SS, chikitsā, 19, 3-24; CD, 40, 1-21; RRS, 18, 28-39.

Classical Prescriptions: Miśraka-sneha; Sukumāra-ghṛta.

Vṛshana-Kacchhu

Causative Factors:

Extrinsic: Uncleanliness

Intrinsic: Kapha

Constituents Affected: Blood

Symptomatology: In an unclean person, the dirt that accumulates around and on the scrotum and the sweat causes itching and watery exudation, which is later followed by the eruption of itching vesicles which are filled with liquid.

Treatment: The patient has to be treated along the same lines as in kushṭha. The pastes of siktha (wax), śatāhva and white variety of sarshapa or of vachā, dāru-haridra and sarshapa or oil extracted from seeds of karanja or sara-taila (oil extracted from simshipa, agaru, sarala, devadāru, etc.,) boiled with drugs of pippalyādi group can be applied externally.

Vyanga

Causative Factors:

Extrinsic: Excessive exertion and emotions such as anger.

Intrinsic: Vāta and pitta.

Constituents Affected: The second layer of skin known as lohita (stratum lucidum), (SS, śārīra, 4, 4).

Pathogenesis and Symptomatology: The deranged doshas localise in the face, and cause circular, blackish or grey, thin (not very elevated), painless patches known as vyanga.

Treatment: The patient is first subjected to bloodletting by venesection. The patches can also be scraped (by pieces of samudraphena, etc.,) and plastered with a paste of milk and bark of kshīri (milk-exuding) trees (like vaṭa), or with the paste of balā, atibala, yashṭi-madhu and haridra, or of payasya, agaru, kaliyā (kṛshṇa-chandana) and gairika, or of kapittha and rājādana.

Related Diseases: Nyaccha, Nīlika

Ref.: SS, nidāna, 13, 45-46; chikitsā, 20, 33-36.

Yava-prakhyā

Causative Factors:

Extrinsic: Factors that aggravate kapha and vāta.

Intrinsic: Kapha and vāta.

Constituents Affected: Flesh or muscles.

Symptomatology: Eruptions that are hard, knotty, and resemble barley (grains) (i.e. which are elevated at the centre and depressed in the periphery), and are found in the fleshy regions are known as yava-prakhyā.

Treatment: The affected area is first fomented, and later plastered with the paste of manahaśila, haritāla, kushṭha, and deva-dāru (or daru-haridra). After the eruptions have suppurated, remedial measures that are useful in vraṇa are to be employed.

Ref.: SS, nidāna, 13, 5; chikitsā, 20, 5-6.

Yoni-vyāpat

Western Nosology: Diseases of the female genital organs

Causative Factors:

Extrinsic:

1. Sexual intercourse by a young girl who is weak and dried up with a man who has a very large penis. The disease can also occur due to unclean and improper habits, due to menstrual disorders or they may be congenital, (SS).

2. These diseases in general may be congenital or may occur due to unclean and improper habits or menstrual disorders, (CS).

Classification:

1. There are twenty such diseases. Of these, the aggravated vāta causes five diseases known as udāvarta, vandhyā, vipluta, paripluta and vātalā. The aggravated pītta causes five diseases, namely, pittala, rudhirāksharā, vāmini, sramsini and putraghni, while the vitiated kapha engenders five diseases, known as śleshmala, ātyānanda, karṇini, and two kinds of charaṇa. The three doshas combined cause five diseases, shaṇḍi, phalini, mahati, sūchi-vakra and sarvaja, (SS).

2. There are twenty diseases of yoni. Of these, rakta-yoni and arajaskā are caused by vitiated pitta. The aggravated vāta and pitta cause paripluta and vāmini. The deranged vāta and kapha engender karṇini and upapluta. The aggravated pitta and kapha cause pittaja-yoni-roga and kaphaja-yoni-roga, while all the three deranged doshaṣ cause one type of yoni-roga. The rest are all caused by the aggravated vāta, (CS).

Causes and Symptoms:

Vātaja-yoni-roga:

1. The vāta is aggravated in a woman with a vatala constitution, is localised in the genital organs, and causes pricking pain, rigidity or stiffness, numbness, formication, roughness, exhaustion and other vāta disorders. The menstrual discharge is painful, and frothy, thin, un-unctuous and accompanied by sound, (CS).

2. The disease is attended by roughness, rigidity, local pain, and pricking pain, (SS).

Pittaja-yoni-roga:

1. The pitta is aggravated by excessive intake of pungent, sour, salty and alkaline food, localises in the genital organs, and causes burning, suppuration, fever and heat. The menstrual discharge will be blue, or yellow or blackish in colour. There will also be a copious hot, offensive discharge from the vagina, (CS).

2. The disease is attended by suppuration, burning and fever, (SS).

Kaphaja-yoni-roga:

1. The kapha is aggravated by abhishyandi food, and causes sliminess, coldness, itching, dull pain, and pale-yellow or white discolouration. The menstrual discharge will be slimy and whitish, (CS).

2. The condition is characterised by sliminess, extreme coldness and itching, (SS).

Tridoshaja-yoni-roga:

1. The three doshas are aggravated, localise in the genital organs and produce their characteristic signs and symptoms. There will be burning and pain, and discharge that is white and slimy, (CS).

2. The three aggravated doshas produce characteristic symptoms, (SS).

Rakta-yoni (Lohita-kshara, according to SS)

1. The blood is vitiated by the pitta which is aggravated by factors responsible for rakta-pitta, and as a result there is excessive discharge of blood, even after conception, (CS).

2. The aggravated pitta causes excessive discharge of blood with burning pain, (SS).

Arajaska (Amenorrhoea): The aggravated pitta that is localised in the genital organs vitiates the blood, and causes amenorrhoea with emaciation and discolouration (of skin, mucous membrane, etc.), (CS).

Vandhyā: The aggravated vatā is responsible for the cessation of menstruation (or ovulation), (SS).

Acharaṇā (Nymphomania):

1. Due to unclean habits, and failure to wash the genital organs, the parts are infested with parasites which cause itching. Due to the itching, the woman craves sexual intercourse, (CS).

2. The woman has an intense desire for intercourse, surpassing the desire of the male partner (this is due to the internal itching, NiS), (SS).

Ati-charaṇā:

1. The vāta is aggravated due to excessive sexual intercourse, and produces swelling, pain and numbness in the female genital organs, (CS).

2. In spite of repeated sexual intercourse, the woman fails to conceive, (SS).

Prāk-charaṇā: If a young girl indulges in coitus, the aggravated vāta causes pain in the back, waist, thighs and groin, (CS).

Upaplutā (Dysmenorrhoea):

1. Due to the disease udāvarta, reversal of the course of uterine contractions occurs. There is thus painful menstruation, and menstruation takes place with difficulty. However, there is relief after menstruation, (CS).

2. The woman suffers from difficult menstruation, and the discharge is frothy, (SS).

Karṇini:

1. The vāta, kapha and the blood are vitiated if the pregnant woman strains to expel the foetus prematurely, and as a result a growth (tumefaction) shaped like an ear is formed, which obstructs the passage of blood, (CS).

2. A fleshy growth shaped like the ear is formed in the genital organ (vagina) due to the vitiation of kapha and blood, (SS).

Putraghnī (Habitual Abortion):

1. The aggravated vāta vitiates the blood by its quality of dryness, and causes repeated abortion, (CS).

2. The woman suffers from repeated abortion as a result of the aggravated pitta causing flow of blood from the uterus, (SS).

Antar-mukhi (Prolapse of the Uterus): The vāta is aggravated and localises in the genital organs due to the woman indulging in coitus just after partaking of a heavy meal, and due to her assuming unnatural positions during coitus, and causes displacement of the vaginal orifice. There is severe pain in the bones and fleshy parts, and due to the pain, the woman is unable to take part in sexual intercourse, (CS).

Sūchī-mukhi (Vaginal Atresia):

1. The aggravated vāta by its quality of dryness causes a congenital narrowing of the vaginal orifice, (CS).

2. The vaginal orifice is extremely narrow, (SS).

Śushkā: The vāta is aggravated by suppressing the natural urges during sexual intercourse, and causes dryness, pain, constipation and retention of urine, (CS).

Vāmini (Female Sterility):

1. The semen that is deposited in the uterus is expelled with or without pain after six or seven days, (CS).

2. The semen that is deposited in the uterus is expelled out along with the menstrual blood, (SS).

Shaṇḍi (Developmental Abnormality):

1. The aggravated vāta affects the normal development of the female genital organs, and causes aversion to the male sex and absence of breasts. This condition is congenital, (CS).

2. This is a condition characterized by absence of both breasts and menstruation and roughness of vagina during coitus, (SS).

Mahā-yoni:

1. The vata is aggravated in the woman employing unnatural postures in bed or during coitus and dilates the vaginal orifice and cervix. There will be pain in the joints and groins, discharge of dry, frothy blood, pain and fleshy growth, (CS).

2. The vaginal orifice and cervix will be highly dilated, (SS).

Viplutā: There is constant pain in the genital organs, (SS).

Sramsinī (Prolapse): The woman suffers from prolapse on exertion and difficult parturition, (SS).

Atyānanda (Frigidity): The woman does not derive any pleasure from sexual intercourse, (SS).

Phalini: The condition where a young girl indulges in sexual intercourse with a person with an abnormally large penis, (SS).

Complications: A woman suffering from these diseases is unable to conceive and suffers from various diseases such as abdominal tumours, haemorrhoids, pradara, etc., (CS).

Prognosis:

1. The five diseases caused by the aggravation of all three doshas are incurable, (SS).

2. The disease known as shaṇḍi is incurable, (CS).

Ref.: CS, chikitsā, 30, 7-40; SS, uttara, 38, 3-20.

Treatment:

1. The diseases caused by aggravated vāta are to be treated by oleation, sudation, enemata and other measures. The diseases engendered by vitiated pitta are treated by measures useful in rakta-pitta and medications that are cooling. The ailments caused by kapha are treated by dry and hot measures. In diseases caused by all three doshas, treatment should be judiciously given depending on which dosha is mainly involved.

In conditions of displacement of the uterus, the part should be oleated, fomented and replaced in the normal position. The position can be changed by manipulation with the hand. If the orifice is narrow, it should be dilated. If the uterus has prolapsed, it should be established in its normal position. If the uterus is completely prolapsed and exposed, it should be considered and treated accordingly as a foreign body.

In almost all cases, the woman should be administered oleation and sudation, followed by mild purificatory procedures.

In vāta-diseases, the patient should partake of meat of aquatic and wet-land animals, milk, tila seeds and rice. The nāḍi and kumbhī types of fomentation can be given using drugs that alleviate vāta. The patient can be massaged with oil mixed with rock-salt, and subjected to aśma, prastara and sankara types of fomentations. She should then take a bath in warm water and partake of meat-juices medicated with drugs that alleviate vāta. The medicated ghee known as balā-ghṛta and kāśmaryādi-ghṛta can be administered. The pastes of pippali, kṛshṇa-jīraka, ajāji, vāsā, rock-salt, vachā, yava-kshāra, ajamoda, sugar and chitraka are fried with ghee and administered with prasannā wine. The paste of vāsā, mātulunga roots, madayantika, pippali and kṛshna-jirāka can be given with rock-salt and wine. If there is severe pain, the patient can partake of milk boiled with rāsna, gokshura and vāsā. The part can be affused with the decoction of triphala, guḍūchi and danti. Oil medicated with rock-salt, tagara, kushṭha, bṛhatī, and devadāru can be used locally. One prastha of oil is boiled with double the quantity each of cow's urine, and milk and one tola each of guḍūchi, mālati, rāsna, balā, yashṭi-madhu, chitraka, kaṇṭakāri, devadāru and yūthika. A tampon impregnated with the oil is inserted into the vagina. The part can be massaged with oil, and the paste of himsra can be applied within.

In diseases caused by the aggravated pitta, ghee can be used for oleation, while cold substances and drugs that alleviate pitta should be used for administering effusions, massages and for preparing tampons. The paste of pancha-valkalas can be applied locally. The preparation known as bṛhat-śatāvari-ghṛta and jīvanīya-ghṛta can be administered internally.

In diseases caused by kapha, the paste of śyāmadi drugs can be applied locally. A sam-śodhana-varti (plug) rubbed with hog's bile or a tampon prepared from barley flour, rock-salt, and milky exudation of arka can be inserted (the latter only for a short while). The part can be washed with warm water. A tampon prepared from pippali, maricha, māsha, śata-pushpa and rock-salt can also be used.

A tampon dipped in udumbarādi-taila should be inserted in the vagina. A cold decoction of drugs mixed with sugar can be used for washing the part (as douche). This is useful in slimy, dilated and chronically diseased genital organs. Oil extracted from tila seeds which have been soaked six times in the milky exudation of udumbara should be medicated with the decoction of udumbara and used in the aforesaid manner. A tampon can be dipped in dhātakyādi-taila and inserted into the vagina in case of slimy discharge, viplutā, upaplutā, cases of ulceration and pain, and prolopsed, elevated and swollen vagina, (or uterus). The waist, back and sacral region should be massaged with oil. Unctuous-enemata can also be given. The patient can be administered douches with the decoction of karīra dhava, nimba, arka, veṇu, kośūmra, jambu, jingini, and vāsā roots, mṛdvīka, sīdhu-wine, and vinegar, or with the decoction of triphala mixed with butter-milk, cow's urine and vinegar (śukta).

The person suffering from diseases of kapha can be administered pippali, pulverised iron, and harītaki with honey. Enema of cow's urine and pungent drugs can also be given.

The powder known as pushyānuga-chūrṇa is also very efficacious in yoni-roga. Ghee medicated with the decoction of kāśmari and kuṭaja can be used as a vaginal douche in rakta-yoni, arajaskā and putraghnī. Milk medicated with drugs of the jīvanīya group or the blood of hog, deer, goat or sheep can be drunk with curds, juice or sour-fruits and ghee in arajaska. Oil medicated with drugs of the jīvanīya group can be used as a douche in karṇini, acharaṇa, śushka-yoni, prak-charaṇa and diseases caused by kapha and vāta. A piece of silk cloth soaked twenty-one times in cow's bile or fish-bile or the powder of yeast (kiṇva) mixed with honey can be kept in the vagina, in acharaṇa. It relieves itching, softening and swelling and cleanses the part.

In prāk-charaṇa and ati-charaṇa, oil that has been boiled with drugs that alleviate vāta should be used for administering āsthāpana and anuvāsana enema. The patient should then be fomented, given upanāha (poultice-sudation) and food consisting of substances that alleviate vāta. A paste or lump consisting of śātapushpa, barley, wheat, kiṇva (yeast), kushṭha, priyangu, ākhu-parṇi and śryāhva can be kept in the vagina. In vāmini and upa-pluta, the woman can be subjected to oleation, sudation, etc., and nourishing treatment. An unctuous tampon should be inserted in the vagina. A tampon dipped in the decoction of śallaki, jingini, jambu, dhava, dālchini and the five-barks (pancha-valkala) can be used in viplutā. In karṇini, measures that alleviate kapha are to be employed. A plug or tampon prepared from kushṭha, pippali, arka-sprouts, rock-salt and goat's urine can be inserted.

In udāvartā, the patient can be oleated with traivṛta-ghṛta, fomented and given meat-juices of aquatic and domesticated animals. Milk medicated with daśamūla drugs should be used for giving enema. In mahā-yoni and srasta-yoni (prolapse) traivṛta-sneha should be used for administering anuvāsana-enema and vaginal douche. In mahā-yoni, the uterus should be filled with fat of bear and hog and ghee medicated with sweet drugs, and should be bandaged with a piece of silken cloth. The prolapsed uterus should be massaged with ghee, fomented with milk, gently replaced into its normal position and bandaged with the padding of a lump of vesavāra until the time for micturition.

All yoni-rogas, especially mahā-yoni should be first treated with measures that alleviate vāta. These diseases do not occur unless vata is aggravated.

In conditions where the vagina, etc., have become slimy and softened, the paste of palāśa, sarja, jambu, dālchini, samanga, mocha-rasa and dhātaki can be applied. If these organs have become rough and stiff, either vesavāra or pāyasa or kṛśara can be kept in the vagina. In cases of offensive smell, the decoction or paste of tuvāra or the powders of aromatic drugs can be used, (CS).

2. In all cases of yoni-rogas, measures such as snehana (oleation), sudation, etc., should be employed depending on the dosha that is involved. Vaginal douches (uttara-basti) are also very useful.

In cases where the genital organs are rough, cold, rigid and numb during coitus, the patient can be given kumbhi type of sudation with flesh of aquatic and wet-land animals. Vesavāras medicated with sweet drugs can be kept in the vagina. A tampon dipped in oil can also be inserted. The parts have to be kept clean. The diet has to consist of articles that alleviate vāta.

Cases where there is burning pain, etc., are to be treated with cooling measures. In cases where the genital organs are slimy and offensive, the powders of nyagrodha, udumbara, plaksha, aśvattha and gardabhāṇḍa are dusted within. The decoction of drugs of the āragvadhādi group should be used for washing the parts. In conditions marked by discharge of pus, balls made of śodhana (disinfectant) drugs mixed with cow's urine and rock-salt should be inserted into the vagina.

In conditions marked by itching and loss of sensibility, drugs such as bṛhati-fruits, haridra and dāru-haridra should be used for fumigation and in the form of tampons. In karṇini, tampons prepared from śodhana drugs are inserted. In pra-sramsini, the uterus should be anointed with ghee fomented with milk, replaced in the normal condition and should be pasted with vesavāra and bandaged.

The diet should consist of surā, āsava and arishṭa depending on the dosha affected. The expressed juice of laśuna should be administered every morning. Milk and meat-juices can also be taken, (SS).

3. The pastes of lodhra, and tumbi-fruits or of vachā, nilotpala, kushṭha, maricha, aśvagandha and haridra or of madana-fruits, yashṭi-madhu and kharjūra are useful in strengthening or imparting firmness to the genital organs. The sexual organs can also be washed with a decoction of vetasa-roots.

The following prescriptions are useful in

inducing conception: ghee boiled with milk and aśvagandha which should be taken after the menses; ghee medicated with pippali, nāgara, maricha and nāga-kesara; the paste of svarṇa-bhasma, rajata-bhasma and tāmra-bhasma with ghee, etc.

A tampon prepared from ikshvāku seeds, danti, pippali, jaggery, madana, kiṇva (yeast), yashṭi-madhu and milky exudation of snuhi is useful in bringing on the menses. The flower of japā is made into a paste with kānji, fried with leaves of jyotishmati and is administered in cases of amenorrhoea.

The powders of āmalaki, anjana and harītaki if administered with water or the paste of leaves of śelu will stop the menstrual flow. The drug known as dūrva is very useful in arresting the flow of blood from vagina, and in the early stages of abortion.

The formulations known as phala-ghṛta, and bṛhat-śatāvari-ghṛta, are also useful in yoni-roga (when administered internally), (CD).

4. The person suffering from yoni-śula (pain in the genital organs or dysmenorrhoea) should be administered the leaf-juice of nirguṇḍi with jaggery, followed by wine. After this has been digested, butter-milk can be drunk. The prolapsed uterus (pra-sramsini) should be replaced and plastered with the paste of kārali-kanda. In a case of vivṛta-yoni (where the orifices are dilated), the paste of mākanda-roots, karpūra and honey will make them as narrow as is found in a young girl. The oil known as śrī-parṇi-taila is very efficacious in restoring sunken breasts to their original condition.

The paste of somarāji, devadāru, nimba, dāru-haridra, āsava and butter-milk is very useful in yoni-roga, when applied locally. The paste of rasona, soot, viśāla, viḍanga, and kaṇṭakāri-fruits is applied externally in cases of local pain and parasite infestation.

A woman suffering from amenorrhoea should be administered tri-yoni-rasa with old jaggery and powder of harītaki, followed by black tila seeds and cold water. The powders of lāngali root or apāmārga roots or indra-vāruṇi roots are also useful. The decoction of tila roots and bhārngi roots administered with powder of yashṭi-madhu and trikaṭu are also useful. The dish prepared from chaṇaka-juice, milk and ghee, mixed with sugar and honey is also useful. The powders of tila, bhārngi, jaggery and trikaṭu can be taken with a decoction of tila.

The paste of tila oil and rock-salt if kept within the vagina (or uterus) after the menses will induce abortion. The stalk of castor leaves can be inserted for eight angulas into the vagina in order to induce abortion. The paste of expressed juice of nirguṇḍi, chitraka roots and honey can be administered internally for the same purpose.

The roots of śārapunkha can be administered with rice-water in excessive bleeding.

Ref.: CS, chikitsā, 30, 41-127; SS, uttara, 38, 21-30; CD, 62, 21-53; RRS, 22, 123-128; 25, 79-98.

Classical Prescriptions: Kalyāṇaka-ghṛta; Sahacharādi-taila; Phala-ghṛta; Śatāvari-guḍa.

Yoni-ruja

Aśokārishṭa; Aśoka-ghṛta; Sukumāra-ghṛta.

Appendices

APPENDIX-I

Groups of drugs according to Charaka-samhita, sūtra, 4

1.Jīvanīya drugs (nutrients) include jīvaka, ṛshabhaka, meda, mahāmeda, kākoli, kshrirakākoli, mudgaparṇi, māsha-parṇi, jīvanti and madhuka.

2. Bṛmhaṇiya drugs (roborants) include kshirini, rajaksavaka, aśvagandha, kākoli, kshirakakoli, vatyayani, bhadraudani, bhāradvaji, payasyā and ṛshyagandha.

3. Lekhaniya drugs (attenuants) include mustā, kusṭha, haridrā, dāruharidra, ativisha, vachā, kaṭurohiṇi, chitraka, chira-bilva and haimavati.

4. Bhedanīya drugs (laxatives) include suvah, arka, urubuka, agnimukhi, chitra, chitraka, chira-bilva, śankhini, śakulādani and svarṇaksīriṇi.

5. Sandhűnīya drugs (synthesizers) include madhuka, madhuparṇi, pṛśniparṇi, ambasṭhaki, samanga, mocha-rasa, dhātaki, lodhra, priyangu and kaṭphala.

6. Dīpanīya drugs (digestive, stimulants or appetizers) include pippali, pippali mūla, chavya, chitraka, śṛngavera, amlavetasa, maricha, ajamoda, stone of bhallātaka and hingu niryāsa.

7. Balya drugs (which promote strength) include aindri, atirasa, ṛshabhi, ṛshyaprokta, payasyā, aśvagandha, sthirā, rohiṇi, balā and atibalā.

8. Varṇaja drugs (which promote complexion) include tunga, chandana, padmaka, uśīra, madhuka, manjishṭha, sāriva, payasyā, sitā and lata.

9. Kaṇṭhya drugs (which enhance the voice) include sāriva, ikshu-mūla, madhuka, pippali, drāksha, vidāri, kaiṭarya, hamsa-padi, bṛhati and kaṇṭakārika.

10. Hṛdya drugs (cordials) include āmra, āmrātaka, lakucha, karamarda, vṛkshāmla, amlavetasa, kuvala, badara, dāḍima and mātulunga.

11. Tṛptighna drugs (which remove satiety) include tagara, chavya, chitraka, viḍanga, murva, guḍūchi, vachā, musta, pippali and paṭola.

12. Arśoghna drugs (anti-haemorrhoidals) include, kuṭaja, bilva, chitraka, nāgara, ativisha, abhayā, dhanvayāsa, dāru-haridra, vachā and chavya.

13. Kushṭhaghna drugs (which cure kushtha) include khadira, abhayā, āmalaka, haridra, ārushkara, saptaparṇa, āragvadha, karavīra, viḍanga and jati-pravāla.

14. Kaṇḍughna drugs (which relieve pruritus) include chandana, nalada, kṛtamāla, naktamāla, nimba, kuṭaja, sarshapa, madhuka, dāru-haridra and musta.

15. Kṛmighna drugs (anthelminthics) include akshīva, maricha, gaṇḍhīra, kebuka, viḍanga, nirguṇḍi, kiṇihi, svadamśtra, vṛksha-parṇi and ākhu-parṇika.

16. Vishaghna drugs (anti-toxic) include haridra, manjishṭha, suvaha, sūkshma-ela, palindi, chandana, kataka, sirīsha, sindhuvāra and śleshmāntaka.

17. Stanya-janaka drugs (galactagogues) include virana, śāli, shasṭika, ikshu-vālika, darbha, kuśa, gundra, itkaāa and kattrna.

18. Stanya-śodhana drugs (galacto-purificators) include pāṭha, mahaushadha, sura dāru, musta, mūrva, guḍūchi, vatsaka fruit, kirātatikta, kaṭu-rohiṇi and sāriva.

19. Śukra-janana drugs (spermatopoietics) include jīvaka, ṛshabhaka, kākoli, kshīra-kākoli, mudgaparṇi, műshaparṇi, meda, vṛddhāruha, jaṭila and kulinga.

20. Śukra-śodhana drugs (spermato purificators) include kushiha, elavāluka, kaṭphala, samudraphena, kadamba gum, kāṇḍekshu, ikshu, ikshuraka, vāsuka and uśīra.

21. Chardi-nigrahaṇa drugs (anti-emetics) include jambu, tender leaves of āmra, mātulunga, badara, dāḍima, yava, yashṭika, uśīra, mṛt and lājā.

22. Tṛshṇā-nigrahaṇa drugs (which relieve thirst) include nāgara, dhanvayāsa, musta, parpaṭaka, chandana, kīratatikta, guḍūchi, hrīvera, dhānyaka and paṭola.

23. Hikka-nigrahaṇa drugs (which relieve hiccough) include śaṭi, pushkaramūla, badara stone, kaṇṭakāri, bṛhati, vṛkshāruha, abhayā, pippali, durālabha and kulīra śṛngi.

24. Purīsha-sangrahaṇīya drugs (intestinal astringents) include priyangu, anantā, āmra stone, katvanga, lodhra, mocharasa, samanga, dhātaki flowers, padma and filaments of padma.

25. Purīsha-virajaniya drugs (faceal pigment restorers) include jambu, śallaki bark, kacchūra, madhuka, śālmali, śrīveshṭaka, fried earth, payasya, utpala and tila grains.

26. Mūtra sangrahaṇīya drugs (ischuretics) include jambu, āmra, plaksha, vaṭa, kapītana, udumbara, aśvattha, bhallātaka, aśmantaka and soma-valka.

27. Mūtra-virajanīya drugs (urine pigment restorers) include padma, utpala, nalina, kumuda, saugandhika, puṇḍarīka, śatapatra, madhuka, priyangu and dhātaki flowers.

28. Mūtra-virechanīya drugs (diuretics) include vṛkshādani, svadamśtra, vāsuka, viśira, pāshaṇabheda, darbha, kuśa, kāśa, gundra and root of itkaṭa.

29. Kāsa-hara drugs (drugs which cure cough) include drāksha, abhayā, āmalaka, pippali, durālabha, śṛngi, kaṇṭakārika, vṛschīra, punarnava and tāmalaki.

30. Śvāsa-hara drugs (which cure śvāsa) include śaṭi, pushkara-mūla, amla-vetasa, ela, hingu, agaru, surasā, tāmalaki, jīvanti and chaṇḍa.

31. Śvayathu-hara drugs (which cure śvayathu) include pāṭala, agnimantha, śyonaka, bilva, kāśmarya, kaṇṭakari, bṛhati, śālaparṇi, pṛśniparṇi and gokshura.

32. Jvara-hara drugs (which are anti-pyretic) include sāriva, sugar candy, pāṭha, manjishṭha, drāksha, pīlu, parūshaka, abhayā, āmalaka and vibhītaka.

33. Śrama-hara drugs (which relieve fatigue) include drāksha, kharjūra, priyāla, badara, dāḍima, phalgu, parūshaka, ikshu, yava and shashṭika.

34. Dāha-praśamana drugs (which relieve burning pains) include lājā, chandana, kāśmarya fruit, madhuka, sugar candy, nilotpala, usira, śāriva, guḍūchi and hrīvera.

35. Śīta-praśamana drugs (which cure chill) include tagara, agaru, dhānyaka, śṛngavera, bhūtika, vachā, kaṇṭakāri, agnimantha, śyonaka and pippali.

36. Udara-praśamana drugs (which cure udara) include vidārigandha, pṛshniparṇi, bṛhati, kaṇṭakārika, eraṇḍa, chandana, usira, ela, madhuka and kākoli.

37. Śūla-praśamana drugs (which cure śūla) include pippali, pippali root, chavya, chitraka, śṛngavera, maricha, ajamoda, ajagandha, ajāji and gaṇḍhīra.

38. Śonitāsthapana drugs (which are haemostatic) include honey, madhuka, rudhira, mocha rasa, lodhra, pieces of earth, gairika, priyangu, sugar and fried paddy, (lājā).

39. Vedanā-sthāpana drugs (which are sedatives or pain killers) include śūla, kaṭphala, kadamba, padmaka, tumba, mocha rasa, sirīsha, vanjula, elavāluka and aśoka.

40. Sanjnā-sthāpana drugs (which restore consciousness) include hingu, kaiṭarya, arimeda, vachā, choraka, vayastha, golomi, jaṭila, palankaśa and aśoka-rohiṇi.

41. Prajā-sthapana drugs (fertility promoters) include aindri, brāhmi, śatavīrya, sahasra-vīrya, amoghā, avyathā, aśiva, arisṭha, vāṭyapushpi and vishvaksena-kānta.

42. Vayasthāpana drugs (which promote longevity) include amṛta, abhayā, dhātri, mukta, śveta, jīvanti, atirasa, maṇḍūka- parṇi, sthirā and punarnava.

APPENDIX-II

Group of drugs according to Susruta-samhita, sūtra, 38

1. Vidārigandhādi group - consists of vidārigandha (śālaparṇi), vidāri, viśvadeva, sahadeva, gokshura, pṛthakparṇi (pṛśni parṇi), śatāvari, sāriva, kṛshna-sāriva, jīvaka, ṛshabhaka, mahāsaha (māshaparni), kshudrasaha (mudga parṇi), bṛhati, kaṇṭakāri, punarnava, eraṇḍa, hamsapadi, vṛschikāli and ṛshabhi (kapi-kacchu).

These drugs alleviate pitta and vāta, and are useful in tuberculosis, gulma, body ache, dyspnoea and cough.

2. Āragvadhādi group - consists of āragvadha, madana, gopa-ghaṇṭa, kaṇṭaki (vikankaṭa), kuṭaja, pāṭha, pāṭala, mūrva, indra-yava, sapta parṇa, nimba, kuruṇṭaka, dāsī-kuruṇṭaka, guḍūchi, chitraka, śarngeshṭa, two types of karanja, paṭola, kirātatikta and śushavi.

These drugs alleviate kapha, are anti-toxic, purify and cleanse ulcers and wounds and are useful in prameha, skin diseases, fever, vomiting and pruritus.

3. Sālasārādi group - consists of sāla-sāra, ajakarṇa (sarja), khadira, kadara, kālaskandha, kramuka (pūga), bhūrja, mesha-śṛnga (karkaṭa-śṛnga), tinisha, chandana, ku-chandana (rakta-chandana), simshipa, sirīsha, asana, dhava, arjuna, tāla, śākā, nakta-māla, pūtika (chirabilva), aśvakarṇa, agaru and kalīyaka.

These drugs alleviate kapha, reduce the medas (fatty tissues), and relieve skin diseases, prameha and anaemia.

4. Varuṇādi group - consists of varuṇa, ārtagala, śigru, madhu-śigru, tarkāri (araṇi), mesha-śṛngi (karkaṭaśṛngi), pūtika (chira-bilva), nakta māla (bṛhat-karanja), moraṭa, agni-mantha, the two types of saireyaka, bimbi, vāsuka (vāsā or arka), vaśira (apāmārga), chitraka, śatāvari, bilva, aja-śṛngi, darbha (kuśa), bṛhati and kaṇṭākari. These drugs reduce kapha and medas (fatty tissues) and are useful in headache, gulma and internal abscesses.

5. Vīratarvādi group - consists of vīrataru, the two types of sahachara (kaṇṭa-śelu), darbha, vṛkshādani, gundra, nala, kuśa, kāśa, aśmabheda (pāshāṇa-bheda), agnimantha, moraṭa, vāsuka (baka), vaśira (āpāmārga), bhallūka (śyonāka), kuranṭika, indīvara, kapota-vanka and gokshura. These drugs alleviate vāta and are useful in urinary calculi (aśmari), gravel (śarkara), dysuria, mutrāghūta and pain (renal colic?).

6. Lodhrādi group - consists of lodhra, sāvara-lodhra (with thick, white bark), palāśa, kuṭannaṭa (śyonāka), aśoka, phanji (bhārngi), kaṭphala, elavāluka, śallaki, jingini, kadamba, śāla (sarja) and kadali.

These drugs alleviate kapha, reduce medas (fatty tissues), are anti-toxic and stambhi (styptic, block discharges), enhance the complexion and relieve menstrual complaints and uterine diseases (yoni-dosha-hara).

7. Arkādi group - consists of arka, alarka, the two types of karanja, nagādanti (dantini), mayūraka (āpāmārga), bhārngi, rāsna, indra-pushpi, kshudra-śveta (sveta-syanda), mahā-sveta, vṛschikāli, alavana (jyotishmati), and tāpasa-vṛksha (inguda or putranjiva).

These drugs alleviate kapha, reduce medas, are antitoxic, are very efficacious in cleansing and purifying ulcers and wounds and relieve worm infestation and skin diseases.

8. Surasādi group - consists of surasa, śveta-surasa, phaṇijjaka, arjaka, bhūstṛṇa, sugandhaka, sumukha, kālāmala, kuṭheraka, kāsamarda, kshavaka, kharapushpa, viḍanga, khaṭphala, surasi, nirguṇḍi, kulāhala, unduru-karṇika, phanji, prāchibala, kākāmachi and visha-mushṭi.

These drugs alleviate kapha, are antheminthic, purify and cleanse ulcers and are useful in coryza (catarrh), anorexia, dyspnoea and cough.

9. Mushkakādi group - consists of mushkaka, palāśa, dhava, chitraka, madana, vṛkshaka, śimshapa, vajra-vṛksha and triphala.

These drugs are useful in urinary diseases (including diabetes), defects in semen, haemorrhoids, anaemia, urinary calculi, and gravel and reduce medas.

10. Pippalyādi group - consists of pippali, pippali mūlam, chavya, chitraka, śringavēra, maricha, hasti-pippali, hareṇuka, ela, ajamoda, indrayava, pāṭha, jīraka, sarshapa, mahā-nimba-phala, hingu, bhārngi, madhurasa, ativisha, vachā, viḍanga and kaṭurohiṇi.

These drugs alleviate kapha and vāta, digest the āma (improperly digested macro-molecules of food), are appetising and are useful in anorexia, nasal catarrh, gulma and śūla.

11. Elādi group - consists of ela, tagara, kushtha, māmsi, dhyamaka, tvak, patra, nāga-pushpa, priyangu, hareṇuka, vyāghranakha, śukti, chaṇḍa, sthauneyaka, shriveshṭaka, chocha, choraka, bālaka, guggulu, sarjarasa, turushka, kunduruka, agaru, sprikka, uśīra, bhadradāru, kumkuma, punnāga and kesara.

These drugs alleviate kapha and vāta, are anti-toxics, improve the complexion and relieve itching, eruptions and urticaria.

12. Vachādi and haridrādi group - consists respectively of vachā, musta, ativisha, abhayā, bhadradāru, nāgakeśara (vachādi); and haridra, dāruharidra, kalashi, kuṭaja seeds and madhuka (haridrādi). These drugs are appetizing, digestive, purify the breast milk and are useful in āma-atisāra.

13. Śyāmadi group - consists of śyāma, mahā-śyāma, trivrit, danti, śankhini, tilvaka, kampillaka, ramyaka, kramuka, putrashroni, gavākshi, rājavriksha, the two kinds of karanja, guḍūchi, saptala, chhagalantri, sudhā and suvarnakshiri.

These drugs are anti-toxic, purgative, and are useful in gulma, ānāha, ascites and udāvarta.

14. Bṛhatyādi group - consists of bṛhati, kaṇṭakāri, kuṭaja-phala, pāṭha and madhuka.

These drugs alleviate pitta, kapha and vāta, are digestive and are useful in anorexia, heart diseases and dysuria.

15. Paṭolādi group - consists of paṭola, chandana, kuchandana, murva, guḍūchi, pāṭha and kaṭurohini.

These drugs alleviate pitta and kapha, are anti-toxic and are useful in fevers, ulcers, vomiting and itching (pruritus).

16. Kākolyādi group - consists of kākoli, kshīra-kḱoli, jīvaka, rishabhaka, mudga-parṇi, māshaparṇi, meda, mahāmeda, chhinna-ruha, karkaṭa-sṛngi, tugākshīri, padmaka, prapauṇḍarika, riddhi, vṛddhi, mridvīka, jīvanti and madhuka.

These drugs alleviate pitta and vata, increase kapha, are galactagogue, nourishing, jīvanīya, aphrodisiac and relieve ailments of vitiated blood.

17. Ūshakādi group - consists of ūshaka (alkaline earth), saindhava salt, śilājatu, the two kinds of kāsīsa, hingu and tutthaka.

These drugs alleviate kapha, reduce the medas, and are useful in urinary calculi, gravel, dysuria and gulma.

18. Sārivādi group - consists of sārīva, madhuka, chandana, kuchandana, padmaka, kāśmari phala, madhūka-pushpa and uśīra.

These drugs relieve thirst, rakta-pitta, pitta-jvara and daha.

19. Anjanādi group - consists of anjana, rasānjana, nāgapushpa, priyangu, nilotpala, nalada, nalina, kesara and madhuka.

These drugs relieve rakta-pitta, antidote poison and are useful in internal burning sensation (dāha).

20. Pārūshakādi group - consists of parāshaka, drākshā, kaṭphala, dāḍima, rājādana, kataka-phala, śaka-phala and triphala.

These drugs alleviate vata, are a heart tonic, appetizing and relieve thirst and urinary troubles (mūtra-dosha-hara).

21. Priyangvādi group - consists of priyangu, samanga, dhātaki, nāga-pushpa, chandana, kuchandana, mocharasa, rasānjana, kumbihka, srotonjana, padma-keśara, jojanvalli and dīrghamūla.

22. Ambashtṭādi group - consists of ambashṭha, dhātaki flowers, samanga, kaṭvanga, madhuka, bilva-peshika, rodhra, sāvara-rodhra, palāśa, nandī-vriksha and padma keśara.

Drugs belonging to the above two groups alleviate pitta and are useful in pakva-atisāra and in speeding up healing of fractured bones and ulcers.

23. Nyagrodhādi group - consists of nyagrodha, udumbara, aśvattha, plaksha, madhuka, kapītana, kakubha, āmra, kośāmra, chorakapatra, the two sorts of jambu, piyāla, madhuka (maula), rohiṇi, vanjula, kadamba, badari, tiṇḍuki, śallaki, rodhra, sāvara-rodhra, bhallātaka, palāśa, and nandi-vṛksha.

These drugs reduce medas, are constipative (sangrāhi), speed up healing of fractures and ulcers, and are useful in rakta-pitta, yoni-dosha and dāha.

24. Guḍuchyādi group - consists of guḍūchi, nimba, kustumburu, chandana and padmaka.

These drugs are appetizing and are useful in all fevers, nausea, anorexia, vomiting, thirst and dāha.

25. Utpalādi group - consists of utpala, raktotpala, kumuda, saugandhika, kuvalaya, puṇḍarīka and madhuka. These drugs alleviate pitta and vitiated blood, and relieve dāha, thirst, poisoning, heart diseases, vomiting and syncope.

26. Mustādi group - consists of musta, haridra, dāru-haridra, harītaki, āmalaki, vibhītaka, kushṭha, haimavati, vachā, pāṭha, kaṭurohiṇi, śārngaeshṭa, ativisha, drāviḍi, bhallātaka and chitraka.

These drugs alleviate kapha, are digestive, purify breast-milk and relieve yoni-doshas.

27. Triphala group - consists of harītaki, āmalaki and vibhītaki.

These drugs alleviate kapha and pitta, are anti-toxic, beneficial to the eyes, appetizing and are useful in prameha and vishama-jvara.

28. Trikaṭu group - consists of pippali, maricha and śṛngavera.

These drugs alleviate kapha, reduce medas, are appetizing and relieve skin diseases, gulma, pīnasa and loss of appetite.

29. Āmalakyādi group - consists of āmalaki, harītaki, pippali and chitraka.

These drugs alleviate kapha, are aphrodisiac, appetizing, beneficial to the eyes, and relieve all fevers and anorexia.

30. Trapvādi group - consists of trapu, śīsa, tāmra, rajata, kṛshṇa-lauha, suvarṇa and lohamala.

These drugs antidote gara-visha, are anthelminthic, and relieve thirst, poisoning, heart diseases, anaemia and prameha.

31. Lākshādi group - consists of lāksha, arevata, kuṭaja, aśvamāra, kaṭphalam, haridra, dāru-haridra, nimba, saptachchhada, mālati and trāyamāṇa.

These drugs are astringent, bitter and sweet, alleviate kapha and pitta, purify ulcers (dushṭa-vraṇa) and are useful in skin diseases and worm-infestation.

32. Svalpa (or laghu) panchamūla group-consists of the roots of medicinal plants known as the trikaṇṭaka, the two species of bṛhati, pṛthakparṇi and vidārigandha.

These drugs are astringent, bitter and sweet, alleviate vāta and pitta, are nourishing and strength giving.

33. Mahā panchamūla group - consists of roots of such trees as bilva, agnimantha, tuṇṭuka, pāṭala and kashmari.

These drugs alleviate kapha and vāta, are appetizing and are bitter, with a sweet anu-rasa.

34. Daśamūla group- consists of both laghu-panchamūla and mahā-panchamūla drugs.

These drugs alleviate all three doshas, help in digesting the āma, and are useful in dyspnoea and all fevers.

35. Vallī-panchamūla group - consists of the roots of the five creepers-vidāri, sāriva, rajanī, guḍūchi and ajaśṛngī.

36. Pancha-kaṇṭaka group - consists of the five (thorny) shrubs-trikaṇṭaka, karamarda, saireyaka, śatāvari and gridhranakhi.

These drugs alleviate kapha, and are useful in all types of prameha, in the three kinds of śopha, in rakta-pitta and defects of semen (śukra-dosha).

37. Tṛṇa-pañcha group - consists of kuśa, kāśa, nala, darbha and kāṇḍekśuka.

These drugs if administered with milk relieve rakta-pitta and urinary troubles (mūtra-doṣha) speedily. They also alleviate pitta.

Glossary of Disease Terms

Abdomen, flatulent distension of,—adhmana
Abdominal pain—sula
Abscess—irivallika
Acne—mukha-dushika
Adenitis—gandamala
Alchoholism—panatyatya
Allergic respiratory disease—svasa
Allergy—sita-pitta
Alopecia—indralupta, khalitya
Amenorrhea—yoni-vyapat
Anemia—pandu-roga
Anorexia nervosa—karshya
Anorexia—arochaka
Anus, pain in, —pratituni
Arthritis—vata-rakta
Ascites—udara
Asthma—svasa
Bell's palsy—ardita
Breast abscess—stana-vidradhi
Bubonic plague? —agnirohini
Calculi,renal—asmari
Callosities—kadara
Carbuncles—nadi-vrana
Carbuncle—valmika
Cardiac ailments—hrdroga
Cellulitis—jala-gardabha
Children, diseases of, —balaroga
Coma—sanyasa
Condylomata—charmakilaka
Constipation—sanniruddha-guda
Corns—kadara
Coryza—nasa-roga
Cough—kasa
Dehydration—daha
Diabetes—prameha
Diaper rash—ahiputana
Dislocations—bhagna
Dyspepsia—ajirna
Dysuria—mutra-krcchra
Ear, diseases of, —karna-roga
Elephantiasis—slipada
Emaciation—karshya
Emprosthotonus—abhyantarayama
Enteritis—atisara
Epilepsy—apasmara
Erythema anulare? —vivrta
Erythema multiforma—mashaka
Eyes, diseases of, —netra-roga
Facial palsy—ardita
Felon—chippa
Fevers—jvara
Fissures—pada-dari
Fistula in ano—bhagandara
Flatulence—anaha
Flatulence—mudha-vata
Flatulent gastritis—pratyadhmana
Foot drop—vata-roga
Fractures—bhagna
Furunculosis—arumshi
Gastritis—annadrava-sula
Gastritis—parinama-sula
Gastro-enteritis—visuchika
Goiter—galaganda
Gonorrhoea—aupasargika-meha
Gout—vata-rakta
Grandmal—apatantraka
Granuloma—yava-prakhya
Gravel—asmari
Guinea-worm infestation—snayuka
Gums, diseases of, —mukha-roga
Haemorrhage—rakta-pitta
Haemorrhoids—arsas
Hair, graying of, —palita
Headaches—siro-roga
Helminthiosis—krmi
Hemiplegia—paksha-vadha
Hernia—bradhna,vrddhi
Herpes zoster—indra-vrddha, kaksha, visarpa
Hiccough—hikka
Hydrocele—bradhna, vrddhi
Hydrocephalus—mastishka-apachaya
Hypochondriasis—gadodvega
Impetigo—masurika
Indigestion—ajirna
Inflammation—sotha
Intertrigo—ahiputana
Intestinal obstruction—udara
Jaundice—halimaka
Jaundice—kamala
Lactose intolerance—kshiralasaka

Laryngitis—svara-bheda
Leprosy—kushtha
Linea albicans—kikkisa
Lips, diseases of, —mukha-roga
Liver enlargement—udara
Lupus vulgaris—vyanga
Lymphadenopathy—apachi
Lymphadenosis—gandamala
Malabsorption syndrome—grahani
Mandibular dislocation—hanu-graha
Mandibular joint, arthritis of, —pashana-gardabha
Measles—romantika
Menorrhagia—asrgdhara
Menstrual disorders—yoni-vyapat
Mercury poisoning—parada-vikara
Metrorrhagia—asrgdhara
Mole, non-elevated, —tila-kalaka
Mole—nyaccha
Mycetoma—valmika
Neurofibroma—jatu-mani
Nose, diseases of, —nasa-roga
Obesity—sthaulya
Obstructive uropathy—mutraghata
Onychomycosis—ku-nakha
Osteo-arthritis of knee—kroshtuka-sirsha
Osteomalacia?—bahyayama
Palate, diseases of, —mukha-roga
Para-phimosis—parivartaka
Pellagra—kushtha
Pemphigus vulgaris—visphotaka
Perforation—udara
Peripheral neuritis—pada-harsha
Peripheral neuritis—vata-roga
Phimosis—niruddha-prakasa
Phlegmonous abscess—andhalaji
Piles—arsas
Pleural effusion—urastoya
Poliomyelitis—vata-roga
Postpartum abscess—makkalla
Proctitis—guda-paka
Prolapsus ani—guda-bhramsa
Prostate enlargement—ashthila
Prostate, enlargement of, —pratyashthila
Puerperal sepsis—makkalla
Pyoderma—kushtha
Pyothorax—kshata-kshina
Pyrexia—jvara
Pyrosis—amlapitta
Rheumatism—amavata
Rickets—khalli
Rickets—phakka
Salivary glands, swelling of—gandalaji
Sciatica—grdhrasi
Scrotum, swellings of, —vrddhi
Sebaceous cysts—granthi
Seminal concretions—asmari
Sinuses—nadi-vrana
Skin diseases—kushtha
Spastic neuralgia—dandalasaka
Spleen, enlargement of, —pliha-roga
Status epilepticus—apatanaka
Stomatitis—mukha-roga
Sunstroke—amsughata
Suppurative lung disease—kshata-kshina
Swellings, inflammatory, —granthi
Syncope—murccha
Syphilis—phiranga-roga
Taenia capitis—darunaka
Taenia corporis? —padmiini-kantaka
Taenia nigra—vrshana-kacchu
Teeth, diseases of, —mukha-roga
Tetanus—akshepaka
Throat, diseases of, —mukha-roga
Thyrotoxicosis? —bhasmaka
Tongue, diseases of, —mukha-roga
Trachoma—kukunaka
Tuberculosis—raja-yakshma
Tumours—arbuda
Ulcers—vrana
Urinary calculi—tuni
Urinary disorders, —prameha
Urticaria—kotha
Uterine prolapse—yoni-vyapat.
Venereal diseases—upadamsa
Vertigo—bhrama
Vitiligo—kilasa
Vomiting—chardi
Warts—arakilaka
Warts—charmakilaka
Whitlow—chippa
Worms—krmi
Wounds—sadyo-vrana
Wry neck—manya-stambha

Popular Prakashan